Pharmaceutical
PRACTICE

Dr Arthur Winfield

Qualifications: BPharm (Hons) (London External), studied at Bradford, PhD (Bradford), MRPharmS.

Academic and professional positions held: Senior Lecturer and Head of Pharmacy Practice at Robert Gordon Institute of Technology (later Robert Gordon University); First Local Postgraduate Tutor for Scottish Centre for Postqualification Pharmaceutical Education; Academic Advisor and External Examiner for new Faculty of Pharmacy, University of Kuwait and first Chairman of Department of Pharmacy Practice, University of Kuwait.

Professor R. Michael E. Richards OBE (awarded for 'Services to Pharmacy')

Qualifications: BPharm Hons (London) PhD (London) DSc (Strathclyde) DPharmSc (Honorary Khon Kaen Thailand) DPharm (Honorary Mahasarakham Thailand) FRPharmS (awarded for 'Distinction in the Profession of Pharmacy') Registered Thai Pharmacist by full Examination.

Academic and professional positions held: Lecturer in Pharmacy Herriot Watt University Edinburgh; Inaugural Professor of Pharmacy to establish the Department of Pharmacy, University of Rhodesia, and first Head of the Department of Pharmacy, University of Rhodesia; Senior Lecturer in Pharmacy, Strathclyde University; Professor and Head of School of Pharmacy The Robert Gordon University, Aberdeen; Professor Emeritus The Robert Gordon University; Chairman of the Project to Establish the Faculty of Pharmacy at the University of Mahasarakham, Thailand; Inaugural Dean of the Faculty of Pharmacy and Health Sciences, University of Mahasarakham, Thailand.

THIRD EDITION

Pharmaceutical
PRACTICE

Edited by

A. J. Winfield BPharm PhD MRPharmS

Chairman, Department of Pharmacy Practice,
Faculty of Pharmacy, Kuwait University,
Kuwait

R. M. E. Richards OBE BPharm PhD DSc DPharmSc DPharm FRPharmS

Professor and Dean, Faculty of Pharmacy and Health Sciences,
University of Mahasarakham, Thailand

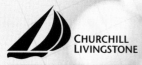

CHURCHILL
LIVINGSTONE

EDINBURGH LONDON NEW YORK OXFORD PHILADELPHIA ST LOUIS SYDNEY TORONTO 2004

CHURCHILL LIVINGSTONE
An imprint of Elsevier Science Limited
© 2004, Elsevier Science Limited. All rights reserved.

Commissioning Editor: Ellen Green
Project Development Manager: Siân Jarman
Project Manager: Frances Affleck
Designer: Erik Bigland

First edition 1990
Second edition 1998
Third edition 2004

ISBN 0-443-07206-X
International Student Edition 0-443-07205-1

British Library Cataloguing in Publication Data
A catalogue record for this book is available from the British
Library

Library of Congress Cataloging in Publication Data
A catalog record for this book is available from the Library
of Congress

Notice
Medical knowledge is constantly changing. Standard safety
precautions must be followed, but as new research and
clinical experience broaden our knowledge, changes in
treatment and drug therapy may become necessary or
appropriate. Readers are advised to check the most current
product information provided by the manufacturer of each
drug to be administered to verify the recommended dose,
the method and duration of administration, and
contraindications. It is the responsibility of the practitioner,
relying on experience and knowledge of the patient, to
determine dosages and the best treatment for each
individual patient. Neither the Publisher nor the editors
assumes any liability for any injury and/or damage to
persons or property arising from this publication.
The Publisher

The
publisher's
policy is to use
**paper manufactured
from sustainable forests**

Printed in Spain

Preface

This new third edition of *Pharmaceutical Practice* has been undertaken by the same editors as the previous edition. Already very successful in English, the second edition achieved wide international acceptance, with translations into Chinese and Thai. The same overall philosophy has guided the editors in the preparation of this new edition. A wide range of authors, often with an international background, has contributed. Each has been chosen because of their expertise in their field and their ability to communicate. Some new chapters have been introduced and existing chapters have been revised or completely rewritten to cover developments that have taken place since the writing of the last edition. The editors have striven to provide the reader with an up-to-date knowledge base for all aspects of good pharmacy practice. It has been presented wherever possible in such a way as to encourage a professional attitude of always seeking to provide the highest standards of pharmaceutical care for the patient. Material is again included to provide the knowledge and skills necessary for the continued developing roles of the pharmacist. At the heart of these new roles is contributing to and taking responsibility for the maximizing of patient benefits from their medication. This is best accomplished by the pharmacist interacting and communicating effectively both with patients and colleagues as part of an integrated, efficient and cost-effective health care team. It also requires a sound scientific knowledge of the wide range of pharmaceutical products available. Indeed, product knowledge remains vital for the pharmacist and represents a body of knowledge which is unique to pharmacy. Core information has been carefully selected to provide the sound knowledge base necessary for the competent practice of pharmacy both in the UK and internationally.

This volume of *Pharmaceutical Practice* has two companion volumes: *Pharmaceutics: The Science of Dosage Form Design* (2002) 2nd edition edited by ME Aulton (Churchill Livingstone) provides greater detail on the scientific principles which underpin dosage form design; *Clinical Pharmacy and Therapeutics* (2003) 3rd edition edited by R Walker and C Edwards (Churchill Livingstone) considers in greater detail aspects of treatment with drugs and clinical practice by pharmacists. The three books complement each other. Students should realize that information cannot be compartmentalized. It is detrimental to patients to ignore any aspect of the total knowledge base – all must be integrated in optimizing pharmaceutical care.

A.J.W.
R.M.E.R.

Acknowledgements

The editors would like to take this opportunity to thank the many people who have helped to make this third edition possible. Since publication of the second edition, both of us have spent time working overseas. This has, in some ways, made the process more difficult, but at the same time has added new perceptions which have influenced some of the decisions made during the planning of this edition.

Many new authors have been recruited for this edition. We are deeply grateful to all the authors for their willingness to contribute to this volume and for the time and effort they have spent researching their subjects and in preparing text – and for the way they have responded to e-mails!

Our special thanks are due to our wives, Jean Winfield and Joan Richards, for their continued encouragement, support and assistance, without whom it would not have been possible to set aside the time to produce this book.

Those companies, organizations and individuals who have given permission to use or modify their materials or who have helpfully answered queries or provided information to our authors are thanked. Without this type of cooperation, any textbook cannot hope to present a worthwhile overview.

Thanks are also expressed to the publishers, in particular Ellen Green and Siân Jarman, for their guidance and timely support throughout the preparation of this third edition. Professional guidance is always necessary. It was provided by them and made our life much easier.

Finally, a thank you to our students in the UK, in Kuwait and in Thailand. Staff learn all the time from students – we hope that some of this is reflected in this book.

A.J.W.
R.M.E.R.

Contents

PART 1
PHARMACY IN SOCIETY

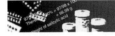

PART 2
PRINCIPLES OF PHARMACY PRACTICE

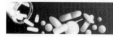

PART 3
PHARMACEUTICAL PRODUCTS 161

PART 4
USING PHARMACEUTICAL SKILLS IN CARING FOR PATIENTS

PART 5
APPENDICES

Contributors

Joanne Barnes BPharm PhD MRPharmS
Lecturer in Phytopharmacy, Centre for
Pharmacognosy & Phytotherapy,
School of Pharmacy, University of London,
London, UK
Ch 41 Complementary/alternative medicine

Christine M Bond BPharm MSc MEd PhD FRPharmS MFPHM
(Hon) ILTM
Professor of Primary Care (Pharmacy),
Department of General Practice and Primary
Care, University of Aberdeen, Aberdeen, UK
and Consultant in Pharmaceutical Public Health,
NHS Grampian, Aberdeen, UK
*Ch 1 The contribution of pharmacy to today's health care
provision*
Ch 31 Clinical pharmacy practice
Ch 40 Concordance and compliance
Appendix 1 Current UK pharmaceutical legislation
Appendix 2 NHS dispensing

Derek G Chapman BSc (Pharm) PhD MRPharmS
Lecturer in Pharmacy Practice, School of
Pharmacy, Robert Gordon University,
Aberdeen, UK
Ch 6 The principles and applications of quality assurance
Ch 9 Packaging
Ch 13 Sterile production areas
Ch 25 Parenteral products

Ivan O Edafiogho BPharm MSc PhD RPh
Associate Professor, Department of Pharmacy
Practice, Faculty of Pharmacy, Kuwait University,
Kuwait.
Ch 8 Pharmaceutical calculations

Clive Edwards BPharm PhD MRPharmS
Primary Care Group Pharmaceutical Adviser,
Newcastle and North Tyneside Health Authority,
Newcastle upon Tyne, UK
Ch 37 Responding to symptoms

K Hannes Enlund MSc (Pharm) DSc (Pharm)
Professor, Department of Pharmacy Practice,
Faculty of Pharmacy, Kuwait University, Kuwait
and Professor of Social Pharmacy, Department of
Social Pharmacy, University of Kuopio, Kuopio,
Finland
Ch 2 Social and behavioural aspects of pharmacy
Ch 3 Communication skills for the pharmacist

Martha M Everard BSc (Pharm) MSc(Pharm) MSc (LSHTM)
MRPharmS
Technical Officer, Essential Drugs and Medicines
Policy, World Health Organization, Geneva,
Switzerland
Ch 4 WHO and the essential medicines concept

Ian F Jones MSc PhD DMS FRPharmS FIPharmM
Professor of Pharmacy Practice,
School of Pharmacy and Biomedical Sciences,
University of Portsmouth, Portsmouth, UK
Ch 5 Pharmacy management

Janet Krska BSc PhD MRPharmS MCPP
Practice pharmacist, Tayside Primary Care NHS
Trust, Scotland and Governor, The College of
Pharmacy Practice, Coventry, UK
Ch 32 Adverse drug reactions
Ch 34 The evaluation of medicines
Ch 36 Formularies and guidelines
Ch 37 Responding to symptoms
Ch 43 Clinical governance

Anne Lee MPhil MRPharmS
Principal Pharmacist, Area Medicines Information
Centre, Glasgow Royal Infirmary, Glasgow, UK
Ch 33 Medicines information

Judith A Rees BPharm MSc PhD MRPharmS
Senior Lecturer, School of Pharmacy and
Pharmaceutical Sciences, University of
Manchester, Manchester, UK
Ch 15 The prescription
Ch 38 Counselling
Ch 39 Health promotion

Peter M Richards BPharm MRPharmS
Asthma Clinic Provider, Consultant and Locum
Pharmacist, Lincoln, UK
Ch 24 Inhaled route

R Michael E Richards OBE BPharm PhD DSc DPharmSc
DPharm FRPharmS
Professor and Dean, Faculty of Pharmacy and
Health Sciences, University of Mahasarakham,
Thailand
Ch 12 Principles and methods of sterilization
Ch 14 Sterility testing
Ch 26 Ophthalmic preparations
Appendix 6 Presentation skills

Kamal Sabra BPharm PhD FPSI FBSE MCPP
Director of Pharmaceutical Services, St. James's
Teaching Hospital, Dublin, Ireland and Professor
of Clinical Pharmacy, Faculty of Health Sciences,
Trinity College Dublin, Dublin, Ireland
Ch 27 Specialized services
Ch 28 Parenteral nutrition and dialysis

Jennifer Scott BSc (Pharm) PhD MRPharmS
Lecturer in Pharmacy Practice, Department of
Pharmacy and Pharmacology, University of Bath,
Bath, UK
Ch 42 Substance use and misuse

Jonathan Silcock BPharm MSc MRPharmS
Research Practitioner, Leeds Teaching Hospitals
and University of Leeds, Pharmacy Practice and
Medicines Management Group, School of
Healthcare Studies, University of Leeds, Leeds, UK
Ch 35 Pharmacoeconomics

Megan R Thomas BSc (Med Sci) MB ChB DRCOG MRCP
FRCPCH
Consultant Community Paediatrician,
Blenheim House Child Development and Family
Support Centre, Blackpool, UK
Appendix 3 Medical abbreviations

Margaret Watson BSc (Pharm) MSc PhD MRPharmS
MRC Fellow, Department of General Practice
and Primary Care, University of Aberdeen,
Aberdeen, UK
Ch 31 Clinical pharmacy practice

Arthur J Winfield BPharm PhD MRPharmS
Chairman, Department of Pharmacy Practice,
Faculty of Pharmacy, Kuwait University,
Kuwait
Ch 3 Communication skills for the pharmacist
Ch 7 Dispensing techniques
Ch 8 Pharmaceutical calculations
Ch 10 Storage and stability
Ch 11 Labelling of dispensed medicines
Ch 16 Routes of administration and dosage forms
Ch 17 Solutions
Ch 18 Suspensions
Ch 19 Emulsions
Ch 20 External preparations
Ch 21 Suppositories and pessaries
Ch 22 Powders and granules
Ch 23 Oral unit dosage forms
Ch 29 Wound management, stoma and incontinence
Ch 30 Medical gases
Ch 40 Concordance and compliance
Appendix 4 Pharmaceutical Latin
Appendix 5 Systems of weights and measures

Jean H Winfield BPharm PhD MRPharmS
Technical Consultant, Faculty of Pharmacy,
Kuwait University, Kuwait
Ch 29 Wound management, stoma and incontinence

Some contributions made to the second edition
have also been used in the current edition.
The following contributors are acknowledged:
DM Collett, JA Cromarty, D Graham, JG Hamley,
SL Hutchinson, EJ Kennedy, MM Moody.

About this book

The last edition indicated that pharmacy was going through a time of rapid change. Students were urged to 'keep up to date' by reading professional journals. Against that background, it is not surprising that there are many changes in this third edition. There are changes amongst the authors and there are changes in the chapters. This led the editors to revise the layout of the book as a whole. The section format has been retained, but the order of the chapters and the emphasis of these have changed to reflect the way the profession has developed. The four sections are:

1. Pharmacy in society
2. Principles of pharmacy practice
3. Pharmaceutical products
4. Using pharmaceutical skills in caring for patients
5. Appendices.

Part 1

The attempt here is to give background information which will be used in later chapters. The book opens with an overview of the current role of pharmacy and how the pharmacist interacts with other health care professionals. Aspects of social and behavioural science are now a core element of the undergraduate curriculum. Chapter 2 gives a broad-brush appreciation of these subjects. Throughout the book there are references to the need for effective communication skills. These cannot be learned from reading a book, but have to be learned through practice. However, Chapter 3 covers key aspects to achieving effective communication. The next two chapters are completely new. Chapter 4 presents information about the WHO and its essential medicines concept. This is important for many countries including 'developed' countries. Many pharmacy students will have to manage a business. How to do this completely is beyond the scope of this book, but Chapter 5 gives some of the terminology and basic skills required.

Part 2

This section develops more specific pharmaceutical skills which will be used in different contexts in this book and in everyday practice as a pharmacist. The assurance of quality is becoming more and more important in all aspects of society, but especially in health care. Chapter 6 considers the meaning of 'quality' and some of the ways in which it can be incorporated into practice at all levels. Some of the ideas included are developed in later chapters. The medicine supply function is still important in pharmacy, so Chapter 7 deals with the basic principles of dispensing, including the assurance of quality in the processes used. Whilst students do not in general appreciate it, the ability to perform calculations is an essential skill. Chapter 8 is an expanded chapter dealing with this. To assist, there is an extensive section of 'exercises' to give further practice. Chapters 9, 10 and 11 cover three important requirements – packaging of medicines, the storage of medicines and their correct labelling for the patient. Then Chapters 12, 13 and 14 cover the more specialized areas concerned with sterile medicines: the principles and methods of sterilization, sterile production areas and aseptic manipulation and sterility testing. These relate to the preparation of injections, ophthalmic products and to some other specialized products.

Part 3

Pharmacists handle a wide range of different types of medicines and appliances. These are ordered on a prescription – the subject of the first chapter in this section, in which the different types of prescriptions and how they are processed is described. Chapter 16 gives an overview of the main routes by which drugs can be administered to patients and the different dosage forms which can be used. Then follows a systematic covering of the different types of medicines. Chapters 17 to 23 concentrate mostly on extemporaneously prepared medicines, which pharmacists still need to be able to make. From Chapter 24, the emphasis changes to more specialized medicines and the role of the pharmacist in ensuring their effective use. Chapter 24 discusses how medicines are given by inhalation, Chapter 25 by injection and Chapter 26 deals with ophthalmic products. In Chapters 27 and 28 there is information on hospital-based services such as centralized intravenous additives, reconstitution of cyctotoxics and other drugs, radiopharmaceuticals, total parenteral nutrition and dialysis. This section ends with 'supportive' treatments – wound management, stoma and incontinence in Chapter 29 and medical gases in Chapter 30.

Part 4

Patient aspects have already been referred to in some of the preceding chapters, but this section more widely demonstrates how the knowledge of those chapters is applied to patients. Chapter 31 looks back over the development of clinical pharmacy in the UK and considers some of the ways in which it is currently put into practice. Other aspects of medicines management are then considered. Chapter 32 deals with adverse drug reactions and how to minimize their impact. Accessing accurate information is vital in the modern world, especially in medicine. Chapter 33 provides valuable guidance of how to locate and use that information. A specialized aspect of this is the evaluation of medicines, the subject of Chapter 34. Whether we like it or not, cost is an important factor in modern health care, so Chapter 35 gives information about pharmacoeconomics and how it can inform decisions. Allied to this is the development of formularies which is reviewed in Chapter 36. The next four chapters deal with other important aspects of the day-to-day practice of pharmacy – responding to symptoms, counselling patients, health promotion and concordance and compliance. Alternative medicines are being increasingly demanded and used by the public, many being supplied through pharmacies. Aspects of this large topic are dealt with in Chapter 41. It is a sad fact of modern society that drugs are misused. Chapter 42 has been written to give an overview of this somewhat controversial subject and also highlight the pharmacist's role in harm reduction. To end this section there is a chapter on audit and related tools – which are useful to assure professions that they are delivering quality in their service to the public.

Part 5

As in the previous edition, there are a number of appendices. These give useful information which does not require a full chapter. Those on legislation and the NHS are mostly of UK relevance. Medical abbreviations increasingly have to be understood by pharmacists as they work closely with medical staff and have access to patient medical notes. Some of these abbreviations have been included in Appendix 3. Pharmaceutical Latin and weights and measures are the topics in the next two appendices. Presentation skills are needed by students and pharmacists throughout their professional careers. Guidance is given on making a presentation in Appendix 6.

It is a daunting task to produce a textbook that thoroughly covers a whole subject. This is the case with this current edition of *Pharmaceutical Practice*. We have attempted to provide an overview and supply key information. Students who wish (and need) to know more should go to other, more specialized, sources.

We acknowledge that there will be changes taking place between the writing and publishing of this book which will mean that by the time this book appears in print some of it will already be out of date. This process of obsolescence will continue with time. It is, therefore, again necessary to invite students to develop the habit of keeping up to date with the pharmaceutical and medical literature. There is no substitute for a regular reading of professional journals.

Further reading

A book of this size cannot cover every subject in detail. For this reason we have collected together suggestions for further reading. These key references and further reading are collected together by chapter and are given in Appendix 7. This appendix begins with a list of the most frequently used references.

PART 1

PHARMACY IN SOCIETY

1

The contribution of pharmacy to today's health care provision

C. M. Bond

After studying this chapter you will know about:

An outline of the position of pharmacy within the National Health Service in the UK

Recent developments in the services being provided by pharmacists

The need for lifelong learning

Introduction

Pharmacists are experts on the action and uses of drugs, including their chemistry, the formulation of medicines and the way in which drugs are used to manage diseases. Pharmacists' raison d'être is to use this expertise to improve patient care. Pharmacists are in close contact with patients so that they have an important role in assisting patients to make the best use of their prescribed medicines, and in advising patients on the appropriate self management of self-limiting and minor conditions. Increasingly this latter aspect includes over-the-counter prescribing of effective and potent treatments. Pharmacists are also in close working relationships with other members of the health care team— doctors, nurses, dentists and others—where they are able to give advice on a wide range of issues surrounding the use of medicines.

Pharmacists are employed in many different areas of practice. These include the traditional ones of hospital and community practice, as well as newer advisory roles at health authority/health board level, and working directly with general practitioners as part of the core, practice-based, primary health care team. Additionally, pharmacists are employed in the pharmaceutical industry, and in academia.

The general public are most likely to meet pharmacists in high street pharmacies or on a hospital ward. However, pharmacists also visit residential homes, make visits to patients' own homes and are now involved in running chronic disease clinics in primary and secondary care. In addition, pharmacists will also be contributing to the care of patients through their dealings with other members of the health care team in the hospital and community setting.

Historically pharmacists and general practitioners have a common ancestry as apothecaries who both dispensed medicines for physicians and recommended medicines for those members of the public unable to afford physicians' fees. As the two professions emerged this remit split so that the pharmacists became primarily responsible for the technical, dispensing aspects of this role. With the advent of the National Health Service (NHS) in the UK in 1948, and the philosophy of free medical care at the point of delivery, the advisory function of the pharmacist further decreased. As a result pharmacists spent more of their time in the dispensing of medicines—and derived an increased proportion of their income from it. At the same time, radical changes in the nature of dispensing itself, as described in the following paragraphs, occurred.

In the early years, many prescriptions were for extemporaneously prepared medicines, either to recipes from the standard formularies such as the *British Pharmacopoeia* (BP) or *British Pharmaceutical Codex* (BPC), or to recipes written by the prescriber. The situation was similar in hospital pharmacy, where prescriptions were prepared on an individual basis. There was some small-scale manufacture of a range of commonly used items. In both situations, pharmacists required manipulative and time-consuming skills to produce the medicines. Thus a wide range of preparations were made, including liquids for internal and external use, ointments, creams, poultices, plasters, eye drops and ointments, injections and solid dosage forms such as pills, capsules and moulded tablets.

Scientific advances have greatly increased the effectiveness of drugs, but they are also more complex, potentially more toxic, and require more sophisticated use than their predecessors. The pharmaceutical industry developed in tandem with these drug developments, contributing to further scientific advances and producing manufactured medical products. This had a number of advantages. For one thing, there was an increased reliability in the product, which could be subjected to suitable quality assessment. This led to improved formulations, modifications to drug availability and increased use of tablets which have a greater convenience for the patient. Some doctors did not agree with the loss of flexibility in prescribing which resulted from having to use predetermined doses and combinations of materials. From the pharmacist's point of view there was a reduction in the time spent in the routine extemporaneous production of medicines, which many saw as an advantage. Others saw it as a reduction in the 'mystique' associated with the professional role of the pharmacist. Some aspects of what it means to be 'professional' are dealt with in Chapter 2. There was also an erosion of the skill base of the pharmacist. A look through copies of the BPC in the 1950s, 1960s and 1970s will show the reduction in the number and diversity of formulations included in the Formulary section. That section was omitted from the most recent editions.

Some extemporaneous dispensing is still required and pharmacists remain the only professionals trained in these skills. For this reason, Part C of this book deals with the types of medicine used, the ingredients employed in them and describes some of the practical skills required to make products suitable for use by patients.

The changing patterns of work of the pharmacist, in community pharmacy in particular, led to an uncertainty about the future role of the pharmacist, and a general consensus that pharmacists were no longer being utilized to their full potential. If the pharmacist was not required to compound medicines, and was not required to give general advice on diseases, what was the pharmacist to do?

THE EXTENDED ROLE

The need to review the future for pharmacy was first formally recognized in 1979 in a report on the NHS which had the remit to consider the best use and management of its financial and manpower resources. This was followed by a succession of key reports and papers which repeatedly identified the need to exploit the pharmacist's expertise and knowledge to better effect. Key amongst these reports was the Nuffield report of 1986. This report, including nearly 100 recommendations, led the way to many new initiatives,

both by the profession and by the Government, and laid the foundation for the recent developments in the practice of pharmacy, which are reflected in this book.

Radical change, as recommended in the Nuffield report, does not necessarily happen quickly, particularly when regulations and statutes are involved. In the 25 years since Nuffield was published there have been several different agendas which have come together, and between them facilitated the paradigm shift for pharmacy envisaged in the Nuffield report. These three agendas referred to above will be briefly described below. They have finally resulted in extensive professional change, most recently articulated in the definitive statements about the role of pharmacy in the NHS plans for pharmacy in England (2000), Scotland (2001) and Wales (2002).

THE PROFESSION

The Council of the Royal Pharmaceutical Society of Great Britain (RPSGB) decided that it was necessary to allow all members to contribute to a radical appraisal of the profession, what it should be doing and how to achieve it. The 'Pharmacy In A New Age' consultation (familiarly referred to as PIANA) was launched in October 1995, with an invitation to all members to contribute their views to the Council. These were correlated and a follow-up document was produced by the Council in September 1996 called 'Pharmacy in a New Age: the New Horizon'. This indicated that there was overwhelming agreement from pharmacists that the profession could not 'stand still'. Four main areas in which pharmacy should make a major contribution to health outcomes were identified:

- *The management of prescribed medicines.* This covers drug development, provision of medicines, information and support, and ensuring patient needs are met safely, efficiently and conveniently so that they can get maximum benefit from their medicines.
- *The management of chronic conditions.* Here the need is to improve the quality of life and outcomes of treatment for the patient. Pharmacists may help by supplying medicines and advice, helping to develop local 'shared care' protocols, ensuring that patients are taking or using their medicines properly and working as part of the health care team.
- *The management of common ailments.* Patients require reassurance and advice, with or without the use of non-prescription medicines, and referral to other professionals if necessary.

- *The promotion and support of healthy lifestyles.* Pharmacists can help people protect their own health through health screening, giving advice on healthy living and providing educational materials.

During the consultation process, pharmacists expressed their views on the way the profession should change. These, too, may be summarized under four main headings.

- *The strengths of pharmacy.* There was a high level of consensus that the knowledge base of pharmacy was very important. This is based on both the study of and experience with medicines and also in managing the medicines and handling relevant information. A second strength which was seen as important was pharmacists' availability and accessibility in a wide range of different locations in the heart of the community, such as conventional high street premises, health centres, supermarkets, hospitals and in people's homes. This accessibility is strengthened by easy communication with both patients and other professionals, giving pharmacists a pivotal position. The growth of information technology could be a potential threat to this, although pharmacists are noted for their adaptability.
- *Demonstrating the value of pharmacy.* Pharmacy must claim its rights as a profession and accept the responsibilities which come with this. Thus high standards must be set and achieved. Additionally, evidence must be produced which demonstrates clearly the value of pharmacy in health care. This will require research and professional audit (this is dealt with in Ch. 43). Further support for this development will come from increased continuing education and recognition achieved by effective promotion of the profession.
- *Changes in practice.* Three main areas where there could be an increase in services were identified. These are the enhancement of services to patients (advice, counselling, domiciliary visits, health promotion and non-prescription medicine sales), improved relationships with other health care professionals (closer support for prescribers, medicine management, liaison between hospital and community pharmacy and different community pharmacists, training for other professionals and carers), practice research and audit, continuing education and better use of information technology (all required to support the other developments). There was also a high level of support for a reduction in the mechanical aspects of dispensing, sale of non-health-related products and routine paperwork associated with the NHS and business activities.

- *A sustainable future.* These elements could make up a sustainable future for the profession. In particular, pharmacy would be concerned with advice and counselling, dispensing, health promotion, the sale of non-prescription medicines, medicines management and as a 'first port of call' for health care. Some of these may require changes in the setting of pharmaceutical provision and others may require different types of employment for pharmacists. Other changes which would be required included changes to the system of payment under the NHS, a rationalization of pharmacy distribution and at least two pharmacists being employed per community pharmacy.

Whilst the profession endorsed the need for change, the current pharmacy contract continues to reflect the now historical, core dispensing role of community pharmacy, and mitigates against the newer professional roles. Although pharmacists are increasingly providing these under the auspices of the Professional Allowance (Appendix 2), and some services are recognized through local arrangements with individual boards and trusts, change throughout the profession will only become a reality once the remuneration package recognizes the newer services. The most recent Government documents now contain clear directives for a new contract to be negotiated.

THE NHS DRUGS BUDGET

Health services are expensive to run. Governments try to reduce expenditure as far as possible through a range of methods. In the UK some medicines have been identified as being ineligible for prescribing on the NHS and the so-called 'Black List' was introduced in 1984 to reduce the size of the NHS bill. Furthermore the introduction of computer technology into prescription pricing has enabled far more data to be produced than was previously possible. Doctors now receive a regular breakdown of the drugs they have prescribed and their prescribing costs. Chapter 34 considers the use of prescribing data (PACT or SPA) by pharmacists when advising doctors about reducing their prescribing costs.

However despite these moves, and in common with other developed countries, UK drug costs are inexorably rising due to the greater availability of new effective treatments, patient demand and changes in patient demography (more older people). This has made many governments look at other ways of controlling this item of expenditure, and there are two ways in which pharmacists can have a role.

Firstly, it is recognized that not all prescribing follows the current best evidence for cost-effective practice. Pharmacists are seen as a profession with the necessary knowledge to support quality in prescribing at a strategic and practice level. At a strategic level they can appraise the evidence and make recommendations for the inclusion of a drug in a formulary. At a general practice level pharmacists can advise prescribers on the best drugs to prescribe for individual patients, and community pharmacists are well placed to monitor and review repeat prescriptions—which account for 80% of all prescriptions in primary care.

Secondly, in a move to promote self care, encourage patients to be responsible for their own health care, and by implication remove the costs of treating what is known as 'minor illness' from the NHS, many drugs previously only available on prescription (POM) are now available over-the-counter (P) (Appendix 1). This has resulted in many potent drugs now being available for sale from community pharmacies and the advisory role of the pharmacist has therefore been greatly enhanced. In 1983, ibuprofen and loperamide were the first of many drugs to be deregulated in the following decades, and there is no obvious end to the process. Recent high profile deregulations in the UK include emergency hormonal contraception, and conversely the return to prescription control of the non-sedating antihistamines, terfenadine and astemizole, as the safety of drugs when taken in the wider population is constantly reviewed. These moves have implications for the pharmacist's role potentially as a diagnostician and a return to the traditional pre-NHS advisory role (see Ch. 37).

The NHS workforce

As demand for health care grows, it is not only budgets that are stretched—increasingly there are insufficient trained professionals to deliver services, and innovative ways of working need to be introduced to maximize the skills of the different professionals in the health care team. This has resulted in a recognition that many of the tasks previously undertaken by the medical profession, in both primary and secondary care, can be undertaken by other professions such as pharmacists and nurses. Thus some of the professional roles originally identified by the profession, such as the management of chronic disease, and a greater role in responding to symptoms, are now supported by the wider health care community because they can contribute to more effective health care for the population.

THE CURRENT AND FUTURE ROLES OF PHARMACISTS

There are currently 43 000 UK member pharmacists working in all sectors of the profession both in Britain and overseas. About 22 000 members work in community pharmacy, 5500 in hospitals and 1600 in the pharmaceutical industry. The rest are employed in a range of pharmacy- (including other NHS roles) and non-pharmacy-related posts. This section will summarise the community, hospital and other NHS roles as they are practised today, with indications of likely changes and challenges in the near future.

Community pharmacy

Dispensing

Because of the current remuneration contract, dispensing remains the core role of community pharmacy, but the preponderance of original pack dispensing means that, compared to even a decade ago, whilst the name may remain the same the similarity ends there. The focus of dispensing now rests not only on accurate supply of medication, but on checking that the medication is appropriate for the patient, and counselling the patient on its appropriate use (see Ch. 38). All community pharmacists maintain computerized patient medication records which are a record of previous prescriptions dispensed (see Ch. 31). Whilst not necessarily complete, as to date patients are not registered with an individual pharmacy, in practice the vast majority of patients do use one pharmacy for the majority of their supplies. Thus pharmacists have a database of information which will allow them to check on issues such as accuracy of the new prescription, compliance, and potential drug interactions.

In the future the dispensing role will be further enhanced as connection of community pharmacy into the NHS net becomes a reality, opening up the opportunity for electronic transmission of prescriptions, currently being piloted in selected sites in England and Scotland. Ultimately this electronic link should allow access by the pharmacist to at least a selected portion of the patient's medical record, further enhancing the pharmacist's ability to assess the appropriateness of the prescription. It is hoped that there will also be a facility for pharmacists to write to the patient record, so that GPs will know whether or not prescriptions have been dispensed and what OTC drugs have been purchased.

A further enhanced dispensing role is in the management of repeat prescriptions, which until recently have been issued from GP surgeries with little clinical review. Again pilot sites are currently exploring the logistics of allowing pharmacists to have responsibility for the issuing of repeat prescription, which should improve convenience for patients, and improve their care. Research projects testing out this role have demonstrated that when given this responsibility, community pharmacists can identify previously unrecognized side effects, adverse drug reactions and drug interactions, as well as saving almost a fifth of the costs of the drugs prescribed.

This opportunistic clinical input at the point of dispensing is also being developed in a more systematic way, such that patients with targeted chronic conditions, such as coronary heart disease, have formal regular reviews with the community pharmacist of their medication and other disease related behaviours. Again schemes like this, with research evidence of benefit in small studies, are currently undergoing widespread national pilots to confirm their feasibility as a service innovation. This is often referred to as pharmaceutical care, or medicines management (see Ch. 31).

Responding to symptoms

Provision of advice to customers presenting in the pharmacy for advice on self care is now an accepted part of the work of a pharmacist, which as described earlier has been enhanced by the increased armamentarium of pharmacy medicines. Advertising campaigns, particularly those by the National Pharmaceutical Association (NPA), have brought to the public attention the advice which is available from the pharmacist, as have the commercial adverts from the pharmaceutical industry for their deregulated products. The increased emphasis on the provision of advice from community pharmacies has also extended to the counter staff, who require special training and must adhere to protocols. Some of the principles of responding to symptoms are dealt with in Chapter 37.

The full contribution of this advisory role to health care has been limited, to some extent, to the more advantaged sections of the population; those on lower incomes, and particularly those who are exempt from prescription charges, may in the past have attended their doctor only for the purpose of obtaining a free prescription. In the future this will be circumvented, as the introduction of pharmacist protocols and pharmacist prescribing will allow pharmacists to supply medication on the NHS free to those normally exempt from payment.

Health promotion and health improvement

A large number of people pass through the nation's pharmacies in any one day; on the basis of prescription numbers this is frequently said to be 6 million people per day in the UK. Thus the pharmacist is one of the best placed health care professionals to provide health promotion information and health education material to the general public. This has now become part of the pharmacist's NHS contract, and formalized as a requirement to provide a range of leaflets, but there are increasing opportunities for extensive health promotion in pharmacies. The development of cancer and cardiovascular disease are both closely linked to diet. Pharmacists can give out patient information leaflets on healthy nutrition, which may reduce the development of disease which would otherwise occur and lead to the need for expensive treatment. Likewise smoking is the single biggest cause of preventable ill health, and pharmacists have a successful record in supporting smoking cessation through tailored face-to-face advice, and the supply of smoking cessation products such as nicotine replacement therapies (see Ch. 39).

Services to specific patient groups

Certain groups of patients have particular needs which can be met by community pharmacists more cost effectively than by any other health professional. Such specific patient services often cause the remit of a profession to change almost overnight in response to an unexpected national issue. One such example is drug misuse and the spread of blood borne diseases such as hepatitis and AIDS. Drug misuse is an increasing problem in society today, and it is now generally accepted that drug misusers have a right to treatment both to help them come off their addiction, and to reduce the harm they may do, either to themselves or to society, until such time as they are ready to undergo detoxification. The vast majority of pharmacists will be involved to a greater or lesser extent in a number of ways, as discussed in Chapter 42. In particular, pharmacists have become involved in needle exchange schemes and in instalment dispensing of methadone. Because of the urgent need for these important services, and to some extent because of the unwillingness of some community pharmacists to become involved on the grounds of professional responsibility alone, these services have unusually been recognized by specific, locally negotiated, remuneration packages.

Domiciliary visiting

Pharmacists have traditionally delivered oxygen to a patient's home, and many pharmacists will visit a small number of patients to deliver medicines and provide advice on their use. This will now be extended to include other situations where patients could benefit, such as on discharge from hospital, including highly specialized services, often called the 'hospital at home', where patients may be on palliative care, cytotoxic agents, intravenous antibiotics or artificial nutrition. These topics are discussed in more detail in Chapter 28. Extension of the medicines management projects described above to housebound patients will also mean more domiciliary visits, and the development of services to residential and nursing homes has also increased the involvement of pharmacists.

Personal control

One of the requirements of the current regulations is that a pharmacist has to be in personal control/supervision of registered community pharmacy premises, and that in his/her absence, professional activities such as dispensing or the sale of 'P' medicines cannot be undertaken. The principle is that the pharmacist should be aware of any transaction in which a medicine is provided to a member of the public and be able to intervene if deemed necessary. The RPSGB Code of Ethics covers some interpretation of this requirement. However whilst the requirement was intended to protect the public, it has been a barrier to innovative practice, and means that for single-handed pharmacists any professional activities undertaken outwith the pharmacy premises have to be done outside normal working hours. This issue is unresolved, but possible solutions include the formation of group community pharmacy practices, or the training and recognition of pharmacy technicians for short-term cover. In practice a single pharmacist cannot be involved in all sales in a busy shop and should ensure that all the staff are adequately trained to know when a referral to the pharmacist is necessary. The Statutory Committee has considered the situation a number of times and has suggested that it is a matter of degree, and at the moment it therefore remains a decision for professional judgment.

A further challenge to established practice will also come from the increasing use of the Internet for personal shopping and the acquisition of medicines, whether prescribed or purchased, will not be immune to such developments. Already mail order pharmacy and e-pharmacy are making small inroads into medicines distribution and supply and challenging some of the principles of the Code of Ethics and professional practice points which encourage personal counselling wherever possible. Although probably more developed in North America, such changes to practice are inevitable and need to be managed professionally, remembering that best care of the patient, rather than professional self interest, must be the rationale of any decision making.

Out of hours services

The NHS call centres, NHS Direct (England and Wales) and NHS 24 (Scotland) handle health-related telephone enquiries from the general public and triage them onto appropriate services. Referral to community pharmacy is one of the formal dispositions included in the algorithms used by the call handlers, and it is intended therefore that the community pharmacist will not be bypassed by the new telephone helplines. It should also serve to educate the public about the role of the community pharmacist and to increase general awareness that the community pharmacy is just as much a part of the NHS as is the general practice.

Primary care pharmacy

During the 1990s there was increasing evidence of close working between pharmacists and the rest of the general practice-based primary health care team. Doctors realized that pharmacists had many possible additional clinical roles in primary care, beyond their traditional community pharmacy premises. Many pharmacists now provide doctors with advice on GP formulary development (see Ch. 36) and undertaking patient medication reviews, either seeing patients face to face or through review of patient records—globally or on an individual basis. They may also take responsibility for specific clinics following agreed protocols, such as anticoagulant and *Helicobacter pylori* assessment clinics. These pharmacists are known as primary care pharmacists. However as community pharmacy develops along the lines described above, and IT links become the norm, it is envisaged that many of the tasks now done by primary care pharmacists will ultimately be carried out from the community pharmacy base.

Pharmaceutical advisers

As new NHS structures emerge in primary care, services are being delivered in an integrated way, involving the wider health care team as well as local authority managed services such as social work, and other community workers. In

England these organizations are called Primary Care Trusts, in Scotland, Local Health Care Co-operatives, in Wales, Local Health Groups, and in Northern Ireland, Health and Social Services Trusts. Management teams for these organizations generally include a senior pharmacy adviser who will coordinate pharmaceutical care for the organization, integrating community pharmacy into the delivery of core health care, and co-coordinating the primary care pharmacist workforce, to achieve area wide goals in prescribing.

Pharmaceutical public health

Larger geographical areas are administered by strategic health authorities in England and NHS Boards in Scotland. Most of these also have a senior pharmacist adviser, operating at consultant level, as part of the public health team. They have a specific responsibility for local pharmacy strategy development, compliance with statutes, and the managed entry of new drugs, as well as providing local professional leadership, and advice on professional governance, alongside their senior pharmacy colleagues in the trusts. Increasingly as professional boundaries begin to merge, they are also seen as public health professionals and take their share of the generic public health workload.

Hospital pharmacy

Clinical pharmacy services have been established in the hospital setting for some time; indeed many of the innovations identified for community pharmacy come from earlier experience in hospitals. In general there is already a greater working together of the professions in the hospital setting compared to primary care, including pharmacists' involvement in medication history taking, for pharmacists to be more actively involved in research, and for the provision of 24-hour services. In 1988, the NHS Circular 'Health Services Management: the Way Forward for Hospital Pharmaceutical Services' laid down the government policy aim as 'the achievement of better patient care and financial savings, through the more cost effective use of medicines, and improved use of pharmaceutical expertise obtained through the implementation of a clinical pharmacy service'. Two main components were identified. One is the overall management of medicines on the hospital ward. This is achieved through the provision of advice to medical and nursing staff, formulary management and ensuring the safe handling of medicines. The other component is the development of individual patient care plans. This is achieved through the provision of drug information and assisting patients with problems which may arise. In practice there are many stages and activities involved in these processes. A working group in Scotland published 'Clinical Pharmacy in the Hospital Pharmaceutical Service: a Framework for Practice' in July 1996 (Steering Group and Working Group 1996). The framework advocates a systematic approach to enable the pharmacist to focus on the key areas and optimize the pharmaceutical input to patient care. Some of the thinking behind this document is discussed in detail in Chapter 31.

There is a growing awareness of the problems which arise at the interface between community (primary) and hospital (secondary) care. Patients move in both directions. Their medical and pharmaceutical problems also move with them. Over the next few years it is hoped that a large proportion of these problems will have been resolved through the greater involvement of pharmacists at admission and discharge with effective (ultimately electronic) transfer of information, from hospital pharmacist to community pharmacist.

A quality assured NHS

Some high profile examples of substandard health care, most particularly the investigation into the standards of children's heart surgery at Bristol Royal Infirmary, have focused attention on the need to identify and learn from mistakes, and to systematically assess and manage risk. There is now an increasing understanding of the components of a quality assured NHS, and the systems that need to be in place to support this.

Clinical effectiveness

Clinical effectiveness is a term often used to describe the extent to which clinical practice meets the highest known standards of care. Clinical governance is a term used to describe the accountability of an organizational grouping for ensuring that clinical effectiveness is practised by all functions for which it is responsible. Central to this is the use of evidence-based guidelines and protocols, which has increased dramatically in the past decade. An overview is provided in Chapter 31. These guidelines are a way of increasing the quality of service because they are developed after systematic searches of the research evidence, and make recommendations for 'best practice', which are easily understood and widely accepted.

The extent to which guidelines are actually applied in particular situations should be measured by clinical audit.

Chapter 43 aims to give the background to the need for audit and the different ways in which it may be carried out. Audit is also an important tool in the raising of standards of service delivery.

Training, research and development are also all important strands of clinical effectiveness as are professional reflection and development. Structures established to deliver this agenda for pharmacy are described in more detail in the next paragraph.

CONTINUING EDUCATION AND CONTINUING PROFESSIONAL DEVELOPMENT

In such a rapidly changing profession, there is a need for continual updating of knowledge. The College of Pharmacy Practice (CPP) to some extent mirrors the Royal Medical Colleges, providing a further professional qualification, specialist faculties and inculcating a general ethos of reflective practice and continued personal learning. The RPSGB, through *The Pharmaceutical Journal*, has established a regular pattern of continuing education (CE) articles on a wide range of topics, and is currently piloting a formal portfolio-based Continuous Professional Development (CPD) initiative. The Council of the RPSGB, through the Code of Ethics, requires that all pharmacists undertake at least 30 hours of continuing education each year.

Continuing education is further supported by the Centres for Postgraduate or Postqualification Pharmaceutical Education (CPPE). They are located in Manchester (England), Cardiff (Wales) and Belfast (Northern Ireland). The Scottish centre has recently been amalgamated with sister organizations in medicine, dentistry, psychology and nursing to create a new special Health Board, the NHS Education for Scotland Board. This is an exciting development once again reflecting new approaches to health care delivery, and facilitating teamwork across professional boundaries. Courses from all four centres are provided free to pharmacists who are employed in the provision of pharmaceutical services to the NHS.

There is, therefore, good provision for CE, which pharmacists use to good effect. At the moment there is no requirement for a further assessment of competence once the pre-registration year is successfully completed, but it is unlikely that this will remain the case for much longer.

The role of the RPSGB

The RPSGB has an unusual dual role as a professional body and a regulatory body. For the latter function it is responsible for the registration of pharmacists and premises, the maintenance of standards through a network of inspectors, and for disciplining those who do not meet the required standard through the statutory committee. With increasing public concerns about standards of health care in general, the regulatory function is increasingly open to public scrutiny and there are ongoing proposals to review the Society's remit and to ensure it meets the requirements of the newly established Council for the Regulation of Healthcare Professionals.

PHARMACY EDUCATION

Undergraduate education

Teaching of pharmacy was traditionally under four subject headings: pharmaceutical chemistry, pharmaceutics, pharmacology and pharmacognosy. This was seen as a restraint on the development of new ideas of teaching to make the course more relevant to the profession. The course has to have a firm science-base building on knowledge acquired in secondary school, but be relevant to practice. Pharmacognosy is no longer a core part of the undergraduate curriculum. Pathology and therapeutics, law and ethics, the teaching of dispensing practice all have their place alongside clinical pharmacy which is now accepted as a subject in its own right and one of the most important parts of the course. The course also includes social and behavioural science, a broad subject area which covers many sociological and psychological aspects of disease and patients, and communication skills. Although communication cannot be 'learned' solely by studying a book, it is still useful to have an understanding of the underpinning theoretical framework when learning about good professional communication in practice. In this book chapters have been included dealing with social and behavioural science (see Ch. 2), communication skills (see Ch. 3) and counselling skills (see Ch. 38).

Most schools of pharmacy involve both primary and secondary care pharmacy practitioners in undergraduate teaching. The aim of utilizing these teacher–practitioners is to ensure that the university course is relevant to current professional practice. This reflects the situation in other health care professions such as medicine. Other ways of fostering current practice as part of course provision are also used—

such as visiting lecturers, organizing GP practice and hospital visits, using part-time teaching staff, staff secondment to practice and joint academic/practice research studies.

As a result of the need to harmonize the undergraduate courses across the EU as far as possible, all UK courses are now four years with a further year of structured preregistration training in a practice situation.

Preregistration training

The purpose of the preregistration year is for the recent graduate to make the transition from student to a person who can practise effectively and independently as a member of the pharmacy profession. Preregistration training is normally carried out, in either hospital or community pharmacy practice, in a structured way with a competency-based assessment after 12 months. The recommendation to include both hospital and community practice in the preregistration year has not yet been acted upon. Some of the differences between community and hospital practice are becoming less distinct as pharmacists in the community take on roles which in the past have been common in hospital practice, such as prescribing advice to doctors. In the future, it may be that a combined preregistration year may be introduced and interchange between the two areas of practice will become easier to achieve than it is at present.

Higher degrees and research

As recently as the 1980s only a few taught MSc degrees were available. A wide range of postgraduate courses is now offered. Some are relatively short, others offer a postgraduate diploma, others a master of science. Subject matter may be very specialized or more general. Study may be full time or part time. There are also distance learning courses for those who have limited opportunity to be away from their place of work. Research has also developed, and research articles appear regularly in *The Pharmaceutical Journal*, and the *International Journal of Pharmacy Practice* as well as other academic journals from medicine and primary care. There are practice research sessions at the British Pharmaceutical Conference each year, and there is an annual dedicated Health Service and Pharmacy Practice Research Conference. Many students are now graduating with a doctorate for studies undertaken in aspects of pharmacy practice. Reflecting the integrated multidisciplinary delivery of

care, many pharmacists are carrying out research in multidisciplinary primary care research teams. The development of the discipline of pharmacy practice research has a lot to be proud of. The generation of research evidence of the clinical and cost-effective contribution which pharmacists can make to health care has had a key part to play in the innovations in professional practice we have seen in the past decade, and which have been summarized in this introductory chapter.

CONCLUSION

During the 20th century, pharmacy has undergone major changes. This process has accelerated since the introduction of the NHS in 1948, the Nuffield report in 1986, and most recently in the new plans for the NHS published at the turn of the century. Thus pharmacists now deal with more potent and sophisticated medicines, requiring a different type of knowledge than was previously the case. At the same time, the public have become more aware of the services which are available from pharmacists. They are making increasing use of the pharmacist as a source of information and advice about minor conditions and non-prescription medicines. This is now extending to the general public regarding pharmacists as a source of information and advice about their prescribed medicines and seeking help from pharmacists with any medication problems which they may encounter. This process is likely to develop further as society moves into the 21st century. We are also likely to see further changes reflecting the merging of professional boundaries and competency-based delivery of health care. Thus generic health care professionals may emerge, and tasks traditionally undertaken by one profession may be undertaken by many. In addition, in order to free up professional time we can expect to see pharmacy technicians taking on greater responsibility for the technical aspects of the pharmacist's role, whilst qualified pharmacists concentrate on cognitive functions, and interact directly with the patient.

Pharmacists need to have the knowledge and adaptability to take a lead in these processes, so that they can have a key role in ensuring that the health care of the public can be delivered as efficiently as possible. The undergraduate pharmacy courses must reflect these changes to ensure that their graduates meet the demands of the future NHS workforce.

Key Points

- The UK NHS came into being in 1948.
- Early developments in the NHS were in hospital services, but this has gradually changed to focus on community practice.
- Publication of the Nuffield Report in 1986 marked a watershed for pharmacy in the UK.
- Nuffield made nearly 100 specific recommendations for change in all aspects of pharmacy practice, many of which have been implemented.
- In community pharmacy, use of IT, links with GPs, responding to symptoms, health education, meeting patients' needs, re-regulation of POM to P medicines have all developed.
- Changes to a more patient-oriented undergraduate curriculum which began in the 1980s has provided a knowledge base for changing roles in pharmacy practice.

2

Social and behavioural aspects of pharmacy

K. H. Enlund

After studying this chapter you will know about:

Why social and behavioural sciences are important in pharmacy
The meanings of health and illness
Factors incorporated into models of health
How people behave when they are ill
Behavioural aspects of health care
Factors affecting the treatment process
Sociological and behavioural aspects of drug treatment
A sociological perspective of pharmacy
Measuring outcomes

Introduction

Social and behavioural aspects of drug use and pharmacy are still rather new areas within pharmacy education and research. Therefore our understanding of these aspects is still limited. Understanding and resolving drug-related problems that result in suboptimal outcomes need a broad scientific basis. Earlier attempts to solve drug-related problems using 'common sense' approaches have been only partially successful. Therefore there is a need to broaden our perspectives by incorporating relevant social and behavioural theory and research. The purpose of this chapter is to give a broad overview of the health-related issues within a social and behavioural framework to show the importance of 'non-biological' factors in understanding health and medical care, pharmaceutical services and drug-related problems. A common view is that the pure biomedical model underemphasizes the human aspects of patient care and neglects important psychosocial issues. The social sciences have a shared focus on understanding patterns and meaning of human behaviour, which distinguishes them from the physical and biological sciences.

Pharmacists have to deal with many social and behavioural issues in their daily work either directly or indirectly. The contribution of social sciences to pharmacy and pharmacy practice can be summarized in the following three areas:

- Analysing pharmacy, i.e. helping in identifying important questions related to medicines and the use of medicines, the practice of pharmacy and pharmacy services, and pharmacy as a profession.
- Providing conceptual and explanatory frameworks for understanding pharmacy and use of medicines.
- Providing tools and techniques to study pharmacy and the use of medicines.

Many of the subjects presented could fill a book on their own, so it is evident that only a brief introduction to each subject is possible in this chapter. This chapter will focus on the definitions, dimensions and determinants of health and illness. For a pharmacist it is also very important to understand the different processes involved in illness behaviour and medical treatment. There is also an attempt to mention the major concepts and theories in each context. An overall framework is presented in Figure 2.1. The interested reader is referred to specialized textbooks, other books and articles on the topic that are included in the further reading.

HEALTH AND ILLNESS IN A SOCIOBEHAVIOURAL CONTEXT

Illness can be seen either as a purely biophysical state or more comprehensively as a human societal state where behaviour varies with culture and other social factors. The process of medical care normally starts with a recognition of need, i.e. an individual perception of something being wrong. This is usually triggered by the experience of abnormal symptoms. The dominant biomedical model of the

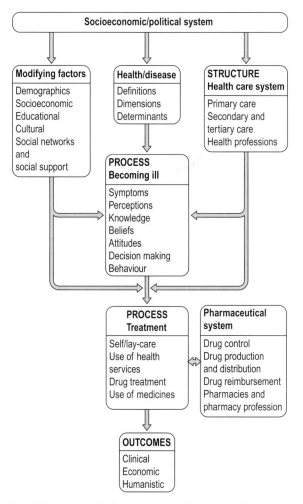

Fig. 2.1 A model of the social and behavioural factors involved in health and illness.

causes of ill health is expanded to include a comprehensive view which includes different definitions and determinants of health as presented in the following text.

DEFINING HEALTH AND ILLNESS

Health and illness mean different things to different people. Most young people take health for granted. We commonly think about health as the absence of signs that the body is not functioning properly or absence of symptoms of disease or injury. There is a tendency to dichotomize health, either you are healthy or not. However, health is not merely the absence of disease, but rather a continuum of different

states. There are degrees of wellness and of illness. Disease in contrast to illness is something professionally defined and therefore also perceived to be more accurate. This has also become the essential framework for the organization we call health care. However, research shows that physicians and other experts vary to a great extent in their views on both physical and mental disorders and their connections. Therefore we can ask whether disease is well defined or even definable.

Illness is more a state defined by a layman or a reaction to a perceived biological alteration of the body or mind. It has both physical and social connotations. Illness is also highly individual. Illness is influenced by cultural, social and other factors. It is important to note that a person may have a disease and not be ill, might be ill but not have a disease or might have both an illness and a disease. Sickness is also a socially defined condition, a social status conferred on an individual by other members of the society. This will be further elaborated in the context of the sick role.

The most widely used definition of health or wellness is that of the World Health Organization (WHO) stating that: 'Health is a state of complete physical, mental and social well-being and not merely the absence of diseases and infirmity'. This definition has been widely quoted, but is less used in daily practice in health care. The definition has to be seen more as a goal that is actively sought through positive actions and not merely as a passive way of avoiding disease-causing agents. Different definitions and models of health also have practical relevance, as they are needed to guide policymakers in their allocation of resources.

Dimensions of health

The WHO definition distinguishes physical, mental and social health. In some narrower definitions only physical and mental health are included, thus implicitly excluding resource allocation for other areas. A broader definition may emphasize social and other dimensions as well. One of the dangers is that the broader the definition, the more we tend to medicalize our society as we include more and more everyday things as part of the responsibility of clinical medicine and public health (e.g. loneliness, attention deficit disorders, domestic violence). On the other hand, these broad definitions allow us to examine health issues more comprehensively. The definition used will also have economical and other consequences.

Most of us see physical health as being free from pain, physical disability, acute and chronic diseases and bodily discomfort, i.e. as the normal functioning of the body's cells, organs and systems. However, prior experiences of disease, age, education and a variety of other personal and social factors will influence our perception of physical health.

Mental health is composed of the ability to deal constructively with reality and adapt to change without feeling threatened by it. A positive self image and an ability to cope with stressors and develop intimate relationships is also part of mental health. Furthermore, enjoying the pleasures of ordinary life and making plans for the future are important aspects of mental health.

The role of spiritual health has raised less research interest. Some might consider this as merely part of the mental health dimension, while others argue that it is a separate dimension. It should not be confused with religion or religiousness. A sense of spiritual well being is possible without belonging to an organized religion. Spiritual health has been characterized by Miller and Price as the ability to articulate and act on one's own basic purpose of life, giving and receiving love, trust, joy and peace, having a set of principles to live by, having a sense of selflessness, honour, integrity and sacrifice and being willing to help others achieve their full potential. By contrast, a negative spiritual health can be described by loss of meaning in one's life, self-centeredness, lack of self-responsibility, and a hopeless attitude.

The impact of social health on the well being of the individual has been widely demonstrated. Lack of social support is closely related to poor health. A low socioeconomic status defined by educational level, income and occupation is closely related to higher morbidity and mortality.

Determinants and models of health

The history of medicine contains several theories or frameworks for the origins of disease. One of the earliest explanations was that mystical forces like evil spirits could cause physical and mental illness. The father of medicine Hippocrates (460–370 BC) developed the humoral theory to explain why people get sick. According to this theory the body contains four fluids (blood, phlegm, yellow and black bile) called humors, and when these are in balance we are in a state of health and accordingly when there is an imbalance we are sick.

In the Middle Ages illness was closely related to religious beliefs; sickness was often interpreted as God's punishment for doing evil things. Priests led most of the practice of medicine and became more involved in treating the ill, sometimes torturing the body to drive out evil spirits. After

the Renaissance different scholars became more human-centred, one of the most influential in the 17th century being René Descartes. His impact on scientific thought has been extensive and lasted for centuries. His main health-related ideas can be summarized in three points: firstly he saw the body as a machine and described how action and sensation occurs, secondly he proposed that body and mind, although separate, could communicate and thirdly that the soul in humans leaves the body at death.

In the following centuries scientists learned more and more how the body functions with the help of the microscope and other technical advances. New theories, like the germ theory, tried to explain disease by microbes, etc. All these advances led to the foundation of the current biomedical disease model, which proposes that all diseases or physical disorders can be explained by disturbances in physiological processes, which result from injury, biochemical imbalances and bacterial or viral infections. The biomedical model assumes that disease is an affliction of the body and is separate from the psychological and social processes of the mind.

A more recent and comprehensive model is the biopsychosocial model that involves the interplay of biological, psychological and social aspects of a person's life.

Some of the ancient beliefs are still prevalent among primitive tribes and in certain cultures. They also continue surprisingly strongly in industrialized countries alongside conventional medicine. Wrong behaviour, diet and dirty water, weather, accidents, black magic or witchcraft, spirits and God are all mentioned as causes of diseases. 'Don't wet your feet or you'll catch a cold' typifies certain superstitious thinking.

Genetic and biological determinants

In current medicine there is much interest in the genetic basis of disease. The origin of most health problems seems to lie in human genes. The newspapers have declared the finding of the alcoholism, antisocial behaviour and obesity genes among others. This leads to the lay impression that once the genetic code has been solved all health problems will also be solved without any need to pay attention to, for example, health habits. This of course is a far too simplified way of thinking. The scientific interest in this field is more in the possibility of a genetic predisposition with individual exposures to trigger factors accounting for individual differences in disease. For example, is there a genetic factor which explains why some smokers get lung cancer and others do not? This is a relevant question, but it is only part of the picture. We should also ask whether it can explain differences in risk of disease between populations not just between individuals.

Behavioural determinants

The leading causes of death today, heart disease, cancer, stroke and accidents, are all associated with behavioural risk factors. The origin of many chronic diseases, like diabetes and hypertension, can be found in lifestyle factors. Sedentary lifestyle explains a lot of the causes of these diseases, without the need to go to the gene level. It is also remarkable that the remedy for most of these lifestyle diseases can be found in simple behavioural remedies like increased physical activity, reduced stress, balanced diet and quitting smoking.

Behaviour and mental processes are the focus of psychology and they involve cognition, emotion and motivation. Cognition involves perceiving, knowing, learning, remembering, thinking, interpreting, believing and problem solving. Emotion is a subjective feeling that affects and is affected by our thoughts, behaviour and physiology. Emotions can be positive/pleasant or negative/unpleasant. People whose emotions are more positive are less disease prone and more likely to recover quickly from an illness than those with more negative emotions. Motivation applies to explanations of why people behave the way they do, e.g. why they start a health-related activity or why they don't take their medicines as prescribed. Psychology is also interested in interpersonal relationships, which includes thinking, feeling and doing with someone else. Descriptions of cognition, affect, behaviour and interpersonal interactions overlap and it may be difficult to separate them, e.g. in a situation causing anxiety the person may think he is not in control of the situation (cognitive component), he is afraid (affective) and his hands are sweating (behavioural) and he may ask somebody to help support him (interpersonal).

Stress is a condition that results when personal/environmental transactions lead the individual to perceive a discrepancy (real or not) between the demands of a situation and the resources of the person's biological, psychological or social system. The connection between body and mind is also reflected in how people react to stress. It can produce changes in the body's physiology and cause illness. Stress can release hormones, especially catecholamines and corticosteroids, by the endocrine system through arousal. Effects on the cardiovascular system can be important and stress-related emotions such as anxiety and depression can

play a critical role in the balance of the immune system. Stress can be described as a stimulus. Events and circumstances that are perceived as threatening or harmful, and produce feelings of tension, are called stressors. However, stress can also be seen as a response to stressors. The person's physiological and psychological response to a stressor is called strain. Stress can be seen as a process including stressors and strain and the relationship between the person and the environment as continuous interactions and adjustments.

Stress can also affect health through the person's behaviour. People who experience high levels of stress tend to behave in a way that increases their chances of becoming ill or injured. They consume more alcohol and drugs and smoke more than people who experience less stress. The accident rates are also higher among those with elevated stress.

Environmental determinants

The role of environmental factors (biological, chemical, physical, mechanical) in influencing human health is widely accepted. The main pathways into the human body are air (outdoor and indoor), water, food and soil. The role of these environmental factors in the pathogenesis of asthma, hay fever and others are clear. However, environmental factors have a much broader impact, e.g. starting in the prenatal phase (the use of some drugs like thalidomide during pregnancy has lead to severe birth defects).

The importance of the environment has been demonstrated in migrant and time-trend studies of disease. When people change environment their disease risk patterns change. One interesting demonstration is the case of Japanese migrants. The further they went across the Pacific the higher their incidence of coronary heart disease and the lower their rate of stroke. Japanese in Hawaii have rates of heart disease intermediate between those in Japan and those in California. Environment and lifestyle are the most probable explanations of these differences. There is also a distinction between individual risk factors and environmental causes of disease. Differences in individual risk factors explain only a part of the variation in the occurrence of disease. While reducing high risk factors might be beneficial for the individual concerned, it makes a limited contribution to reducing disease rates in the whole population. Rose has suggested that the causes of individual differences in disease may be different from the causes of differences between populations. A risk factor does not necessarily cause the disease even if it is associated with it.

Socioeconomic determinants

These factors are also 'environmental', but their role can be debated as to whether they are genuine factors determining health or whether they only represent predisposing factors. Society establishes certain health values, which are often reflected in the media. These values can be both positive and negative. Being fit and healthy is 'good' and exemplifies a positive value, whilst celebrities smoking cigarettes or marijuana exemplifies a negative value. The family is the closest and most continuous social relationship for most people. Therefore, many health-related habits, behaviours and attitudes are learnt and modelled from this context. The degree of support or encouragement received from family members and friends for partaking in a health-related activity might be an important factor. This is dealt with in more detail in a later paragraph.

In developing countries factors such as poverty, poor nutrition and poor resistance to pathogens are all interrelated with a poor health status of the population. Similarly, historical statistics from industrialized countries show that over the last two or three centuries there is a strong positive correlation between improved health, life expectancy and improved economy. In most countries the relationship between socioeconomic status and disease runs across the social hierarchy. This shows that the relationship between socioeconomic status and health is a question of relative deprivation rather than absolute deprivation. This linear association can only partially be explained by lifestyle factors. Usually people with a higher socioeconomic status have healthier habits than those from lower socioeconomic groups. Similarly there are huge differences in life expectancy between western and eastern European countries that can be attributed to socioeconomic factors.

Interaction of different factors

It is evident that no factor alone can explain the health of a nation, demographic group or individual. It is difficult to capture all the relevant features and their relationships. Having good genes can prevent some people from getting a disease and, on the other hand, somebody with poor genes can get ill regardless of a healthy lifestyle and other positive factors. Considering the impact of all aspects of a person's life as a total entity in understanding health and illness is called holism.

One comprehensive attempt to describe/model the interactions between different factors is the 'Nested Model of Health'. This model consists of two levels of activity, the individual and the community level. The individual level is composed of five different categories:

- Psychosocial environment (e.g. personal housing)
- Microphysical environment (e.g. chemicals and noise)
- Work environment (e.g. work stress)
- Behavioural environment (e.g. smoking, alcohol use, exercise)
- Race/class/gender environment.

These environments are thought to affect each other and to affect and be affected by the individual. The individual level is nested/located in the centre of the community level. This community level, which is the main focus of health policy decision makers, is composed of four components, the political/economic climate (e.g. unemployment level), the macrophysical environment (e.g. air quality), social justice/ equity (e.g. social security system) and local control/ cohesiveness (e.g. local planning efforts). These four components are interrelated and changes in them are expected to lead to changes in the health of individuals.

PROCESS OF ILLNESS

Becoming ill

Understanding illness behaviour can help pharmacists appreciate and accept why patients respond differently to seemingly similar pain or discomfort. The general criteria by which people view themselves as 'well' include a feeling of well being, an absence of symptoms and an ability to perform normal functions. This is the baseline situation against which any changes are judged. When studying health-related behaviour it is important to consider how behaviour changes with the health status of the individual. Kasl and Cobb defined three types of behaviour that characterize three stages in the progress of disease:

- Health behaviour, which refers to any activity undertaken by people believing themselves to be healthy for the purpose of preventing disease or detecting it at an asymptomatic stage.
- Illness behaviour, which involves any activity undertaken by people who feel ill, to define the state of their health and to discover a suitable remedy.
- Sick-role behaviour refers to the activity undertaken for the purpose of getting well by those who consider themselves ill.

Ways of identifying and reacting to symptoms

Symptoms can be classified into three broad groups, those symptoms noted by the patient, symptoms noted by behavioural changes and patient complaints. A behaviour, which in some situations is regarded as normal, can in other situations be regarded as a sign of illness. Not all symptoms can be regarded as medical, as they may have a natural explanation, like tiredness. Different symptoms may be perceived very differently, depending on the person, setting and situation. Differences in illness behaviour occur as a function of the immediate experience, past experiences and the patient's information processing, organizing and recall. The significance of symptoms are judged according to the degree of interference with normal activities, the clarity of symptoms, the person's tolerance threshold, familiarity of symptoms, assumptions about cause and prognoses, interpersonal influence from the lay-referral system and other life crises making the symptoms appear more severe. The subjective and psychosocial aspects of an incident can be more important in determining decision and action than the symptoms themselves.

The experience of illness involves affective and cognitive reactions to illness, in which the patient undergoes emotional changes and attempts to understand the illness. Bernstein and Bernstein have described these emotional reactions to illness and treatment in the following ways:

- Emotional reactions directly related to illness or treatment, including fear, anxiety, and a feeling of damage and frustration caused by loss of habitual gratification and pleasure.
- Reactions determined primarily by life experience before or during illness, such as anger, dependency and guilt.
- Complications like depression and loss of self-esteem.

Women are more likely than men to interpret discomfort as a medical symptom; they also recall and report more symptoms. These differences may partly be explained by a higher interest in and concern with health issues among women than men. The family often plays an active role in the symptom identification process. Other family members may recognize some symptoms before the person does. The family also takes part in the interpretation process of symptoms. The culture is also an important factor influencing the process of symptom identification and evaluation. Some cultures describe more readily common symptoms as medical, while others tend to suppress signs of medical symptoms. There might also be differences between generations in this respect. What was earlier considered as normal may today be seen as something requiring medical attention. The individual's feeling of anxiety may also explain the symptom levels, since high anxiety has been associated with the identification of many symptoms.

Sick-role behaviour

When people perceive themselves to be sick they adopt the so-called 'sick-role behaviour'. According to Parsons this includes the following components:

- The patient is not blamed for being sick.
- The patient is exempt from work and other responsibilities.
- The illness is seen as legitimate as long as the patient accepts the undesirability of it.
- The patient is expected to seek competent help to get well again.

It has been found that not all people follow these patterns of the sick role and it should be seen more as a general framework for understanding illness behaviour. However, this framework is not able to explain variations within illness behaviour; it is not applicable to chronic disease and often not mental illness. There are also certain diseases where there might be some unwillingness to grant the exemptions from blame. These include certain conditions related to smoking, overuse of alcohol and AIDS. But even epilepsy has been stigmatized in many cultures.

The role of personality in illness

Personality has been shown to be associated with illness. People who have high levels of anxiety, depression and anger/hostility traits seem to be more disease prone than others. These emotions are part of reactions to different types of stress. People handle stressful situations in different ways. People who approach stressful situations more positively and hopefully are less disease prone and also tend to recover more quickly if they get ill. People who are ill need to overcome their negative thoughts and feelings in order to recover more quickly.

The cardiologists Friedman and Rosenman were the first ones to describe differences in behavioural and emotional style, when studying the behaviour of heart patients. These patterns have been named as Type A and Type B behaviour. The Type A behaviour pattern is characterized by:

- A competitive achievement orientation, including a high level of self-criticism and striving towards goals without feeling a sense of joy in achievements.
- Time urgency, e.g. tight scheduling of commitments, impatience with time delays and unproductive time.
- Anger/hostility which is easily aroused. This component, especially, seems to be detrimental to good health. Type A individuals respond more quickly and strongly to stress, often seeing stressors as threats to their personal control.

The Type A pattern may also increase the person's probability of getting into stressful situations. The relationships between Type A behaviour and psychosocial factors are very complex, involving multiple levels of human experience. Type B behaviour pattern is opposite to Type A, taking life more easily with little competitiveness, time urgency and hostility. Interestingly the overall evidence for an association between Type A and B behaviour and general illnesses is weak and inconsistent. However, many studies, but not all, have shown a clear association between Type A behaviour and coronary heart disease.

HEALTH KNOWLEDGE, BELIEFS AND ATTITUDES

There are different definitions of what this knowledge is. Sometimes it may include a variety of things such as beliefs, expectations, norms and cognitive perceptions. If this is the case, knowledge has to be considered in a wider framework than merely having some factual knowledge about diseases and treatment. One of the goals in current health care is to improve the patient's problem-solving capacity. The starting point is providing the necessary information and improving the factual knowledge of the patient. It has been shown several times that knowledge alone is not sufficient to ensure change in behaviour, which is often the goal. Preventive behaviours, the treatment process, taking medications all require a certain amount of knowledge. The current trend emphasizing guided self-care in chronic diseases like asthma, diabetes and hypertension requires a well-informed patient. The aim is to produce patients who actively participate in their own treatment. In research settings, the narrow approach towards knowledge, usually involves using a knowledge index (set of questions) that the patient has to answer before and after an educational intervention.

Attitudes have been defined as states of readiness or predisposition, feeling for or against something, which predisposes to particular responses. They involve emotions (feelings) and knowledge (or beliefs) about the object and emanate in behaviour. Attitudes are not inherited but learnt and though relatively stable are modifiable by education.

The Health Belief Model

The Health Belief Model, which was originally developed by Rosenstock and his colleagues to predict the use of preventive health services, has been extensively used during the last two decades to try to explain various health behaviours. The model was further developed for predicting health behaviour in chronic diseases and reformulated for predicting compliance with health care regimens.

The elements of the model are subjective perceptions which can be modified, at least in theory. According to the model the probability that a person will take a preventive health action—that is, perform some health, illness or sick-role behaviour, is a function of:

- The perceived susceptibility to the health problem or disease
- The perceived severity of medical and social consequences of the disease
- The perceived benefits and barriers (costs) related to the recommended behaviour.

According to the model the more vulnerable the person feels and the more serious the disease the more likely it is the person will act. Furthermore, various factors that result from the perceptions are expected to modify this motivating force. These factors include demographic, socioeconomic and therapy-related factors as well as the illness itself and the prescribed regimen. Prior contact with the disease or knowledge about the disease may modify the behaviour. Some incidents, so-called 'cues to action', are also expected to trigger the behaviour. These include, for example, a mass media campaign, magazine article, advice from significant others or illness of family member or friend.

The concept of perception is important in the Health Belief Model. It is the patient's and not the pharmacist's perceptions that drive the decisions and behaviours of the patient. In studies of compliance with prescribed medications the concept of personal susceptibility has been modified because the illness has already been diagnosed. One approach includes examining the individual's estimate of or belief in the accuracy of the diagnosis. This concept has also been extended to estimating resusceptibility or measuring the individual's subjective feelings of vulnerability to various other diseases or to illness in general. Studies show that in hypertension, for example, the threat posed by hypertension and the perceived effectiveness of treatment in reducing this threat seem to be important predictors of compliance. Likewise the perceived control over one's own health is important. There is some controversy about the chronology of these beliefs and whether they precede or develop simultaneously with health behaviour.

The Health Belief Model and commonsense might tell us that the patient's decision to seek health care, accept a diagnosis and engage in health-related behaviours would be related to the seriousness of the disease. Research indicates this may not always be the case. Patients' health behaviours are a function of many psychosocial variables. Reasons why humans may behave illogically are dealt with in more detail in the section 'Decision analysis and behavioural decision theory' below.

The theory of reasoned action

According to the theory of reasoned action by Ajzen and Fishbein, a person's intention is the best predictor of what he will do. The person's intention is determined by his attitude regarding the behaviour and whether he thinks it is a good or bad thing to do. This assessment is based on behavioural beliefs about possible outcomes of the behaviour and evaluations of whether these outcomes would be rewarding. The other attitude represents the impact of social pressure or influence. These are based on normative beliefs regarding others' opinions about the behaviour and the person's motivation to follow those opinions, i.e. what do other people think I should do? The theory proposes that the subjective norm and the attitude regarding the behaviour combine to produce an intention, which leads to the behaviour.

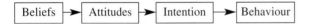

Beliefs → Attitudes → Intention → Behaviour

If behaviour is determined by beliefs, this raises the question what factors determine beliefs? These factors would include things like age, sex, education, social class, culture and personality traits. These variables influence behaviour indirectly rather than directly. One of the problems with the theory is that people do not always do what they plan, i.e. intentions and behaviour are only moderately related. Another problem is that people do not always act rationally. Irrational decisions like delaying medical treatment when symptoms exist cannot be explained by the model. Neither does the model include prior experiences with the behaviour, which might be an important factor to consider, since past behaviour is a strong predictor of future practice of that behaviour.

The conflict theory

The conflict theory has been used to explain rational and irrational decision making. According to the model the process a person is using in arriving at a health-related decision involves five stages. It starts when something challenges the person's current course of action. It can be a threat (e.g. symptom) or a mass media alert about the danger of narcotics or an opportunity (e.g. free membership to a health club). The different stages of the conflict theory model are:

1. Assessing the challenge, i.e. whether the risk is serious enough. The assessment may involve thoughts like, the risk is not real, it is irrelevant or inapplicable. If the risk is not considered serious enough, the behaviour continues as before and the decision-making process stops.
2. Assessing alternatives, i.e. the search for alternatives for dealing with the risk starts when the risk is acknowledged. This stage ends when the suitability of available alternatives has been surveyed.
3. Weighing alternatives, i.e. the pros and cons of each alternative are weighed to find the best alternative.
4. Making a final choice and committing to it.
5. Adhering despite negative feedback, i.e. after starting a new behaviour people may have second thoughts about it if the environment is not supportive or it gives negative feedback.

The decision process can be aborted at any point. Errors in decision making are often caused by stress, information overload, group pressure and other factors. The way people cope with stress has an important role in health, illness and sick-role behaviour. According to the conflict theory a person's coping with a conflict is dependent on the presence and absence of risks, hope and adequate time. Different combinations of these may result in different types of behavioural response. For example, when there are perceptions of high risk in changing the behaviour and no hope in finding a better alternative, a high level of stress is experienced. Denial and shifting responsibility to someone else are typical responses, with delays in seeking care when needed. The perception of serious risk, and belief in a better alternative, but also a perception of running out of time, also creates high levels of stress. People search desperately for solutions and may choose an alternative hastily if promised immediate relief. Different untested cancer quacks are good examples where unscrupulous people try to make use of this kind of situation. The perception of serious risk, with a belief that a better alternative will become available and there is time to search for it, results in low levels of stress and rational choices.

Locus of control

It has been claimed that how individuals perceive their ability to influence disease and the treatment is an important determinant of health behaviour. People have been categorized into two groups: those with an internal locus of control and those with an external locus of control. Those who have an internal locus of control tend to perceive that they are in control of their own health by their actions and behaviour, while the second group perceives that health is externally determined and their actions have little or no effect. Therefore those with a strongly internal locus of control should tend to practise behaviours that prevent illness and promote health. Research has shown that this is the case, but the relationship is not very strong. This shows that the locus of control is just one factor among many others that determine health behaviour. Belief in internal control is likely to have a greater impact among people who place a higher value on their health than among those who do not.

Self-efficacy and social learning

Sometimes performing a health action is hard to do because it is technically difficult or it may involve several steps. Therefore the belief in the success in doing something—called self-efficacy—may be an important determinant in choosing or not choosing to change behaviour. People develop a sense of efficacy through their successes and failures, observations of others' experiences and assessments of their abilities by others. People assess their efficacy based on the effort that is required, complexity of the task and situational factors, e.g. possibility of receiving help if needed. People who think they are not able to quit smoking will not even try, while people who believe they can succeed will try and eventually some may even succeed.

Those with a strong sense of self-efficacy show less psychological strain in response to stressors than those with a weak sense of efficacy. People differ in the degree to which they believe they have control over the things that happen in their lives. Those who experience prolonged, high levels of stress and lack a sense of personal control tend to feel helpless. Having a strong sense of control seems to benefit health and adjustment to sickness.

As environmental factors and expectations directed towards the individuals change, they must either intensify their activities or change their environment. Individuals have different capabilities of coping and coping strategies. According to the social learning theory, people change their environment with the help of symbols they choose in accordance with their values, norms and goals. On the other hand, the environment changes the individual's behaviour by rewarding beneficial activities and punishing or not rewarding activities that harm the environment. Through the socialization process the individual adopts the values and norms of the community, is socialized as its member and gains identity. Through this process the individual has learnt to act efficiently in social systems.

Antonowsky has used the 'sense of coherence' concept, which is an extensive and constant feeling of an individual's internal and external environment being in harmony with each other. Every individual has characteristic psychosocial potentials that include material resources, intelligence, knowledge, coping strategies, social support, arts, religion, philosophy and health behaviour. Antonowsky calls a sense of coherence 'salutogenic' or health generating. Disease–health is a continuum at one end of which is a high degree of coherence and health (ease) and at the other end a low degree of coherence and illness (dis-ease). External factors that the individual considers threatening mobilize the defence mechanisms and cause stress conditions in the individual. Prolonged stress is disease generating and causes the condition dis-ease.

Coping

Because of the emotional and physical strain that accompanies it, stress is uncomfortable and people are motivated to do things that reduce their stress. The concept of coping is used to describe how people adjust to stressful situations in their life. Coping is the process by which people try to manage the perceived discrepancy between the demands and resources they appraise in stressful situations. Coping means the ability to meet the demands of new situations and solve the problems with which one is confronted. Coping is determined by situational and personal determinants. At the individual level, external factors turn into stress factors if previous experiences together with personality traits, consciously or unconsciously, are considered as threatening or diminish self-esteem. Coping efforts can be quite varied and do not necessarily lead to a solution of the problem. It can help the person to alter his perception of a discrepancy, tolerate or accept the harm or threat and escape or avoid the situation. The coping process is not a single event.

Coping mechanisms

Coping can alter the problem or it can regulate the emotional response causing the stress reaction to the problem. Behavioural approaches include using alcohol or drugs, seeking social support from friends or simply watching TV. Cognitive approaches involve how people think about the stressful situation, e.g. changing the meaning of the situation. Emotion-focused approaches are used when people think they cannot do anything to change the stressful situation. Problem-focused coping is used to reduce the demands of the stressful situation or to expand the capacity and resources to deal with it. The two types of coping can also be used together. Sarafino has summarized commonly used methods of coping as follows:

- The direct method, i.e. doing something specifically and directly to cope with a stressor, e.g. negotiating, consulting, arguing, running away.
- Seeking information and acquiring knowledge about the stressful situation.
- Turning to others, i.e. seeking help, reassurance and comfort from family and friends.
- Resigned acceptance, i.e. the person comes to terms with the situation and accepts it as it is.
- Emotional discharge, i.e. expressing feelings or reducing tension by taking, for example, alcohol or drugs, smoking cigarettes.
- Intrapsychic processes, i.e. cognitive redefinition, e.g. the 'things could be worse' attitude.

DECISION ANALYSIS AND BEHAVIOURAL DECISION THEORY

Decision analysis is a systematic way of studying the process of decision making among patients, pharmacists and physicians. This is a widely used tool in pharmacoeconomics today (see Ch. 35). It usually involves assigning numbers to perceived values of the therapeutic outcomes and the probability that the outcome will occur. This gives a utility of each outcome and the one with the highest utility would be chosen. One problem is that humans do not always make decisions logically or treat information value free.

Why don't humans behave logically? One explanation that has been offered is that humans are biased when making decisions under uncertainty because we fail to appreciate randomness. We believe that there are known causes and effects for all phenomena and we have a need to be able to explain outcomes. It is easier to explain, even incorrectly, than to have to deal with uncertain situations. People also tend to be inconsistent in judgment, often because of difficulties in remembering how a judgment was made. Another reason is that we seldom receive feedback from negative decisions, e.g. if we decide not to take the medicine we do not know how effective it would have been.

Behaviour decision theory has been used to understand how patients make decisions about their medicine and health-related behaviour. These include acquisition of information, information processing, making decisions under uncertainty and interpreting outcomes of that decision. It has been found that patients are more likely to take a health risk to avoid an aversive situation, rather than to gain a positive health outcome. Patients are also more likely to choose a certain outcome rather than an outcome with a high probability of occurrence, even if the certain outcome is less valued than that one with a high probability of occurrence. When a person has already invested time and money on a product or activity they are likely to continue it, even if it does not appear to be effective.

Hogarth has described different biases that people tend to have in decision making, which may be helpful in understanding patient choices about health behaviour. We tend to believe more in well-publicized events than in those that are less publicized. This has direct links with the consumer's choice of well-advertised over-the-counter (OTC) medicines. There is a tendency to believe what matches our existing beliefs. This selective perception has direct implications to health education in pharmacies. We also tend to believe real incidents more than abstract statistics. Positive experiences from a family member quitting smoking is more likely to be effective than showing statistics about future (uncertain) consequences of smoking. Two incidents occurring close in time and place tend to be regarded as causal. Becoming ill after having taken a medicine (regardless of cause and effect) would usually trigger a response of aversion next time seeing the same medicine. We are reluctant to change our beliefs, even when given new data, and tend to discount the new information rather than discount our belief. Very few instances of an occurrence are needed for us to form a new belief if it has a strong effect upon us. This has direct implications to the experience of side effects of drugs. We also believe something is more likely to happen if we want it to happen. A decision that was successful is more likely to be considered to be due to the knowledge and wisdom of the decision maker. On the other hand, a decision resulting in bad outcomes is likely to be blamed on others.

Theory into practice—the process of behaviour change

A lot of pharmacists' activities will focus on changing the behaviour of patients. Without going into the ethical aspects of behaviour change, we will concentrate on the process of change. It has been proved several times that merely using commonsense is not enough to reach permanent behaviour change. Using a commonsense approach would assume that, by giving the facts, people are able to change their behaviour in a direction anticipated by the health care professional. A simple example illustrates the limits of this approach. Why do so many people still smoke cigarettes despite knowing all the negative consequences of smoking?

Even if many of the behavioural theories are far from complete or comprehensive, they may guide us in improving the outcome of behavioural interventions. Behaviour change includes a long list of steps that need to be taken before it is finalized.

- The process starts with 'attention'. The person needs to be exposed to the message, which might be a counselling session by the pharmacist or a health campaign in the mass media. If the same message is repeated from different sources and these sources are regarded as credible, the likelihood of change grows. Therefore it is important that the information received from physicians and pharmacists are congruent. If the patients receive mixed messages they are more likely to ignore them.
- The attention is followed by 'motivation'. The person must feel motivated to change their behaviour. It is well known that immediate rewards are more motivating than anticipated rewards after several years.
- Next the person has to 'comprehend' the message to be able to act upon it, but they also need to learn some facts, i.e. improve their knowledge base. These facts need to be simple and match the local culture.
- The following step is persuasion, i.e. the person needs to 'change their attitude'.
- Furthermore they might need to learn some new techniques and skills in how to take or handle the medication. Demonstration and guided practice is the best way of handling this step.
- The person must also be able to perform the skills and maintain the learned skills, which includes self-efficacy training and feedback of success. Many experiments with a long enough follow-up show that positive results can be achieved with pharmacists' interventions, but when the experiment is over, the results soon deteriorate to pre-experiment levels.

- 'Continuous reinforcement' is necessary to maintain good results in any intervention, be it changing medicine-taking behaviour or modification of preventive health behaviour.

THE TREATMENT PROCESS

Self- and lay-care

During the 1970s and 1980s a new trend emphasizing the role of the individual and patient emerged as a part of a more general trend called consumerism. People have become more committed to getting and taking control of their own lives and assessing the impact of their behaviour on their health. Different self-care and self-help movements were a direct result of this trend. The same trend has been obvious in most countries although the starting time and speed of it has varied. At the same time the dominant role of the health care personnel has diminished. With new information sources, and especially the Internet, the trend continues to grow and spread to countries where physicians and other health care personnel still dominate. This new trend has included a much more critical attitude towards what is being done in health care and the quality of care given. Patients are asking more questions, seeking more information and taking a more active role in their health care. They have a better basic education and knowledge especially about their own disease and treatment of that disease.

The new trend has also put increasing demands on pharmacists regarding their knowledge base especially in therapeutics but also in communication. The priorities in treatment goals may differ between the patient and the treating physician and this calls for negotiation. One aspect is that patients' views have to be taken seriously.

According to the self-care philosophy people should be given more responsibility for their own health. One way this can be achieved is to emphasize the role of self-care in treating minor ailments using home remedies and an increased number of self-medication products. Especially in the 1980s and early 1990s this trend was obvious in many countries. The most common 'action' in response to a perceived health problem has been to ignore the problem or wait for a few days. It is estimated that some 30–40% of health problems are dealt with in this way. Of those who take some action 75–80% self-diagnose and use self-treatment, while only 20–25% seek professional care. Therefore a seemingly small change in this ratio (towards using more professional care) has a substantial impact and burden on the official health care system. Of those who use self-treatment some 70–90% are self-medicating and of those self-medicating some 80% are using OTC drugs. Home remedies like onion, garlic, warm drinks, in addition to different herbal products, vitamins and minerals, are widely used all over the world. Some of the newly emerging preparations are marketed with high promises of eternal youth and health, the evidence base being nonexistent or weak.

Before people decide to seek medical care for their symptoms they get and seek advice from friends, relatives and coworkers. These advisors form a lay-referral network that provides its own information and interpretation regarding the symptoms, recommending home remedies, self-medication, professional help or consulting another 'lay expert' who may have had a similar problem.

The pharmacy is often the first place where people come to seek help within the health care system. Increased self-care includes also potential risks in that lay people may not be able to distinguish between serious and non-serious symptoms. Certain situations may demand professional care without further delay caused by inappropriate self-medication practices. The lay-referral network can in some cases be guilty of causing the delay in seeking care. This treatment delay has been divided into three stages, i.e. appraisal delay, illness delay and utilization delay. Appraisal delay is the time it takes to interpret a symptom as a part of an illness. Illness delay is the time between recognizing the illness and the decision to seek care. Finally utilization delay is the time between the decision and actually using a health service.

There has also been concern about misuse of OTC drugs, like laxatives, codeine-containing cough medicines, etc. The other side of the coin is saved resources in health care when there is less reliance on professionals. This seems to be an important aspect as health care budgets tend to increase more rapidly than the general inflation rate.

Primary care

Simultaneously with emerging self-care, the concept of primary health care was introduced. In 1977 the World Health Assembly of the WHO adopted the concept of Health for All by the Year 2000. The following year this concept was translated into the so called Alma Ata declaration at the Alma Ata conference on primary health care. The focus was on making health care more accessible and lowering the health care costs and thus improving the quality of life for the whole population. According to the declaration primary health care should include:

- Education about prevailing health problems
- Methods of identifying, preventing and controlling them
- Promotion of food supply and proper nutrition
- Adequate water supply and basic sanitation
- Maternal and child health care including family planning
- Immunization against the major infectious diseases
- Prevention and control of locally endemic diseases
- Appropriate treatment of common diseases and injuries
- Promotion of mental health
- Provision of essential drugs.

Primary health care focuses on principal health problems and must be part of the national health policy and planning. The conference recommended a re-evaluation of health priorities, putting less emphasize on curative facilities especially in third world countries. The conference also called for cooperation and commitment in striving for an acceptable level of health for all people by the year 2000.

The scope of public health is population based rather than individually based. Public health problems are not a series of individuals presenting diseases to a health care provider for cure, alleviation or prevention, but they are considered in the context of the community. It is a public health problem to determine the prevalence of a disease in the community, compare that with figures from previous years and plan health services to reduce the prevalence. Public health includes enumeration, analysing and planning, but also specific actions to be taken. Public health exists on two levels, the microlevel, i.e. performing some public health function like immunization or preventing inappropriate use of illicit drugs, and on the macrolevel with activities like planning or policy formulation.

Factors influencing the use of health services

The structures of the health care systems in different countries have a lot of similarities, but also a lot of differences. The system is the sum of historical development, culture and economic factors. In some countries there are actually several different systems in place within the health care system. It is not within the scope of this chapter to describe these different systems, rather to highlight some of the current issues in organizing the health care of the citizens and to highlight some sociobehavioural factors influencing the provision of care. It may seem obvious that when having bad angina you will need hospital care and you will be provided with all the technical know-how and help in dealing with the problem. However, the country you happen to live in, the insurance policy you have, the services available, quality of care, etc. will all influence the outcome of the disease. The organization and financing of health care, the environment of medical care, social and cultural factors all influence the care that you will receive.

Demographic factors

Several important differences have been reported between different age groups and gender. However, there are few that have been able to validate the reasons. As mentioned before it is well known that women report more symptoms, they have a lower threshold of pain and discomfort and they are more likely to seek care. Men are more hesitant than women to admit having symptoms and seek medical care for these symptoms. This can be a result of perceived sex-role stereotypes—men should be tough and independent and ignore and endure pain. Women use physician services more than men in all age groups except for the first few years of life. Regardless of this, men have a higher mortality and shorter life expectancy at all ages.

In general young children and the elderly use physician services more often than adolescents and young adults. Age differences in health behaviour cannot be explained by biological ageing alone. Elderly people have different views on health and illness, symptoms, health care use and drugs. There is a danger in labelling all elderly as having similar attitudes concerning health issues, but, as with younger persons, among the elderly there is also a big variety of views on health and treatment. Certain ideas are more prevalent among the elderly than young. The differences can partly be explained by so-called cohort effects, people of the same age have been disposed to the same kind of experiences and attitudes in society and therefore are also likely to share certain behavioural characteristics.

Cultural and socioeconomic factors

Ethnic and cultural background may explain some differences in symptom experience, how people seek medical care and how they take their medicines. In the 1950s a classic study about how people deal with pain found big differences between Italian, Jewish, Irish and Yankee (Old American) hospitalized patients. Italian and Jewish patients were more likely to respond emotionally and expressively to pain than Irish or Yankee patients, who tended to deny pain. Italian and Jewish patients showed their pain by crying, complaining and demanding, while the Irish and Yankee patients preferred to hide their pain and withdraw from others. More recent

studies among immigrants in the USA found that the differences in willingness to tolerate pain diminish in succeeding generations. Other similar studies have shown cultural differences among European countries and the USA, e.g. in perception of fever and the need to medicate children's fever.

There are also differences in seeking care according to social class, education and income. These factors all point in the same direction, those who are better off also use more health services. Different models of why people seek or do not seek health services have been proposed. The Health Belief Model has also been used in this context.

Social support

Social environments and networks are important in the growth, development and health of people. Social support is an important factor in all phases of the process of illness and the treatment process. Social support relates directly to the general and universal needs of people. The best known theory is that by Maslow. According to his theory human needs are hierarchical, starting with basic physiological needs, followed by safety needs, belongingness and love needs, esteem needs and finishing with the highest—self-actualization needs. A slightly modified and simplified model is that by Allardt; according to him people's needs include standard of living (having), social relations (loving) and forms of self-actualization (being). Social relations include social networks and belonging to them is the basis of one's identity and social existence. Social support is the term used for different forms of emotional and material support. The nature of social support is reciprocal. It can be support provided directly by one person to another or indirectly through the system or community.

Forms and levels of social support:

- Material or instrumental support includes money, goods, auxiliary appliances and medicine.
- Operational support includes service, transportation and rehabilitation.
- Informational support includes advice, directions, feedback, education and training.
- Emotional support involves the expression of caring, empathy, love and encouragement.
- Mental support involves a common ideology, belief and philosophy.

Social support has two dimensions, a qualitative and a quantitative dimension. It can also be subjective and objective in nature. The quality of social support can be measured only by subjective assessments. When providing material support the quantitative aspect is more prominent (medicines an exception) and in the other support forms the qualitative aspect (including timing) is more important than the quantitative aspect. Thus a small functioning support network is better than a broad but passive one.

Social support has been divided into primary, secondary and tertiary levels based on the intimacy of the social relationships. The primary level includes family and close friends, the secondary level includes friends, colleagues and neighbours and the tertiary level acquaintances, authorities, public and private services. Social support can be provided by a lay person (usually on the primary and secondary level) or a professional (usually on the tertiary level). Recently different organizations have started training courses for lay providers of support aiming at strengthening the second level of support. Social support has both direct effects on health and well being and indirect stress-buffering effects on coping in stressful situations.

The research on the effects of social support on health goes back to the late 1940s and early 1950s. The first studies in this area showed that lack of social support exposes people to recurrent accidents, suicide and risk of catching tuberculosis. In the 1970s the emphasis was on relationships between social support structures and health in communities. It was shown that the lack of social support increases the incidence of coronary heart disease, mortality due to myocardial infarction and total mortality in the population. It has also been shown that social support is important in perceived health and in reducing hypertension. Social support also has a positive effect on physical, social and emotional recovery. It reduces the need for medication and speeds up symptom amelioration. The positive effects of social support in different stages of illness can be summarized:

- In the prevention of illness it can reduce insecurity and anxiety.
- In the acute stage of illness it has a calming effect giving a sense of security.
- In the rehabilitation phase it can improve adherence to medical regimens.

The side effects to the patient of excessive social support or poor quality support may include increasing the passiveness of the patient, creating dependence, reducing self-confidence and self-esteem and causing feelings of shame and guilt.

DRUG TREATMENT

In understanding the drug treatment process we can partially apply the same theoretical models as for illness behaviour. When explaining patient behaviour in taking or not taking medicines and the interaction with the environment we can, for example, use the social learning theory and the concept of self-efficacy. The Health Belief Model has been used to explain patients' adherence in taking medicines. In addition, we need to understand the behaviour of the physician when prescribing the medicines and dealing with the patient. Likewise our interest is to understand the behaviour of the pharmacist and the interactions between patient–physician–pharmacist. Different models and theories provide a slightly different perspective on the use of medicines, and the adequacy of the theory often depends on the question being addressed. Because this is a relatively new research area there are still many gaps in our understanding of the different processes involved and their interactions.

It is also feasible to regard the drug treatment process from a micro- and macroperspective. The microperspective includes the patient level and the interaction between patient and practitioner. The macroperspective includes an analysis of the different systems and structural components in place to ensure a rational use of drugs, which is one of the primary goals of the system.

Defining rational use

Rational use of drugs has been defined as the safe, effective, appropriate and economic use of drugs. The definition as such seems to be clear and straightforward, but how do we define 'safe' and the other components of the definition. Safety relates to aspects like relative and absolute safety. It is well known that all drugs have side effects, some less and some more. The safety aspect has to be assessed from many different angles, e.g. the severity of the disease, the available treatment options including drug and non-drug options, long-term or short-term treatment, is the drug to cure or control symptoms, any risks of overdoses and other possible factors.

Effectiveness relates to the question of how well the drug works in daily practice when used by unselected populations and patients having comorbidities and other medications. Efficacy relates to a clinical trial type of situation, where we want to know the maximum effect of the drug in a particular disease and when it is optimally used in selected patients with as few as possible confounding factors like comorbidities and other drugs used simultaneously.

Appropriateness refers to how a drug is being prescribed and used in and by patients, including aspects such as appropriate indication, with no contraindications, appropriate dosage and administration. Duration of treatment should be optimal and the drug should be correctly dispensed with appropriate and sufficient information and counselling. To achieve the intended effects, the drug also needs to be correctly used by the patient.

The economic aspect does not refer merely to price, rather a cost-effectiveness approach needs to be applied, where all factors are assessed. A somewhat more expensive drug may be preferable to a less expensive drug, because it has better treatment outcomes or it may have fewer side effects. We should also be aware of hidden costs, such as a need for more extensive laboratory tests, which may increase the total costs of a particular treatment (see Ch. 35).

Functions of drugs

Social and behavioural scientists have proposed that drugs and drug use also serve important latent functions for the individual and society. In this context it is important to have a wide definition of the word 'drug'. The functions may be the same as the approved medical uses or hidden functions. Barber and later Svarstad have identified the following functions of drugs:

- Therapeutic function—the conventional use of drugs to prevent, treat and cure disease
- Placebo function—show concern and satisfy patient
- Coping function—to relieve feelings of failure, stress, grief, sadness, loneliness
- Self-regulatory function—to exercise control over disorder or life
- Social control function—to manage behaviour of demanding or disruptive patients, hyperactive children
- Recreational function—relaxation, enjoying company of others, experience of pleasurable feelings
- Religious function—to seek religious meaning or experience
- Cosmetic function—to beautify skin, hair and body image
- Appetitive function—to allay hunger or control the desire for food
- Instrumental function—to improve academic, athletic or work performance
- Sexual function—to increase sexual ability
- Fertility function—to control fertility

- Research function—to gain knowledge and understanding of human behaviour
- Diagnostic function—to help make diagnosis
- Status-conferring function—to gain social status, prestige, income.

Prescribing

The process of prescribing has gained a lot of interest lately because of ever increasing drug costs and the concern for rational prescribing from a clinical point of view. Before this, social scientists had studied aspects such as the decision-making process in prescribing and the adoption of new drugs, using the 'diffusion of innovations' theory. Concern about prescribing habits is not new. In 1752 the famous Swedish physician and botanist Carl von Linne mentioned in a paper 21 different reasons for irrational prescribing, including factors like outdated knowledge, wrong diagnosis and chemical incompatibility, which are still relevant aspects when assessing rationality of prescribing. It is noteworthy that he used pharmacy records as his source of information.

Today, irrational prescribing would include things such as prescribing a drug that has no significant medical effects or whose expected side effects exceed the benefits of the drug, prescribing of irrational combination drugs, drugs that interact with each other, prescribing excessive quantities or improper dosage. Also writing expensive drugs when cheaper alternatives are available could be considered irrational, as would continuing an unnecessary medication for years. Several studies have tried to find typical characteristics of the prescribing physicians and their work setting that would explain both irrational prescribing and prescribing in general. Basically three types of models and approaches have been used:

- Models focusing on demographic and practice variables, which give descriptive information about what and how physicians tend to prescribe. These variables are often difficult or impossible to change, but these type of studies point to where the focus should be put and possible points for intervention.
- Models focusing on psychosocial issues related to physician–patient interaction.
- Models focusing on cognitive theories behind prescribing decisions. These studies focus on how physicians evaluate the available information and their decision-making process.

There seems to be no general competency to prescribe rationally, since a physician may prescribe rationally in one area and irrationally in another. This could be expected if, for example, an ophthalmologist prescribed for cardiac conditions. Younger and more recently graduated physicians usually seem to prescribe more rationally than older physicians. It has been found that physicians with a negative attitude towards the use of drugs for social problems tend to prescribe fewer psychotropics. The availability of non-drug alternatives, e.g. cognitive therapy, reduces benzodiazepine prescribing. Also the social environment may be important in prescribing, e.g. during the Gulf War benzodiazepine prescribing doubled in Israel compared with the period before and after the conflict. A more cosmopolitan attitude and a more critical attitude towards commercial information were associated with more careful prescribing of risky drugs in one study. Another study showed that 'less rational prescribers', defined as those with a high rate of benzodiazepine prescriptions, rely more on commercial information from the drug industry than others. Professional satisfaction and reading professional material seem to translate into better prescribing.

Many physicians base their selection of medicine on their own experience, which may not be an accurate base for rational selection. The probability of observing rare but important side effects is very small for an individual physician. The same biases that were mentioned earlier affecting patients' decision making also affect physicians' decision making. If they have high initial positive expectations before starting a new treatment, the outcomes will be interpreted in a way that meets these expectations. Negative aspects will not be accounted for. Only positive aspects transform into writing more new prescriptions. Irrational prescribing is also often legitimized by positive personal experiences from prescribing or using that medicine. High medical uncertainty may also contribute to irrational prescribing. On the other hand it also may result in seeking information from many sources to reduce this uncertainty.

Certain patient factors also influence the probability of receiving a prescription for psychotropics. The most widely studied factors have been age and gender. The elderly are usually prescribed more than younger people, which may be a reflection of a higher rate of symptoms and psychological distress. There is also a tendency to write more repeat prescriptions for the elderly, partly reflecting the type of medication being prescribed. Women are prescribed psychotropics more often, which is partly explained by a higher consultation rate. The sex of the physician does not seem to influence this tendency to prescribe more for women. Physicians' expectations that women have more psychological-emotional disorders that can be treated

successfully with benzodiazepines may also partly explain the difference.

Besides the pharmacological-therapeutic use, physicians may sometimes use drugs knowingly or unknowingly for other reasons too. According to Smith these can be either patient or physician centred. He has also presented a long list of latent functions of prescriptions in addition to their intended and recognized functions (method of therapy, legal document, record source and means of communication). Medicines may be used to stimulate the patient's expectations for recovery and to meet patient's expectations, e.g. the use of antibiotics for viral infections or boosting a patient's morale in intractable diseases. The physician may also want to gain some time to diagnose the condition more precisely. The medicine also legitimizes the physician–patient relationship. The prescription is a sign of the physician's power to heal and his efforts to try to heal and care for the patient. For the patient the prescription is a sign and symbol that they really are ill. Thus it also legitimizes their sick-role and confirms that they have fulfilled one of the obligations of the sick-role to try to become well again. Finally the physician uses the prescription to communicate to the patient that the office visit is over. Sometimes it may be difficult to distinguish between rational/pharmacological and non-pharmacological use of drugs. It can also raise ethical dilemmas like when purposely using placebos. Is the physician in this case cheating and/or behaving in a paternalistic way, when he should have an honest and trustful physician–patient relationship?

Choosing the right drug

Therapeutic effect is the most important criterion when the physician tries to choose the right drug. When treating severe cases this aspect is even more important. A second aspect is a low incidence and severity of side effects. It has been shown that physicians tend to concentrate on a few serious side effects. The medical situation often determines the level of acceptable side effects. Economic aspects have a lower priority than the first two dimensions. Low drug cost or actual amount paid by the patient, has a minor role due to reimbursement systems in place in most industrialized countries. If patients pay, the physician gives more attention to cost. Patient convenience and compliance may be decision criteria in situations when medically similar preparations are available, e.g. suppositories not being recommended when oral preparations are feasible. When prescribing for children taste may be an important factor to consider.

In studies concerning the adoption of new drugs, it was shown that those physicians at the centre of a professional network tended to be innovators and started prescribing the new drug at an early point. An early adopter in one therapeutic area might not necessarily be an early adopter in another therapeutic area. The opinion of colleagues is important; two physicians in close contact with each other tend to start a new drug at the same time. Also the type of practice is an important factor. Physicians working alone adopt a new preparation more slowly than those working in group practices.

Barber has shown the dilemma the physician faces when choosing drugs. The problem is summarized in the question of how to find the right balance between (Fig. 2.2):

- Maximizing the effectiveness of treatment
- Minimizing the side effects
- Minimizing costs and finally
- Taking into account patient's wants and wishes.

Influencing drug prescribing

Providing drug information and employing educational programmes to change physicians' prescribing behaviour has become an integral part of the pharmacist's new role. Pharmacists participate in this kind of activity as part of their daily work, but also in formal trials or programmes in community and institutional settings. Several experimental studies have shown that pharmacists providing information and educating physicians produce positive effects on knowledge and attitudes, but the effects on prescribing behaviour have usually been modest. Providing physicians with printed material alone will not influence prescribing habits.

Individual feedback, coupled with one-to-one education, is the most likely method to be successful. Educational outreach or academic detailing has been studied and practised

for the last 20 years. It follows the same principles as do medical representatives for drug companies in their promotional activities. The basic principles are that doctors need to be interviewed in their own office where they are most receptive, the facilitators (often pharmacists) should be well presented and briefed, and the messages should be concise, clear and relevant to the prescriber. The programme should also be ongoing with repeat visits on a regular basis to maintain the contact and keep the messages up to date. The second major strategy includes managerial and regulatory activities such as limited lists, hospital or regional drug committees and formularies, structured drug order forms (e.g. special forms for narcotics), drug utilization review (DUR) and treatment guidelines (see Ch. 36).

USE OF MEDICINES

Drug use or utilization studies and pharmacoepidemiological studies during the last 25 years have basically tried to describe who are using the drugs and how much are being used. On a macrolevel factors influencing drug consumption include among others: size of population, age and gender distributions, occupational structure, income levels (Gross National Product), availability of health services, number and type of health facilities, number and type of personnel, social insurance and reimbursement mechanisms. Chapter 36 describes in more detail some of the methodological aspects related to drug utilization studies.

Drug use studies have also been used to identify different types of 'irrational use', e.g. overuse of psychotropics and antibiotics in the 1970s and 1980s (such as people using them when not indicated, for too long periods, habitual use of analgesics every morning without a medical reason). There has also been a lot of interest in the 'underuse' of drugs for major chronic diseases, like hypertension, diabetes and elevated lipids (not starting or stopping treatment, 'drug holidays', taking only half of what is prescribed). Underuse together with misuse or erratic use (wrong way of administration, taking with contraindicated drugs/food, etc.) has been one of the main focuses of patient compliance studies. From these studies we know something about the use of medicines, and its clinical, social and economic consequences (see also Ch. 41).

Attempts to understand the drug use behaviours of patients have been less common. However, more recently, a new research line has emerged using qualitative research methods like indepth interviews. These studies have focused more on what people think about their medicines, their

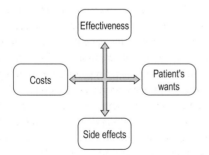

Fig. 2.2 The factors which must be balanced in treating patients (after Barber).

motives when taking or not taking them, attitudes and beliefs about medicines, and their experiences and expectations.

Some general consumer behaviour models have been used to explain non-prescription and prescription purchases. In one American study the drug attributes that consumers rated as important included possible side effects (97%), physician recommendation (90%), strength (73%), prior use (72%), price (58%) and the availability of generic version (51%). Drugs are not ordinary goods and the consumers acknowledge this, as recommendations by physicians and pharmacists are important as well as rational product attributes. According to one purchase theory, purchase motivations can also be characterized as being either transformational (positive) or informational (negative). Positive purchases are made to enhance or generate a positive situation or state of mind (e.g. clothes, music) and negative purchases to minimize or prevent negative situations (e.g. car service). Negative purchases are based on (rational) choices like perceived benefits and convenience (and therefore require more information), while positive purchases are more emotional and based on subjective appeal and positive shopping experience. Research has shown that OTC medicines and vitamins are neutral on the positive–negative dimension and oral contraceptives highly negative. This type of research is still not very well developed within the pharmaceutical field.

Like general illness behaviour, drug use occurs in a social context. Choosing self-medication or consulting a physician to obtain prescription medicines is not based solely on symptoms or clinical aspects. The concept of social knowledge has been used to describe collective understanding, which is based on available information and nature of prior experiences. Family members, friends, work colleagues and their experiences, books and the media in addition to own experiences, form the basis of social knowledge of drugs. Montagne has described some interesting social conceptions or fundamental principles about drugs in peoples' minds, which he calls 'pharmacomythologies'. It is a common belief among lay people that a specific drug produces only one 'main' effect, which is positive. Other effects are considered as negative or 'side' effects. Likewise it is believed that a drug produces the same main effect every time it is taken and in each person who takes it. This means that drug effects are caused by the taken drug and the drug effects are a property residing inside the chemical compound and are not a function of some change in a living organism. This may lead to the belief that drugs cure the disease.

The general illness behaviour models and theories previously presented, like the Health Belief Model, theory of reasoned action, social learning theory, conflict theory and behavioural decision theory can all be used to explain certain types of behaviour related to taking medicines. Basic decision-making and problem-solving skills are important components of patients' seemingly rational and irrational behaviours. As presented earlier, the choices do not always follow the criteria of medical rationality, but may seem quite rational to the patient themselves. It may be useful to consider rationality more as a continuum rather than either/or. The degree of rationality is also influenced by the social knowledge, micro- and macroenvironment as described earlier, as well as the actual health problem.

Improving public understanding of drugs

During the last few years there has been different attempts both in developed and developing countries to improve the knowledge and understanding about drugs among the general public. This can be seen as an attempt to influence and improve (from a medical point of view) the social knowledge related to drugs and health in general. Campaigns, like 'Ask about your medicines', are good examples of this kind of activity. A more balanced partnership between consumer-patients and health care providers is one of the goals in such activities. Also a better appreciation of the limits of medicines and a lessening of the belief that there is a 'pill for every ill' are examples of the goals of such efforts.

The general public also needs to develop a more critical attitude toward advertising and other commercial information, which may often fail to give objective information about drugs. Drug use should be seen within the context of a society, community, family and individual, recognizing cultural diversity in concepts of health and illness or how drugs work. Improvement of the public's knowledge about drugs should start at school. To facilitate informed choices on drug use, public education should be accompanied by supportive legislation and controls on drug availability. Non-governmental organizations, community groups and consumer and professional organizations should be involved in the planning and implementation of such programmes. Effective public education requires a commitment to and understanding of the need for improved communication between health care providers and patients. This should also be reflected in the basic and continuing education of health care personnel.

A SOCIETAL PERSPECTIVE ON RATIONAL DRUG USE

Ensuring rational drug use requires that there are appropriate structures in place and that the processes involved are functioning well. The starting point and frame of reference is the National Drug Policy (NDP). The role of a National Drug Policy is usually discussed in the context of drug issues in developing countries. In industrialized countries it has received much less attention, because many key issues and policies regarding drugs and their rational use are already in place. However, the global crisis in health care financing, especially the drug budget, has created a momentum to look more closely at drug policies in industrialized countries too. When trying to understand the general principles that can be applied to all countries it is helpful to use the guidelines that have been proposed for developing countries, and from there try to understand how the system works and what might be the strong and weak points in each particular country.

The NDP can be seen as a guide for action, including the goals and priorities set by the government, the main strategies and approaches. It also serves as a framework in the coordination of different activities. Depending on cultural, historical and socioeconomic factors there are differences in objectives, strategies and approaches between countries, but some common components can be distinguished. The goals for a NDP can be divided into:

- Health-related goals, which entail making essential drugs available, ensuring the safety, efficacy and quality of drugs, and promoting rational prescribing, dispensing and use of drugs.
- Economic goals, which may include lowering the cost of drugs and providing jobs in the pharmaceutical sector.
- National development goals, which may include increasing the skills of personnel in pharmacy, medicine, etc. and encouraging industrial activities in drug manufacturing.

There is further discussion of these issues in Chapter 4.

Ensuring safety of drugs

Why is it important to regulate and control the drug sector with special laws and regulations? The drug sector is of concern to the whole population. Most citizens will use medicines and related services on a regular basis and therefore the functioning of the sector is of common interest. There are also many parties involved—patients, health care providers, manufacturers and salespeople—requiring detailed rules for interaction and functioning. The consequences from the lack of medicines or their misuse might be serious. History has shown that informal controls are not sufficient or respected. Generally there is little disagreement about the need to regulate the drug sector; the disagreement rather lies in to what extent the sector should be regulated.

Legislation and regulation include different health-related laws, pharmacy law, trademark and patent laws, criminal law, international treaties (e.g. on narcotic and psychotropic drugs) and governmental decrees. Sometimes there may be a lack of political will or a weak infrastructure to enforce the laws. When looking at the legal situation in the drug sector in different countries the problems seem to be more often in the enforcement of legislation than in the lack of legislation.

Drug registration is a key tool in assuring the safety, quality and efficacy of a new drug being introduced on the market. In this connection the new medicine will also be scheduled to a certain category such as prescription or OTC drug. The infrastructure that will assure drug quality, safety, and efficacy can be ascertained by licensing and inspection of manufacturers, distributors and the premises, but also by setting some standards on the professionals working there. There is wide international cooperation in this field among the different competent authorities. Nevertheless every now and then the media have reports about counterfeit products and toxic products sold to the public, sometime with disastrous consequences. News such as somebody having replaced glycerin with diethyleneglycol in paracetamol syrups intended for small children should not be possible with all the controls in place today.

Pharmacoepidemiological studies are used to assure the safety of new medicines after they have been accepted on the market. This kind of information can supplement that available from premarketing studies, it can also give a better quantification of the incidence of known adverse drug reactions (ADRs) but also of the beneficial effects. For ethical and other reasons it is not always suitable to perform clinical trials on certain patient groups such as children, elderly, and pregnant women in the early phase of a new product. It is also important to establish how other medicines and diseases may alter the positive effects. New types of information not available from premarketing studies such as rare undetected ADRs, long-term effects that manifest only after long use or after long latency periods, and effects with low frequency are also the concern of pharmacoepidemiological studies. Further aspects on the safety and evaluation of medicines are dealt with in Chapters 32 and 34.

Ensuring the availability of medicines

Availability of medicines is one of the key requirements in a functioning drug service system. This includes a functioning manufacturing and importation system of medicines, good procurement and distribution practices. These functions are often taken for granted in industrialized countries, while in developing countries they are key issues for a functioning system. In developing countries the maintenance of a constant supply of medicines, keeping them in good condition, minimizing losses due to spoilage and expiry, are issues that need to be solved to assure the availability of medicines to the population.

With more and more sophisticated new medicines the prices of new products are beyond reach for a large part of the population if no mechanisms like price control or drug reimbursement/insurance systems are in place. Economic availability of medicines will be a major drug policy issue in all countries during the next few years. With national drug budgets increasing annually by more than 10%, there is a doubling of the budget every 5–6 years.

PHARMACIES AND THE PHARMACY PROFESSION

Historically a pharmacy has been the place for storing drugs, making medicines and supplying and distributing them to the customers. The first known pharmacy was established in the year 766 in Baghdad. In Europe the first pharmacies date back to the 11th century. In ancient times the same person acted as both doctor and pharmacist, i.e. diagnosed, prescribed and prepared the medicines for the patient. But in 1231 the German emperor and king of Sicily, Frederick II of Hohenstaufen in the edict of Palermo, legally separated the professions of medicine and pharmacy. Physicians were to diagnose and prescribe drugs, while pharmacists were to be responsible for making the drugs and providing these to the patients. Pharmacies were also designated to certain areas, where they had the monopoly of selling drugs. Certain physicians were also to oversee the work of pharmacists. Frederick also gave rules about the education of health professionals. These and other provisions given by him have been the basis of legislation and practice of pharmacy in many European countries until the 20th century.

In some other countries the distinction between the medical and pharmaceutical profession has not been so clear and today we still find dispensing doctors. However, in most countries through the last centuries pharmacists have acted as the 'poor man's doctor' diagnosing and prescribing. It should be remembered that the classification of drugs into prescription and OTC drugs has happened fairly recently. In some other countries there might be similar legislation in place, but it is not enforced. The system of dispensing doctors has been defended based on availability and grounds of patient convenience. The problems related to the system are an apparent conflict of interest, which is present when the income of the physician depends on the volume and price of medicines prescribed. This problem has been highlighted in Japan, which has also one of the highest costs of medicines per capita in the world and prescription drugs are mainly distributed by physicians. The same conflict of interest is often mentioned in the context of the professional and business roles of the pharmacist, especially concerning the sales of non-prescription medicines.

There has been much discussion about the occupational status of pharmacists. Is pharmacy a true profession or not? Two major approaches have been used by academics in trying to answer the question. One approach is to look at the functions pharmacists perform for the society, asking if they are vital for the society? The second approach is to look at certain characteristic traits of the occupation and determine whether they fulfil typical traits of a profession. During the last 50 years different traits have been mentioned by different academics, but there are some common ones. In the 1950s Lewis and Maude mentioned the following traits that characterize a profession:

- Registration or state certification embodying standards of training and practice in some statutory form
- A fiduciary practitioner–client relationship
- An ethical code
- A ban on the advertising of services
- Independence from external control.

Most authors agree that the basic traits of a learned profession are advanced and lengthy training in a highly specialized body of knowledge. This knowledge is to be used in the service of society and mankind. Research and abstract reasoning are the ways of expanding this unique body of knowledge. The services provided by a profession are also related to the degree of impact or danger they may have on individuals or society. Besides the expert knowledge the professional possesses he must also exert his professional judgment to the benefit of the client. Coworkers in the same or related occupations acknowledge the level of expertise of the profession, which is also important in legitimating the practice. There is also a certain level of trust that the public must place in the work performance of the professional.

Professionals themselves define which kind of activities are allowed and what privileges members may claim. They also define, through ethical codes and legislation, which they have often themselves had an opportunity to draw up, the type of controls that guarantee the social privileges given to them (like autonomy of action, monopoly of practice, remuneration) are not abused.

Role of pharmacists

The origin of the pharmacy profession was in the unique knowledge base and skills needed to compound a drug product. With the growth of the pharmaceutical industry this function decreased throughout the 20th century, especially in the 1950s and 1960s. Today it is impossible for the individual pharmacist in the pharmacy to compound similar products to those of the pharmaceutical industry. Also the pharmacist's traditional role of procuring and storing crude drugs has vanished. As the pharmacist's knowledge about the proper preparation, storage and handling of medicines is still greater than any other professional group, the quality assurance aspects of medicines are still their responsibility. Both the society and the profession have defined that the duty of the profession is to ensure that the drugs provided to patients are safely and accurately dispensed. The question raised in the 1960s was whether the status of pharmacy as a profession could be maintained if it was based solely on storing and distributing drugs. The discussion was referred to as 'the profession in search of a role'. This discussion was one contributory factor in the rise of the clinical pharmacy movement in the USA starting in the 1960s. The debate about the pharmacist's role has continued ever since, with new developments like the pharmaceutical care movement and the 'extended role' of the pharmacist in the 1990s. Today there seems to be some kind of consensus among pharmacy spokespersons that the future of pharmacy as a profession lies in pharmaceutical care. In different countries, however, there seem to be different interpretations about what pharmaceutical care is all about. Another question is to what extent has the profession at the grass-root level embraced this philosophy and to what extent is it being practised in everyday pharmacy practice.

International guidelines for Good Pharmacy Practice by the FIP

The International Pharmacy Federation (FIP) has issued its guidelines for Good Pharmacy Practice (GPP), stating that the mission of pharmacy practice is to provide medications and other health care products and services and to help people and society to make the best use of them. The concept of GPP is based mainly on the concept of pharmaceutical care. The patient and community are the primary beneficiaries of the pharmacist's actions and the pharmacist's first concern must be the welfare of the patient in all settings. The core of pharmacy activity is the supply of medication and other health care products, of assured quality, appropriate information and advice to the patient, and monitoring the effects of their use. From an international perspective a rather new aspect is the quest for the pharmacist's contribution to the promotion of rational and economic prescribing and appropriate medicine use. According to GPP the objective of each element of pharmacy service should be relevant to the individual, clearly defined and effectively communicated to all those involved.

In satisfying GPP requirements, professional factors should be the main philosophy underlying practice. Economic factors are also important, but they should not be the driving force. Pharmacists should give their input to decisions on medicine use and a therapeutic partnership with physicians and good relationships with other pharmacists are important. Pharmacists are also responsible for the evaluation and improvement of the quality of services given. There is a need for keeping patient profiles and to record pharmacists' interventions (see also Ch. 31). Pharmacists need independent, comprehensive, objective and current information about drugs. They should also accept personal responsibility for life-long learning and educational programmes should address changes in practice. National standards of GPP need to be put in place and adhered to.

According to the guidelines there are four main elements of GPP; promotion of good health, the supply and use of medicines, self-care and influencing prescribing and medicine use. It also encompasses cooperation with other health professionals in health promotion activities, including the minimization of abuse and misuse of medicines. Professional assessment of promotional materials for medicines should also be carried out and evaluated information about medicines and health care disseminated to the public. The involvement in all stages of clinical trials is also recommended. The guidelines include further areas within the four main elements that need to be addressed, like national standards for facilities for confidential conversation, provision of general advice on health matters, involvement in health campaigns and the quality assurance of equipment used and advice given in diagnostic testing. In the supply and use of prescribed medicines, standards are needed for facilities, procedures and use of personnel.

Assessment of the prescription by the pharmacist should include therapeutic aspects (pharmaceutical and pharmacological), appropriateness for the individual and social, legal, and economic aspects.

Furthermore, national standards are needed for information sources, competence of pharmacists and medication records. Advice should be given to ensure that the patient receives and understands sufficient oral and written information. It is also important to have standards on how to follow up the effect of prescribed treatments and the recording of professional activities. When trying to influence prescribing and medicine use, general rational prescribing policies and national standards are needed. In research and practice documentation, pharmacists have a professional responsibility to document professional practice experience and activities and to conduct and/or participate in pharmacy practice research and therapy research. These guidelines form an international consensus on current practice of pharmacy and point to the direction for national guidelines and efforts to improve it.

OUTCOMES OF MEDICAL TREATMENT

Evaluation and outcomes research

Evaluation and outcomes research are fairly new topics within pharmacy. They are integral elements of pharmaceutical care and much more effort needs to be put into these aspects of pharmacy practice and research in the future. Evaluation has been defined as making a comparative assessment of the value of the invention, using systematically collected and analysed data, in order to make informed decisions about how to act or to understand causal mechanisms and general principles. One important aspect from society's point of view is the question—'What are we getting for our money?' According to the model originally proposed by Donabedian, evaluation of health care can focus on:

- Structure such as facilities, equipment, money, number and qualification of personnel
- Process such as activities by the staff and patients, prescribing, counselling
- Outcomes which include intermediate outcomes like patients' knowledge and behaviour, and final outcomes such as cure of the disease.

Traditionally evaluation has focused on structure and process and to a lesser extent on outcomes. More recently a whole new research field has emerged within health care called 'outcomes research'.

One difficulty in health-related outcomes research is to demonstrate the linkages between the three elements of the model: structure–process–outcome. For example, will a new computer-based patient medication record system in the pharmacy (structure) improve the follow-up of a patient (process), so that the pharmacist is able to detect more efficiently a drug-related problem in the use of the antihypertensive medicine with the outcome of lowered blood pressure and the patient feeling better and living a healthier, longer and happier life (outcome). Even if there is little empirical evidence, it is the general view that good structure leads to a more appropriate process resulting in better outcomes.

A general observation in the health care field is that we still lack evidence of many widely used procedures and interventions. Since the mid 1960s new medicines have undergone clinical trials and an official evaluation through the registration process. This does not mean that all drugs currently on the market or being marketed are safe, effective, economic or appropriate. Furthermore, even if we have only high-quality medicines on the market the outcome of medical treatment is ultimately dependent on how the medicines are being prescribed and used by the patients.

Within the pharmaceutical field a more comprehensive framework has been proposed by Kozma and his colleagues. This model has been named ECHO, which classifies outcomes in three categories: economic, clinical and humanistic outcomes. Clinical outcomes have been defined as medical events that occur as a result of the condition or its treatment. Economic outcomes are the direct, indirect and intangible costs compared with consequences of medical treatment alternatives. Humanistic outcomes include well being, health-related quality of life and patient satisfaction.

Health-related quality of life

The primary objective of health care is to improve patients' quality of life. To what extent this objective is achieved often remains unanswered. This may be due to lack of proper measures, the knowledge and attitudes of health care providers or some other factor. The central feature and objective of pharmaceutical care is to achieve outcomes by identifying, solving and preventing drug-related problems that will improve a patient's quality of life. In experimental settings this has been shown to be the case. To what extent it is achieved in ordinary everyday practice is still an open question.

A classic list of outcomes in medical care has been crystalized in the five Ds, i.e. death, disease, disability, discomfort and dissatisfaction. These include a wide range of different aspects, but are all negative terms. They will give partial answers to the questions about the quality of life of the patient, but are not sufficient to cover all aspects of quality of life. The term 'health-related quality of life' has been used quite differently in the literature and daily practice. Explicit definitions are quite rare because of the multidimensionality of the concept. The domains of health-related quality of life usually include functional health (physical activity, mobility and self-care), emotional health (anxiety, stress, depression, spiritual well being) social and role functioning (personal and community interactions, work and household activities), cognitive functioning (memory), perceptions of general well being and life satisfaction, and perceived symptoms.

Health-related quality of life has been measured with disease-specific instruments and general or generic instruments, e.g. health profiles and measures based on utilities. Disease-specific instruments provide a greater detail concerning functioning and well being in that particular disease. The disease-specific measures (e.g. those used in hypertension and asthma) can also be further categorized as population specific (e.g. elderly), function specific (e.g. sexual) and condition specific (e.g. pain). Examples of these instruments include Asthma Quality of Life Questionnaire and Diabetes Quality of Life Questionnaire.

The generic measures include health profiles, which constitute a number of questions covering the different aspects giving separate scores for each domain of life mentioned earlier. Examples of these health profiles include the Nottingham Health Profile, Sickness Impact Profile, McMaster Index and SF-36. The advantage of health profiles is that they provide a comprehensive array of scores that is multidimensional. If the measure used is sensitive enough, through the profile we may be able to distinguish, for example, when a medicine influences the emotional domain while having no effect on the functional health domain.

The utility-based measures incorporate specific patient health states while adjusting for the preferences (utilities) for the health state. The outcome scores range from 0 to 1, where 0 represent quality of life associated with death and 1 represents perfect health. The preferences have been empirically tested in different populations and been through a validation process. These utility-based measures have been extensively used in pharmacoeconomics research and more specifically in cost–utility analysis (see Ch. 35).

The most accurate and comprehensive end-result may be achieved by using both a generic and disease-specific measure when possible. The focus in current medicine is more on patient-perceived impact on long-term morbidity than on limiting mortality. It is good to remember that medicines can both increase and decrease the quality of life. The goal of drug therapy is to improve health and make patients feel better. Physiological measures may change without people feeling any better. Treatment of mildly elevated blood pressure is a good example of this. Nevertheless, treatment may improve subjective health without any measurable changes in clinical parameters. There may also be a trade-off between positive treatment outcomes and adverse drug events.

Client and patient satisfaction

An important aspect when measuring the outcomes of pharmacy practice and pharmaceutical interventions is the satisfaction of clients and patients. Measurement of client satisfaction can be an important tool in quality assurance of pharmacy practice (see also Ch. 43). There are difficulties in defining the quality of pharmacy services. One approach is to divide the quality into a technical dimension (i.e. what is offered) and a functional dimension (i.e. how it is offered). Different proposals have been made to cover different aspects of service provision in general. One comprehensive model is that by Parasuram. He distinguishes between 10 different dimensions: reliability, responsiveness, competence, access, courtesy, communication, credibility, security, understanding/knowing the customer and tangibles. Hedvall has presented a somewhat simplified model. She has proposed four dimensions: professionalism, commitment, confidentiality and milieu, which also contain the essence of what Parasuram has proposed. Customers may have difficulties in distinguishing between all 10 dimensions and some of them tend to overlap. The proposed dimensions represent important aspects to both prescription and self-care clients visiting the pharmacy. These aspects also have a direct linkage to communication skills and pharmaceutical care.

Measurement of patient satisfaction has usually focused more specifically on aspects in providing care. Cleary and McNeil have listed the following dimensions that are typically covered in the measurements of patient satisfaction: accessibility and availability of care, convenience, technical quality, physical setting, efficacy, personal aspects of care, continuity and economic aspects. In these dimensions we can distinguish a technical or cognitively based evaluation of the services offered and also an emotional or affective aspect—how well they are offered. The significance of client satisfaction can be correlated to patronage, patient compliance, and ultimately to the survival of the pharmacy profession.

Key Points

- Social and behavioural issues can help explain non-biological aspects of health.
- Illness is a person's reaction to a perceived alteration of body or mind, whilst disease is something which is professionally defined.
- Health has been defined by the WHO as a 'state of complete physical, mental and social well being and not merely the absence of disease and infirmity'.
- Apart from biophysical factors, health is also affected by behavioural, environmental and socioeconomic determinants.
- People react differently to symptoms as a consequence of many factors.
- Family, culture, gender and age influence response to symptoms.
- Type A behaviour is more closely associated with illness than Type B behaviour.
- The knowledge which a person has will affect his response to illness.
- According to the Health Belief Model, the patient's perception is most important in determining patient behaviour and decisions.
- The Theory of Reasoned Action suggests that beliefs give rise to attitudes, which form intentions which lead to behaviour.
- The Conflict Theory can be used to explain rational and irrational decision making.
- People use a wide range of coping mechanisms when under stress.

- Humans may not reach decisions logically for many reasons, with biases being particularly important.
- Behaviour is seldom changed as a result of providing facts, but results from a long series of stages.
- Through the self-care philosophy, patients are increasingly encouraged to be responsible for their own health, placing increasing demands on pharmacists.
- The 1978 Alma Ata Declaration defines the content of primary care which should be available to all.
- Demographic, cultural and socioeconomic factors influence the use of health services.
- Social support networks may be primary, secondary or tertiary and are important for the health of individuals.
- Drugs have a wider function than treating disease and their use is not always rational.
- Selection of medicines is often based on subjective information rather than unbiased data about therapeutic effects.
- Prescribing is a complex process in which the prescriber has to balance cost, effectiveness, side effects and the patient's wants.
- Patients' drug use behaviour is influenced by complex social and behavioural factors.
- Society expects safety of the drugs used and attempts to achieve this by employing legislation and regulation supported by pharmacoepidemiological studies.
- The professional status of pharmacy can be determined from its role in society and the service characteristics of pharmacists in society.
- Pharmacy is changing from a 'storage and supply' function only, to include an advisory and monitoring role in the context of pharmaceutical care.
- Evaluation of health care is achieved by measuring structure, process and outcomes.
- Outcomes may be economic, clinical or humanistic.
- Health-related quality of life can be assessed using disease-specific questionnaires or general health profiles.

3

Communication skills for the pharmacist

A. J. Winfield and K. H. Enlund (original authors M. M. Moody, S. L. Hutchinson and E. J. Kennedy)

Introduction

Almost everything we do in life depends on communication. Pharmacists spend a large proportion of each working day communicating with other people; patients, doctors, other health care professionals, staff and others. Advertising campaigns over recent years have alerted the public to the availability of advice from the community pharmacy. General practitioners are seeking advice from community pharmacists. The role of pharmacists in hospitals has an increasing emphasis on talking to patients and medical staff. Poor communication has the potential to cause a range of problems. For example, if there is incomplete communication with health care professionals on correct drug dosage or inappropriate or incomplete advice on the use of medication, potential harm to a patient may occur.

Thus there is a need for effective communication skills for pharmacists, but how effective is our communication? Many are able to talk at length, but do our listeners benefit from our words? Others may find talking to strangers difficult. Good communication demands effort, thought, time and a willingness to learn how to make the process effective. Good communication is difficult to achieve and an awareness of this fact is an important first step to improving it.

This chapter will consider some of the elements of successful communication. Firstly we shall consider the ways in which we assume things about other people and how this can influence our attitudes. Next follow sections considering the ways in which non-verbal communication occurs and behaviour patterns in communication and empathy. This leads to a consideration of questioning and listening skills and barriers to effective communication. The importance of confidentiality and the needs of special groups are considered. Finally there are some difficult situations to consider and practise with.

To a large extent good communication is based on commonsense. However, no two people are the same and our personalities influence our communication abilities. As you work through this chapter it will help if you can identify your strengths and build on them, whilst working to correct your weaknesses. Achieving this will increase your personal and professional fulfilment.

ASSUMPTIONS AND EXPECTATIONS

It is said that 'You never get a second chance to make a first impression'. When we meet somebody for the first time we make assumptions about that person. We often put people into categories and the assumptions lead to expectations of their behaviour, jobs and character.

This initial judgment of a person is often based purely on what we see and hear and includes appearance, dress, age, gender, race and physical disabilities. It is important that we are aware of these assumptions in order to avoid stereotyping people. For example, the impression we have of a person wearing a denim jacket may be very different from that of the same person wearing a suit. Conversely, people will make assumptions about us based on initial impressions; e.g. a pharmacist wearing a white coat in a clean, clinical environment may inspire more confidence than a pharmacist wearing a scruffy jumper and working in a cluttered, untidy environment.

It is well documented that age and gender affect our communication because of assumptions and expectations. We should not assume that people in wheelchairs cannot communicate effectively. Likewise, we must ensure that we direct our communication at an appropriate physical level and to the appropriate person (that is, to the patient in the wheelchair, not the person pushing it).

Demeanour

The way in which people present themselves will lead to certain judgments being made. For example, people who stride aggressively towards someone else may make the person being approached feel defensive because the assumption may be made that they have come to make a complaint. However, people who approach hesitantly may lead to the assumption that this person needs help and advice, perhaps on a potentially embarrassing matter. Both will affect our behaviour and attitude in subsequent communication with this person.

Tone of speech, accents, common expressions

All of these have an impact on communication. Our response to a person speaking with a whining, complaining tone will differ from our response to someone who greets us in a friendly welcoming manner. Similarly, a cultured, 'BBC' English accent may invoke a different response from that to someone with a strong local accent.

No one experiences the same situation in the same way. Whilst people may appear to be doing similar things, they will have different feelings about them. We can only guess what people are thinking or feeling from how they look and from their behaviour. For example, we may think that people are nervous if they move restlessly or twitch, but that may not be the case. It is also useful for us to consider how aware we are of our own behaviour and appearance and what message this may give to other people.

NON-VERBAL COMMUNICATION

The meaning of what a person says is made up of several component parts. These are the words which are spoken, the

---

EXERCISE 3.1

To test your awareness of communication and assumptions there is a simple exercise. To be effective, you must not read the questions which follow just yet. Spend about 5 minutes talking to a person who you do not know very well—there is no particular topic, just let the conversation flow. After this time, turn away from each other and each write down your answers to the following questions:

1. What did you notice about your partner? What type of facial expression did he/she have? What was his/her posture (or gestures) like? How did he/she speak—tone, speed, volume? What does this tell you about him/her?
2. How aware were you of your own non-verbal communication? What was your facial expression? How were you sitting (posture, position in relation to your partner), gesturing, and speaking?
3. What assumptions did you make about your partner? For example, what is his/her taste in food, political persuasion, favourite TV programmes, family background.
4. How accurate were the assumptions that you made? Ask your partner.
5. Do these assumptions say anything about you and the initial judgments you make of people based on sex, age, class, dress, etc.?

Now come back together and share your answers about each other—do they surprise you? If you complete this exercise without 'cheating' you will realize just how many assumptions we make about other people with no evidence for them—and how wrong some of them are!

---

tone of voice used, the speed and volume of speech, the intonation and a whole range of body postures and movements. It is generally agreed that in any communication the actual words convey only about 10% of the message. This is called verbal communication. The other 90% is transmitted by non-verbal communication which consists of how it is said (about 40%) and body language (about 50%).

Vocal communication

Vocal communication, sometimes called paralanguage, concerns the vocal characteristics; the quality and fluency of the voice. The quality of the voice refers to the tone, pitch, volume and speed. Tone in particular can convey more meaning than actual words. 'Thank you for asking the question' said in a harsh voice contradicts the words and indicates that it is not meant. The same words in a warm tone show sincerity. The volume must be adjusted to the circumstances and can emphasize key words. The speed of speaking must enable the listener to understand. Varying the speed and pitch can make the words more interesting and hold the listener's attention.

We have all heard people who use interruptions such as 'er', 'you know' or 'like' every few words. It makes following the message difficult and can be annoying. This often indicates nervousness, uncertainty or a lack of confidence, which may also show as nervous giggles, long pauses or similar interruptions.

Effective use of vocal communication requires that we become proficient at speaking with a warm confident tone of voice at an appropriate speed and volume and without interruptions or vocal mannerisms.

Body language

It is well documented that our impression of another person is very often created at first glance. As you get to know a person better, initial impressions are either reinforced or discarded. In many situations in life the opportunity does not present itself to get to know someone better and the first impression is the one which remains. This will not necessarily detract from communication if the impression which was first given is a favourable one. However, if a poor image was created, it may cause problems at future meetings or even prevent future encounters taking place. In a pharmaceutical context, pharmacists who create a friendly approachable impression are more likely to find customers, patients and doctors receptive to what they say. Pharmacists who make negative impressions will have to work considerably harder to gain other people's confidence. If customers perceive the pharmacist as being unfriendly and unhelpful they will probably go elsewhere for advice or will be unreceptive to any information or advice the pharmacist offers.

Body language can be broken down into several component parts which include gestures, facial expression, eye contact, physical contact, body posture and personal space. It is the combination of all these components which gives the overall impression. It is important to ensure that they are all compatible. If a mixture of messages is portrayed it will cause confusion to observers.

Gestures

Hand gestures in particular are useful when emphasizing a point or to help to describe something. Used appropriately, they can greatly enhance communication and improve the listener's understanding. However, it is important not to overuse them, as this can detract from the spoken word and become a distraction to the listener. Pharmacists should use gestures, where appropriate, to emphasize a point or describe a particular procedure. Observing other people's gestures can give useful information on how concerned, agitated or confused they may be. Do some 'people watching'! It is amazing how much information about people you can pick up just by quietly observing their gestures.

Facial expression

It has been suggested that, after the spoken word, facial expression is the most important part of communication. The facial expression of the pharmacist at the start of the conversation may very well determine how receptive the patient will be to any advice or information offered. Facial expression says a lot about mood and emotion, with the eyes and the mouth giving the dominant signs. As well as ensuring that facial expression is encouraging and welcoming, it is important for pharmacists to be able to read the meaning of facial expressions. In this way important points regarding a patient's level of comprehension or receptiveness can be judged.

Eye contact

Avoiding eye contact is a very successful way of avoiding communication. This can be very well illustrated by observing a class of students who have just been asked a question by a lecturer!

The maintenance of eye contact during a conversation is vital to ensure the continuation of the process, because it indicates interest in the subject and is also useful as a means of determining whose turn it is to speak. However, care must be taken. An uninterrupted stare can be rather off-putting and may reduce the success of the communication.

Physical contact

This is an important aspect of any communication process and can be used to enhance verbal communication. A sympathetic touch on an arm can often say far more than any number of words. However, physical contact is governed by broad social rules which vary greatly between cultures. The British are identified as one of the least 'touching' nations, whilst in many cultures touching between the sexes is unacceptable. An awareness of this is important for pharmacists who will come into contact with people from a wide variety of social and cultural backgrounds. What is considered acceptable behaviour in one culture could be unacceptable in another.

Body posture

We can usually control the words we say, but we are not so good at controlling our body language. Thus although we may be giving a positive verbal message, our body posture may be giving a negative message. The listener may pick this up and the verbal message will be lost.

Body posture can have a major influence on how well communication progresses, or even if it gets started at all. There are several classic body postures which have been identified as having significant meanings.

- *The closed position*. A person standing with his arms folded would illustrate this. This is seen as a rather negative posture and not one likely to encourage initiation of communication.
- *Feet position*. It is often found that a person's feet will be pointing in the direction in which he wants to go. This can be used to check whether the listener is giving you his full attention or would rather be elsewhere.
- *Positive body posture*. Leaning towards the person who is talking, or sitting in a relaxed fashion, are both examples of non-verbal language which can encourage good communication.

As pharmacists, we are constantly trying to build up a complete picture of a patient's problems. In many instances, one of the most important information sources at our disposal is the patient. Good communication will provide much useful information which can then be used to the benefit of the patient.

Personal space

We all have our own space in which we feel comfortable. Personal space varies between cultures and its extent depends on the situation. The different space zones are generally divided into four main areas.

General area

This is approximately 3 m or more. This is the space we would normally prefer to have around us if we are addressing a group of people or are working alone.

Sociable area

This is approximately 1–3 m and is the type of distance used when communicating with people we do not know very well.

Personal area

This is approximately 0.5–1 m. This is the space we would normally feel comfortable with, when at a business or social meeting with people we know reasonably well. It is sufficiently close to allow friendly and meaningful communication without any individuals feeling threatened by having their intimate zone invaded.

Intimate area

This is usually 0–50 cm. This space is reserved for people we know very well. Husbands, wives, children, close friends and family are examples of the kind of people with whom we would be comfortable at these distances. If anybody else enters this so-called 'intimate zone' we feel threatened and will generally withdraw into ourselves. There are occasions when we find ourselves in these sorts of situations. Next time you are in a crowded lift watch the behaviour of the people around you. They are all having their personal space invaded. It is unlikely that anyone will talk and eye contact will be avoided.

An awareness of personal space is important for pharmacists as it can play an important role in the success or otherwise of communication. If you carry on a conversation with someone at too great a distance it may be difficult to build up any rapport. However, if you are so close to people that they feel uncomfortable and threatened, no meaningful dialogue will occur. A simple enquiry, which is perfectly acceptable when asked in the general area, can feel like an accusation when asked in the personal area.

PATTERNS OF BEHAVIOUR IN COMMUNICATION

A number of terms are used in connection with behaviour during communication:

- Assertiveness may be defined as standing up for personal rights and expressing thoughts, feelings and beliefs in direct, honest and appropriate ways, which do not violate another person's rights. Being assertive involves listening to others and understanding their feelings. An assertive communicator will find a mutually acceptable solution. An important part of being assertive therefore is to formulate your aims and objectives clearly. People who behave assertively deal with other people as equals.

- Aggressive behaviour violates others' rights as the aggressive person seeks to achieve goals at the expense of others. Aggressive behaviour is often frightening, threatening and unpredictable. It will bring out negative feelings in the receiver and communication will be difficult.
- Passive–aggressive behaviour usually involves a person giving a mixed message; that is, he may agree with what you are saying but then raise his eyebrows and pull a face at you behind your back.
- Submissive behaviour is portrayed by people who behave submissively, have very little confidence in themselves and poor self-esteem. They often allow others to violate their personal rights and take advantage of them.

Assertiveness is a positive way of relating to other people— a means of communicating as effectively as possible, particularly in potentially awkward situations. Assertive behaviour is useful when dealing with conflict, in negotiation, leadership and motivation, when giving and receiving feedback, in cooperative working and in meetings. Assertive communication can give the user confidence, a clearer self-image and leads to a feeling of more control over situations, especially those of conflict.

People who behave assertively usually achieve what they set out to do. This does not necessarily mean that the other person does not also achieve what they set out to do. This is in comparison to those who act aggressively, who think that they have achieved their goal, but this is usually at the cost of respect and loyalty from those around them. Submissive people rarely achieve what they want.

Part of assertiveness is recognition of personal rights and the rights of others. The following list includes examples of personal rights:

- To state my own needs and priorities
- To be respected as an intelligent and capable equal
- To express my feelings
- To express my own opinions and values
- To say 'Yes' or 'No'
- To make mistakes
- To change my mind
- To say 'I don't understand'
- To ask for what I want (realizing that the other person has the right to say 'No')
- To decline responsibility for others' problems

- To deal with others without being dependent on them for their approval.

Techniques in assertive communication

Use of 'I' and 'You' statements

Using 'I' rather than 'You' in a statement places the responsibility with the asserter rather than attempting to place the responsibility on the other person. Use of 'I' statements can minimize negative reactions such as anger. For example, compare the following two statements which are effectively saying the same thing. 'You appear to have been arriving rather late for work, recently.' 'I have noticed that you have been arriving rather late for work, recently.' The first statement gives an impression of accusation while the second is more observational and less threatening.

Repeating the message

If a request for information is not being answered directly by the receiver, a useful assertive technique would be to repeat the request. If this is done firmly and without aggression, the message can be repeated until a reply is obtained. However, there are situations when this technique would not be appropriate, e.g. when an answer to the request has been given, even though it may not be the desired response (such as when children repeatedly ask for sweets and the parent has already said 'No!'). Repeating this request will not be helpful and will aggravate the situation.

Clear communication

To communicate we use both verbal and non-verbal language. Both are important and it is essential that they match or we will send mixed and confusing messages. An example of a mixed message in a community pharmacy may arise when asking a patient if she understands how to take her dispensed medicine. An affirmative reply may be given verbally by the patient but non-verbal signs such as close examination of the label and a creased forehead may indicate some confusion which would need to be clarified.

Extracting the truth

Strong emotions can get in the way of clear communication. Communicators who are angry or upset may cloud the message they are trying to convey with other issues. They may exaggerate or become emotional. It is important, as the receiver, to accept this in an assertive manner. Acknowledge true criticisms but do not be distracted by side issues.

Self-talk

In a situation of conflict we can often 'work ourselves up' to an angry or emotional state which can then lead to unclear and unsuccessful communication. If we use self-talk (i.e. talk to yourself) and clarify the issues in a situation, considering the points of view and rights of all those involved, not just ourselves, we can often defuse the situation inside ourselves. We can then be ready to undertake clear, unconfused communication which will lead to a more successful outcome. Self-talk does not have to involve 'giving way' to the other person. Rather it is a way of controlling naturally felt emotions and then, instead of 'letting fly', expressing yourself in a manner which is more likely to produce the desired result.

There are a number of steps which you could follow to increase your assertiveness.

- *Choose the right situation.* Choose situations where you believe you have a reasonably good chance of maintaining your assertion, and achieving a mutually acceptable outcome. Changes in behaviour come in small steps, e.g. making requests or giving praise.
- *Prepare for situations.* Spend a short time before an important situation working through the following steps: clarify your objectives, clarify your own and other people's rights, turn 'faulty' dialogues into sound ones, self-talk the assertive statements with which you want to start the interaction and consider your response to anticipated hassles.
- *Behave assertively during the situation.* To overcome unexpected hassles, buy brief thinking time, e.g. 'Have I got this right? What you're saying is ... ', or 'I'd like to think about that for a moment'.
- *Review the situation afterwards.* Analyse what happened and learn from it. Be honest. Do not play down or exaggerate your success. Never berate yourself. Remember that some people may have a vested interest in your not becoming more assertive.

EMPATHY

Illness is often associated with different emotional aspects, like uncertainty, stress, fear and dependency. The ability to enter into the life of other people and to accurately understand both their meaning and feelings is called empathy. It involves an accurate perception and identification of both the actual words and underlying feelings contained in what a person is saying. Pharmacists need the skill to respond in a way that communicates this understanding convincingly. Empathy is one of the cornerstones in communication skills and is an essential part of assertiveness. It is needed in information gathering, when interviewing customers and patients and when educating and counselling. Furthermore, the resolution of conflict situations requires empathic understanding. There are three elements to empathic communication.

Facilitating empathy

Being empathic requires that pharmacists are able to communicate their readiness and willingness to listen to other people and to establish a safe non-threatening atmosphere where they can express themselves. Much of this communication is nonverbal in nature, like eye contact, tone of voice and body posture. There is also a need to express respect and assurance that there is no need for embarrassment or fear of being criticized. People often speak intellectually about a problem rather than saying how they feel. Pharmacists should encourage them to describe their feelings. This does not mean that we should force people to say things they are not ready for.

Perceiving feelings and meaning

The correct identification of feelings and their meaning is important for pharmacists in their work. Patients often experience a combination of feelings, like being unfairly treated, hurt, depressed and angry. These need to be identified in order to respond properly. It is also important to pay attention to non-verbal communication and how closely it agrees with the verbal communication. Facial expressions and body movements may communicate more accurately how the person feels than is being verbally expressed initially. Some words commonly used to express different intensity of feelings are shown in Table 3.1. When trying to identify meanings and feelings of others it is necessary to be aware of our own personal biases, prejudices, stereotyped impressions or a preoccupation with personal concerns. We have our own assumptions about how people, such as those with depression, feel and behave, or stereotyped views, e.g. that all drug addicts are the same.

Table 3.1 Feeling vocabulary				
Feeling	**Very strong**	**Strong**	**Moderate**	**Mild**
Anxiety	Panic-stricken	Tense	Nervous	Worried
Fear	Terrified	Frightened	Fearful	Uneasy
Happiness	Elated	Joyful	Happy	Pleased
Depression	Suicidal	Depressed	Unhappy	Low
Sadness	Grief-stricken	Distressed	Sad	Sorry
Desire	Craving	Longing	Desirous	Wishful
Confusion	Chaotic	Disorganized	Bewildered	Uncertain
Confidence	Bold	Self-assured	Secure	Adequate

Responding

The third component, responding, involves the verbal and non-verbal expression of how much we understood and that we are interested to hear more. Often, it may be tempting to just use the phrase 'I understand how you feel'. This may generate the answer 'No, you don't!' It is better to respond by restating and reflecting feelings, i.e. to restate what was said in slightly different words. Another way is to try to help people focus and clarify their own feelings on what is most important for them. You can also verbalize implied meanings or ask for further clarification.

How we communicate empathic listening is important. The most likely way to be effective is by understanding and focusing. Other helpful approaches include quizzing and probing, analysing and interpreting, advising, placating and reassuring. All of these include potential pitfalls but when used appropriately they can be effective. One technique that is rarely effective is generalizing the problem; e.g. when trying to give comfort you say that the problem is 'not serious' or 'everybody has it'. Other ineffective techniques include judging people or their actions, and warning or threatening them.

Just as with all other communication skills, some people are more empathic than others, but empathy and empathic listening can be practised and improved. This requires an active willingness to learn from experience and analyse different situations and our own actions and reactions with an open mind.

QUESTIONING SKILLS

It is said that 'questioning' is one of the most widely used social skills. Good questioning skills are an asset to any pharmacist.

What are the functions of questions? In a pharmacy setting questions are normally asked to encourage the listener to provide information. For example, pharmacists need to be able to respond to patients' enquiries and to try to resolve problems or difficulties they may have in taking prescribed medicines, or to give advice on over-the-counter (OTC) medicines. In these situations, communication between two individuals will only be effective if it succeeds in solving the problem or providing the right medicine. This will require asking questions to obtain essential information. However, the type of question and the way in which it is asked will dictate the level of response given.

Use of open and closed questions

There are two main types of questions: open and closed.

A closed question is one which is direct and close-ended. It requires the respondent to give a single word reply such as 'yes' or 'no'. Such questions do not include a 'feeling' component, but do provide specific information on a subject area. Examples of closed questions used in a pharmacy setting include:

- Are you taking any medicine at present?
- Have you ever taken this medicine before?
- Do you understand how to take it?
- Do you have any questions about the medicine?
- Did the medicine work for you?
- Will you work in the dispensary for me next Sunday?

Open questions are open-ended and often allow people to respond in their own way. They do not set any 'limits' and generally allow the person to provide more detailed information. Open questions encourage elaboration and help people expand on what they have started to say. Examples of open questions include:

- Describe your symptoms to me.
- Tell me about any over-the-counter medicines you are taking just now.
- How do you relieve the symptoms of headache?
- What do you do when that sensation occurs?

The above examples show that open questions are often built around words like 'what' and 'how' and generally allow an element of 'feeling' to be introduced by the patient in the reply.

Pharmacists can also encourage patients to explain more about their symptoms or condition by using open questions which require elaboration, e.g. 'What can you tell me about the symptoms you have after taking the medicine?' There is a tendency to use too many closed questions, but a balanced combination of both open and closed questions is more beneficial.

The funnelling technique

A funnelling technique can be used to allow direction and focusing of ideas on a specific topic. This involves initially asking background open questions to provide basic information, then asking specific closed questions to provide specific detail and clarify points. In these circumstances, it can be useful to paraphrase comments made, to ensure that the understanding of the information being obtained from the patient (doctor, etc.) is accurate. Without this checking procedure the listener may misinterpret something and a misunderstanding can occur. It is possible during any one conversation to use

---

EXAMPLE 3.2

Now imagine an industrial pharmacist dealing with other staff in a small working group, responsible for quality assurance:

'Please explain about the sampling techniques used.' (background open question)

'Who sampled the sterile water batch yesterday?' (specific closed question)

'Where were the quality control samples taken from?' (specific closed question)

'How many samples were taken?' (specific closed question)

'Now I would like to discuss ways of validating the sampling techniques.' (this starts a new funnel)

---

more than one 'funnel', e.g. establishing a patient's current medical condition, then going on to suggest appropriate action or medication available. In a pharmacy setting, where time can be a limiting factor, using the funnelling technique can be useful for directing and focusing a conversation to enable an end point to be achieved more quickly.

The use of open and closed questions in a pharmacy setting

If we consider the situation of a pharmacist responding to symptoms, the pharmacist has a number of options available in order to obtain information from the patient. Choosing the correct type of question can prove to be a difficult decision, particularly bearing in mind the circumstances under which the conversation may be taking place, such as in a busy pharmacy where other customers are waiting for prescriptions or OTC advice. It is tempting to ask a number of closed questions which will provide information, albeit limited to one-word answers. However, this could result in the patient being 'bombarded' with many questions, makes patients feel as if they have been through an 'interrogation' and takes a great deal of time to establish the patient's condition. It could also mean a vital piece of information was missed because no specific question was asked about it. Pharmacists must learn to develop good questioning skills to enable them to build up an accurate picture of the patient's condition. This is achieved by using a combination of open and closed questions which can ensure that accurate and complete information is obtained. It also allows patients

---

EXAMPLE 3.1

Imagine a hospital clinical pharmacist, on a ward round, speaking to a patient. A conversation could be as follows:

'Please tell me about the insulin products you have used in the past.' (background open question)

'What type of insulin do you currently use?' (specific closed question)

'How long have you been using this?' (specific closed question)

'Now that we have established a little about your medicine, can we discuss what action we will take in the future to prevent problems with your medicine?' (this starts another funnel)

time to elaborate certain points and builds their confidence in the pharmacist.

Time pressures may make us reluctant to use open questions. However, although interviews using open-ended questions can take longer than interviews based upon protocols of closed questions, they typically elicit more information.

Application of questioning skills

Questioning skills do not only apply to the communication between pharmacists and patients, although a large part of their work will be in this area. Good questioning skills are required in staff training and implementation of procedures, dealing with other health care professionals and in ordering and supplying goods.

Questioning skills are not only required for face-to-face communication. Often a pharmacist has to communicate by telephone with, e.g. a GP, a dentist, a district nurse, nursing home staff, hospital staff or patients' relatives. The major drawback of this type of communication is that reliance is put solely on good verbal communication skills (see p. 39) and not on the non-verbal aspect of communication. In these circumstances, it is vital to obtain the information as quickly and efficiently as possible. At the same time, the pharmacist must remain professional, give out accurate advice and offer reassurance if necessary. For example, a GP phones to order a prescription for a patient, the pharmacist is required to ask specific questions to ensure that all information is accurate. As another example, a patient phones to ask about a prescription item that may have been incorrectly dispensed, and using good questioning skills, the pharmacist would check the prescription information, identify the patient's concerns and be able to take appropriate action.

Often people feel awkward answering questions, so it is important to encourage them. This is usually done using non-verbal communication (see p. 37). Position, posture and eye contact are important to give a relaxed, open appearance. We should avoid using a counter or desk as a barrier or getting too close and invading a patient's 'intimate zone'. The voice should be warm and friendly, and nodding or using vocal signs such as 'Mm' or 'Ah-ha' can give further encouragement.

LISTENING SKILLS

Asking questions is only part of communication. Listening to the answers is of equal importance! True listening involves the eyes as well as the ears. For example when someone is describing an illness, their facial expression and body posture may reveal more than their actual words.

Inattention is the most obvious problem in listening. Sometimes we pretend to be listening, but this is usually obvious to the speaker and leads to a failure to communicate. Distractions occur in any busy setting and can be reduced, to some extent, by having a 'quiet area'. We should always look for the hidden meaning of the words used. For example a reply of 'Just like the doctor said' in response to a question about how a medicine is used, might hide a compliance problem.

Being effective at listening is hard work. When it is fully developed it will involve attempting to reflect back to the patient what you think the patient was trying to say, including their feelings. This was developed earlier in this chapter in the section 'Empathy'.

BARRIERS TO COMMUNICATION

In a pharmacy setting there are a number of factors which can be of benefit to, or can detract from, the quality of any communication. Common barriers which exist can be identified under four main headings:

- Environment
- Patient factors
- The pharmacist
- Time.

Environment

Community pharmacies, hospital outpatient pharmacies and hospital wards are all areas where pharmacists use their communication skills in a professional capacity. None of these areas is ideal, but an awareness of the limitations of the environment goes part of the way to resolving the problems. Some examples of potential problem areas are illustrated below:

- *A busy pharmacy*. This may create the impression that there appears to be little time to discuss personal matters with patients. The pharmacist is supervising a number of different activities at the same time and is unable to devote his full attention to an individual matter. It is important that pharmacists organize their work patterns in such a way as to minimize this impression.

- *Lack of privacy*. Some pharmacies, both in community and hospital outpatient departments, have counselling rooms or areas, but many have not. Many hospital wards could be likened to a busy thoroughfare. For good communication to occur and rapport to be developed ideally the consultation should take place in a quiet environment, free of interruptions. Lack of these facilities requires additional skills.
- *Noise*. Noise levels within the working environment are an obvious barrier to good communication. People strain to hear what is said, comprehension is made more difficult and particular problems exist for the hearing impaired (see p. 46). The opposite may also be true, where a patient feels embarrassed having to explain a problem in a totally quiet environment where other people can 'listen in'.
- *Physical barriers*. Pharmacy counters and outpatient dispensing hatches are physical barriers and also may dictate the distance between pharmacist and patient. This in turn can create problems in developing effective communication. A patient in bed (or in a wheelchair) and a pharmacist standing offers a different sort of barrier which will create a sense of inferiority in the patient. Ideally faces should be at about the same level.

Patient factors

One of the main barriers to good communication in a pharmacy can be patients' expectations. In today's world people have busy and hectic lifestyles. In many cases they have become used to seeing a 'good' pharmacy as one where their prescription is dispensed quickly. They are not expecting the pharmacist to spend time with them checking their understanding of medication or other health-related matters. However, once the purpose of the communication is explained, most patients realize its importance and are quite happy to enter into a dialogue.

- *Physical disabilities*. Dealing with patients who have sight or hearing impairment will require the pharmacist to use additional communication skills. Practical suggestions on help which can be given to patients with sight impairment can be found in the chapter on counselling (see Ch. 38). Dealing with the hearing impaired is discussed in this chapter (p. 46).
- *Comprehension difficulties*. Not all people come from the same educational background and care must be taken to assess a patient's level of understanding and choose appropriate language. In some cases the lack of ability to comprehend may be because English is not the patient's first language. Pharmacists working in areas where there is a high proportion of non-English speakers may find it useful to stock or develop their own information leaflets in appropriate languages.
- *Illiteracy*. A significant proportion of the population, in the UK and other countries, is illiterate. For these patients written material is meaningless. It is not always easy to identify illiterate patients as many feel ashamed and are unlikely to admit to it, but additional verbal advice can be given and pictorial labels can be used. For example the United States Pharmacopoeia has designed a range of pictograms for this purpose.

The pharmacist

Not all pharmacists are natural, good communicators. Identifying strengths and weaknesses will assist in improving communication skills. Some of the weaknesses which can be barriers to good communication are:

- Lack of confidence
- Lack of interest
- Laziness
- Delegation of responsibilities to untrained staff
- A feeling of being under pressure, especially time pressure
- Being preoccupied with other matters.

If any of these characteristics is present the reason for it should be identified and resolved, if possible.

Time

In many instances time, or the lack of it, can be a major constraint on good communication. Try developing a meaningful conversation with someone who constantly looks at his watch! Similarly, if the person who has initiated the conversation is short of time, the wrong kind of questions may be used or little opportunity for discussion will be allowed. It is always worthwhile checking what time people have available before trying to embark on any communication. That way you will make the best use of what time is available.

Not all barriers to good communication can be removed, but an awareness that they exist and taking account of them will go a long way towards diminishing their negative impact.

CONFIDENTIALITY

Matters related to health and illness are highly private affairs. Therefore it is important that privacy and confidentiality are assured in the practice of pharmacy.

According to the public, lack of privacy is one of the most important issues when developing pharmacy services. The public expects pharmacists to respect and protect confidentiality and have premises that provide an environment where you can communicate privately without fear that private matters will be disclosed. There is a need to maintain the trust of the public by communicating in such a way that no doubts about lack of privacy or confidentiality arise. This concerns the whole staff of the pharmacy not just the pharmacists.

Physical privacy can be assured by providing facilities (not necessarily always private counselling rooms) that allow communication without somebody else overhearing a private conversation. In addition there is a need to provide psychological privacy and this has much to do with how things are perceived. It is possible, by appropriate communication, to minimize the impact of distracting factors. The techniques are often non-verbal, such as proper use of the voice (not too loud, not to low), eye contact, leaning forward and concentrating on the person and their problem.

Ethical guidelines and privacy laws set the rules about confidentiality in pharmacy. Any information relating to an individual which the pharmacist or any other staff member acquires in the course of their professional activities has to be kept confidential. When communicating with other health care professionals it may be difficult to draw the line between what is acceptable and what is not acceptable. Without the consent of the person, only information to prevent serious injury or damage to the health of the person can be shared. We must act in the interests of patients and other members of the public. When communicating with patients/customers it is also important to respect patients' rights to participate in decisions about their care and to provide information in a way in which it can be understood.

SPECIAL NEEDS

Patients with special needs must be considered carefully when adopting questioning skills. We need to be non-patronizing, avoid the use of jargon and adopt a procedure for obtaining information which is acceptable to the patient. Blind people will not be able to read any written material, unless it is in Braille. Special labels are available. They may also require some compliance aids to assist with measuring doses.

Many customers who come into pharmacies will suffer from a degree of hearing impairment. Studies have shown that one in six of the adult population in the UK has clinically significant hearing loss. By retirement age (61–70 years old), around 34% of people have significant hearing loss; this increases to 74% in people aged over 70. Considering that people in these age groups present the highest number of prescriptions, it is evident that pharmacists must implement appropriate communication skills.

Recognizing the profoundly deaf is usually simpler than recognizing those who have hearing impairment. The following guidelines may be useful for identifying these customers.

How to recognize the hearing impaired

A person with hearing difficulty is likely to do one or more of the following:

- Speak in an unusually loud or soft voice
- Turn their head to one side or cup a hand to their ear whilst listening
- Concentrate on lips whilst being spoken to
- Give inappropriate responses to questions
- Have a blank or confused expression during conversation
- Frequently ask speakers to slow down or repeat information
- Be unable to hear a conversation when they cannot see the speaker's mouth
- Be unable to carry on a conversation in a noisy environment.

Having recognized a customer with hearing impairment, the following guidelines are helpful.

Guidelines when speaking to the hearing impaired

- Ask them how they wish to communicate
- Make sure that background noise is at a minimum
- Look directly at the person and do not turn away
- Make sure sufficient light is on your face
- Do not hide your face or mouth behind hands, pens, etc.
- Do not shout
- Keep the normal rhythm of speech but slow down slightly
- Articulate each word carefully and exactly, particularly emphasizing consonants
- If a sentence is not heard, rephrase it or write it down
- Do not change the subject in mid-sentence.

Listening, and being able to demonstrate that you are listening, is very important using non-verbal responses for the deaf.

DIFFICULT SITUATIONS IN PHARMACY

There are times in all our lives when we have to deal with 'difficult situations'. Good communication skills may not always produce the perfect result but can help prevent making a situation worse.

EXERCISE 3.2

Read through the following scenarios and think carefully how you would react and deal with such a situation in 'real life'. Consider how the other person would be feeling. Remember, there will no one perfect answer. Discuss the scenarios with a friend or group of friends. This will also allow you to identify the different ways people react to the same situation.

1. A young girl returns to your pharmacy to purchase laxatives. You notice that she has been buying them fairly regularly, and decide to tackle the situation. How would you approach this as the pharmacist? How do you think the young girl will react?

2. A drug addict asks to purchase some 1 mL 'insulin' needles. You know that there is a needle exchange scheme at a pharmacy on the other side of town. How do you give this advice to the addict, or advise him on the safe disposal of the needles? How do you think the addict would react?

3. A hospital prescription for morphine, written for pain relief in a terminally ill patient, has been written incorrectly by a junior doctor. The doctor has already been on duty for 40 hours. How do you approach her? How do you think she will react?

4. You are working on the production of a batch of drug in industry. Your boss is pressing you to release the drug onto the market; however, you feel that it has not fully met all of the quality assurance requirements. How would you present your case to a board of managers?

5. Worried parents ask for your advice as a pharmacist. They have found some tablets in their son's bedroom. You identify them, and they are drugs that have the potential for misuse and abuse. How do you handle this situation? How do you think the parents will react? Consider the feelings/reaction of the son. Where does confidentiality come into this?

6. A middle-aged man comes storming into your pharmacy. You have given him the wrong strength of tablets and he is very angry. How do you deal with this situation? How do you think the man will react?

7. An older lady wishes to purchase some codeine linctus 'for someone else'. After much soul searching and questioning, you decide to sell her a 100 mL bottle. She returns 10 minutes later with a broken bottle (and not much evidence of codeine linctus). She claims she has dropped it, and wants a replacement. What do you do?

Further examples of difficult situations in pharmacy can be found in Table 3.2.

Table 3.2   Types of patients' problems and the communication difficulties which they present

Problem type	Examples	Communication difficulties
Embarrassing problems	Contraception, disorders of the reproductive system, hyperhydrosis, skin conditions	Obtaining privacy in the pharmacy. Establishing a common language of understanding. Demonstrating empathy and understanding. Establishing trust and confidentiality. Not exhibiting negative non-verbal behaviour
Emotional/psychological problems	Anxiety, depression, marital problems, drug abuse and dependence, stress	Demonstrating empathy and understanding. Insufficient time for counselling. Evaluating patient's immediate needs. Establishing the nature and amount of advice to be given. Establishing two-way listening
Problems of handicap Sensory Physical Communicative Mental Psychological Social	 Blindness, deafness Paralysis, congenital deformity Speech impairment Educationally subnormal Personality disorders Introversion	Making inaccurate judgments regarding personality, intellect, etc. Providing effective explanations. Listening, taking sufficient time with patient. Overcoming social barriers
Terminal illness		Knowing what to say and how to say it. Establishing patient's feelings
Financial problems		Interpreting cues given off by patient regarding cost of medicines. Not embarrassing the patient

SUMMARY

Good communication is not easy and needs to be practised. We all have different personalities and skills which means we have strengths in some areas and weaknesses in others. If we can become aware of, and maximize, our strengths and work to minimize our weaknesses, we will become better communicators. Being articulate and able to explain things clearly is of great importance to a pharmacist. However, listening with understanding and empathy is of equal, and in certain situations of greater, importance. We may all hear the words being said but are we really listening to the complete message?

This chapter has emphasized communication skills for pharmacists, particularly in the workplace, but remember, good communication is a life skill to be used at all times.

Key Points

- Non-verbal communication is made up of vocal communication (paralanguage) and body language.
- Body language includes gestures, expression, eye and physical contact, body posture, space and proximity.
- After the spoken word, facial expression is probably the most important part of communication.
- Eye contact must be maintained, but must not become a stare.
- An awareness of personal space is needed to allow effective communication.
- Assertive behaviour treats other people as equals, and is not to be confused with aggressive behaviour which violates other people's rights.
- Assertive communication will tend to use 'I' rather than 'You', repeat messages, employ clear verbal and non-verbal communication and clarify issues without emotion.

- Empathy (active listening) involves understanding other people's feelings and reflecting this back to them.
- Questions may be open or closed and in most situations a balanced combination is required.
- Questioning skills also involve listening to answers.
- In the working environment there are many potential barriers to effective communication including the environment, patient and pharmacist and the time implications.
- Confidentiality must be assured in the practice of pharmacy.
- The special needs of patients must be met without being patronizing.
- Hearing loss is common in the elderly and will present a barrier to effective communication.
- A number of signs help identify those with hearing loss and many steps can be taken to help the situation.
- Pharmacists need to maximize their strengths and minimize their weaknesses of communication.

WHO and the essential medicines concept

M. M. Everard

After studying this chapter you will know about:

Main functions of WHO
Principles of the essential medicines concept
Description of essential medicines
Key features of the new procedure for updating the Model List of Essential Medicines
Impact of essential medicines

Introduction

The 20th century witnessed revolutionary progress in improving human health, leading to dramatic declines in mortality and equally dramatic increases in life expectancy. Income growth, higher educational levels, improved sanitation and better food all contributed to this progress. The development of pharmaceuticals, particularly essential medicines, also played an important role.[1]

Despite these remarkable achievements, more than one thousand million people, one-fifth of the world's population, have not benefited from the improved economic situation and the advances in medical and pharmaceutical sciences that have increased life expectancy and quality of life. Health is a fundamental human right, still denied to more than one-fifth of the world's population.[1]

The work of the world's leading international public health agency, the World Health Organization (WHO), covers numerous health-related technical areas, supporting its overall objective of 'the attainment by all peoples of the highest level of health'.

Much has been achieved in pharmaceuticals since the essential medicines concept was introduced in 1975. Today, three out of four countries in the world have national essential medicines lists as the basis for public procurement, reimbursement schemes, training, supervision and public information.[2] Perhaps most importantly, in 1977, less than half the world's population had regular access to essential medicines. Today, through a combination of public and private health systems, nearly two-thirds of the world's population are estimated to have access to effective treatments essential for their health needs. It is estimated that the number of people with access to essential medicines increased steadily from 2.1 billion in 1977 to 3.8 billion in 1997.[3] Essential medicines are one of the most cost-effective elements in health care.

WORLD HEALTH ORGANIZATION

WHO, which was established in 1948, is a specialized agency of the United Nations system. It is the technical and professional body concerned with international public health issues. WHO was endorsed on 7 April 1948 by the United Nations and had fewer than 60 Member States; in 2002, it had 191. Its definition of health and its overall objective are provided in Box 4.1.[4]

WHO has 27 disease-control and health-related technical programmes, administratively arranged in seven clusters. Two others represent management and external relations activities. The organization has six regional offices and country representation in the majority of its Member States. This organizational structure allows for close cooperation in the field of health between country, regional office and headquarters' levels.[4]

Box 4.1 The WHO definition of health

WHO's constitution describes health as 'a state of complete physical, mental and social well being and not merely the absence of disease or infirmity'.

Its overall objective is: 'the attainment by all peoples of the highest possible level of health'.

Beside closely cooperating with Member States, WHO is in official relations with almost 200 non-governmental and voluntary organizations involved in health promotion and health care provision. Various public–private partnership initiatives have been established over time.[4]

WHO represents the efforts of international health co-operation that began over 150 years ago. Nations joined forces to combat common health threats such as plague, yellow fever, cholera, leprosy, tuberculosis, smallpox and typhus. Some of these diseases still exist. Smallpox has been eradicated and others diseases are in the process of being eliminated, like polio, measles and leprosy.[5]

The 20th century saw the discovery and further development of pharmaceutical products, like the introduction of penicillin (1928), measles vaccine (1943), streptomycin (1945) and chloroquine (1946). In the 1950s the first clinical use of oral contraceptives, of medicines for diabetes and for mental illness were introduced, and later medicines for cardiovascular diseases.[6]

Also in this century, there were significant gains in life expectancy of 20–40 years worldwide. This was mainly due to declining infant and child mortality rates, maternal mortality ratios and fertility rates, a drastic reduction in the disease burden of infectious diseases caused by effective preventive actions and improved treatment. In addition, general sanitation measures and immunization programmes were implemented. These achievements were the results of dedicated international health efforts.[1,5]

Despite these successes, the current international health situation indicates that not all people have benefited equally from improvements in health status and access to health services. It is estimated that more than one thousand million people are still excluded from adequate health care.[1]

Moreover, the World Bank reported in 2000 that the socioeconomic gaps and health status differences between low- and high-income countries are still growing.[7]

Low-income countries face ill health, mainly through communicable diseases, due to poverty-related conditions, such as inadequate food, water and sanitation, housing, education and health services. The emergence of the HIV epidemic, the resurgence of tuberculosis and malaria, and the tobacco-related diseases are also factors. In high-income countries ill health, mainly non-communicable diseases, results mainly from excessive eating, drinking and smoking, using and abusing narcotic drugs, and from environmental pollution and urbanization.[1,5]

The organization has to consider this diversity of health challenges in order to develop strategies and programmes to meet the needs of its Member States, and to achieve better health for all. WHO's main functions can be divided into normative work and technical cooperation; they are listed below.[1]

WHO has six main functions:

1. Providing guidance and advocacy for health worldwide by articulating consistent, ethical and evidence-based policies
2. Setting global norms and standards for health by developing, validating and monitoring these and promoting their proper implementation
3. Managing information by assessing trends, comparing performance and stimulating research and development
4. Stimulating the development of appropriate health technology by testing, applying and transferring of new technologies, tools and guidelines for disease control, risk reduction, health care management and service delivery
5. Negotiating and sustaining national and global partnerships
6. Cooperating with governments in strengthening their national health programmes by catalysing change through technical and policy support, in ways that stimulate action and help to build sustainable national and local capacity.

Given the scale and complexity of the world's health problems, it is evident that WHO has to set priorities for its work. The organization concentrates mainly on areas in which it can demonstrate a comparative advantage to other partners actively engaged in health, or where there is a need to build or to scale up national capacity.[1]

Essential Drugs and Medicines Policy

The Department of Essential Drugs and Medicines Policy is central to WHO's mission to help save lives and improve health by closing the gap between the potential that essential medicines have to offer and the reality that for more than 20% of the world's population medicines are unavailable, unaffordable, unsafe or improperly used.[2]

WHO sets norms and standards for, among others, biological and pharmaceutical products. It provides guidance on regulatory standards, defines international non-proprietary names, provides therapeutic advice, such as treatment guidelines, and produces a Model List of Essential Medicines. Technical assistance to Member States is also provided on the development and implementation of their national drug policies.

WHAT TRIGGERED THE ESSENTIAL MEDICINES CONCEPT?

During the 1970s a growing number of low-income countries had more than 20 000 different brands of pharmaceutical products circulating in their markets. This situation was similar to that in high-income countries, despite the differences in their prevailing common diseases and their socio-economic situation. Also, pharmaceutical products were promoted and marketed with little concern for the different health needs and priorities of individual countries.[8]

Large amounts of money were spent by governments and consumers on expensive new medicines and on ineffective drug products. Thus, not all pharmaceutical products that they purchased represented value for money or met local health needs. Most of the time the medicines did not reach the places where they were most urgently needed, especially in rural settings.[8]

In the early 1970s some governments of low-income countries (Costa Rica, Cuba and Sri Lanka) started to realize that if medicines should meet the real health needs of the majority of their populations and should be equally available to all, then criteria had to be set, especially for selection of medicines. The concept of essential medicines was born. This concept also proved to have a positive impact on drug procurement, distribution, use and prices.[8]

Essential medicines are one of the most cost-effective elements in health care provision, and their potential health and economic impact is substantial. Access to essential medicines of assured quality is fundamental for the optimal performance of the health care system. Uninterrupted supplies of essential medicines determine the credibility of health services.

THE CONCEPT OF ESSENTIAL MEDICINES

The essential medicines concept was stimulated by three factors:[8]

1. Limited access to medicines essential to meet the health needs of the majority of the population
2. Limited public funding for pharmaceuticals and health
3. The implementation of WHO's Health For All Strategy.

The essential medicines concept underpinned the fact that a limited range of systematically selected essential medicines stimulates better quality of health care provision, improves drug management, prescribing and dispensing, and contains or reduces costs.

The principles of the essential medicines concept are:[8]

- Common health problems of the majority of the population can be treated with a small, carefully selected number of medicines.
- Health professionals routinely use less than 200 medicines. Training and clinical experience should focus on the proper use of these selected medicines.
- Procurement, distribution and other supply activities can be carried out most economically and efficiently for a limited number of drug products.
- Patients can be better informed about the effective use of medicines by the health professionals.

THE MODEL LIST OF ESSENTIAL MEDICINES

In 1977, inspired by the essential medicines concept, a WHO Expert Committee discussed the question of how many medicines were really needed to treat the common health problems. It concluded that approximately 220 medicines and vaccines could be considered essential. All of these medicines were of proven safety, efficacy and effectiveness and possessed well-understood therapeutic properties. Moreover, the majority of drug products were off patent and could be produced at relatively low cost.[2]

The first Model List of Essential Drugs was published by WHO in 1977 and has since been updated every 2 years. It created a revolution in international public health. It was met with a mixture of surprise, opposition and enthusiasm by the medical and pharmaceutical establishment.[2]

Its function should not be seen as an attempt to establish a uniform medicines list, as this is not feasible or realistic. The Model List can therefore be seen as a guide that can assist countries to identify their own priorities, to make their own selection and to develop their national or institutional lists of essential medicines. In addition, national lists can be stratified to better reflect skills and requirements at different levels within the national health care system.[9]

The Model List should thus reflect the priorities in medication needs. This does not imply that no other medicines are useful, but simply that in a given context those medicines selected are the ones most needed for the national health services. They should, therefore, be available at all times in adequate amounts and in the proper dosage forms.[9]

Over the years, national lists of essential medicines were mainly used to guide public drug procurement, health insurance schemes that reimburse costs of medicines, medicines donations, and local pharmaceutical manufacturing in the public sector. Recently, there has been a trend to use national treatment guidelines as the starting point for medicines selection and for preparing the national list of essential medicines. These lists, closely linked to national treatment guidelines, can be decision-making tools for drug procurement, educational tools, especially for training and supervision of health workers, and used as informational tools for consumers[9] (Fig. 4.1).

Nowadays, many new treatments and medicines for second-line therapies are costly and mostly unaffordable for consumers and many governments, especially those of low- and middle-income countries. Health care managers and policy makers in these countries have to make difficult financial decisions regarding the various recommended treatments for multidrug-resistant tuberculosis and malaria, for HIV/AIDS and for other infectious diseases, so that care and treatment can be offered to their citizens. Moreover, several European countries have difficulties in matching their allocated public health budgets with their peoples' medication needs and expectations.[10]

This has consequences for the role of the Model List and has necessitated the revision of its selection process and updating procedures.

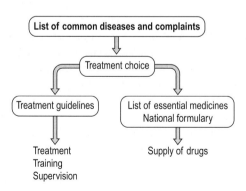

Fig. 4.1 Relationship between treatment guidelines and a list of essential medicines. (From World Health Organization June 2002: 'WHO's policy perspectives on medicines. The selection of essential medicines'.[14])

NEW PROCEDURES FOR UPDATING THE MODEL LIST OF ESSENTIAL MEDICINES

The process of developing the Model List is intended as an example of a model drug evaluation procedure for national drug and therapeutic committees. It should be a systematic and transparent process.[11]

In 1999, the WHO Expert Committee on the Use of Essential Medicines reviewed the current procedures for updating the Model List of Essential Medicines. They concluded that these procedures did not define the range of conditions covered with adequate specificity, nor were the reasons for inclusion recorded in sufficient detail. In addition the updating process was mainly consensus based. The Expert Committee also pointed out that the Model List and WHO's treatment guidelines should be better linked. They recommended to WHO that the methods for updating the Model List should be revised because of:[11]

- Advances in the science of evidence-based decision making
- The increasing link between essential medicines and guidelines for clinical health care
- The high cost of many new and effective medicines.

KEY FEATURES OF THE NEW PROCEDURE

As a result of a comprehensive consultation process, a new procedure for updating the Model List has been developed and adopted. The main components of the revised procedure are:[11]

- Strengthening the evidence-based approach rather than the consensus-based approach
- Broadening the global review process
- Linking selection to clinical guidelines
- Ensuring the independence of the Expert Committee in its scientific, normative and public health functions
- Creating an essential medicines library which links the Model List with WHO's clinical guidelines, the WHO Model Formulary, and other normative drug-related information
- Using the term 'essential medicines' as an alternative to 'essential drugs' with immediate effect.

Selection criteria

The updated criteria for the selection of essential medicines are based on several factors, such as: the disease burden; up-to-date and relevant data on the pharmacokinetic properties; safety and efficacy of the proposed medicine; cost-effectiveness; stability in various conditions; the need for special diagnostic or treatment facilities; the cost of the total treatment (and not only the unit cost of the medicine); single compounds (fixed-ratio drug combinations are selected only when the combination has a proven advantage in therapeutic effect, safety or compliance over single compounds administered separately). When adequate scientific evidence is not available on current treatment of a priority disease, the Expert Committee may either defer the issue until more evidence becomes available, or choose to make recommendations based on expert opinion and experience. Cost and cost-effectiveness comparisons may be made among alternative treatments within the same therapeutic group.[9,11]

At the beginning of 2002, the 11th Model List of Essential Medicines was revised by the Expert Committee applying the new procedure. The 12th Model List contains 325 individual medicines for the treatment of infectious and chronic diseases, which affect populations worldwide.[11] Over the last 25 years, 192 new medicines were added to and 70 medicines deleted from the Model List.

The updated Model List has a 'core' list indicating the minimum drug needs for a basic health care system, and a 'complementary' list including mainly essential medicines for priority diseases which may be cost effective but not necessarily affordable.[11]

The latest Model List reflects a model product, developed through a model process, and both models can be used for advocacy purposes.[11]

The Expert Committee reviewed the definition of essential medicines and recommended that:[11]

> *Essential medicines are those that satisfy the priority health care needs of the population. They are selected with due regard to public health relevance, evidence on efficacy and safety, and comparative cost effectiveness. Essential medicines are intended to be available within the context of functioning health systems at all times in adequate amounts, in the appropriate dosage forms, with assured quality and adequate information, and at a price the individual and the community can afford.*

> *The implementation of the concept of essential medicines is intended to be flexible and adaptable to many different situations; exactly which medicines are regarded as essential remains a national responsibility.*

IMPACT OF ESSENTIAL MEDICINES

Cost effective tools for fighting ill health worldwide are available. Essential medicines are one of those tools, when they are properly used. The following impacts of essential medicines have been identified and are discussed below.[2]

Health impact

Essential drug treatments are available for most prevailing communicable diseases, including acute respiratory infections, diarrhoeal diseases, malaria, tuberculosis, sexually transmitted infections and HIV/AIDS.[5] Essential life-saving medicines exist for non-communicable diseases such as ischaemic heart disease and cerebrovascular disease.[5] Poor and disadvantaged populations are hardest hit by these prevailing diseases. The availability of essential medicines has been found to attract patients to health facilities, where they can also benefit from preventive services. However, patient attendance dropped when essential medicines were out of stock at the health facility.[12] A community's health situation may then stagnate or worsen.

Economic impact

In high-income countries, two-thirds of medicines are prepaid through government revenues and social health insurance programmes.[12,13] This means that the cost of medicines is not directly borne by the patient. For most ministries of health in low- and middle-income countries, public spending on medicines represents the largest health expenditure after staff salaries. In many low-income countries, 50–90% of medicines are paid for out-of-pocket at the time of illness. This means that medicines represent the largest non-budgeted household expenditure.[12,13] By focusing pharmaceutical expenditure on essential medicines, the cost effectiveness of government and personal outlay drug expenditure can be improved and health impact strengthened. Increasing access to essential medicines would therefore contribute markedly to poverty reduction.

CONCLUSION

Over the years, the essential medicines concept has become a global concept and is a powerful tool to promote health equity. Although originally intended for low-income countries, an increasing number of high-income countries also use its key components. Health systems, from basic health systems in the poorest countries to highly developed national health insurance schemes in the industrialized countries, have recognized both its therapeutic and economic benefits. This recognition has been triggered by the introduction of many new and often expensive drug therapies, increasing drug costs and by observed quality variations in health care provision.[11]

The essential medicines concept is now widely accepted as a highly pragmatic approach to providing the best of modern evidenced-based and cost effective health services. It is as valid today as it was when first introduced in 1975. The concept does not exclude all other medicines but focuses on those medicines that have the best balance of quality, safety, efficacy and cost for a given health service.[9] It has also been adopted by international and bilateral aid agencies, and non-governmental organizations that include strategies on rational drug selection, supply and use in their programmes of work.[9]

Moreover, the concept is forward looking.[9] It promotes the need to regularly update drug choices when new therapeutic options and improved quality, safety and efficacy profiles of medicines become available. It also stimulates research and development for better pharmaceutical formulations and for more efficient responses to new or re-emerging diseases.

By the end of 1999, 156 Member States had officially published national lists of essential medicines, often in combination with standard treatment guidelines and stratified according to the level of care, and 127 of these lists had been updated during the last 5 years.[11] Many countries have also successfully applied the essential medicines concept to teaching hospitals and facilities providing specialized care. Health insurance schemes increasingly use national lists of essential medicines as a reference. Throughout the six WHO regions, a total of 88 countries have introduced the essential medicines concept into the curricula of medicine and pharmacy training programmes.[2] Moreover, the Model List has also resulted in greater international coordination in health care development, and in health emergency situations.[9]

These achievements show clearly what can be done when governments, public interest groups, the private sector and international organizations cooperate together.

Key points

- WHO was founded in 1948 and has 191 Member States (2002).
- Health is described as 'a state of complete physical, mental and social well being and not merely the absence of disease or infirmity'.
- The essential medicines concept was launched in 1975, and was triggered by factors such as limited access to the most needed medicines, limited public funding, and the implementation of WHO's Health For All Strategy.
- The first Model List of Essential Drugs was published by WHO in 1977 and included around 220 medicines.
- The Model List, updated in 2002, consists of 325 essential medicines divided into a 'core' and 'complementary' list.
- The Model List reflects a model product and a model process, which can both be used for advocacy.
- The health and economic impacts of essential medicines are considerable.
- By the end of 1999, 156 countries had published national lists, often in combination with standard treatment guidelines.

5

Pharmacy management

I. F. Jones

After studying this chapter you will know about:

The basic principles of financial management in community pharmacy
Profit and loss accounts
Balance sheets and their interpretation
Some tools used in financial control including gross margin and stockturn

Introduction

Management is about making decisions. The decisions are concerned with the efficient use of economic resources which, by definition, are in short supply and comprise capital (money), buildings, stocks and personnel. Decisions also have to be made on how and where the manager's time is spent. In pharmacy that is particularly important as the 21st century gets underway and the profession, particularly in community pharmacy, grapples with change in the nature and extent of NHS pharmaceutical services.

The model posed in Figure 5.1 identifies most of the skills required by the efficient manager. The various categories shown appear independent of one another, but that is too simplistic. For instance 'human resource' denotes employment which, in turn, includes recruitment, training and other matters but knowledge of employment law and finance are also relevant. Similarly 'premises' and 'marketing' are related because of the desire in merchandising to use space effectively.

Inspection of the model implies that the current MPharm. degree programme does not help very much to develop skills in management. This is because management skills have their roots in social sciences as opposed to the traditional pharmaceutical sciences that underpin much of the MPharm. programme. The Nuffield Report in Pharmacy (1986) advocated, amongst many other recommendations, that the undergraduate programme in pharmacy develops

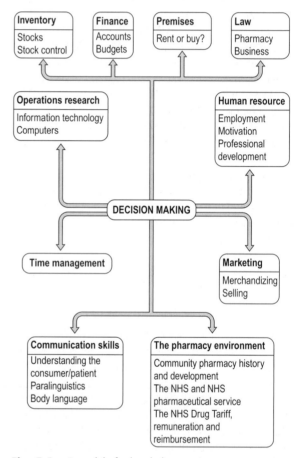

Fig. 5.1 A model of related elements in management in community pharmacy.

this area of curriculum. Clearly social and behavioural skills relate to people and in the context of pharmacy, their fears and aspirations about health, ill health and health promotion (see Ch. 2). A vital part of social skill development is in understanding what is meant by communication and of learning how to be a good communicator. A good manager will be a good communicator. In pharmacy a good manager will understand the customer and what that customer wants from the pharmacy and from the pharmacy staff.

Because schools of pharmacy devote only a small time to these subjects, management has to be a separate and post-pharmacy graduation exercise. A management qualification like an MBA/Diploma in Management Studies is helpful, particularly to the younger pharmacist to broaden the intellectual outlook that is narrowed considerably by concentration on traditional science in the current undergraduate programme.

Pharmacy is about people as much as it is about drugs. Management is particularly about people. But it is also about finance. The pharmacy scene in the developed countries of the world is fundamentally about profit. The profit motive underpins the provision of pharmaceutical services. Without profit there would be no community pharmacy as we know it today. Government and health authorities depend on the existence of private capital to fund the provision of primary care services in pharmacy. For instance, very little public capital is tied up in providing premises for the traditional NHS pharmaceutical service. Should investors and entrepreneurs decide not to invest capital in pharmacy then the state would have to provide alternative arrangements like setting up public 'dispensaries' or nationalizing existing pharmacies—or groups of them.

Nevertheless there is currently considerable investment in pharmacy, particularly by the multiple pharmacy groups and the supermarket chains. Satisfaction of the profit motive would be fundamental to this. So good managers have to have a working knowledge of financial accounting data and budgets.

Strictly speaking, managers are those individuals who are skilled at looking after someone else's economic resources. A pharmacy manager will have dealings with cash and NHS prescriptions that become 'invoices' once the clinical job is done. Managers control staff and look after premises and stock. Young pharmacists become managers very quickly after registration, principally because their membership of the Royal Pharmaceutical Society is mandatory in taking 'personal control' of dealing with medicinal products as per Part IV of the Medicines Act 1968.

This chapter will focus on finance in community pharmacy with reference to the profit and loss account, balance sheet, their interpretation and a brief analysis of the former which can help managers assess how well the pharmacy is progressing. The model accounts for an imaginary community pharmacy, called the 'Exemplar Pharmacy', shown in Figures 5.2 and 5.3 are compiled exclusive of VAT (the usual practice) and have a simplified presentation to demonstrate essential features.

Turnover		£	£	£
	NHS		480 644	
	OTC		174 208	654 852
Cost of goods sold				
Opening stock		70 444		
Purchases		501 201		
		571 645		
Closing stock		83 877		487 768
Gross (trading) profit				167 084
Expenses:				
Rent			12 000	
Wages			50 000	
Light/heat			2300	
Depreciation			6500	
Insurances			2000	
Advertising			1000	
Telephone			1200	
Professional and				
trade subscriptions			650	
Repairs			2000	
Motor expenses			2000	
Bank charges			1000	
Accountancy fee			1500	
Sundry expenses			1500	83 650
Net operating profit				83 434

Fig. 5.2 Model profit and loss account for the Exemplar Pharmacy: year ended 31 March 2002.

THE PROFIT AND LOSS ACCOUNT

This account, preferably called the 'trading and profit and loss account' measures the amount of profit or loss that accrues over a defined period of time. That time has to be no longer than one year, for tax purposes. The more frequently the account is compiled the better as far as using it for management purposes is concerned, as will be seen later. The main problem in regular, accurate assessment of profit (or loss) would be the necessity to count the stock remaining in the pharmacy at the end of the period. This can be an unavoidably time consuming and costly exercise, particularly if undertaken by a professional stocktaker; however it is a very necessary exercise as will be seen later.

In efficient business a balance is struck between the costs and upheaval of stocktaking with the need for accurate management information on which decisions can be made. It is usual for the larger company pharmacies to make up their

Liabilities	£	£	Assets	£	£
Owners liability			Fixed assets	Cost	NBV
Brought forward	85 290		Fixtures and fittings	15 300	10 340
+ Profit	83 434	168 724	Computers	3 000	1 887
Less drawings		68 390	Company vehicle	11 000	4 641
		100 334			16 868
Current liabilities			Current assets		
			Stock (at valuation)	83 877	
Total creditors	51 506		Debtors (NHS)	48 106	
Expense creditors	1 206	52 712	Cash (in hand)	560	
			Cash (at bank)	3 635	136 178
		153 046			153 046

(NBV = Net book value (often referred to as Written down value, WDV): the amount still to be depreciated)

Fig. 5.3 Model balance sheet for the Exemplar Pharmacy: year ended 31 March 2002. NBV = net book value (often referred to as written down value (WDV)); the amount still to be depreciated.

accounts twice a year. Most proprietor-operated pharmacies produce their accounts annually and then use them principally for assessment of income/corporation tax purposes as opposed to using them for financial control purposes.

Turnover

A model trading and profit and loss account is shown in Figure 5.2. Turnover is the first item. The turnover shows the mixed business of community pharmacy, that of the over-the-counter (OTC) retailing of traditional (and sometimes non-traditional) chemists' merchandise and the supply of prescription medicines to the National Health Service. Total turnover, as shown, of around £650 000 would be typical of a so-called 'average' pharmacy in 2002. Indeed pharmacies with turnover levels of less than, say, £400 000 are increasingly less viable and less attractive as 'going concerns' for prospective purchasers, unless a shrewd investor can see a potential opportunity to develop rapid financial growth.

The turnover represents the goods that have been sold for cash or 'sold' in some form of contractual obligation where cash will ultimately be generated. The NHS 'sales' is such an example.

The profit and loss account measures the profit or loss accruing between the time of opening the business on the first day of the accounting period to the close of business on the last day of the period. The turnover then includes payment for prescriptions dispensed during the last month

of the trading year (or period). As payment through the appropriate pricing authority (see Appendix 2) takes several weeks to reach the pharmacy the account is not usually made up until the final payment for the last month's prescriptions is received, usually around 3 months after the end of the period.

Similarly, goods sold by credit at the end of an accounting period should be included in the turnover figure, although actual payment will be made in the next accounting period.

Gross profit

Once the turnover is established, the cost of the goods which have been sold (or supplied) will be deducted to arrive at the gross (or sometimes called 'trading') profit. The model account shows how this is calculated. The opening stock is the stock present in the pharmacy at opening time on the first day of the period. It is, of course, the closing stock that is taken as the value of the stock at the end of the previous period. The stock is measured at cost, or other lower realizable value. This means that stock that has become unsuitable for sale during the year will be excluded from the closing sum. So, for example, stock that is damaged or out of date is 'written off'. The final closing stock figure then reflects good saleable stock. The figure for purchases reflects the value of all the goods entering the pharmacy during the year irrespective of whether or not their suppliers have been paid.

There has to be a principle to deal with credit and debit issues, and to be consistent in accounting terms it is assumed that all goods 'sold' or acquired under a contractual obligation are 'realized' in the accounts to which they relate. In this way meaningful comparisons can be made from one year to the next and from one pharmacy to another.

The gross profit is the measure of 'profit on trade' (hence the equivalent and perhaps preferable term 'trading profit') and is simply the difference between selling price and cost price of goods leaving the pharmacy during the year. The amount of gross profit particularly in relation to the turnover is a very important parameter and is discussed later in this chapter.

Expenses and depreciation

The profit and loss account then charges the expenses that have been incurred during, and because of, the operation of the business in that accounting period. The most notable are the wages and salaries paid to employees and the rent (if the business premises are leasehold, as opposed to freehold). All expenses that have been incurred should be charged so that a true level of 'net' profit is obtained. Most of the items shown in the model account will be self-explanatory. However, the term 'depreciation' deserves special mention.

This financial sum represents the wear and tear and/or obsolescence of fixed assets, that is those possessions of the business which are tangible, not purchased with a view to selling them, but are used in one way or another to assist in selling goods/collecting revenue. Fixtures and fittings, computers and motor vehicles are good examples. The problem with the technique of depreciation is estimating how much a particular asset wears out or becomes obsolete in a particular period so as to charge this cost against the corresponding revenues collected. Depreciation is a necessary but unsatisfactory technique because a charge is to be made for the 'use' of these assets but the amount estimated is at best a guess, based on what the principals of the business (or their accountants) estimate as their useful life and what they are worth at the time of disposal. Almost invariably an 'adjustment' is made at disposal to recognize the difference between disposal price (if an asset is disposed at a price) and the 'value' of the asset quoted in the balance sheet.

Traditionally in a proprietor-pharmacist operated pharmacy the 'salary' of the proprietor is not found in the profit and loss account. This is because the proprietor will draw cash from the business instead of a 'salary' as such. After all it is the proprietor's business and he/she will draw money from the business in the light of its financial success (or

otherwise). A proprietor's drawings from capital would be shown in the balance sheet. In a managed branch the manager's salary would be included in payroll costs and if the business is operated as a company incorporated under the Companies Acts, the principals of the business, as shareholders, would be regarded as employees and their 'salaries' would be included in this section of the account. Payments made to locum pharmacists and casual labour would also be included.

Once all the measurable operating costs are noted, the net operating profit (the profit accruing from the operation of the business) can be declared.

THE BALANCE SHEET

This is a statement of the overall financial position of the business at a certain instant in time. The balance sheet shows, in financial terms, the possessions of the firm—the assets on one side and the claims of various parties to these assets (known as liabilities) on the other. The liabilities can also be regarded as the sums owed by the business both to its owner(s) and to creditors. The description that follows relates to the model balance sheet presented in Figure 5.3 which, in turn, reflects the trading shown in the model profit and loss account. A simple, and traditional, presentation is made with the 'assets' on the right and the 'liabilities' on the left. The principle of the balance sheet is clearly shown—that the claims to the assets of the business can only equal the value of those assets. By definition then, balance sheets must balance!

Assets

Assets are the possessions of the firm. They may be tangible or intangible. Tangible assets can be either fixed or current assets. Fixed assets are used in one way or another to help collect revenue. They are not purchased with the intention of resale. From time to time when their useful life in the business is over, new ones that are more efficient or up to date replace them. Many accounting periods will derive benefit from these assets. An important task for management will be to work out a realistic charge to be made each accounting period to reflect their usage. That charge is the depreciation found in the profit and loss account. The decision about the level of depreciation is essentially one for management based on how long the asset can be used for optimum effect. Clearly fixtures and fittings can be regarded as lasting for a number of years in pharmacy before, say, a shop refit would be desirable. Motor vehicles and, particularly, computers might need more frequent replacement. Methods of depreciation are important issues but beyond the scope of this brief chapter.

Current assets are those tangible items that consist of cash or goods which, in theory, can be converted rapidly into cash. In pharmacy two items are particularly important: stock and debtors. Stock is there from a business point of view with the sole intention of rapid conversion into cash. However, from a purely professional perspective stocks such as traditional merchandise of cosmetics, toiletries, chemist sundries (including dressings and appliances) and OTC/NHS medicines are present in order to provide a comprehensive pharmaceutical service. Therefore, a balance has to be drawn between a pharmacy having a reputation for always having comprehensive stock levels and the need for business efficiency in realizing the money tied up on shelves. In management terms stock must be viewed as cash lying idle. The subject of stockturn (see below) helps to further consider this subject.

Debtors are not a welcome sight in accounts, on the basis that ordinarily any business debtors can become bad debts and not be realizable. A balance sheet like the one shown would cause considerable disquiet in general retail business for this reason. However, debts are a traditional part of community pharmacy business because of the monies owed by the NHS for dispensing. If money has to be owed there is some compensation in knowing that the NHS (as a government agency) will pay and so pharmacy debtors, in this respect, are considered as good debts and will be realized. Creditors are well aware of this.

Cash is clearly important for the business to pay its operating expenses and to purchase new assets. Arrangements with banks to provide overdraft facilities are often necessary to provide short-term loans, to meet demands by creditors while the monthly payment from the NHS is outstanding. Too much cash in a current account is another problem. With the principle of business to make a profit the concept that 'capital needs to be remunerated' is fundamental. Any spare cash must attract an interest. In times of high inflation, stocks increase in value at a rapid rate and any 'extra cash' would be wisely invested in good saleable stock. During times of low inflation extra cash might be placed in other investment opportunities.

The other main asset in pharmacy is goodwill. It is an intangible asset and of little value in the day-to-day management of the pharmacy and for this reason is not included in the model balance sheet. It is important when the business is valued before it is sold. In the current climate suitable pharmacy businesses can attract considerable goodwill values. While the modern tendency is to base goodwill values on the total turnover, such a narrow vision may be too simplistic and, in any event, a goodwill figure will eventually be a matter of agreement between a willing seller and a willing buyer. In a premier pharmacy business the goodwill payment would be expected to be the largest part of the purchase price. So perhaps hundreds of thousands of pounds could change hands for something that can't be seen but is there. What the buyer pays for in goodwill is the likelihood that he/she will inherit the proceeds and reputation enjoyed by the previous owner and that those customers who previously patronized the pharmacy will continue to do so under the new ownership.

The restriction in 1987 in granting NHS contracts by local health authorities to potential new (or existing) proprietors saw a significant increase in goodwill values. Of course, the possibility that such limitation of contract may be revoked (as is under consideration at the time of writing this chapter) would see the opposite effect.

Liabilities

On the left hand side of the balance sheet are the liabilities. This defines those who can rightfully justify that they are owed money from the business. Current liabilities consist of creditors. In pharmacy, trade creditors, wholesalers and other suppliers who provide goods on a credit basis, mainly take up this section. Occasionally expense creditors are seen such as the landlord who is owed rent, perhaps because of a dispute.

The remaining quarter section of the balance sheet is the owner's capital (or in the case of a pharmacy operated as a limited company this would be referred to as the shareholders' account or the shareholders' equity). It consists of the owner's claim to the assets of the business brought forward from the last period to which the net operating profit is added. This is the financial reason for proprietorship—that profits gained accrue to the entrepreneur who takes the risk of investing capital in the first place. Profit is the reward for the proprietor's effort and skills in business. A loss has to be viewed as also accruing to the proprietor and similarly relates to the risks associated with business.

The proprietor's drawings from capital are expressed here. The sum shown will be inclusive of all drawings including the payment of income tax. The resulting sum, in this case £100 334, is regarded as the 'net worth' of the business to the owner. Should the owner wish to sell and a new prospective purchaser make an acceptable offer for goodwill of, say, £200 000 then the net worth would be increased automatically to £300 334. In this case the right hand side of the balance sheet would show a goodwill figure of £200 000 to acknowledge the increased value of the pharmacy business. This would, of course, make the balance sheet balance.

FINANCIAL CONTROL

The question that might be posed is 'why are accounts required in the first place'? There are several answers. Self-employed pharmacists, including proprietors, would need accounts to arrive at fair and reasonable calculations of profits prior to income tax (or corporation tax) assessment. Accounts are also necessary by law if the pharmacy is operated as a company registered under the Companies Act. A requirement under the Act is to submit an Annual Return, and part of it would include some details of profit and loss and a balance sheet. Sometimes accounts are needed to convince creditors, or potential creditors, for example a bank manager, that loans given will be repaid. The fourth and most important reason as far as this chapter is concerned, should be that accounts are available to provide vital management information about what is happening in the business.

The remaining section of this chapter is restricted to an analysis of the trading account. This focus of attention is chosen, and is particularly appropriate, because of the immediate relevance to day-to-day issues in the management of the pharmacy.

TURNOVER

This figure is easily recorded and monitored because it is derived from daily OTC sales and revenue from NHS dispensing. Turnover for one particular accounting period is relatively unimportant. The main issue is: is it (or its components) increasing, and by how much? Two factors are important. Firstly, inflation needs to be considered. NHS receipts are not monitored in figures for the Index of Retail Prices (used as a measure of inflation) and so NHS and OTC elements need to be separately considered. If OTC sales this year are 10% above that achieved in the previous year the initial reaction of management might be one of satisfaction. The question is 'how much has the cost of buying those goods increased'? If the 'cost' has also risen by 10% then the 'real' increase is zero as there is no volume increase. The

following simple, but exaggerated, example helps to understand this situation. Assume OTC sales are made only from, say, soap. If the sales of soap are 10% up on last year, i.e. there is 10% more money in the cash register from sales, but the cost of soap has gone up by 10%, then the same number of bars of soap have been sold. There is no 'real' increase in volume. No more business has been achieved this year. Therefore taking account of inflation is important. In order to monitor this situation good management will be aware of the monthly publication by government of the Index of Retail Prices. The overall Index this last 10 years or so has shown small, modest increases as inflation appears within government-defined acceptable limits. For a proprietor the 'All Items Index' published in the national press is a useful guide for assessing net operating profit (NOP). If NOP increases outstrip 'inflation' it means generally that his standard of living is improving.

Perhaps more important for all pharmacy management is a subordinate index which refers solely to chemists' OTC merchandise. This index can be found together with other information in the government's National Statistics Website http://www.statistics.gov.uk/rpi. Monitoring this index and its changes enables a far more accurate assessment of OTC performance. At the present time (2002) inflation in chemists' OTC goods is similar to the 'all items' index.

A second critical and related issue is the performance of competitors. How are other businesses of a comparable type performing? This can be addressed to some extent by considering the Index of Retail Sales for retail business published in the Business Monitor Series. The relevant publication for pharmacy is Business Monitor SDM28. This covers many aspects of retail trade including chemists' OTC trade. If all chemists are seen to be achieving a 10% increase then the previously mentioned 10% increase achieved by the Exemplar Pharmacy is typical of business generally— whether or not it matches inflation. If the pharmacy more than matches the performance of similar businesses this can be cause for celebration. If all other relevant businesses were better than an individual pharmacy that would be the cause of serious inquiry and management would be required to provide an explanation.

In most pharmacies the NHS receipts make the biggest contribution to turnover. Increases in NHS receipts are closely associated with increases in the number of prescriptions. National, Regional and NHS health authority/primary care area totals for prescription numbers and costs are monitored in documentation produced by the various prescription processing authorities in England, Scotland, Wales and Northern Ireland. Local Pharmaceutical Committee (LPC) secretaries might have access to some data for their own health authority/primary care area. Information will also be available in annual reports of the prescription processing agencies and also from the Pharmaceutical Services Negotiating Committee (for England and Wales) and Scottish Pharmaceutical General Council. Prescription numbers (and costs) are increasing significantly at the time of preparing this chapter and pharmacy proprietors will be monitoring these closely to compare individual performance with national/local trends.

GROSS MARGIN

Gross margin is defined as:

$$\text{Gross margin} = \frac{\text{gross (or trading) profit}}{\text{turnover}} \times 100\%$$

Inspection of the profit and loss account for the Exemplar Pharmacy shows the margin to be:

$$\frac{\pounds167\ 084}{654\ 852} \times 100 = 25.5\%.$$

This is, perhaps, the most important financial ratio as far as day-to-day management is concerned. A margin of 25.5% means that of every £100 of turnover £25.50 is left after paying for the goods. So £25.50 is left to contribute to the operating expenses and net operating profit.

The margin in pharmacy reflects the mixed business of OTC trade and NHS dispensing. Careful monitoring of stocks and purchases enables a separate margin calculation for NHS and OTC activities to be made. Managers can then start to identify from precisely where, in the mixed business of community pharmacy, the profit comes from.

Clearly the higher the gross margin the greater the opportunity for a higher net margin—meaning more net operating profit. Traditionally OTC merchandise in pharmacy has a wide range of margin. Baby foods and photographic film, for example, have relatively low margins while agency cosmetics, costume jewellery and developing and printing photographic film have much higher margins. In providing a comprehensive pharmaceutical service proprietors of pharmacies will offer a wide range of goods and the OTC margin will reflect this. Of course management might choose to diversify the range of goods to include higher margin merchandise but this might have some adverse consequences (like 'dead' stock which is eventually 'written off'). Because the NHS side of pharmacy business has been, for the last 25 years or so (for the average independent pharmacy), the most prominent contribution to turnover in most pharmacies, the

NHS margin attracts considerable attention. Theoretically, at least, the gross profit from dispensing is the sum of the various professional fees payable according to the NHS Drug Tariff plus the 'payment for additional professional services' (also referred to as the 'professional allowance') divided by the NHS turnover. This NHS turnover is the sum of NHS receipts as computed each month by the prescription processing authority. Accordingly:

$$\text{NHS gross margin} = \frac{\text{Drug Tariff fees + allowances}}{\text{Total NHS receipts}} \times 100\%$$

Calculated nationally for England this theoretical NHS margin (taking all pharmacies, and the total of professional fees/allowances and total prescription costs) was around 12–13% in 2002. Northern Ireland, Scotland and Wales are similar, notwithstanding differences in the fee and allowance structure in Scottish and Northern Ireland drug tariffs. There is variation in NHS margin from one pharmacy to another. While fees and allowances are the same the cost of drugs is a variable depending on local doctor prescribing habits. For the Exemplar Pharmacy the national (and theoretical) NHS average of, say, 12% is a long way from the 25.5% as calculated above for the mixed OTC/NHS business. A 12% margin means that only £12 of every £100 of NHS receipts is available to contribute to operating expenses and net operating profit. In practice the Exemplar Pharmacy, like most others, will derive considerably higher NHS margins. This is because a considerable gross profit accrues in the application of the drug tariff reimbursement prices to dispensed prescriptions. The prices used to reimburse drug costs as found in the Tariff are, in general, much higher than market acquisition prices. Pharmacy contractors (proprietors) to the NHS are generally over-reimbursed, notwithstanding the automatic application of a drug tariff deduction/discount scale to take account of what is often referred to as 'uncovenanted profits'. In practice the NHS margin might well be over 20% thus helping to explain the margin of 25.5% recorded for the Exemplar Pharmacy.

Because of the ability of the multiple chain pharmacies to have a vertically integrated business of manufacture and distribution and to be able to purchase NHS and other goods at more competitive prices than, say, the Exemplar Pharmacy, the NHS gross margin stands to be considerably higher. This has serious implications for pharmacy proprietors. Periodically the Department of Health will organize a discount inquiry of prescription ingredient costs. Such inquiries generally lead to a revision (increase) of the drug tariff deduction/discount scale. Although it is difficult to find absolute documentary evidence, it is generally understood that government regard the application of drug tariff pricing to be based on the principal of 'strict net cost reimbursement'. Thus, any discount on NHS Drug Tariff prices received by the Exemplar Pharmacy (and all others) can be viewed as the property of HM Government and, accordingly, is (potentially, at least) recoverable. The implication of such a policy would then have massive implications for proprietors and the net profitability of their pharmacy business.

Gross margin variation

In most pharmacies where the mix of OTC and NHS business remain essentially the same, little variation in gross margin is expected on a year-to-year basis. There are small erosions of margin due to manufacturers' price increases at cost and recommended retail level not keeping in step. However, in any one pharmacy a margin variation of, say, more than 1% on the year previous would likely be significant and so would demand an explanation. In the Exemplar Pharmacy inspection of the profit and loss account (Fig. 5.2) would show that a fall in margin of 1% would reduce gross (and therefore net) profit by £6548. Margin erosion therefore demands serious attention and pharmacy principals/directors can expect management to account for it. Some explanations can be understandable or predictable although others might have more unpleasant implications.

Some reasons for decline in margin are:

- The identification of items of stock that are no longer saleable either because they are date expired, damaged or obsolete. Such stock should be 'written off' at stocktaking. If, say, £2000 of stock were identified in this way the closing stock valuation would be reduced by this amount—just as though it did not exist.
- Reduction in selling prices. Retail outlets that have a periodic sale, perhaps at the year end, might operate a policy decision to reduce prices to encourage greater sales volume. So, for instance, goods that might have been sold originally for, say, £5000 are sold in a sale for, say, £3000. Clearly sales turnover is reduced with the obvious knock-on reduction in margin. Of course community pharmacies are not well known for having 'sales'. The abolition of resale price maintenance might result in price reductions for proprietary medicines that would reduce margins, just as if they were in a sale. Current evidence is that there is as yet little price competition in operation.
- Reduction in discounts from suppliers and/or an increase in the NHS deduction/discount scale.

- Faulty stocktaking where goods that should have been identified and included in the closing stock have been overlooked or incorrectly valued. Such a problem might not be recognized and corrected until the stocktake the following year.
- If one or more of these above do not provide plausible explanation the spectre of theft has to be considered. Theft of either stock and/or cash has clear implications for margin erosion. The identification of, and dealing with, dishonesty by consumers and/or staff has to be one of the most unpleasant duties that management has to address. The explanation might be customer shoplifting, stocks not being delivered (but charged) and theft by staff members of cash and/or stock items.

Clearly if accounts are compiled only once a year it can be a 12-month wait to find out if a problem affecting margin erosion has been corrected. In multiple-chain pharmacies unexplained margin erosion would be quickly identified and investigated in a few weeks because systems would be set up to monitor just this. In a small pharmacy the problem, if not similarly identified by the owner, might come to light only if the business is subjected to an investigation by HM Inland Revenue. Margin reduction means decreased gross profit and similarly decreased net profit (on which income tax/corporation tax would be assessed).

STOCKTURN

Stockturn is a ratio of sales divided by stocks. There are several definitions in use, perhaps the best and most favoured is:

$$\text{Stockturn} = \frac{\text{cost of goods sold}}{\text{average stock at cost}}$$

The average stock is the average of opening and closing stocks and is chosen for use in this ratio as generally it more closely measures the average investment in stock during an accounting period.

The stockturn ratio gives a measure of how often stock is turned over. Put another way, it is a measure of how quickly the investment in stock is converted back into cash. In many retail businesses the biggest asset on a day-to-day basis is the stock whether on the shelves, in drawers or a stock room. In financial terms stock must be viewed as cash waiting to be taken from a shelf or drawer to be released into the cash register. Stock on shelves should be viewed as the same as cash in a current bank account and so not earning interest. Also cash in a bank is more secure than stock on a shelf.

Ideally stock needs to be at a level to satisfy customer demand and to prevent unnecessary lost sales/prescriptions. Stockturn analysis will help managers to assess if the pharmacy's operating policy on stock is being successful. For instance some multiple company pharmacies operate a policy of keeping 6 week's stock. Such pharmacies will then have a stockturn of approximately eight, that is, turning stock at the rate of eight times a year.

Inspection of the Exemplar Pharmacy stockturn using the definition above shows:

$$\text{Stockturn} = \frac{£487\,768}{77\,161} = 6.3$$

The stockturn of six means turning over stock every 2 months and therefore the Exemplar Pharmacy currently carries approximately 8 weeks' stock. If it were to comply with the policy of, say, 6 weeks' stock then, with other factors remaining unchanged, by using the simple calculation above the average stock would be:

$$\text{Stock} = \frac{£487\,768}{8} = £60\,971$$

This would then, in theory, transfer around £16 000 worth of stock to cash. This paper exercise would indeed be a rapid conversion into cash (as explained earlier in considering the balance sheet current assets). Such a theoretical exercise is most difficult to implement in practice without loss of sales.

The stockturn figure is clearly an average. Some items are turned over almost daily, in which case the stockturn would be around 300. This is balanced against slow-moving lines that might remain on shelves until they are sold eventually or discarded due to date expiry or other reason. An example of slow-moving lines would be agency cosmetics with an extensive product range. A stockturn of say three (or even less) might have to be accepted in order to cater for a select clientele. Managers would have to decide if investing in such stock was worth the financial risk.

Generally stockturn for dispensary items is greater than for OTC goods, particularly if local GPs adhere to a formulary and do not frequently change prescribing habits. It would be usual to expect dispensary stocks to 'turn over' at least once a month (i.e. stockturn = 12 minimum). Town centre pharmacies which cater for a wide GP cohort could expect to experience a broader range of dispensary stock items and an accompanying reduced stockturn or be at increased risk of lost prescriptions. Good pharmacy managers will devote time to a study of the NHS Drug Tariff in order to achieve optimum reimbursement from dispensing. In this context it is of interest to note that the NHS will, in principle, permit claims for broken bulk if slow-moving dispensary stock is not turned over within 6 months (i.e. a stockturn of 2).

As a summary it would be preferable to consider margin and stockturn together. Generally fast-moving lines tend to be low margin and slow-moving lines tend to have the compensation of larger margins. In striving towards optimum profit, managers would wish for the utopia of high margin and high stockturn. Clearly what has to be avoided is a combination of low margin and low stockturn. In attempting to provide a comprehensive pharmaceutical service managers of community pharmacies have to be prepared to accept a balance of high and low margin, high and low stockturn goods. A final comment, then, would be to regard profit as a function of margin and stockturn in the following expression:

Net operating profit $\propto$ gross margin × stockturn − expenses.

Key Points

- Management requires many skills, few of which are dealt with in the undergraduate pharmacy course.
- The trading and profit and loss account shows the accrued profit or loss over a specified time period (often 6 months or 1 year).
- Turnover is the total sales of a business, including NHS income.
- Gross profit is the difference between cost and selling prices of goods sold.
- Depreciation is a method of accounting for 'use' of assets which will wear out or become obsolescent.
- Net profit is the difference between all income and all expenses.
- A balance sheet displays the overall financial position of a business.
- Assets are possessions of the business, whilst liabilities represent what the business owes to others.
- Stock levels are important and decisions may be monitored using the stockturn ratio.
- Goodwill is important, but is only necessarily quantified at the time the proprietor is contemplating selling the business.
- Changes in turnover must be measured against inflation and the performance of similar competitors.
- Gross margin is one of the most important financial ratios in day-to-day management. Sudden reductions not brought about by deliberate management policy changes need to be investigated and analysed carefully.
- In pharmacy, gross margin could be affected by government policy on the drug tariff/discount scale. This is likely to be a future problem for management.
- Net operating profit is a function of margin and stockturn.

PART 2

PRINCIPLES OF PHARMACY PRACTICE

6

The principles and applications of quality assurance

D. G. Chapman

After studying this chapter you will know about:

Terminology and definitions associated with quality

The nature of quality assurance systems

Application of quality assurance to:

Good manufacturing practice

Quality control

Standards

Personnel and 'qualified person'

Premises and equipment

Documentation

Production

Complaints and product recall

Quality audits

Sterile product manufacture

Quality in community pharmacy

Introduction

Very complex and potent medicines have been developed in recent times. These medicines have very high research, development and production costs. The special nature of these products requires a high level of product consistency resulting in the need for highly regulated production processes. The consumers of these medicines, namely the patients, rightly have a high expectation of product quality. All of these factors have resulted in the need for advanced quality assurance systems in the batch production of medicines.

Useful definitions

Quality assurance. All systems which ensure that manufactured products are of the required quality for use.

Good manufacturing practice. Ensures that products are consistently produced. The standard of quality must be suitable for use.

Quality control. Ensures that a satisfactory quality of materials and products is used. This will involve sampling, testing, documentation and release procedures. Only when materials and products are of a satisfactory quality are they released for use.

Product design. All factors involved with the design of the product must be selected to achieve a quality product.

Process development. The production process must be designed to produce a quality product. It must allow for any deviations which arise in the production process.

Validation. The procedure which is used to prove that the various production procedures, equipment and materials will produce accurate results.

A QUALITY ASSURANCE SYSTEM

In the large-scale production of medicines quality is not achieved by accident. It is the result of a carefully constructed quality assurance (QA) system. This system must ensure that each medicinal product conforms with its intended use. This applies in terms of safety, therapeutic effectiveness and acceptability. It is important that quality is built into the product. This applies at all stages of the manufacturing process. It is not adequate that the product is only tested retrospectively at the end of the manufacturing process.

A quality assurance system is constructed by merging a series of actions. These actions collectively ensure product quality. As a result, the quality assurance system must:

- Establish specific activities before production begins
- Control factors during production
- Evaluate results following production.

The quality assurance system in a pharmaceutical production unit can be likened to the railings on a suspension bridge (Fig. 6.1). The bridge spans the production process

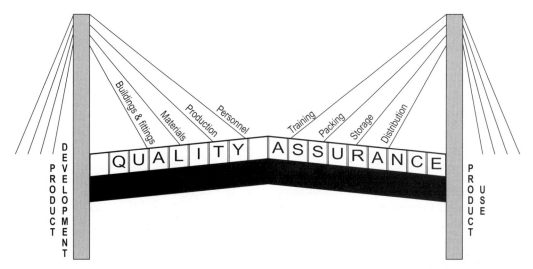

Fig. 6.1 The production bridge. (After Goldberger 1991.)

from the initial stages of product development to the final use of the product. The span of the bridge is supported by suspension wires that represent a range of production functions carried out in the manufacturing plant. Collectively the functions form the complete production process.

The senior management of a manufacturing facility is responsible for obtaining a quality product. However, to obtain total control of quality requires an organized effort by the entire production workforce, suppliers of materials and the final product distributors. It may be beneficial if the manager of quality assurance in the manufacturing unit is involved with the production team as a coach, counsellor or teacher. By adopting these various roles, the manager is promoting quality assurance in the workplace that ultimately results in an improved quality of product.

Differences exist in the organization of a quality assurance system in each manufacturing facility. However, there are certain fundamental features of any quality system. These features include:

- A quality policy which defines the purpose and objectives of the pharmaceutical manufacturing facility; it also outlines the ways in which these objectives will be achieved
- Resources which include materials, equipment and personnel
- Documentation which includes procedures and standards
- An audit process to provide assurance that procedures have been complied with; this process can also be used to improve the quality system.

In a pharmaceutical production process, quality assurance is involved in the following activities:

- purchasing
- dispatching
- warehousing
- operational protocols
- manufacturing
- training
- quality control
- validation
- packaging.

Rigorously designed procedures must be used to achieve a quality system for each of these activities. Each system must be detailed and monitored both during and after the activity. The systems for each of the listed activities must provide:

- Assurance that materials, product, labelling and storage have conformed to an established programme of operation.
- Monitoring to ensure that the system is complied with or updated.

With a system of quality assurance integrated into a manufacturing process, simply making a product well is insufficient. The production processes must be carried out according to good manufacturing practice. All processes must be monitored both during and after the activity. Details of the manufacturing procedures must be entered onto

documents known as records. Records must account for all
the procedures which have been carried out during manufacture. The records form a history of the production process
and are available for further study. Any changes to the manufacturing processes must comply with specified procedures. As a result of these actions in the production process,
the quality assurance system will:

- Ensure quality
- Provide evidence
- Generate confidence.

Implementing a quality assurance system in a manufacturing facility is expensive. However, these costs are greatly
outweighed by the benefits of a quality assurance system.
The benefits of a quality assurance system include:

- Higher standards of production
- Compliance with regulatory requirements
- Reduced waste
- Less risk of product defects.

Quality assurance is an all-embracing function. The concept
includes not only manufacturing but also all the other
factors that affect the quality of the manufactured product.
This extends from the initial stages of product development
to the administration of the product. With the manufacture
of medicines, the quality assurance system is also involved
with product recall from the marketplace if necessary.

Quality assurance must be distinguished from quality
control which is concerned with specifications, sampling
and testing. Quality control is only one component of the
multicomponent quality assurance system. On its own,
quality control cannot provide the necessary assurance of
product quality.

Quality assurance in pharmaceutical manufacturing
encompasses both good manufacturing practice and quality
control systems. It is also involved with product design and
process development. Ultimately, all these areas contribute
to assuring the quality of the product. The concepts of good
manufacturing practice, quality control, product design and
process development are interrelated and encapsulated by
the term 'quality assurance'. This concept is illustrated in
Figure 6.2.

In the evolution of a new product quality assurance
involves product design. This begins in the initial stages of
product development. Factors such as the route of administration, formulation and packaging are incorporated into
product design. All these factors must be carefully considered to produce a quality product. In addition, the product
must be designed to allow for process development.

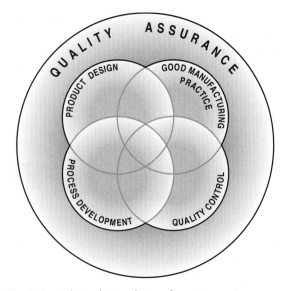

Fig. 6.2 Relationships within quality assurance in
pharmaceutical manufacturing.

Manufacture of a batch must ensure that each product, for
example each tablet, exhibits a consistent quality. To
achieve this objective, the manufacturing systems must have
some flexibility. This will allow for variables which may
arise during the production process, yet produce a consistent
quality of product.

Within the European Union a system of marketing
approvals is designed to ensure that a competent authority
assesses all medicinal products. Authorized manufacturers
must produce these medicines. Within the UK this competent authority is the Medicines Control Agency. This agency
ensures the quality, safety and efficacy of the product. A
licence to manufacture is required by manufacturers of
medicines in the European Union. This applies to products
sold either within or outside Europe.

GOOD MANUFACTURING PRACTICE FOR MEDICINAL PRODUCTS (GMP)

The principles of GMP are applied to the manufacture of
medicines for both human and veterinary use. The principles
of GMP also apply in the hospital production of medicines
for use in clinical trials and for wholesaling.

GMP ensures that manufacturing processes are defined,
validated and reviewed according to laid-down procedures.
This does require certain actions by the manufacturer. It
includes training for personnel and the use of suitable

equipment and premises. Correct materials with suitable transport and storage are also necessary. These procedures result in the consistent production of quality medicines. GMP is continuously evolving due to the ongoing improvement of technology and production processes.

Quality control

There is often confusion about the difference between quality assurance and quality control (QC). Quality assurance has a preventive and wider role than quality control. Quality assurance not only initiates, but also promotes, quality in products. In comparison, quality control carries out an analytical function. It is involved with controlling the quality of components and products. To perform this function, quality control uses physical, chemical and other test methods. In effect, quality control has a verifying role. It acts after an event, but does not prevent errors or poor manufacturing practice occurring in the workplace. For example, quality control must identify a faulty batch of product and avoid its distribution for use. To achieve this, tests must be carried out. As a result of these tests, quality control must provide a verdict on the batch of product by passing or failing it. Quality assurance is involved with quality control in exactly the same way as it is involved with other functions. It approves test methods and standards and ensures that high standards, which must conform with good laboratory practice, are being maintained within the quality control facility.

In small organizations a single manager may be responsible for both quality control and quality assurance. However, workers in the production facility may have trouble accepting a situation where the person who controls quality also assures quality. In the larger organization there may be a separate manager for each of these roles.

Standards

In 1991 the European Union issued directives which laid down principles and guidelines of GMP for medicinal products for human and veterinary medicines. The directive on human medicines came into force on 1 January 1993. The veterinary directive was implemented on 23 July 1993.

The directive for the production of human medicines is detailed in Volume IV of the Rules Governing Medicinal Products in the European Community (Commission of the European Communities 1998). It is entitled 'Good Manufacturing Practice for Medicinal Products'. It is a statutory requirement that manufacturers in the European

Union must ensure that medicines are made, packaged and distributed according to these rules. The European document has been incorporated into the 2002 publication from the Medicines Control Agency. This document is entitled 'Rules and Guidance for Pharmaceutical Manufacturers and Distributors 2002'. As with previous editions, this text is bound in an orange cover. It has thus become known as the 'Orange Guide'. The Orange Guide contains the main regulations, directives and guidance that a manufacturer is expected to follow when making a medicine.

Personnel

Everyone involved with the manufacture of a medicinal product must have quality at the forefront of their thinking. They must build quality into every aspect of their work— 'Quality Rules, OK!'. Each individual must ensure that every step and every component involved with the manufacturing process is rigorously performed. This will help to ensure that the required quality is contained within the product. Most defects in manufactured medicinal products arise through human error or carelessness. This is a clear indication of the need for quality procedures by the workforce. The personnel involved with the production of medicines should be aware of the principles of GMP that affect them. They should be given initial and continuing training to suit their working procedures. Details of the training which the workforce receives should be documented.

All new personnel should receive a medical examination. Persons with potentially infectious diseases or open wounds should not be involved with the manufacture of medicinal products. Personnel working in the manufacturing areas should wear appropriate garments. Care should be taken to avoid contact between the hands of personnel and the exposed product or the equipment which may contact the product. Unhygienic practices by personnel within the production areas must be avoided. Food, drink or smoking materials are excluded from the production areas.

There are three important personnel employed in a manufacturing unit: the production manager, the quality control manager and the qualified person. The production manager and the quality control manager must be different individuals. They must act independently of each other.

The qualified person

The qualified person, commonly known as the 'QP', is the individual who is ultimately responsible for ensuring that each manufactured batch of product has been suitably produced and tested. The QP is responsible for releasing each batch of product for use. It is important that the actions carried out by the QP are detailed on records. Within a manufacturing unit there must be sufficient QPs to carry out all the tasks that are the responsibility of the manufacturer.

Premises and equipment

The premises and equipment must be designed and constructed to suit the manufacturing operations. The premises must also be suitably maintained for the production processes. Both the premises and the production equipment should be designed and positioned to minimize the risks of errors during the manufacturing process. The cleaning and maintenance of the production equipment and premises should be easy. This will reduce the risk of cross-contamination and the build up of dust. As a result of these actions there should be less risk of adverse effects which could affect the quality of the manufactured products.

Documentation

Good documentation of the procedures involved with the production of pharmaceutical products is an essential part of a quality assurance system. All documents involved with the manufacture of medicines must be clearly written. They must also be set out logically and be free of errors. The documents must be approved, signed and dated by authorized personnel such as the head of production. The documents used in the manufacture of medicines provide details of:

- Specifications. These documents detail the materials to be used during the procedures. They will also specify the packaging materials.
- Manufacturing formulae and instructions for processing and packaging.
- Procedures for carrying out processes such as the operation of equipment and the sampling and testing of materials. These documents are commonly known by the self-descriptive term 'standard operating procedures' (SOPs) and specify what should be done, when, where and by whom.
- Production records such as batch manufacturing records and batch packaging records. These documents form a record of the appropriate activity.

The use of these documents avoids potential errors that could arise from verbal communication. The documents used in the manufacturing process should be reviewed and updated at timed intervals such as every 1 or 2 years. The timing for the review is frequently specified on the document. When a document has been revised, it is important that the superseded document is not used. A system should exist to continuously overcome this potential problem.

During the manufacturing processes, it is imperative that the required details are entered onto the appropriate documents at the time of the event and not entered subsequently. With this system of entering data onto a document, the information is then available for subsequent inspection. The entries on documents act as a history of the production process. If a change is required to an entry on a document, the original entry must remain visible. The change must be signed and dated. The reason for the alteration must also be noted on the document.

The documents used in the manufacturing process must be kept for at least 1 year beyond the expiry date of the product. However, manufacturers frequently keep their documents for a longer period.

As an alternative to paper documentation, manufacturing facilities are increasingly using electronic data processing systems. However, it is important that only authorized personnel should be able to access or modify the data contained in the electronic storage system. Access to the electronic data system, which usually employs computer facilities, is frequently regulated using a password entry system. The use of a password also restricts both the type and the amount of data accessible to the operator using the electronic storage system. As with paper documents, any changes to the electronically stored information must be recorded.

Production

Production operations must follow clearly defined procedures. The operations must comply with the principles of GMP. This is necessary to produce the required quality of product and comply with the manufacturing and marketing authorizations. The measures taken to prevent cross-contamination of starting materials and products should be regularly assessed. Validation studies are used to reinforce GMP and are carried out according to specified procedures.

Guidelines are detailed for the purchase, delivery, labelling and storage of starting materials. The purchase, handling and control of starting materials, including primary packaging and printed packaging materials (see Ch. 9), should be carefully examined. The processing and packaging operations are carried out according to defined procedures. Following production, the finished products are held in a pre-release store, also known as 'quarantine' by some manufacturers. The products will remain in the pre-release store until they are released for use or sale. These products must fulfil all the conditions which have been set up by the manufacturer. They are then released for use by the manufacturer.

Rejected materials and products should be clearly identified as 'rejected'. They must be separated from the materials which are suitable for use. This is necessary to avoid any mix-up between the rejected materials and the materials or the products which are suitable for use.

Rejected materials should either be returned to the suppliers or, where appropriate, reprocessed or destroyed.

Quality control in practice

Each manufacturing facility which has a manufacturing authorization should have a quality control department. This department should be independent of other departments. The quality control department operates under the authority of an experienced manager. However, quality control personnel will need to access production areas for sampling and investigation. Certain test procedures may be carried out during production processes by personnel involved with the manufacturing operation, such as 'positioning' settle plates in production areas to establish the microbial contamination of the environment. However, the procedures that these operators carry out must conform with methods that have been approved by quality control.

As detailed above, quality control is concerned with sampling, specifications and testing. It is also involved with the organization, documentation and release procedures. These procedures are established to ensure that the necessary tests are performed.

The tests carried out by quality control ensure that the materials are suitable for use and the products are suitable for sale or supply. All of these quality control tests are carried out according to written procedures using analytical methods that have been validated. The results of these tests require to be detailed on records. Sampling of products or materials for quality control tests should be carried out according to approved written procedures. It is important that the samples of the packaged product should be representative of the entire batch of product. Samples of the product may be tested before release for use. In addition, product samples are stored in their final container in suitable conditions. These samples are kept for at least 1 year after the product expiry date. Samples of the materials used in the production process should be placed into containers which are suitably labelled. Stable sample materials are kept for at least 2 years after release of the product.

Complaints and product recall

All complaints and other information regarding potentially defective products must be reviewed according to written procedures. A designated person should handle these complaints. Records of complaints should be kept and regularly reviewed. Deficiencies arising during the manufacturing process should be reviewed. These deficiencies have narrowly avoided errors in the production process. They are often known as 'near misses' or more appropriately 'near hits'. Both the QP and the quality control manager should be informed of all complaints and deficiencies.

A procedure should be designed to recall products from the market. These products may be either defective or potentially defective. The method of recalling these products is carried out and coordinated by a designated person. Within the manufacturing facility, this person should operate independently of both sales and marketing. Following recall, the products should be identified and stored in a secure area. These products are kept in storage until a decision is made about their fate. The progress of the recall process is recorded and a final report issued. Both the QP and the quality control manager should be aware of all recall operations.

Inspections

Inspections are carried out as internal quality audits of the manufacturing system. The manufacturer may also carry out external inspections. External inspections are typically carried out with suppliers of materials. Inspection is also carried out with contract manufacturers, packagers and contract warehouse and distribution systems.

Internal inspections are carried out at regular time intervals as part of the quality assurance system. Competent personnel from the manufacturer carry them out in an independent and detailed manner. Independent audits by internal or external experts may also be performed. The inspection will check that the principles of good manufacturing practice are being carried out throughout the production facility. Information about each self-inspection should be recorded as a report. This report must detail the observations made during the inspections. The report also gives proposals for corrective measures. The actions which were implemented as a result of the report should be documented. Internal inspections will:

- Determine the level of compliance
- Generate confidence in good manufacturing practice and the quality assurance system

- Promote interdepartmental understanding
- Identify necessary procedures to improve production standards
- Recommend and monitor improvements.

In addition to the functions of the internal inspection, the external inspection will:

- Establish and monitor the capability of suppliers and contractors to deliver suitable goods and services
- Promote understanding between the manufacturer and suppliers of materials or services.

Manufacture of sterile medicinal products

Quality assurance is very important in the manufacture of sterile products owing to the need to avoid particulate and microbial contamination. The manufacture of these products must be carried out using carefully established and validated procedures. The skill, training and attitudes of the personnel involved with the manufacture of sterile products are important. The manufacture is carried out according to established and validated procedures in clean areas as detailed in Chapter 13. Methods of sterilizing these products are detailed in Chapter 12. It is important for the manufacture of sterile products that the method of sterilization is validated.

Samples of the product which are used in a sterility test should be representative of the entire batch. However, it is important that any areas of the batch considered to be at most risk of contamination should be included in the sampling programme. Sterility testing of the finished product is only the last in a series of control measures which give assurance of product sterility. Parametric release, arising through the implementation of quality assurance procedures, has superseded sterility testing in some situations (see Ch. 14).

QUALITY ASSURANCE IN COMMUNITY PHARMACY

Clinical governance will be applied to all organisations within the National Health Service, including hospital and community pharmacies. This will involve changes from current practice. The aim is to improve the quality of service that is provided to patients. These measures to improve on the quality in the health service will result in the need for national standards, implementation of quality assurance

mechanisms and the evolution of multidisciplinary teams. To optimize the outcome from these teams it is important that the team members cooperate and communicate. Good practice should be shared within the team together with information, effort and goals. A pharmacist will be a member of many teams. This will promote the development of clinical governance of community pharmacy services and support the contribution pharmacists make to the clinical governance of other services. All the activities formed as a result of clinical governance will promote a higher quality of patient care. This will also result in improved patient confidence in the health care services that are provided.

The application of clinical governance to community pharmacy will result in several changes including:

- Improved patient services
- Additional staff training
- Effective use of resources
- Developing a more appropriate complaints procedure.

Providing a quality service in community pharmacy that conforms to clinical governance requires ensuring that:

- An identified pharmacist is accountable for all activities
- All staff are suitably trained and competent for the work
- In-use equipment is validated and suitable for its intended purpose
- Risk assessment and risk management procedures are followed
- Adequate records are maintained.

Within community pharmacy many elements of quality assurance exist including procedures, records, documentation, validation, controls, training, complaints procedures and inspection. However these elements of quality assurance are less well developed in community pharmacy in comparison to those in the pharmaceutical industry and hospital pharmacy. This can be evidenced in the tragic case involving the death of a young infant following the administration of peppermint water solution that had been inappropriately prepared in a community pharmacy. This case was detailed in *The Pharmaceutical Journal* of 11 March 2000. Differences existing in the quality procedures operating in hospital and community pharmacy were also highlighted during the report of this incident. The use of an outdated formula book was also noted. This tragic event, together with government requirements for the application of clinical governance throughout the NHS, will ensure the development and use of quality assurance procedures within community pharmacy. An extended time period was required for the development of quality assurance in the pharmaceutical industry and in hospital pharmacy. Improvements to quality will be more rapidly developed in community pharmacy.

The peppermint water case outlined above clarifies the details supplied in the RPSGB Code of Ethics for the preparation of extemporaneous products. This specifies that these products must be accurately prepared and meet acceptable standards for quality assurance. Ingredients must be of suitable quality and sourced from a reliable supplier. The supervising pharmacist is responsible for both the accuracy and quality of these medicines. There is also a requirement that the pharmacist and staff member preparing the product are competent for the task. There must also be suitable facilities and any equipment that is being used must be in good order.

Procedures

From 1 January 2005, the Royal Pharmaceutical Society will require community pharmacists to introduce and operate written Standard Operating Procedures (SOPs). These documents specify what should be done, when, where and by whom. They will have to be written for all the activities that occur from the time that prescriptions are received into the pharmacy until the medicines are supplied to the patient. They should also be written for procedures on giving advice, information and sales of over-the-counter medicines and for policies for referral to other members of the primary care team.

The use of SOPs will:

- Assure the quality and consistency of the service
- Ensure that good practice is achieved at all times
- Use the expertise of all members of the pharmacy team
- Delegate duties and free pharmacists for other activities
- Promote role clarification.

The use of SOPs in pharmacies complies with the requirements for clinical governance in the pharmacy. Their use will support risk management and quality improvement. Changes in legislation arising from the Health Act 1999 may result in the development of procedures that regulate those working in support of a profession. Using SOPs in the community pharmacy also supports this.

In order to write SOPs it is important that pharmacists carefully study current practice and ensure that safe procedures exist. Details of the procedure must be logically arranged on these documents and be error free. Pharmacists must ensure that the procedures are appropriate and are carried out by competent staff. The identity of staff performing these duties in the pharmacy must be stated in the

SOP. All the procedures used within the community pharmacy must comply with the specifications stated in the SOPs. Pharmacists working with trained and competent support staff can use SOPs to safely delegate the technical aspects of the dispensing process. The use of SOPs in pharmacies will directly improve and control the standards of service in the pharmacy, resulting in improved patient safety.

The delegation of procedures in the pharmacy is affected by various factors including:

- Area of practice
- Volume of work
- Complexity of the procedures
- Competency of support staff.

The use of SOPs allow pharmacists to:

- Define and assess practices in the pharmacy
- Train staff in the procedures
- Improve teamwork within the pharmacy
- Increase their available time for clinical services.

The staff member who performs the procedure usually writes the SOP. It is then examined and approved by the pharmacist in charge of the pharmacy. This pharmacist will be accountable for the SOP and for the dispensing process. Each of these documents must state the date of writing and be reviewed at timed intervals. The significance of avoiding the use of outdated documents can be evidenced by the peppermint water case previously detailed. These documents must also be updated to allow for changes in practice or staff. There is variation in the operation of community pharmacies and in the competency of staff. These factors will affect the content of SOPs used in each pharmacy.

Records

These are completed shortly after a procedure has been carried out. A second checker should countersign the record confirming results or execution of a process. Details of extemporaneous products prepared in a community pharmacy must be recorded: the details of the formula used, the ingredients and their source, the quantities used and their batch number. The record also includes patient and prescription details. The records of the procedure must be kept for at least 2 years. In practice validation records are also kept by some pharmacies. An example of these records is the recorded daily refrigerator temperatures and details of the cleaning protocol. Retention times for these records should also be specified. Procedures for the analysis of the recorded data must be established, as should action levels if the recorded results are outwith recommended specification.

Validation

To ensure that the equipment being used in the pharmacy is in good order requires validation at timed intervals. In practice, pharmacies often use an external agency to perform this work with a validation certificate being supplied after the tests. The pharmacy could also perform interim internal validation of its equipment at more frequent time intervals. The results of these validation tests must be recorded and retained. The internal temperature of pharmacy refrigerators are determined daily. The storage temperature within the fridge together with the maximum and minimum daily temperatures should be recorded and retained.

Validation should also apply to computer hardware and software. System failure that could affect the stored data could be significant. As a result there should be documented evidence that the computer consistently operates as intended.

Audit

This is a part of quality assurance and is involved with the monitoring of procedures and is a form of inspection. Clinical audit in hospital pharmacy is well developed, with pharmacists taking part in uniprofessional and multiprofessional clinical audit (see Ch. 43). Clinical audit has not similarly developed in the community pharmacy where uniprofessional audits with a focus customer services such as prescription waiting times are more common. It should be noted that only selected services are audited. Some community pharmacy chains have developed in-house clinical audit structures. The audit process generates data that is then collected, analysed and appropriate improvements implemented. Audits are repeated to produce an audit cycle where the results of the audits are compared over time. In order to perform the process correctly the composition of the audit team must be carefully selected to comprise only suitably trained and competent personnel. The team must work within defined aims and objectives. The standards within the pharmacy premises could be audited or the services that are provided compared with best practice.

The results of audits performed in community pharmacy must be recorded. These are then analysed and changes for improvement implemented. To ensure that improvements have been made the changes must be monitored and recorded. Records are collected to allow staff to review

performance and compare it with the set standards. To complete the audit cycle, there should be re-audits.

Training

From the 1 January 2005 all community pharmacy staff must have a minimum level of competency. This requires training to improve knowledge and skill of these staff. This will result in quality benefits for patients. Introductory training should be provided for new staff but additional ongoing training is required to maintain the improved standards of the pharmacy staff. The outcome of the training programme is affected by the content and standard of the training together with the competency of the trainer. Records of staff training must be maintained.

An audit process can determine the learning needs of pharmacists. This will result in appropriately structured continuing professional development that will provide greatest benefit to the individual. In the future pharmacists will take part in multidisciplinary training. This training may be provided as structured courses that result in updated skills. Continuing professional development improves the adaptability of the individual and increases the distribution of knowledge yielding a higher quality of health care. The individual must maintain records of personal training.

Monitoring

Quality pharmaceutical care of patients requires accurate information in the form of patient medication records (see Ch. 31). This is usually held on an electronic data processing system in the pharmacy. Only authorized persons should be able to access or modify the computer data. This information must be accurate and up to date in order to be meaningful. Monitoring of procedures should also be carried out on the dispensing processes together with the clinical patient assessment and advice. Procedures in the pharmacy can be monitored in house or by external inspectors.

Inspections

The inspectorate of the Royal Pharmaceutical Society of Great Britain (RPSGB) assesses dispensing and additional services. However, little assessment is made of the procedures for advice, information and sales of over-the-counter medicines or for developing policies on referral to other members of the primary health care team. It would seem that NHS inspectors will examine the content and application of SOPs. These inspectors will also determine appropriate implementation of clinical governance in the community pharmacy. Inspectors must determine that quality assurance procedures are implemented in pharmacies and ensure compliance with these documents. The need for inspection and enforcement can be anticipated to increase with the development of quality assurance procedures in the community pharmacy.

Risk assessment

This is another requirement for implementing clinical governance in community pharmacy. Risks should be assessed and then robust, regularly reviewed, procedures for managing the risk implemented. This relates easily to the implementation and use of SOPs in community pharmacies. Risk assessment and risk management should be a component of the training for continuous professional development. Risk assessment should apply to many procedures in the community pharmacy, including:

- Dispensing and checking procedures
- Incident reporting
- Examination of product expiry dates
- Removal of short and outdated products.

Complaints

A complaints system is required for the implementation of good clinical governance. Each community pharmacy should have an established and operating complaints procedure. In practice the community pharmacist will address most complaints. Alternatively, the drug company, the health authority or the RPSGB could address the complaint. A procedure to listen to the complaints of patients, families and caregivers provides a platform for implementing improvements.

Improving performance

Errors arising in the pharmacy can directly affect the patients and the provision of poor advice to prescribers or patients can cause similar harm. In secondary care, errors occur in about 5% of drug administrations, of which about 0.1% cause serious harm. Unfortunately, figures for the rate of medication errors in primary care are limited. However, the UK government is committed to reducing the incidence of errors by 40% by 2005. How this will be measured in primary care remains unclear.

Clinical governance requires community pharmacies to report serious medication errors and near misses to their NHS organization. Near misses are dispensing errors that are rectified before the error reaches the patient. Medication errors are a serious problem for both the affected patients and the health care professionals involved. Errors may be related to procedures involving professional practice including prescribing, product labelling, packaging and nomenclature, compounding, dispensing, distribution, administration, education, monitoring and use. Patients and health care workers usually identify medication errors while pharmacists or pharmacy staff recognize 'near misses'.

Errors and near misses should be written up in a report. It is important that the reporting of errors is carried out in an open manner without fear of personal recrimination. After details about the error are documented the reports are analysed and the cause of the error established. Remedial procedures are then implemented for an improved quality of pharmacy service. Alternatively feedback could be provided to the prescriber.

A pharmacist should carry out an assessment of each prescription. In this process the pharmacist applies knowledge to establish the safety, quality, efficacy and cost-effective use of the medicinal treatment specified by the prescriber. This does not remove the risk of a dispensing error occurring. A second competent person should carry out dispensing accuracy checks. This may be an accredited checking technician or pharmacist. An individual in this situation can make errors but a suitable checking procedure significantly reduces the incidence of errors.

If there is human involvement in any procedure it is widely recognized that errors are inevitable and this problem is increased during periods of great activity. This is the situation that can arise in the community pharmacy where activity can be complex with intermittent periods of intense activity. In order to minimize or eliminate the potential problem of errors arising in this situation appropriate systems need to be established within the pharmacy. This applies to the existence of adequate staff to deal with the intense activity and the presence of work systems that avoid the errors. The dispensary work area should provide:

- Segregation from the intense activities of the pharmacy with minimization of dispenser distractions
- An area designed for smooth workflow
- Suitable illumination, with an uncluttered work area
- Comfortable temperature and humidity for the work personnel
- Suitable storage of medicines

• A suitably positioned telephone with trained staff to answer calls.

The implementation of quality assurance mechanisms in the community pharmacy will significantly contribute to decreasing errors and ultimately provide an improved health care service for the patients.

Key Points

- QA systems ensure that medicinal products conform with intended use.
- A QA system will normally include a quality policy, resources, documentation and audit.
- Making a product well is insufficient to ensure quality—GMP must be followed.
- GMP ensures quality, provides evidence and generates confidence.
- QC alone cannot assure quality.
- Quality begins with product design.
- Manufacturing procedures must be capable of allowing for variables and still produce consistent quality.
- In the UK, the Medicines Control Agency grants licences to manufacture.
- GMP is evolving as technology advances.
- QC has the role of verifying quality.
- The 'Orange Guide' contains regulations, directions and guidance which a manufacturer is expected to follow.

- Errors by people are the cause of the majority of defects which occur.
- All personnel need to be trained for their part in the production process.
- The production manager and quality control manager should be different individuals.
- A wide range of documentation is required as part of QA, covering specifications, formulae, procedures and production records.
- Documents may be paper based or electronic.
- Quality control is concerned with sampling, specifications and testing and with release procedures.
- Procedures must exist for systematically dealing with complaints and effecting product recall if this is required.
- All procedures need to be audited on a regular basis.
- QA is important in producing sterile products.
- Clinical governance will produce improved quality care in community pharmacy.
- Implementing QA in community pharmacy will decrease risk and the incidence of errors.

7

Dispensing techniques (compounding and good practice)

A. J. Winfield (original author M. M. Moody)

After studying this chapter you will know about:

Good dispensing practice to ensure quality
The working environment and procedures
Extemporaneous dispensing equipment and its correct use, including:
  Balances
  Liquid measuring
  Mortar and pestle
  Tared containers
Heat sources
  Mixing and grinding
Identification and use of materials
Problem solving
Methods of counting tablets and capsules

Introduction

The previous chapter has dealt with the importance of 'quality' in all aspects of pharmacy. This chapter deals with some of the practical aspects of good pharmacy practice. It will concentrate on the small-scale manufacture of medicines from basic ingredients. This process is called compounding or extemporaneous dispensing. In addition, good practice which applies to all aspects of dispensing will be considered and current methods for counting solid dosage forms evaluated.

In modern practice, most medicines are manufactured under well-controlled conditions (see Ch. 15, which deals with the way in which they should be dispensed). Therefore, extemporaneous dispensing, which cannot be as well controlled, should only be used when such products are not available. The pharmacist has a responsibility to maintain equipment in working order, ensure that the formula is safe and appropriate and that all materials are sourced from recognized pharmaceutical manufacturers. There are also requirements concerning calculations, records and labelling.

These are all to be incorporated within Standard Operating Procedures (see Ch. 6).

It is important to remember in any dispensing process that the end product is going to be used or taken by a person or an animal who is ill. It is therefore important that the medicine is of the highest achievable quality. This, in turn, means that the highest standards must be applied during the preparation process. We expect quality assurance procedures to be important in the pharmaceutical manufacturing industry (see Ch. 6). The same careful attention to detail must be applied to small-scale production.

ORGANIZATION

The environment in which you work will have considerable influence on your efficiency and therefore it is important to develop a tidy and organized method of working. The pharmacist who works with a dispensing bench cluttered with several containers all containing different ingredients is more likely to select the incorrect one. Always return ingredients to their appropriate shelf when you have measured out the required quantity.

Cleanliness

The bench that you work at, the equipment and utensils you use and the container which is to hold the final product must all be thoroughly clean. Lack of cleanliness can cause contamination of the preparation with other ingredients. A spatula, which has been used to remove an ingredient from one container, will adulterate subsequent containers if not washed before being used again. Cleanliness will also minimize microbial contamination.

Appearance

A clean white overall should be worn. It should be kept buttoned up since open lab. coats are a potential hazard and cannot prevent outdoor clothes becoming stained if any spillages occur. Hair should be tied back and any skin lesions covered with a dressing.

Documenting procedures and results

Keeping comprehensive records is an essential part of the dispensing process. Records must be kept for a minimum of 2 years (ideally 5 years) and include the formula, the ingredients and quantities used, their sources, batch numbers and expiry date. The record for a prescribed item should also include the patient and prescription details and date of dispensing. A record must be kept of the personnel involved, including the responsible pharmacist. It is best to develop a methodical approach. Being untidy or disorganized can lead to errors. In an attempt to produce neat and tidy lab. books many students do calculations and write details of ingredients on scraps of paper intending to copy the information into the lab. book at a later time. This practice should be discouraged. Information may get lost or mixed up and errors made when transferring details. Good habits learned as an undergraduate should be continued into professional practice.

EQUIPMENT

Not only is the selection of the correct equipment or 'tools' for the job essential, but the tools must also be used in the correct way.

Weighing

Balances

Three types of balance have traditionally been used in dispensing, Class A, Class B (the most commonly used, see Fig. 7.1) and Class C.

New legislation categorizes balances as Class I, Class II, Class III and Class IV. The Class II balance is its nearest equivalent to the Class B balance. All balances, including Class B balances, must be calibrated in metric units. All new balances must now be marked with both maximum and minimum weights that can be weighed. The weights previously allowable are shown in Table 7.1. The move is now to use electronic top-pan balances, where typically the smallest weighable quantity is 10–20 mg and a maximum capacity of about 300 g.

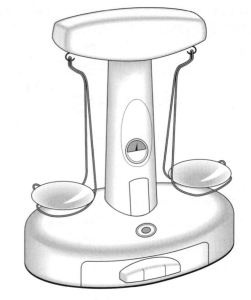

Fig. 7.1 Dispensing balance.

Rules for the use of a Class B dispensing balance:
- Ensure that the balance and pans are clean.
- Check that it is sited in a draught-free area and the pointer is swinging freely.
- Place a piece of paper under the right-hand pan to protect the balance from any spillages.
- Remove the appropriate weights from the drawer, using the tweezers provided, and place them on the left-hand pan. (Never handle weights, as this will affect their accuracy and risks contamination.)
- Immediately close the drawer after removal of the weights. If it is left open there is a possibility that ingredients to be weighed will fall into the drawer, contaminating the weights and affecting their accuracy.
- A solid material to be weighed should then be placed carefully onto the right-hand scale pan. Do not weight ingredients onto a piece of paper as this introduces a

Table 7.1 Classes of balances with their weighing capabilities

Type	Minimum weight	Increment weight	Normal maximum
Class A	50 mg	1 mg	1 g
Class B	100 mg	10 mg	50 g
Class C	1 g	100 mg	2 kg

potential inaccuracy. The exception is when weighing greasy or semisolid material, e.g. white soft paraffin, when a counterbalanced piece of paper should be used.

- When the correct weight has been achieved the pan should be carefully removed from the balance and the material transferred to a suitable container.

- Errors in this transference stage may occur if care is not taken to ensure that all the weighed material has been removed from the scale pan. If the drug is to be dissolved or incorporated into a suspension it can be washed from the scale pan using some of the appropriate liquid vehicle.

- Do not become overzealous when removing material from a pan. Tapping the glass pan against the side of the container can cause it to become chipped. This will affect the accuracy of the balance and slivers of glass will not improve the health of the patient!

- The scale pan should then be washed and dried thoroughly, before any other substance is weighed. A second substance must never be weighed on the remains of the first.

- The weights should be returned to the drawer. Drawers are normally organized in four sections. The weights should be kept together with those of a similar size, e.g. a 10 mg weight should not be placed in the same section as a 10 g weight.

Use of top-pan balance:
- Ensure that the balance is level, in a draught-free environment and working properly.
- Place an appropriate container (such as a weighing boat) or piece of paper on the pan and use the auto-zero to cancel its weight.
- Add the material to be weighed until the correct weight is shown on the display.
- Carefully remove the weighed material as above.

In addition to using the balance correctly there are one or two other rules which should be observed, when weighing, to ensure good dispensing practice. These are:

- If using a solid material which requires to be size reduced (ground) or sieved, always ensure that this is carried out before weighing the required quantity. If a quantity of powder is weighed and then size reduced by grinding in a mortar or sieving, there is a strong possibility that some of the material will be lost in the process and the final preparation will not contain the correct proportions of ingredients. The best approach is to roughly weigh an excess quantity, grind or sieve it as required, then accurately weigh off the required quantity.

- As far as possible never split quantities and do two weighings, as this will increase the inaccuracies.

- If a quantity less than the legal minimum is needed, it is necessary to weigh the minimum weight allowable (or more) and make an excess of the product or prepare it by trituration (see Chs 8, 22 and 23).

Measuring liquids

Liquid measures

All measures for liquids must comply with current Weights and Measures Regulations and should be stamped accordingly. Traditionally, conical measures (Fig. 7.2) have been used in dispensing, although, if not used carefully, they can be less accurate than cylindrical measures.

Whichever type of measure is chosen always ensure that:

- The level of liquid is read to the bottom of the meniscus.
- The measure is vertical when reading the meniscus. If this is not done considerable errors in quantities can occur, especially with conical measures, where the error increases with height because of the slope of the sides.
- The measure is thoroughly drained. Even if the ingredient is only slightly viscous it is amazing how much can be left in the measure.

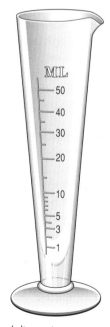

Fig. 7.2 Conical dispensing measure.

- As far as possible, never use more than one measure. Splitting the volume between two measures increases the potential for error.
- Always select the smallest measure which will hold the desired volume, because this gives the greatest accuracy.
- If the substance being measured is so viscous that it would be very difficult to drain the measure effectively, then the volume should be measured by difference. This is done by pouring an excess into the measure and then pouring off the liquid until only the excess volume remains (see Example 7.1).

EXAMPLE 7.1

25 mL of glycerol is required.

Because of the viscosity it is difficult to remove it completely from the measure.

It is therefore advisable to measure, say, 35 mL and pour off the 25 mL required, ensuring that 10 mL is left in the measure. Remember to allow sufficient time for the liquid to drain back down.

When measuring liquids it is important to observe two simple rules which ensure good dispensing practice.

- Always hold the liquid container with the label uppermost so that you pour away from the label. This ensures that any liquid which runs down the side of the bottle will not affect the label. There is nothing worse than bottles where the ingredient name has been obscured because large quantities of the liquid have been allowed to run down the side of the bottle. This is especially true for highly coloured substances (such as amaranth solution) or corrosive substances (like acids). Replace any damaged label immediately.
- If possible, when pouring liquids, hold the cap of the container in your hand, preferably between the fourth finger and the palm of your hand. It is possible you may be measuring more than one liquid and if caps are left lying on the dispensing bench it is easy to mix them up and place the wrong one back on the container.

Measuring small volumes

It is important to select the correct equipment when measuring. The minimum measurable volume for a 10 mL conical measure is 1 mL. Graduated pipettes can be used for volumes from 5 mL down to 0.1 mL. For volumes smaller

than this a trituration should be made. The viscosity of the substance being measured should also be considered.

Correct use of pipettes. Pipettes can be either the 'drainage' or 'blow-out' variety. A rubber bulb or teat should be used. Never use mouth suction.

- A bulb or teat should be placed over the mouth of the pipette, taking care not to push it down too far.
- The container of the substance to be measured should be ready on the bench.
- The top of the container should be removed and held in the hand, between the fourth finger and the palm of the hand.
- The pipette should be put into the container, taking care that only a short length of the pipette is immersed. If a quantity of liquid is allowed to collect on the outside of the pipette the accuracy of the measuring will be affected.
- The correct amount of liquid should then be drawn up the pipette. Take care at this stage as the liquid may shoot up the pipette into the bulb.
- If a pipette bulb is being used the appropriate valve is pressed to prevent the liquid running out of the pipette, the pipette is removed from the container and the liquid then released into the desired container.
- If using a simple teat this should now be flicked off with the thumb and a finger placed firmly over the top of the pipette, taking care not to allow any liquid to be lost. The pipette can then be withdrawn from the container and the liquid measured out by removing the finger from the top of the pipette.

Tared containers

Liquid preparations should as far as possible be made up to volume in a measure. There are, however, instances when accurate transfer of the preparation to the final container is difficult. With some suspensions it can be almost impossible to remove all the insoluble ingredients when pouring from one container to another. Emulsions and viscous preparations can also be difficult to transfer accurately. In these cases a tared container should be used.

To tare a bottle

A volume of water identical to the volume of the product being dispensed is accurately measured. This is then poured into the chosen medicine container and the meniscus marked with the upper edge of a small adhesive label, effectively making the bottle into a single-point measure. The container is then emptied and allowed to drain thoroughly. The preparation is then poured into the container and made up to volume, using the tare mark as the guide.

This procedure should be used with discretion and only in situations when major inaccuracies would occur in the transfer of liquids. It should also only be used when water is present as one of the ingredients. Putting medicines into a wet bottle is generally considered bad practice.

MIXING AND GRINDING

Mortar and pestle

The mortar (bowl) and pestle (pounding device) are used to reduce the size of powders, mix powders, mix powders and liquids, and make emulsions. Two types, each available in a range of sizes, are used.

Glass mortar and pestle

These are generally small and therefore cannot be used for large quantities of material. The smooth surface of the glass reduces the friction which can be generated, so they are only suitable for size reduction of friable materials (such as crystals). They are useful for dissolving small quantities of ingredients, for mixing small quantities of fine powders and for the mixing of substances such as dyes which are absorbed by and stain composition or porcelain mortars.

Porcelain or composition mortars and pestles

These are normally larger than the glass variety and have a rougher surface. They are ideal for size reduction of solids and for mixing solids and liquids, as in the preparation of suspensions and emulsions.

Size reduction using a mortar and pestle

Selection of the correct type of mortar and pestle is vital for this operation. A flat-bottomed mortar and a pestle with a flat head should be chosen. A flat-headed pestle in a mortar with a round bottom, or vice versa, will mean a lot of wasted effort.

Using a mortar and pestle for mixing powders

Adequate mixing will only be achieved if there is sufficient space. Overfilling of the mortar should therefore be avoided. The pestle should be rotated in both right and left directions to ensure thorough mixing. Undue pressure should not be used, as this will cause impaction of the powder on the bottom of the mortar.

Filters

There are occasions when clarification of a liquid is required. Pouring the liquid through muslin can carry out coarse filtration, or 'straining'. Where a finer degree of filtration is required, filter paper or sintered glass filters should be used. Filter paper comes in different grades and selection of the correct grade is determined by the size of the particles to be removed. Details of grades of filter paper are found in Table 7.2. Filter paper has the disadvantages of introducing fibres into the filtrate and may also absorb significant amounts of active ingredient.

Sintered glass filters

These do not shed fibres, are easy to clean and can be used for substances which attack filter paper such as potassium permanganate and zinc chloride. A filter with a pore size 15–40 μm (grade 3) is suitable for most solutions. They will

Table 7.2	Filter paper characteristics		
Number (Whatman series)	**Filtration rate**	**Size of particle removed**	**Average pore size (mm)**
54	1 (fast)	Coarse	3.4–5.0
1	4 (medium fast)	Medium	2.1–2.8
50	23 (slow)	Fine	0.4–1.1

pass through by gravity, although large volumes may be slow and need the assistance of a vacuum. A grade 4 filter (pore size 5–15 µm) requires a vacuum.

Heat sources

Bunsen burners

Bunsen burners should always be placed on a heat-resistant mat on the dispensing bench. When heating with a Bunsen burner, the flame control should be rotated to produce a blue flame. In most dispensing exercises only gentle heat is required, so only use a fierce blue flame if excessive heat is called for. When not in use the Bunsen burner should be turned to a yellow flame or turned off.

Water-baths

These are used when melting ointment bases or preparing suppositories. Normally the materials to be heated are placed in a porcelain evaporating basin and placed over the hot water in the water-bath. In most melting exercises the materials should be melted gently. There is no necessity to have the water boiling vigorously, this does not increase the heat, but does increase the risk of scalding.

Electric hot plates

Electrically heated hot plates can be used and have the advantage of thermostatic controls, although there is a time lag involved in heating and cooling the plate.

MANIPULATIVE TECHNIQUES

Selection of the correct equipment and using it appropriately is fundamental to good compounding. There are, in addition, several basic manipulative techniques which must be practised.

Mixing

The goal of any mixing operation should be to ensure that even distribution of all the ingredients has occurred. If a sample is removed from any part of the final preparation it should be identical to a sample taken from any other part of the container (see Ch. 13; Aulton, 2002).

Mixing of liquids

Simple stirring or shaking is usually all that is required to mix two or more liquids. The degree of stirring or shaking will be dependent on the viscosities of the liquids. Thus mixing liquids of low viscosities will require only minimal stirring, while mixing two liquids, both with a high viscosity, will need more vigorous agitation.

Mixing solids with liquids

Particle size reduction is also of paramount importance. This will either speed up the dissolution process or improve the uniform distribution of the solid throughout the liquid. When a solution is being made, a stirring rod will be adequate. However, a suspension will require a pestle and mortar.

Mixing solids with solids

As well as the correct use of a mortar and pestle, the amounts of material being mixed together must be considered. Where the quantity of material to be mixed is small and the proportions are approximately the same, the materials can be added to an appropriately sized mortar and effectively mixed. Where a small quantity of powder has to be mixed with a large quantity, in order to achieve effective mixing, it must be done in stages.

- The ingredient with the smallest bulk is placed in the mortar.
- A quantity of the second ingredient, approximately equal in volume to the first, is added and carefully mixed, using the pestle.
- A further quantity of the second ingredient, approximately equal in volume to the mixture in the mortar, is now added.
- This process, known as 'doubling-up', is continued until all the powder has been added.

Mixing semi-solids

This usually occurs in the preparation of ointments where two or more ointment bases may be mixed together. If all the ingredients are semi-solids or liquids, they can be mixed together by rubbing them down on an ointment slab, using a spatula. If there is a significant difference in the quantities of the ingredients, a 'doubling-up' process should be used. An alternative method is the fusion method.

Table 7.3 Some substances which occur in a variety of forms	
Substance/form	**Use**
Light magnesium carbonate	Because of its lightness and diffusible properties, it is used in suspensions
Heavy magnesium carbonate	Normally used in bulk or individual powders
Light kaolin	Used in suspensions
Heavy kaolin	Used in the preparation of kaolin poultice
Precipitated sulphur	This has a smaller particle size than sublimed sulphur and is preferred in preparations for external use, e.g. suspensions, creams and ointments
Sublimed sulphur	Slightly gritty powder which does not produce such elegant preparations as precipitated sulphur
Yellow soft paraffin	Used as an ointment base
White soft paraffin	Bleached yellow soft paraffin normally used when the other ingredients are not strongly coloured

The fusion method

- Place the bases in a porcelain evaporating basin and gently heat them over a water-bath until they have just melted. Excess heat should not be used as overheating may cause physical or chemical changes in some materials.
- The basin is then removed from the heat and the contents are stirred continuously, but gently, until the mixture has cooled and set. Stirring at this stage is of vital importance as otherwise the components may segregate on cooling.

When using the fusion method do not be tempted to add any solid active ingredients to the basin before the bases have set. Addition of any further ingredients is best done by rubbing down on an ointment slab. Further details of methods used in the preparation of ointments can be found in Chapter 20.

SELECTION OF INGREDIENTS

When dispensing, selection of the correct product is vital. Dispensary shelves are filled with an increasing number of products and the label on each container must be read carefully and checked to ensure that it contains the required product. There are many examples of manufactured preparations where names may be misread if care is not taken; examples include Atrovent inhaler and Alupent inhaler, Danol and De-Nol, folic acid and folinic acid, cefuroxime and cefotaxime. Further examples are given in Chapter 15. Problems

and errors can also occur in extemporaneous dispensing. Extemporaneously dispensed medicines may contain several ingredients, so the potential for error is increased.

Pharmacy undergraduates may encounter difficulties when an ingredient occurs in a variety of forms or a synonym is used.

Variety of forms

The following item has to be prepared: Coal Tar Paste BP.

This paste consists of 7.5% strong coal tar solution in compound zinc paste. Coal tar is available as:

Coal tar solution
Strong coal tar solution
Coal tar.

If all three containers are sitting together on a shelf the wrong item may be selected by accident. Some other materials where confusion can occur are listed in Table 7.3. This list is not meant to be comprehensive. The only foolproof method of avoiding errors is to read the container label carefully.

Synonyms

Some substances used in dispensing may be known by more than one name. An awareness of this is useful when selecting ingredients. Some examples of commonly used materials are given in Table 7.4. This table is not intended to be comprehensive.

Table 7.4	Example of substances with synonyms	
Substance	**Synonym**
Wool fat	Anhydrous lanolin
Hydrous wool fat	Lanolin
Hard paraffin	Paraffin wax
Compound benzoic acid ointment	Whitfield's ointment
Macrogol 2000	Polythylene glycol 2000 PEG 2000
Theobroma oil	Cocoa butter

Concentrated waters

Liquid preparations for oral use are often flavoured to make them more palatable for the patient. In extemporaneously prepared products the flavouring is frequently a flavoured water, e.g. peppermint water, aniseed water. These flavoured waters are available in a concentrated form and are either used as such, or are diluted to provide the vehicle for the preparation. All concentrated waters have the same dilution factor, i.e. 1 part of concentrate plus 39 parts of water to give 40 parts of flavoured water.

EXAMPLE 7.2

In 200 mL of a particular suspension there is 100 mL of peppermint water. The peppermint water is only available as concentrated peppermint water. The dilution factor 1 + 39 is used.

1 mL concentrate + 39 mL water =
40 mL peppermint water

If 40 mL of peppermint water contains 1 mL of concentrated peppermint water then:

100 mL of peppermint water will contain 2.5 mL of concentrated peppermint water.

Therefore to 2.5 mL of concentrated peppermint water is added 97.5 mL of water to produce the 100 mL of peppermint water required.

PROBLEM SOLVING IN EXTEMPORANEOUS DISPENSING

For extemporaneous dispensing, it is helpful if a method detailing how to prepare the product is available. Methods for 'official' preparations can sometimes be found in reference sources such as the *Pharmaceutical Codex*. However, on many occasions no method is available. When faced with an extemporaneous preparation and no method, students are often perplexed and unsure of where to start. The application of simple scientific knowledge, especially of physical properties, is often all that is needed. The following gives an example of how this is done.

Putting theory into practice

Solubility

Always check the physical properties of the ingredients being used. This provides some very useful information. Always check the solubility of any solid materials. If they are soluble in the main vehicles, then a solution is likely to be produced. If solubility is limited to one liquid, this will assist in achieving uniform dose distribution. Solution will be achieved more quickly if the particle size is small and so size reduction should be considered for any soluble ingredients which are presented in a lumpy or granular form. If the substance is not soluble, a suspension will be produced. If not already in a finely divided form, it should always be size reduced. Whether a suspending agent will be required should be considered (see Ch. 18). Where one material is an oil and another aqueous, it is likely that an emulsifying agent will be required to produce an emulsion (see Ch. 19).

Volatile ingredients

If an ingredient is volatile then it should be added near the end of the dispensing process. If it is added too early much may be lost due to evaporation.

Viscosity

The viscosity of a liquid will have a bearing on how it is measured, i.e. is a pipette or measure suitable, or should it be measured by difference, and how will it be incorporated?

The following example illustrates how some very simple facts can be applied to develop an accurate method of preparation.

EXAMPLE 7.3

The following prescription is received:

Sodium Bicarbonate Ear Drops BP
Send 10 mL
   Formula:
Sodium bicarbonate   500 mg
Glycerol   3 mL
Freshly boiled and cooled water to   10 mL
   Points to note:
- Solubility of sodium bicarbonate is 1 in 11 of water.
- Glycerol is a viscous liquid.
- The quantity of water in the ear drops is approximately 6.5 mL.
   Method:
1. The sodium bicarbonate should be size reduced in a mortar and pestle, if necessary.
2. 500 milligrams of sodium bicarbonate is then weighed and put into a 10 mL conical measuring cylinder.
3. The sodium bicarbonate is soluble, requiring a minimum of 5.5 mL in which to dissolve. Add about 6 mL of water, ensuring that the volume of ingredients does not go beyond the 7 mL mark.
4. Stir the contents of the measure until the sodium bicarbonate is dissolved.
5. Make the volume up to 7 mL with water.
6. The glycerol is viscous and trying to pour 3 mL from a measure is inaccurate. The 3 mL of glycerol can now be added by pouring it into the 7 mL of sodium bicarbonate solution and carefully making the volume in the measure up to 10 mL.

Expiry date

All extemporaneously prepared products should be awarded an expiry date. Ideally stability studies should be undertaken in order to predict an accurate shelf life for all products. This is not usually possible for 'one-off' preparations and most hospital pharmacies have guidelines based on previous stability studies. Further information on stability and appropriate expiry dates is found in Chapter 10.

COUNTING DEVICES

Tablets and capsules form a large proportion of the medicines which are dispensed today. Many are now presented in patient packs or original packs, but in many instances drugs are supplied in bulk packs and the prescribed amount is counted from them.

Various methods can be used for this counting:

- The manual method
- A counting triangle or capsule counter
- A counting tray
- An electronic counter.

These methods all have their advantages and disadvantages and it is up to each pharmacist to select the most appropriate for the task. Whichever method is selected it must be noted that the medicines must not be touched by hand. The equipment should also be carefully cleaned before use, as powder left from one product could cause contamination of the next one.

The manual method

This consists of pouring the product onto a piece of clean white demy paper which overlaps another piece. The products are then counted off in tens, using a spatula, onto the second piece of paper. This is formed into a small funnel and the tablets or capsules poured into the appropriate container.

Initially this can be a rather slow method but an experienced pharmacist or dispenser can count very quickly. However, concentration must be maintained or the wrong quantity may be counted. The other problem is that white demy paper is becoming increasingly expensive and difficult to obtain.

Counting triangles and capsule counters

Counting triangles

This is a fast, accurate and simple way to count tablets. The triangles are made either of metal or plastic. Two rows of figures are printed or etched along the edge. The top row of figures refers to the number of rows and the numbers below refer to the number of tablets contained in that number of rows. This is illustrated in Figure 7.3. Tablets are poured into the triangle and rows completed using a spatula. Any excess of tablets is returned using the spatula and the correct number poured into a tablet bottle.

Capsule counters

Because of their shape, capsules cannot be counted on triangles. A capsule counter, illustrated in Figure 7.4, is a metal tray which consists of 10 rows of grooves. The capsules are poured onto the tray and using a spatula, lined up in the

Number of tablets   Number of rows

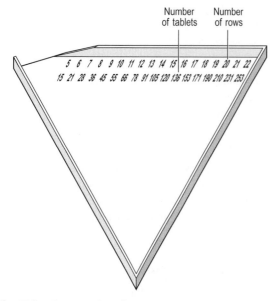

5 6 7 8 9 10 11 12 13 14 15 16 17 18 19 20 21 22
15 21 28 36 45 55 66 78 91 105 120 136 153 171 190 210 231 253

Fig. 7.3   Counting triangle.

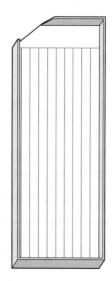

Fig. 7.4   Capsule counter.

grooves. Each complete row will contain 10 capsules so the number of complete rows multiplied by 10 gives the number of capsules.

Capsule counters are not as easy to manipulate as triangles but are an efficient method for counting capsules. Studies testing the accuracy of the various counting methods have shown these two devices to be the best.

Perforated counting trays

These are normally made of clear perspex. They consist of a rectangular box with a sliding lid, on top of which is placed a perforated tray. Each box is supplied with several trays with different-sized perforations to accommodate different sizes and types of products (Fig. 7.5). These trays can be used to count tablets or capsules.

An experienced operator can count quickly and accurately using this type of device. The main disadvantage is the necessity to change the trays for different products.

Electronic counters

There are two types of electronic counter, those which use the weight of the product to count and those which count using a photoelectric cell.

Electronic balances

Between 5 and 20 of the required dosage form is put on a balance pan or scoop. From the weight of this reference sample, a microprocessor within the device calculates the total number of dosage forms, as they are added. The main problem with this type of device is that for accurate counting, it requires consistent uniformity of the weight of the tablets or capsules. There can be problems with accuracy when counting sugar-coated or very small tablets.

Photoelectric cell counters

The product to be counted is poured through a hopper on the top of the machine. The tablets or capsules are then channelled into a straight line and counted as they interrupt the beam of light to the photoelectric cell. This is an efficient method of counting and these devices are widely used. They are not without their problems, however.

- They do not discriminate between whole or broken tablets.
- As the beam of light from the photoelectric cell must be interrupted for counting to occur, these devices cannot count clear capsules.
- The speed at which the dosage forms are poured through the hopper must be controlled. If pouring becomes too fast the system will not cope.
- They are difficult to clean.

Because of this last point the Council of the Royal Pharmaceutical Society of Great Britain issued the following advice concerning the use of electronic counters:

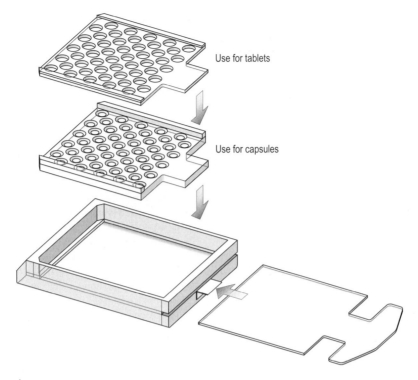

Use for tablets

Use for capsules

Fig. 7.5 Perforated counting tray.

Severe allergic reactions can be initiated in previously sensitized persons by very small amounts of certain drugs and of excipients and other materials used in the manufacture of tablets and capsules. In order to minimize that risk, counting devices should be carefully cleaned after each dispensing operation involving any uncoated tablet, or any coated tablet or capsule from a bulk container holding damaged contents. As cross-contamination with the penicillins is particularly serious, special care should be taken when dispensing products containing those drugs.

This type of device should therefore be reserved for counting only coated tablets or capsules or for prepacking operations.

AUTOMATED DISPENSING SYSTEMS

There are a number of automated dispensing systems available of varying degrees of sophistication. They are linked to a computer, which is used for label production and creation of the patient medication record. The computer 'orders' counting of loose tablets or capsules (using a photoelectric cell counter) into a suitable container, or retrieval of a prepackaged medicine. Some incorporate barcoding technology to improve speed and accuracy. Tests indicate that these machines are less prone to error than human dispensing.

CONCLUSION

Developing good practice takes time and requires attention to detail. During the undergraduate course, students should develop the habit of working on their own. Once established, this can be relied upon throughout your career.

Key Points

- Extemporaneous dispensing should only be used when manufactured medicines are not available.
- Accurate dispensing requires clean, neat methodical work.
- Comprehensive records of extemporaneous dispensing are required to be kept for at least 2 years.
- Class B balances are being replaced by Class II balances.
- Electronic balances are increasingly being used in extemporaneous dispensing.
- Do not use a balance to weigh less than its minimum weighable quantity, which is 100 milligrams for a Class B balance.
- Ensure that liquid measures comply with the Weights and Measures Regulations.
- Always use the bottom of the meniscus when measuring liquids.
- Viscous liquids should be measured 'by difference'.
- Pipettes are used to measure volumes between 0.1 mL and 5 mL.

- Select the smallest measure for the volume of liquid to be measured.
- A glass mortar and pestle can be used for size reduction of friable materials and mixing small quantities of fine powder.
- A porcelain mortar and pestle is used for larger quantities, for mixing solids and liquids, making emulsions and for size reduction.
- 'Doubling-up' is used for mixing a small quantity of powder with a larger quantity.
- Confusion can arise with different forms of the same material and the use of synonyms.
- Concentrated waters are diluted 1 part with 39 parts of water for use as single strength.
- Simple problem-solving techniques can produce a satisfactory method of dispensing a product.
- Tablets and capsules can be counted manually, or by using a triangle, capsule counter, counting tray or an electronic counter.
- Tablets and capsules should not be counted in the hand.

8

Pharmaceutical calculations

I. O. Edafiogho and A. J. Winfield

After studying this chapter you will be able to undertake pharmaceutical calculations dealing with:

Expressions of concentration
Master formulae to working quantities
Changing concentrations
Small quantities (trituration)
Solubility
Calculations related to doses
Reconstitution and rates of infusion

There are some tutorial examples and answers provided to help you assess your progress.

- Write down every step.
- Do not take short cuts; you are more likely to make a mistake.
- Try not to be totally dependent on your calculator. Have an approximate idea of what the answer should be and then if you happen to hit the wrong button on the calculator you are more likely to be aware that an error has been made.
- Finally, always double check your calculation. There is frequently more than one way of doing a calculation, so if you get the same answer by two different methods the chances are that your answer will be correct. Alternatively, try working it in reverse and see if you get the starting numbers.

Introduction

Many pharmacy students approach the calculations involved in dispensing and manufacturing with trepidation. There is no need. Most calculations are simple arithmetic. It is true that there are many steps in the dispensing process where things can go wrong and calculating quantities is one of them. However, careful, methodical working will minimize the risk of errors. Always try to relate the calculation to practice, visualize what you are doing and double check everything.

How to minimize errors

As in all dispensing procedures an organized, methodical approach is essential:

- Write out the calculation clearly. It is all too easy to end up reading from the wrong line.
- If you are transferring data from a reference source double check what you have written down.

EXPRESSIONS OF CONCENTRATION

The metric system is the International System of Units (SI Units) for weight, volume, and length. The basic unit for weight is the kilogram (kg) while the basic unit for volume is the litre (L) and the basic unit of length is the metre (m). Appendix 5 gives information about the weights and measures commonly used in pharmacy. The prefix 'milli' indicates one-thousandth (10^{-3}) and 'micro' one-millionth (10^{-6}).

In some countries, the avoirdupois (or imperial) system (pounds and ounces) is still used in commerce and daily life. The imperial system of volume (pints and gallons) is still a common system for commerce and household measurement. Pharmacists need to know about these systems in order to avoid serious errors in interpretation of prescriptions. It is important to be able to change between the systems. Some conversion factors for the metric, avoirdupois and apothecary systems are shown in Box 8.1.

Box 8.1   Weights and measures

1000 millilitres (mL) = 1 litre (L)
1000 micrograms = 1 milligram (mg)
1000 milligrams (mg) = 1 gram (g)
1000 grams (g) = 1 kilogram (kg)
1 kilogram (kg) = 2.2 pounds (lb)
1 teaspoonful (tsp) = 5 mL
1 tablespoonful = 15 mL (3 teaspoonfuls)
1 grain (Avoir. or Apoth.) = 64.8 mg
1 pint (pt) = 473 mL
1 gallon (gal) = 3785 mL
1 fluid ounce (oz) = 29.57 mL (30 mL)
1 fluid ounce (oz) = 480 minims

EXAMPLE 8.1

Express 85 grains in the metric system.

1 grain = 64.8 mg. Therefore
85 grains = 64.8 × 85 mg

$$64.8 \times \frac{85}{1000} \text{ g} = 5.508 \text{ g} = 5.51 \text{ g (to 2 decimal places)}$$

EXAMPLE 8.2

If 60 minims make 1 fluid drachm, and 8 fluid drachms make 1 fluid ounce, what is the volume of 1 minim in the metric system?

60 minims = 1 fluid drachm; and
8 fluid drachms = 1 fluid ounce (30 mL)

60 × 8 minims = 30 mL; 480 minims = 30 mL

$$\text{Therefore 1 minim} = \frac{30}{480} = 0.06 \text{ mL}$$

EXAMPLE 8.3

Sulfacetamide eye drops contain 200 drops in a 10 mL bottle. Calculate the volume of 1 drop.

200 drops = 10 mL, therefore

$$1 \text{ drop} = \frac{10}{200} \text{ mL} = 0.05 \text{ mL}$$

Expressions of strength

Ratio is the relative magnitude of two like quantities. Thus:

1 : 10 = 1 part in 10 parts or 1 g in 10 g

If 1 g of sucrose is in 10 g of solution, the ratio is 1 : 10. Therefore, 10 g of sucrose is in 100 g of solution. This can be expressed as a percentage, so it is equivalent to a 10% w/w (weight in weight) solution.

Ratio strength is the expression of a concentration by means of a ratio, e.g. 1 : 10. Percentage strength is a ratio of parts per hundred, e.g. 10%.

EXAMPLE 8.4

Express 0.1% w/w as a ratio strength.

$$\frac{0.1 \text{ g}}{100 \text{ g}} = \frac{1 \text{ part}}{y \text{ parts}}$$

$$y = \frac{100 \times 1}{0.1} = 1000$$

Therefore, the ratio strength = 1 : 1000

EXAMPLE 8.5

Express 1 : 2500 as a percentage strength.

$$\frac{1 \text{ part}}{2500 \text{ parts}} = \frac{y \text{ parts}}{100 \text{ parts}}$$

$$\text{Thus, } y = \frac{1 \times 100}{2500} = 0.04\%$$

EXAMPLE 8.6

Express 1 p.p.m. as a percentage strength.

1 p.p.m. = 1 part per million = 1:1 000 000

Let y be the percentage strength:

$$\text{Thus, } \frac{1}{1\,000\,000} = \frac{y \text{ parts}}{100 \text{ parts}}$$

$$y = \frac{1 \times 100}{1\,000\,000} = 0.0001\% = 1 \times 10^{-4}\%$$

Percentage weight in weight (w/w)

Percentage weight in weight (w/w) is the number of grams of an active ingredient in 100 grams (solid or liquid).

EXAMPLE 8.7

How many grams of a drug should be used to prepare 240 grams of a 5% w/w solution?

Let y be the weight of the drug needed.

$$\text{Thus, } \frac{y}{240} = \frac{5 \text{ g}}{100 \text{ g}}$$

$$y = 5 \times \frac{240}{100} = 12 \text{ g}$$

Percentage weight in volume (w/v)

Percentage weight in volume (w/v) is the number of grams of an active ingredient in 100 mL of liquid.

> **EXAMPLE 8.8**
>
> If 3 g of iodine is in 150 mL of iodine tincture, calculate the percentage of iodine in the tincture.
> Let y be the percentage of iodine in the tincture.
>
> $$y/100 \text{ mL} = 3 \text{ g}/150 \text{ mL}$$
> $$y = 3 \times 100/150 = 2\% \text{ w/v}$$

Percentage volume in volume (v/v)

Percentage volume in volume (v/v) indicates the number of millilitres (mL) of an active ingredient in 100 mL of liquid.

> **EXAMPLE 8.9**
>
> If 20 mL of ethanol is mixed with water to make 40 mL of solution, what is the percentage of ethanol in the solution?
> Let y be the percentage of ethanol in the solution.
>
> $$y/100 \text{ mL} = 20 \text{ mL}/40 \text{ mL}$$
> $$y = 20 \times 100/40 = 50\% \text{ v/v}$$

Miscellaneous examples

> **EXAMPLE 8.10**
>
> Express 25 g of dextrose in 500 mL of solution as a percentage, indicating w/w, w/v or v/v.
> Let y grams be the weight of dextrose in 100 mL.
>
> $$y/100 \text{ mL} = 25 \text{ g}/500 \text{ mL}$$
> $$y = 25 \times 100/500 \text{ mL} = 5\% \text{ w/v}$$

> **EXAMPLE 8.11**
>
> What is the percentage of magnesium carbonate in the following syrup?
>
> | Magnesium carbonate | 10 g |
> | Sucrose | 820 g |
> | Water, q.s. | ad 1000 mL |
>
> Percentage is the number of grams of magnesium carbonate in 100 mL of syrup.
>
> $$y/100 \text{ mL} = 10 \text{ g}/1000 \text{ mL}$$
> $$y = 10 \times 100/1000 = 1\% \text{ w/v (grams in mL)}$$

> **EXAMPLE 8.12**
>
> Calculate the amount of drug in 5 mL of cough syrup if 100 mL contains 200 mg of drug.
>
> By proportion, y mg/5 mL = 200 mg/100 mL
> $y = 5 \times 200/100 = 10$ mg

> **EXAMPLE 8.13**
>
> Compute the percentage of the ingredients in the following ointment (to 2 decimal places):
>
> | Liquid paraffin | 14 g |
> | Soft paraffin | 38 g |
> | Hard paraffin | 12 g |
>
> Total amount of ingredients
>   = 14 g + 38 g + 12 g = 64 g.
>
> To find the amounts of the ingredients in 100 g of ointment, each figure will be multiplied by 100/64:
>
> Liquid paraffin = (100/64) × 14 = 21.88% w/w
> Soft paraffin = (100/64) × 38 = 59.38% w/w
> Hard paraffin = (100/64) × 12 = 18.75% w/w
>
> It is useful to double check that these numbers add up to 100% (allowing for the rounding off to 2 decimal places).

Moles and molarity

Concentrations can also be expressed in moles or millimoles (see also Ch. 25). When a mixture contains the molecular weight of a drug in grams in 1 litre of solution, the concentration is defined as a 1 molar solution (1 mol). It has a molarity of 1. Thus, for example, the molecular weight of potassium hydroxide (KOH) is the sum of the atomic weights of its elements i.e. KOH = 39 + 16 + 1 = 56. Therefore a 1 molar solution (1 mol) of KOH contains 56 g of KOH in 1 litre of solution.

A 1 millimole (mmol) of KOH contains one-thousandth of a mole in 1 litre = 56 mg.

> **EXAMPLE 8.14**
>
> Calculate the number of moles (molarity) of a solution if it contains 117 g of sodium chloride (NaCl) in 1 L of solution (atomic weights: Na = 23, Cl = 35.5).
>
> Molecular weight of NaCl = 23 + 35.5 = 58.5 g
> Therefore, 58.5 g of NaCl in 1 litre is equivalent to 1 mole (1 mol) in solution.
> Number of moles of NaCl = 117 g/58.5 g = 2 mol

EXAMPLE 8.15

Calculate the number of milligrams of sodium hydroxide (NaOH) to be dissolved in 1 L of water to give a concentration of 10 mmol (atomic weights: H = 1, O = 16, Na = 23).

Molecular weight of NaOH = 23 + 16 + 1 = 40
1 mmol = 40 mg in 1 L; therefore 10 mmol = 400 mg in 1 L.

EXAMPLE 8.16

Express 111 mg of calcium chloride ($CaCl_2$) in 1 L of solution as millimoles (atomic weights: Ca = 40, Cl = 35.5).

Molecular weight of $CaCl_2$
= Ca + (2 × Cl) = 40 + (2 × 35.5) = 40 + 71 = 111 g

Therefore, 111 mg of $CaCl_2$ = 1 mmol in 1 L.

CALCULATING QUANTITIES FROM A MASTER FORMULA

In extemporaneous dispensing a list of the ingredients is provided on the prescription or is obtained from a recognized reference source where the quantities of each ingredient are indicated. It may be that this 'formula' is for the quantity requested, but more often the quantities provided by the master formula have to be scaled up or down, depending on the quantity of the product required. This can be achieved using proportion or by deriving a 'multiplying factor'. The latter is the ratio of the required quantity divided by the formula quantity. The following examples illustrate this process.

EXAMPLE 8.17

Calculate the quantities to prepare the following prescription:

50 g Compound Benzoic Acid Ointment BPC.

Ingredient	Master formula	Scaled quantity
Benzoic acid	6 g	3 g
Salicylic acid	3 g	1.5 g
Emulsifying ointment	91 g	45.5 g

Double check: the quantities for the master formula add up to 100 g and the scaled quantities add up to 50 g.

EXAMPLE 8.18

You are requested to dispense 200 mL of Ammonium Chloride Mixture BPC. The formula can be found in a variety of reference books such as 'Martindale'. In this example the master formula gives quantities sufficient for 10 mL. As the prescription is for 200 mL the multiplying factor is 200/10. Thus the quantity of each ingredient in the master formula has to be multiplied by 20 to provide the required amount.

Ingredient	Master formula	Scaled quantity
Ammonium chloride	1 g	20 g
Aromatic solution of ammonia	0.5 mL	10 mL
Liquorice liquid extract	1 mL	20 mL
Water	to 10 mL	to 200 mL

Because this formula contains a mixture of volumes and weights it is not possible to calculate the exact quantity of water which is required. However, it is always good practice to have an idea of what the approximate quantity will be. The liquid ingredients of the preparation, other than the water, add up to 30 mL and there is 20 g of ammonium chloride. The volume of water required will therefore be in the region of 150 mL.

In most formulae where a combination of weights and volumes is required the formula will indicate that the preparation is to be made up to the required weight or volume with the designated vehicle. However, occasionally, as can be seen in the next example, a combination of weights and volumes is used and it is not possible to indicate what the exact final weight or volume of the preparation will be. In these instances an excess quantity is normally calculated for and the required amount measured.

EXAMPLE 8.19

Calculate the quantities required to produce 300 mL Turpentine Liniment BP 1988.

Ingredient	Master formula
Soft soap	75 g
Camphor	50 g
Turpentine oil	650 mL
Water	225 mL

When the total number of units is added up for this formula it comes to 1000. However, because it is a combination of solids and liquids, it will not produce 1000 mL. The prescription is for 300 mL so calculate for 340 units and this will provide slightly more than 300 mL. The required amount can then be measured.

Ingredient	Master formula	Scaled quantity for 340 units
Soft soap	75 g	25.5 g
Camphor	50 g	17 g
Turpentine oil	650 mL	221 mL
Water	225 mL	76.5 mL

Calculations involving parts

In the following example the quantities are expressed as parts of the whole. The number of parts is added up and the quantity of each ingredient calculated by proportion or multiplying factor, to provide the correct amounts.

EXAMPLE 8.20

The quantity which is to be prepared of the following formula is 30 g.

Ingredient	Master formula	Quantity for 30 g
Zinc oxide	12.5 parts	3.75 g
Calamine	15 parts	4.5 g
Hydrous wool fat	25 parts	7.5 g
White soft paraffin	47.5 parts	14.25 g

The total number of parts adds up to 100 so the proportions of each ingredient will be 12.5/100 of zinc oxide, 15/100 of calamine and so on. The required quantity of each ingredient can then be calculated. Zinc oxide 12.5/100 of 30 g, calamine 15/100 of 30 g etc., as indicated above.

There are some situations when extra care is necessary in reading the prescription.

EXAMPLE 8.21

Two products are to be dispensed:

Betnovate cream	1 part
Aqueous cream	to 4 parts
Prepare 50 g	

Haelan ointment	1 part
White soft paraffin	4 parts
Prepare 50 g	

At first glance these calculations look similar but the quantities required for each are different. In the Betnovate prescription the total number of parts is 4, i.e. 1 part of Betnovate and 3 parts of aqueous cream to produce a total of 4 parts. However, in the Haelan prescription the total number of parts is 5, i.e. 1 part of Haelan ointment and 4 parts of white soft paraffin.

The quantities required for the prescriptions are as follows:

Betnovate cream	12.5 g
Aqueous cream	37.5 g

Haelan ointment	10 g
White soft paraffin	40 g

Calculations involving percentages

There are conventions which apply when dealing with formulae which include percentages:

A solid in a formula where the final quantity is stated as a weight is calculated as weight in weight (w/w).

A solid in a formula where the final quantity is stated as a volume is calculated as weight in volume (w/v).

A liquid in a formula where the final quantity is stated as a volume is calculated as volume in volume (v/v).

A liquid in a formula where the final quantity is stated as a weight is calculated as weight in weight (w/w).

EXAMPLE 8.22

Prepare 250 g of the following ointment

Ingredient	Master formula	Master formula	Quantity for 250 g
Sulphur	2%	0.2 g	5 g
Salicylic acid	1%	0.1 g	2.5 g
White soft paraffin	to 10 g	to 10 g	242.5 g

The master formula is for a total of 10 g. To calculate the quantities required for 250 g multiply the weight of each ingredient required to prepare 10 g by 25. Remember do not multiply the percentage figure. This always remains the same no matter how much is being prepared.

In the following example a liquid ingredient, the coal tar solution, is stated as a percentage and a weight in grams of final product is requested. The convention of % w/w is applied.

EXAMPLE 8.23

The quantity to be made is 60 g.

Ingredient	Master formula	Master formula	Quantity for 60 g
Coal tar solution	3%	3 g	1.8 g
Zinc oxide	5 g	5 g	3 g
Yellow soft paraffin	to 100 g	92 g	55.2 g

When dealing with preparations where ingredients are expressed as a percentage concentration it is important to check that the standard conventions apply because there are some situations where they do not apply. Two examples are given below:

1. Syrup BP is a liquid—a solution of sucrose and water. If the normal convention applied it would be w/v, i.e. a certain weight of sucrose in a final volume of syrup. However, in the BP formula the concentration of sucrose is quoted as w/w. Therefore Syrup BP is:

Sucrose   66.7% w/w
Water   to 100%

This means that when preparing Syrup BP the appropriate weight of sucrose is weighed out and water is added to the required weight, not volume.

2. A gas in a solution is always calculated as w/w, unless specified otherwise. Formaldehyde Solution BP is a solution of 34–38% w/w formaldehyde in water.

CHANGING CONCENTRATIONS

Sometimes it is necessary to increase or decrease the concentration of a medicine by the addition of more drug or a diluent. On other occasions, instructions have to be provided to prepare a dilution for use. These problems can be solved by the dilution equation:

$$C_1 V_1 = C_2 V_2$$

where C_1 and V_1 are the initial concentration and initial quantity respectively; and C_2 and V_2 are the final concentration and final quantity of the mixture respectively.

When three terms of the equation are known, the fourth term can be made the subject of the formula, and solved.

EXAMPLE 8.24

What is the final concentration if 120 mL of a 12% w/v chlorhexidine solution is diluted to 240 mL with water?

$C_1 = 12\%$, $V_1 = 120$ mL, $C_2 = y\%$, $V_2 = 240$ mL
$12 \times 120 = 240 \times y$, therefore
$y = 12 \times 120/240 = 6\%$ w/v

EXAMPLE 8.25

What concentration is produced when 200 mL of a 2.5% w/v solution is diluted to 750 mL (answer to 2 decimal places)?

$C_1 = 2.5\%$, $V_1 = 200$ mL, $C_2 = y$, $V_2 = 750$ mL
$2.5\% \times 200$ mL $= y \times 750$ mL, therefore
$y = 2.5 \times 200/750 = 0.67\%$ w/v

EXAMPLE 8.26

What volume of 1% w/v solution can be made from 75 mL of 5% w/v solution?

$1\% \times V_1 = 5\% \times 75$ mL
$V_1 = 5/1 \times 75 = 375$ mL

EXAMPLE 8.27

What percentage of atropine is produced when 150 mg of atropine powder is made up to 50 g with lactose as a diluent?

The atropine powder is a pure drug, so its concentration (C_1) is 100% w/w. The initial weight of the atropine powder $(W_1) = 150$ mg $= 0.15$ g. Therefore, we can modify the dilution equation to read:

$$C_1 W_1 = C_2 W_2$$

where C_2 and W_2 are the final concentration and final weight respectively, of the diluted drug. The diluting medium is the lactose.

Thus, $100\% \times 0.15$ g $= C_2 \times 50$ g
$C_2 = 100 \times 0.15/50 = 0.3\%$ w/w

Alligation

Alligation is a method for solving the number of parts of two or more components of known concentration to be mixed when the final desired concentration is known. When the relative amounts of components must be calculated for making a mixture of a desired concentration, the problem is most easily solved by alligation.

EXAMPLE 8.28

Calculate the amounts of a 2% w/w metronidazole cream and of metronidazole powder required to produce 150 g of 6% w/w metronidazole cream (to 2 decimal places).

In alligation, the two starting material concentrations are placed above each other on the left hand side of the calculation. The target concentration is placed in the centre. The arithmetic difference between the starting material and the target is calculated and the answer recorded on the right hand end of the diagonal. The proportions of the two starting materials are then given by reading horizontally across the diagram.

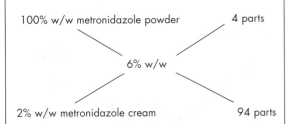

100% w/w metronidazole powder   4 parts

6% w/w

2% w/w metronidazole cream   94 parts

As shown above, the difference between the concentration of the pure drug powder (100%, recorded top left) and the desired concentration (6%) is 94 (recorded bottom right). This is equivalent to the number of parts of 2% cream required (read horizontally across the bottom). Similarly, the difference between the concentration of 2% cream (recorded bottom left) and the desired concentration (6%) is 4 (recorded top right). This is equivalent to the number of parts of 100% drug (metronidazole powder) needed for the mixture (read horizontally across the top).

The total amount (4 parts + 94 parts = 98 parts) is 150 g.

Thus, 1 part = 150/98 g.

Therefore, the amount of 2% cream required = 94 parts × 150/98 g = 143.88 g.

The amount of pure metronidazole (100%) required = 4 parts × 150/98 = 6.12 g.

EXAMPLE 8.29

Thioridazine suspension is available as 25 mg/5 mL and 100 mg/5 mL.

Calculate the quantities to use to prepare 100 mL of 40 mg/5 mL suspension.

Convert all the concentrations to percentages.

Therefore, 25 mg/5 mL is equivalent to 0.025 g in 5 mL = 0.500 g in 100 mL = 0.5% w/v

Similarly, 100 mg/5 mL = 2% w/v; and 40 mg/5 mL = 0.8% w/v

Using the alligation method:

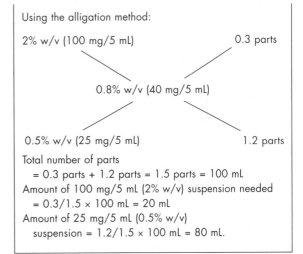

2% w/v (100 mg/5 mL)   0.3 parts

0.8% w/v (40 mg/5 mL)

0.5% w/v (25 mg/5 mL)   1.2 parts

Total number of parts
    = 0.3 parts + 1.2 parts = 1.5 parts = 100 mL
Amount of 100 mg/5 mL (2% w/v) suspension needed
    = 0.3/1.5 × 100 mL = 20 mL
Amount of 25 mg/5 mL (0.5% w/v)
    suspension = 1.2/1.5 × 100 mL = 80 mL.

CALCULATIONS WHERE QUANTITY OF INGREDIENTS IS TOO SMALL TO WEIGH OR MEASURE ACCURATELY

When preparing medicines by extemporaneous dispensing, the quantity of active ingredient required may be too small to weigh or measure, with the equipment available. In these situations a measurable quantity has to be diluted with an inert diluent. The process is called 'trituration'.

Small quantities in powders

EXAMPLE 8.30

Calculate the quantities required to make 10 powders each containing 200 micrograms of digoxin.

Assume that the balance available has a minimum weighable quantity of 100 mg. An inert diluent, in this case lactose, will be used for the trituration. The convenient weight of each divided powder is 120 mg.

The total weight of powder mixture required will be 10 × 120 = 1200 milligrams = 1.2 g.

Quantities for 10 powders:

Digoxin	2 mg
Lactose	1198 mg
Total	1200 mg

The weight of digoxin is too small to weigh. The minimum weighable quantity of 100 mg is weighed and used in the triturate. A 1 in 10 dilution is produced.

Trituration A

Digoxin	100 mg
Lactose	900 mg
Total	1000 mg

Each 100 mg of this mixture (A) contains 10 mg of digoxin.

Trituration B

Mixture A	100 mg	(= 10 mg digoxin)
Lactose	900 mg	
Total	1000 mg	

Each 100 mg of this mixture (B) contains 1 mg of digoxin. This amount of digoxin is less than the required amount, so mixture B can be used to give the required quantity.

200 mg of mixture B provides the 2 mg digoxin required.

Final trituration (C)

Mixture B	200 mg (= 2 mg digoxin)
Lactose	(1200 – 200) = 1000 mg
Total	1200 mg

Each 120 mg of this mixture (C) will contain 200 micrograms (0.2 mg) of digoxin.

The method for preparing divided powders is described in Chapter 22.

Small quantities in liquids

If the quantity of a solid to be incorporated into a solution is too small to weigh, again dilutions are used. In this case a solution is prepared, so the solubility of the substance needs to be considered. Normally a 1 in 10 or 1 in 100 dilution is used.

EXAMPLE 8.31

Calculate the quantities required to prepare 100 mL of a solution containing 2.5 mg morphine hydrochloride/5 mL.

Quantities for 100 mL:

Morphine hydrochloride	50 mg
Chloroform water	to 100 mL

The solubility of morphine hydrochloride is 1 in 24 of water.

The minimum quantity of 100 mg of morphine hydrochloride is weighed and made up to 10 mL with

---

chloroform water (this weight of morphine hydrochloride will dissolve in 2.4 mL).

5 mL of this solution (A) provides the 50 mg of morphine hydrochloride required.

Take 5 mL of solution A and make up to 100 mL with chloroform water.

SOLUBILITIES

When preparing pharmaceutical products the solubility of any solid ingredients should be checked. This will give useful information on how the product should be prepared. Examples of the calculations are given in Chapters 7 and 17. The objective of this section is to clarify the terminology used when solubilities are stated.

The solubility of a drug can be found in reference sources such as the drug monograph in 'Martindale' where it is in the section dealing with physical properties. The method of stating solubilities is as follows:

Sodium chloride is soluble 1 in 2.8 of water, 1 in 250 of alcohol and 1 in 10 of glycerol.

This means that 1 g of sodium chloride requires 2.8 mL of water, 250 mL of alcohol or 10 mL of glycerol to dissolve it. An example of how knowledge of a substance's solubility can help in extemporaneous dispensing can be found in Chapter 7. Some examples of calculating quantities of liquids required to dissolve solids are found in the tutorial section at the end of this chapter.

CALCULATIONS INVOLVING DOSES

A simple calculation which pharmacists sometimes have to make whilst dispensing is to calculate the number of tablets or capsules or volume of a liquid medicine to be dispensed.

EXAMPLE 8.32

The doctor prescribes levodopa capsules, 1000 mg to be taken every 8 hours for 28 days. Levodopa is available as 500 mg capsules. How many capsules should be supplied?

For each dose, 2 capsules are required. Every eight hours means 3 doses per day.

Therefore, the total number of capsules required is $2 \times 3 \times 28 = 168$ capsules.

EXAMPLE 8.33

The following prescription is received:

Sodium valproate oral solution 100 mg to be given twice daily for 2 weeks.

Sodium valproate oral solution contains sodium valproate 200 mg/5 mL.

This prescription is therefore translated as: 2.5 mL to be given twice daily for 2 weeks.

The quantity to be dispensed will be:

2.5 × 2 × 14 = 70 mL.

Calculating doses

An overdose of a drug, if given to a patient, can have very serious consequences and may be fatal. It is the responsibility of everyone involved in supplying or administering drugs to ensure that the accuracy and suitability of the dose are checked. The following are some examples of areas where errors can occur.

The standard way to check whether a drug dose is appropriate is to consult a recognized reference book. One of the commonest used for this purpose is the *British National Formulary* (BNF). When first using any reference source it is important to be aware of the terminology used, to avoid misinterpreting the entries, especially where doses are quoted as 'x milligrams daily, in divided doses'. An explanation of the terminology will usually be given in the introduction to the book.

EXAMPLE 8.34

The following prescription is received:

Verapamil tablets 160 milligrams
Send 56
Take two tablets twice daily

There are a variety of doses quoted for verapamil in the BNF depending on the condition being treated. They are as follows for oral administration:

Supraventricular arrhythmias, 40–120 mg three times daily

Angina, 80–120 mg three times daily

Hypertension, 240–480 mg daily in 2–3 divided doses.

The dose given for hypertension is stated in a significantly different way. Whereas the other doses can be given three times daily, indicating a maximum of

---

360 mg in any one day, the hypertension dose is the total to be given in any one day and is divided up and given at the stated frequencies, i.e. a maximum of 240 mg, given twice daily or a maximum of 160 mg, given three times daily.

The prescription is for a dose higher than recommended, so consultation with the prescriber would be required. Be alert, variation in terminology and a lack of awareness could have very serious consequences.

Calculations of children's doses

Children often require different doses from those of adults. Ideally these should be arrived at as a result of extensive clinical studies, although this is often not possible. When this is the case an estimate of the dose has to be made. This is best carried out using body weight (see next section), but where this is not available, there are three formulas which relate the child's dose to the adult dose.

Fried's rule for infants:

age (months) × adult dose/150 = dose for infant.

Clark's rule: weight (in kg) × adult dose/75 = dose for child.

Body surface area method (BSA):

BSA of child (m^2) × adult dose/1.73 m^2 (average adult BSA) = approximate child's dose.

The BNF also gives a percentage method for calculating paediatric doses of drugs which have a wide therapeutic window, i.e. where accuracy is less critical.

Calculation of doses by weight and surface area

For some drugs the amount of drug has to be calculated accurately for the particular patient. This is normally carried out using either body weight or body surface area. When body weight is being used, the dose will be expressed as mg/kg. In countries, which still use pounds, it will be necessary to convert the patient's weight in pounds into kilograms by dividing by 2.2. The total dose required is then obtained by multiplying the weight of the patient by the dose per kilogram.

Body surface area is a more accurate method for calculating doses and is used where extreme accuracy is required. This is necessary where there is a very narrow range of plasma concentration between the desired therapeutic effect and severe toxicity, such as with the drugs used to treat cancer. The body surface area can be calculated from body weight and height using the equation given below, but it is more usual to use a nomogram for its determination. The actual nomogram is published in many reference sources.

$$\text{Body surface area (m}^2\text{)} =$$
$$\text{Weight (kg)}^{0.425} \times \text{Height (cm)}^{0.725} \times 0.007184$$

RECONSTITUTION AND INFUSION

Some drugs are not chemically stable in solution and so are supplied as dry powders for reconstitution just before use. Many of these are antibiotics, but there is also a range of chemotherapeutic agents used in cancer treatment. The antibiotics may be for oral use or for injection. An oral antibiotic for reconstitution comes as a powder in a bottle with sufficient space to add the water. The powder itself will remain stable for up to 2 years when dry. When reconstituted, a shelf life of 10–14 days is normal, depending on whether it is kept in the fridge or not. Those for injection are equally stable when dry, but are intended to be used within hours of reconstitution. Because they are for injection they are sterile powders and are dissolved in sterile water aseptically (see Ch. 13). There are a number of calculations which may be required around the reconstitution processes.

EXAMPLE 8.35

What dose of antibiotic will be contained in a 5 mL spoonful when a bottle containing 5 g of penicillin V is reconstituted to give 200 mL of syrup?
   For this type of calculation, the simple proportion equation can be used:

$$\text{Wt}_1/\text{Wt}_2 = \text{Vol}_1/\text{Vol}_2$$
$$5 \text{ g} = 5000 \text{ mg}.$$

Substituting we get:

$$5000 \text{ mg}/y \text{ mg} = 200 \text{ mL}/5 \text{ mL}$$
$$y = 125 \text{ mg}.$$

Sometimes, the doctor may request a more or less concentrated syrup to be produced which requires altering the amount of water added from that indicated by the manufacturer.

EXAMPLE 8.36

We have an ampicillin product for reconstitution. It contains 2.5 g of ampicillin to be made up to 100 mL. To what volume should it be made to give 100 mg per 5 mL dose?

The normal mixture will give a dose of:

$$2500 \text{ mg}/y \text{ mg} = 100 \text{ mL}/5 \text{ mL}$$
$$y = 125 \text{ mg per 5 mL}$$

To calculate the amount of water to add, the same equation is used:

$$2500 \text{ mg}/100 \text{ mg} = y \text{ mL}/5 \text{ mL}$$
$$y = 125 \text{ mL}.$$

However, this type of oral mixture is likely to have other ingredients—thickeners, colours, flavours, etc., which will occupy some of the final volume. So this may not be correct and we need to be able to calculate exactly how much water to add.

EXAMPLE 8.37

The label on an ampicillin bottle indicates that 78 mL of water must be added to produce 100 mL of final syrup. How much water must be added to give the 125 mL final volume?

Thus, the volume of powder in the final syrup is
100 mL – 78 mL = 22 mL.

Therefore, the volume to add to give 125 mL is
125 mL – 22 mL = 103 mL.

EXAMPLE 8.38

A child weighing 60 lb requires a dose of 8 mg/kg of ampicillin. Given that a 5 mL dose is to be given, what volume of water must be added when the powder is reconstituted? Instructions on the label indicate that dilution to 150 mL (by adding 111 mL) gives 250 mg ampicillin per 5 mL.

Conversion of weight to kg: 60/2.2 = 27.27 kg
Calculation of amount of ampicillin required:
   $27.27 \times 8 = 218$ mg
Calculation of amount of ampicillin in container:
   250 mg/y mg = 5 mL/150 mL, therefore
   $y = 7500$ mg = 7.5 g
Calculation of amount of water to add to give 218 mg
   per 5 mL: 218 mg/7500 mg = 5 mL/ x mL,
   therefore $x = 172$ mL
Volume occupied by powder: 150 mL – 111 mL = 39 mL
Therefore, volume to be added:
   172 mL – 39 mL = 133 mL.

Drugs for injection solutions do not normally contain ingredients other than the drug (or they make an insignificant contribution to the final volume). However, they are usually packed as a quantity of drug with the final volume left to be calculated by the pharmacist.

EXAMPLE 8.39

Calculate the amount of sterile water to be added to a vial containing 200 000 units of penicillin G in order to produce a solution containing 40 000 units per millilitre.

Again, simple proportion is used:
40 000 units/200 000 units = 1 mL/y mL, therefore
y = 5 mL.

Calculation of infusion rates

Drugs may be given to patients intravenously by adding them to an intravenous (IV) infusion (see Ch. 25). Calculations involve working out how much drug solution should be added, working out how fast, in terms of mL/min, the infusion should be administered, and calculating what this means in terms of 'drops per minute' through the giving set. When an infusion pump is used, this can be set to deliver a specified number of mL/min. The final stage of drops/min is only required for traditional IV 'drips' (see Ch. 25).

EXAMPLE 8.40

An ampoule of flucloxacillin contains 250 mg of powder with instructions to dissolve it in 5 mL of water for injections. What volume of this solution should be added to 500 mL of saline infusion to provide a dose of 175 mg?

250 mg in 5 mL = 50 mg per mL
Therefore, we require: 175 mg/50 mg/mL = 3.5 mL.

When administering intravenous infusions, the rate of addition is first calculated in terms of millilitres per minute.

EXAMPLE 8.41

100 mg of methoxamine hydrochloride are added to 500 mL of saline infusion. What should be the rate of infusion to give a dose of 1 mg per minute? How long will the infusion take?

Using simple proportion: 100 mg/1 mg = 500 mL/y mL
y = 5 mL and contains the required amount of drug
The infusion rate should be 5 mL per minute
The total volume is 500 mL, therefore the time taken at 5 mL/min is:
$$500 \text{ mL}/5 \text{ mL/min} = 100 \text{ min.}$$

Most infusions are administered using a giving set with a dropping device on the tube (called venoclysis set) (see Ch. 25). Partial clamping of the tube can set the rate of dropping. Depending on the drop size—that is the number of drops per millilitre—it is then possible to convert a rate of millilitres per minute into drops per minute which the nurse can adjust.

EXAMPLE 8.42

A doctor requires an infusion of 1000 mL of 5% dextrose to be administered over an 8-hour period. Using an IV giving set which delivers 10 drops/mL, how many drops per minute should be delivered to the patient?

First convert the time into minutes:
8 hour = 8 × 60 min = 480 min

Next calculate how many mL/min are required:
1000 mL/480 min = 2.1 mL/min

Then calculate the number of drops this requires:
2.1 mL/min × 10 drops/min = 21 drops/min.

Alternatively the doctor may specify the duration of the infusion.

EXAMPLE 8.43

20 mL of a drug solution is added to a 500 mL infusion solution. It has to be administered to the patient over a 5-hour period using a set giving 15 drops per millilitre, how many drops per minute are required?

The total volume of infusion is:
20 mL + 500 mL = 520 mL
Then calculate the number of drops which will be administered in total:
520 mL × 15 drops = 7800 drops
The duration of the infusion is to be
5 (hours) × 60 = 300 min
Calculate how many drops are required per minute:
7800 drops/300 min = 26 drops per minute.

Key Points

- Always work methodically and write down calculations clearly.
- Check calculations, using a different method where possible.
- Estimate the answer before you start.
- Try to visualize the quantities you are using in the calculation.
- Look carefully to see if a formula gives the quantities of all ingredients or uses 'to' for the vehicle.
- Equations can be a useful way of carrying out calculations, but care is required to ensure that the correct figures are being used.
- Always check the units being used and be careful not to mix them during a calculation.
- Be very careful to read the wording; small changes in terminology can alter the calculation.
- Triturates with solids and liquids normally use a 1 in 10 dilution per step.
- Be very careful in checking doses, particularly with 'in divided doses' and 'mg/kg' statements in the reference books.
- On completion of a calculation, ask yourself whether the answer is 'reasonable' given the numbers you are using.

SELF-ASSESSMENT QUESTIONS

(Express answers to 2 decimal places where appropriate)

1.1 Express 310 grains in the metric system.

1.2 Express 300 p.p.m. as a percentage strength.

1.3 Express 324 mg in grains.

1.4 What is the total volume to be dispensed when the prescription states:
5 mL twice daily for 1 week?

1.5 Calculate the number of tablets to be dispensed when the prescription states:
1 tablet twice daily 1/52.

1.6 Calculate the volume of each dose and total quantity to be dispensed for a prescription for paracetamol which is available as a 200 mg/5 mL syrup:
50 mg daily for 2/52.

2.1 Express the following as percentages (indicating w/w, w/v, v/v, where appropriate):
a   2 g of drug in 50 mL of solution
b   1 milligram of drug in 200 mL of solution

c   3 mL of drug in 4 L of solution
d   10 g of drug in 250 g of solution
e   6 micrograms of drug in 10 mL of solution
f   2 L of drug in 5000 mL of solution
g   25 000 p.p.m. (parts per million)
h   a 1 in 4000 solution
i   a 3 in 10 000 solution.
j   0.3 mL in 30 mL
k   1 g in 220 mL
l   240 mg/5 mL
m   0.8 mg/mL.

2.2 Express 0.9% w/w as 1 part in …

2.3 The following are examples of concentrations expressed as percentages. Indicate the amount of drug present in:
a   500 mL of a 6% w/v solution
b   30 mL of a 15% w/v preparation
c   2 L of a 0.05% v/v preparation
d   0.5 mL of a 2% w/v preparation
e   20 g of a 0.1% w/w preparation
f   150 mL of a 0.002% w/v preparation.

2.4 What weight of lactose is required to make 70 mL of a 1% w/v solution?

2.5 How much drug is required to prepare 250 g of a 0.08% w/w mixture?

2.6 Express 0.1% w/v as mg/mL.

2.7 How many milligrams of drug are there in 5 mL of 2% w/v solution?

2.8 Calculate the number of milligrams of the following compounds to be dissolved in 1 L of aqueous solution to give a concentration of 10 mmol:
(Atomic weights: H = 1, C = 12, N = 14, O = 16, S = 32, Cl = 35.5, K = 39)
a   Hydrochloric acid (HCl)
b   Sulphuric acid (H_2SO_4)
c   Potassium chloride (KCl)
d   A drug with the molecular formula $C_{12}H_{12}ONCl$.

2.9 Express 222 mg of calcium chloride ($CaCl_2$) in 2 L of solution as millimoles. (Atomic weights: Ca = 40, Cl = 35.5)

2.10 How many grams of azathioprine (molecular weight 277.3) contain 15 mmol of drug?

2.11 How many mmol are there in 5 g of furosemide (frusemide) (molecular weight 330.7)?

3.1 What weight of each ingredient is required for the extemporaneous preparation if 50 g of the following preparation is to be made?

Calamine	7 g
Arachis oil	30 g

	Emulsifying wax	6 g
	Water to	100 g
3.2	Calculate the quantities for:	
a	Benzoic acid	12 g
	Sulphur	20 g
	Coal tar	15 g
	Zinc oxide	45 g
	Yellow soft paraffin	135 g
	Prepare 1 kg	
b	Liquid paraffin	50 mL
	Acacia	12.5 g
	Water	to 120 mL
	Send 90 mL.	
3.3	Calculate the quantities required:	
a	Concentrated anise water	10 parts
	Amaranth solution	15 parts
	Citric acid monohydrate	25 parts
	Chloroform spirit	60 parts
	Syrup	to 1000 parts
	Send 150 mL	
b	Aromatic cascara	1 part
	Liquid paraffin	3 parts
	Milk of magnesia	4 parts
	Send 1 litre	
c	Starch	7 parts
	Zinc oxide	8 parts
	Olive oil	2 parts
	Wool fat	3 parts
	Prepare 60 g	
d	Camphor	0.8 parts
	Calamine powder	8 parts
	Starch	9.2 parts
	Talc	30 parts
	Send 60 g	
e	Coal tar solution	2%
	Zinc oxide	5 g
	Yellow soft paraffin	to 100 g
	Prepare 30 g	
f	Sulphur	3%
	Salicylic acid	2%
	White soft paraffin	to 10 g
	Prepare 60 g	
g	Sodium bicarbonate	0.5%
	Magnesium trisilicate	6%
	Concentrated peppermint emulsion	2.5%
	Water	to 100 mL
	Send 300 mL	
h	Oxytetracycline	3 %
	Zinc oxide	10 g

	Salicylic acid	2.5 g
	Starch	to 50 g
	Send 250 g	
i	Hydrocortisone	1%
	Clioquinol	1.5 g
	Wool fat	5 g
	White soft paraffin	to 50 g
	Prepare 30 g.	

4.1 Calculate the concentration of a solution of potassium permanganate, which, when 1 mL is diluted to 100 mL, produces a solution with a concentration of 100 p.p.m.

4.2 What percentage is produced when 150 mg of powder is made up to 50 g with a diluent?

4.3 What concentration is produced when 200 mL of a 2.5% w/v solution is diluted to 750 mL?

4.4 What concentration is produced when 150 mL of a 1 in 25 solution is diluted to 500 mL?

4.5 What concentration is produced when 60 mL of a 1 in 10 solution is diluted to 250 mL?

4.6 What weight of drug must be added to 150 g of 1% ointment to produce a 4% ointment?

4.7 Sulphur ointment is available as 5% w/w and 8% w/w. Calculate the quantities needed to prepare 30 g of 7% w/w ointment.

4.8 Orphenadrine syrup is available as 25 mg/5 mL and 50 mg/5 mL. Calculate the quantities to use to prepare 50 mL of 30 mg/5 mL syrup.

4.9 What weight of drug must be added to 50 g of 2% ointment to produce a 3% ointment?

4.10 Calculate the amount of drug and 2% w/w ointment required to make 150 g of 3% ointment.

4.11 Calculate the volume of copper sulphate solution 15% w/v which, when diluted to 100 mL, will produce a 1 in 100 solution.

4.12 What volume of normal saline (0.9% w/v NaCl) can be made from 1.5 g NaCl?

4.13 What volume of 0.5 % solution can be produced from 150 mL of 1 in 20 solution?

4.14 What volume of 1% solution can be made from 75 mL of 5% solution?

4.15 What volume of 0.25% solution can be produced from 100 mL of 1 in 25 solution?

4.16 How many grams of ichthammol must be added to 500 g of ointment base to produce an ointment containing 10% w/w ichthammol?

4.17 Calculate the weight of drug which must be added to 1 litre of a 17% w/v solution (density 1.2 g/mL) to make a 20% w/w solution.

4.18 Calculate the volume of 4% solution of Cetrimide required to prepare 200 mL of 1 in 1000 solution.

4.19 Calculate the volume of 5% of potassium permanganate required to prepare 125 mL of a 0.2% solution.

4.20 Calculate the volume of 1 in 20 solution of chlorhexidine solution required to prepare 750 mL of a 0.1% solution.

5.1   Calculate how to make 20 × 120 mg powders, each containing 0.5 mg of colchicine.

5.2   Calculate how to make 25 × 100 mg powders, each containing 2 mg of carbachol.

5.3   Calculate how to make 15 × 100 mg powders, each containing 0.4 mg of atropine sulphate.

5.4   Calculate how to make 20 × 100 mg capsules, each containing 150 micrograms of hyoscine hydrobromide.

6.1   How much water is required to dissolve:
   a   1 g of aminophylline (solubility 1 in 5)?
   b   500 mg of ammonium chloride (solubility 1 in 2.7)?
   c   750 mg of apomorphine hydrochloride (solubility 1 in 50)?

6.2   How much isoniazid will dissolve in 20 mL of water (solubility 1 in 8)? If 300 mg is to be dispensed, will it dissolve in 20 mL of water?

6.3   How much lidocaine (lignocaine) hydrochloride will dissolve in 20 mL of water (solubility 1 in 0.7)? If 50 mg is to be dispensed, will it dissolve in 20 mL of water?

6.4   A drug has a solubility 1 in 50 of water and 1 in 14 of alcohol.
   a   Will 250 milligrams dissolve in 4 mL of water?
   b   Will 4 g dissolve in 60 mL of alcohol?
   c   Will 10 micrograms dissolve in 0.002 mL of water?
   d   Will 1 kg dissolve in 3 L of alcohol?
   e   Will 0.05 g dissolve in 0.2 mL of alcohol?

7.1   For the following prescriptions calculate the dose of active ingredient which the patient will be taking on each occasion and each day.
   a   Sudafed elixir
       Mitte 150 mL
       Sig. 3 mL t.i.d.
       (Sudafed elixir contains pseudoephedrine 30 milligrams/5 mL.)
   b   Codeine linctus half strength
       Mitte 200 mL
       Sig. 2.5 mL t.i.d.
       (Codeine linctus contains codeine phosphate 15 mg/5 mL.)
   c   Ketotifen elixir
       Mitte 300 mL
       Sig. 7.5 mL b.i.d.
       (Ketotifen elixir contains ketotifen 1 milligram/5 mL.
   d   Terfenadine suspension
       Mitte 150 mL
       Sig. 10 mL b.i.d.
       (Terfenadine suspension contains terfenadine 30 milligrams/5 mL.)

7.2   For the following prescriptions calculate the volume of liquid which the patient will take on each occasion.
   a   Hismanal suspension
       Mitte 500 mL
       Sig. 8 milligrams daily
       (Hismanal suspension contains astemizole 5 milligrams/5 mL.)
   b   Dimotane elixir
       Mitte 100 mL
       Sig. 1.5 milligrams q.i.d.
       (Dimotane elixir contains brompheniramine maleate 2 milligrams/5 mL.)
   c   Promethazine elixir
       Mitte 100 mL
       Sig. 12 milligrams daily
       (Promethazine elixir contains promethazine hydrochloride 5 mg/5 mL.)

7.3   What dose of procainamide should be given to a patient weighing 57 kg to provide 50 mg/kg?

7.4   Calculate the dose of zidovudine required to provide 120 mg/m^2 for a patient of estimated surface area 0.32 m^2.

8.1   What is the weight of penicillin V in a 5 mL dose when a bottle containing 5 g penicillin V is made up with water to give 50 mL of syrup?

8.2   A bottle contains 2.5 g of cefaclor. What volume should be made in order to provide 100 mg per 5 mL dose?

8.3   The label on a bottle of ampicillin syrup indicates that 78 mL of water should be added to make 100 mL of syrup. How much water should be added to produce 110 mL of syrup?

8.4   An injection of amphotericin B contains 50 mg/10 mL. What volume must be added to 500 mL of normal saline infusion to produce a 10 mg/100 mL solution?

9.1 An infusion solution contains 50 mg tacrolimus in 500 mL. What rate of infusion should be used to give 90 microgram/min? How long will a 500 mL infusion last?

9.2 In preparing an IV infusion, you have a solution containing 2 g/mL adrenaline (epinephrine) hydrochloride (molecular weight 217.9). What volume must be added to a 500 mL infusion to provide a 10 mmol total dose?

10.1 Paregoric is 4% v/v tincture of opium which is 10% w/v opium. If opium contains 10% w/w morphine what weight of morphine is contained in a 30 mL bottle of Paregoric?

SELF-ASSESSMENT ANSWERS

1.1	310 grains = 64.8 × 310 mg = 20.08 g
1.2	0.03%
1.3	5 grains
1.4	70 mL
1.5	14 tablets
1.6	Dose 1.25 mL, quantity 17.5 mL
2.1a	4% w/v
2.1b	0.0005% w/v
2.1c	0.075% v/v
2.1d	4% w/w
2.1e	0.00006% w/v
2.1f	40% v/v
2.1g	2.5%
2.1h	0.025%
2.1i	0.03%
2.1j	1% v/v
2.1k	0.45% w/v
2.1l	4.8% w/v
2.1m	0.08% w/v
2.2	1 in 111.11
2.3a	30 g
2.3b	4.5 g
2.3c	1 mL
2.3d	0.01 g or 10 mg
2.3e	0.02 g or 20 mg
2.3f	0.003 g or 3 mg
2.4	0.7 g or 700 mg
2.5	0.2 g or 200 mg
2.6	1 mg/mL
2.7	100 mg
2.8a	365 mg
2.8b	980 mg

2.8c	745 mg	
2.8d	2215 mg	
2.9	1 mmol	
2.10	4.16 g	
2.11	15.12 mmol	
3.1	Calamine	3.5 g
	Arachis oil	15 g
	Emulsifying wax	3 g
	Water to	50 g
3.2a	Benzoic acid	52.9 g
	Sulphur	88.1 g
	Coal tar	66.1 g
	Zinc oxide	198.2 g
	Yellow soft paraffin	594.7 g
3.2b	Liquid paraffin	37.5 mL
	Acacia	9.38 g
	Water (approx. 43 mL)	to 90 mL
3.3a	Concentrated anise water	1.5 mL
	Amaranth solution	2.25 mL
	Citric acid monohydrate	3.75 g
	Chloroform spirit	9 mL
	Syrup (approx. 133.5 mL)	to 150 mL
3.3b	Aromatic cascara	125 mL
	Liquid paraffin	375 mL
	Milk of magnesia	500 mL
3.3c	Starch	21 g
	Zinc oxide	24 g
	Olive oil	6 g
	Wool fat	9 g
3.3d	Camphor	1 g
	Calamine	10 g
	Starch	11.5 g
	Talc	37.5 g
3.3e	Coal tar solution	0.6 g
	Zinc oxide	1.5 g
	Yellow soft paraffin	27.9 g
3.3f	Sulphur	1.8 g
	Salicylic acid	1.2 g
	White soft paraffin	57 g

3.3g	Sodium bicarbonate		1.5 g
	Magnesium trisilicate		18.0 g
	Concentrated peppermint emulsion		7.5 mL
	Water (approx. 273 mL)		to 300 mL
3.3h	Oxytetracycline	7.5 g	
	Zinc oxide	50 g	
	Salicylic acid	12.5 g	
	Starch	180 g	
3.3i	Hydrocortisone	0.3 g	
	Clioquinol	0.9 g	

Wool fat   3 g

White soft paraffin   25.8 g

4.1   1% w/v

4.2   0.3% w/w

4.3   0.67% w/v

4.4   1.2%

4.5   2.4%

4.6   Using alligation method:

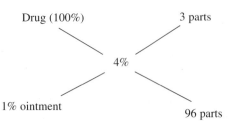

Total amount of drug and 1% ointment = 3 parts + 96 parts = 99 parts

The mass of the 1% ointment is given as 150 g. Thus, 96 parts = 150 g

Mass of drug (100 %) required = 150/96 × 3 parts = 4.69 g

4.7   Using alligation method:

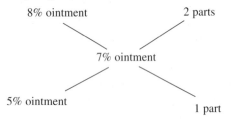

Total number of parts = 2 parts + 1 part = 3 parts which are equivalent to 30 g

Amount of 8% w/w ointment needed = 2 parts/ 3 parts × 30 g = 20 g

Amount of 5% w/w ointment needed = 1 part/ 3 parts × 30 g = 10 g

4.8   40 mL of 25 mg/5 mL syrup and 10 mL of 50 mg/ 5 mL syrup

4.9   0.52 g

4.10   Drug 1.53 g and 2% w/w ointment 148.47 g

4.11   6.67 mL

4.12   166.67 mL

4.13   1500 mL

4.14   375 mL

4.15   1600 mL

4.16   55.56 g of ichthammol

4.17   The weight of drug to be added = 87.50 g

      17% w/v solution = 14.167% w/w

      Weight of 1 litre of 17% w/v solution is 1200 g

4.18   5 mL

4.19   5 mL

4.20   15 mL

5.1   Weigh 100 mg, dilute with 900 mg of lactose, take 100 mg and make up to 2.4 g by adding 2.3 g of lactose

5.2   Weigh 100 mg, dilute with 900 mg of lactose, take 500 mg and make up to 2.5 g by adding 2 g of lactose

5.3   Weigh 100 mg, dilute with 900 mg of lactose, take 100 mg, dilute with 900 mg of lactose, take 600 mg and make up to 1.5 g by adding 900 mg of lactose

5.4   Weigh 100 mg, dilute with 900 mg of lactose, take 100 mg, dilute with 900 mg lactose, take 300 mg and make up to 2 g by adding 1700 mg of lactose

6.1a   5 mL

6.1b   1.35 mL

6.1c   37.5 mL

6.2   2.5 g. Yes

6.3   28.57 g. Yes

6.4a   No, because 250 milligrams of drug requires 12.5 mL of water in which to dissolve

6.4b   Yes, because 4 g of drug requires 56 mL of alcohol in which to dissolve

6.4c   Yes, because 10 micrograms of drug requires 0.0005 mL of water in which to dissolve

6.4d   No, because 1 kg of drug requires 14 L of alcohol in which to dissolve

6.4e   No, because 50 milligrams of drug requires 0.7 mL of alcohol in which to dissolve

7.1a   18 mg per dose, 54 mg per day

7.1b   3.75 mg per dose, 11.25 mg per day

7.1c   1.5 mg per dose, 3 mg per day

7.1d   60 mg per dose, 120 mg per day

7.2a   8 mL of the suspension

7.2b   3.75 mL of the elixir

7.2c   12 mL of the elixir

7.3   2.85 g

7.4   38.4 mg

8.1   500 mg

8.2   125 mL

8.3   88 mL

8.4   10.2 mL

9.1   0.9 mL/min. 556 min (9.26 hours)

9.2   0.55 mL

10.1   12 mg

9

Packaging

D. G. Chapman

After studying this chapter you will know about:

Definition of a container
Considerations made in selecting a container
The difference between primary and secondary packaging
The materials used for packaging, including glass, plastics, metal and paper
Types of container in common use
Child-resistant closures and tamper-evident seals
Patient pack dispensing

Introduction

Pharmaceutical formulations must be suitably contained, protected and labelled from the time of manufacture until the patient uses them. Throughout this period the container must maintain the quality, safety and stability of the medicine and protect the product against physical, climatic, chemical and biological hazards. The *British Pharmacopoeia* (BP 2001) identifies the closure as part of the container.

To promote good patient compliance the container must be user friendly. This is particularly significant for the elderly who have to take more medicines than the general population and have a greater need for improved compliance (see Ch. 40). Thus containers should be easy to open and reclose, most notably for elderly or arthritic patients. However, other factors must also be considered in the selection of the container used to package a pharmaceutical formulation, including the cost and the need for both child-resistant closures and tamper-evident seals.

Repackaging is performed in the community pharmacy for dispensing purposes (see Chs 7 and 10), in hospital pharmacy and in specialized production facilities. Bulk medicines are repackaged into smaller quantities in dispensing containers for distribution to hospital wards, clinics and general practitioners for direct supply to patients. This is mostly carried out with tablets and capsules that are transferred from bulk quantities into smaller amounts that are more suitable for patient use. In the UK this process is performed in the hospital pharmacy where the Medicines Control Agency allows the repackaging of small batches of up to 25 containers. Larger batches must be packed in licensed manufacturing premises. The facilities used for these repackaging operations are designed to maintain the quality of the medicine and avoid product contamination and mix up.

Medicines originally contained in patient packs are subdivided into small amounts by transferring small quantities of the medicine in strip or blister packs into secondary cardboard containers. The composition of containers and closures used for the repackaging of bulk medicines must be carefully selected and must be of a quality as good as the original container. Both glass and plastic containers are used for repackaging but glass containers are often preferred due to the more inert qualities of glass.

Primary containers used for repackaging must not:

- Allow product leakage
- Chemically react with the product
- Release components
- Uptake product components.

The container used in the repackaging process must protect the product from:

- Physical damage
- Chemical and microbial contamination
- Light, moisture and oxygen as appropriate.

As the medicine has been transferred into a new container, the expiry date of the repackaged medicine must not exceed 12 months unless the stability of the repackaged product justifies a longer shelf life. The details of these repackaging processes must be recorded.

Each container of the repackaged batch is labelled with the:

- Identity and quantity of the medicine
- Batch number
- Appropriate storage instructions
- Product expiry date
- Requirements for handling and storage.

There are some situations where the repackaging is limited, such as with glyceryl trinitrate tablets, owing to the potential loss of the volatile drug (see Ch. 10). Sterile products cannot be easily repackaged and require effective closure systems to minimize the risk of microbial contamination of the contents within the container. In addition, the pack itself must withstand sterilization procedures. Consequently, care must be applied to the selection of the container and its closure for the packaging of sterile products (see also Chs 13, 25 and 26).

PRIMARY AND SECONDARY PACKAGING

Primary packaging materials are in direct contact with the product. This also applies to the closure which is also part of the primary pack. It is important that this container must not interact with the medicine. It must protect the medicine from damage and from extraneous chemical and microbial contamination. In addition, the primary packaging should support use of the product by the patient. Secondary packages are additional packaging materials that improve the appearance of the product and include outer wrappers or labels that do not make direct contact with the product (Table 9.1). Secondary packages can also supply information about the product and its use. They should provide evidence of tampering with the medicine.

The following terms are used to describe containers:

Single-dose containers hold the medicine that is intended for single use. An example of such a container is the glass ampoule.

Multidose containers hold a quantity of the material that will be used as two or more doses. An example of this system is the multiple dose vial or the plastic tablet bottle.

Well-closed containers protect the product from contamination with unwanted foreign materials and from loss of contents during use.

Airtight containers are impermeable to solids, liquids and gases during normal storage and use. If the container is to be opened on more than one occasion it must remain airtight after reclosure.

Table 9.1 Types of primary and secondary packaging materials and their use

Material	Type	Examples of use
Glass	Primary	Metric medical bottle, ampoule, vial
Plastic	Primary	Ampoule, vial, infusion fluid container, dropper bottle
Plastic	Secondary	Wrapper to contain primary pack
Board	Secondary	Box to contain primary pack
Paper	Secondary	Labels, patient information leaflet

Sealed containers such as glass ampoules are closed by fusion of the container material.

Tamper-evident containers are closed containers fitted with a device that irreversibly indicates if the container has been opened.

Light-resistant containers protect the contents from the effect of radiation at a wavelength between 290 nm and 450 nm.

Child-resistant containers, commonly referred to as CRCs, are designed to prevent children accessing the potentially hazardous product.

Strip packs have at least one sealed pocket of material with each pocket containing a single dose of the product. The pack is made of two layers of film or laminate material. The nature and the level of protection that is required by the contained product will affect the composition of these layers.

Blister packs are composed of a base layer, with cavities that contain the pharmaceutical product, and a lid. This lid is sealed to the base layer by heat, pressure or both. They are more rigid than strip packs and are not used for powders or semi-solids. Blister packs can be printed with day and week identifiers to produce calendar packs. These identifiers will support patient compliance.

Tropicalized packs are blister packs with an additional aluminium membrane to provide greater protection against high humidity.

Pressurized packs expel the product through a valve. The pressure for the expulsion of the product is provided by the positive pressure of the propellant that is often a compressed or liquefied gas (see Ch. 24).

Original packs are pharmaceutical packs that are commercially produced and intended for finite treatment periods. These packs are dispensed directly to the patient in their original form. Manufacturer's information is contained on the pack but the pharmacist must attach a dispensary label.

An important consideration when selecting the packaging for any product is that its main objective is that the package must contribute to delivering a drug to a specific site of effective activity in the patient.

The selection of packaging for a pharmaceutical product is dependent on the following factors:

- The nature of the product itself: its chemical activity, sensitivity to moisture and oxygen, compatibility with packaging materials
- The type of patient: is it to be used by an elderly or arthritic patient or by a child?
- The dosage form
- Method of administering the medication
- Required shelf life
- Product use, such as for dispensing or for an over-the-counter product.

See also chapter 36 in *Pharmaceutics: the science of dosage form design* (Aulton 2002).

PACKAGING MATERIALS

Glass

Historically, glass has been widely used as a drug packaging material. It continues to be the preferred packaging material for many pharmaceutical products.

Glass does have several advantages:

- It is inert to most medicinal products
- It is impervious to air and moisture
- It allows easy inspection of the container contents
- It can be coloured to protect contents from harmful wavelengths of light
- It is easy to clean and sterilize by heat
- It is available in variously shaped containers.

The disadvantages of glass:

- It is fragile: glass fragments can be released into the product during transport or contaminants can penetrate the product by way of cracks in the container

- Certain types of glass release alkali into the container contents
- It is expensive when compared to the price of plastic
- It is heavy resulting in increased transport costs.

The chemical stability of glass for pharmaceutical use is given by the resistance of the glass to the release of soluble minerals into water contacting the glass. This is known as the hydrolytic resistance. Details are given in the BP (2001) for four types of glass.

Type I glass

This is also known as neutral glass or borosilicate glass. It possesses a high hydrolytic resistance due to the chemical composition of the glass. It is the most inert type of pharmaceutical glass with the lowest coefficient of thermal expansion. As a result, it is unlikely to crack on exposure to rapid temperature changes. Type I glass is suitable for packing all pharmaceutical preparations. However, it is expensive and this restricts its applications. It is widely used as glass ampoules and vials to package fluids for injection. In addition, it is used to package solutions that could dissolve basic oxides in the glass. This would increase the pH of the formulation and could affect the drug stability and potency.

Type II glass

This is made of soda-lime-silica glass with a high hydrolytic resistance due to surface treatment of the glass. Type II glass is used to package aqueous preparations. In general, it is not used by manufacturers to package parenteral formulations with a pH less than 7. This glass has a lower melting point than Type I glass. It is thus easier to produce and consequently cheaper. It is the glass used to produce containers for eye preparations and other dropper bottles.

Type III glass

This is made of a soda-lime-silica glass. It has a similar composition to Type II glass but contains more leachable oxides. Type III glass offers only moderate resistance to leaching and is commonly used to produce dispensary metric medical bottles. It is also suitable for packaging non-aqueous parenteral products and powders for injection.

Type IV glass

This is made of a soda-lime-silica glass with a low hydrolytic resistance. This glass must not be used to package parenteral products but it is suitable for packaging solid, liquid and semi-solid formulations.

Types of glass containers

Bottles. These are commonly used in the dispensary as either amber metric medical bottles or ribbed (fluted) oval bottles. Both types of bottle are available in sizes from 50 mL to 500 mL and are supplied with a screw closure.

Amber metric medical bottles have a smooth curved side and a flat side (Fig. 9.1). The bottle was designed to permit the curved side of the bottle to fit into the palm of the hand when pouring from the bottle. The flat side was intended to permit the attachment of a label. In practice, however, the label is commonly attached to the curved surface of the bottle. Amber metric medical bottles are used for packaging a wide range of oral medicines.

Ribbed oval bottles have flutes down one side of the container (Fig. 9.2). The characteristic feel of the flutes warns the user that the contents are not to be taken. A label is attached to the plain front of the bottle. Ribbed oval bottles are used to package various products that should not be taken orally; this includes liniments, lotions, inhalations and antiseptic solutions.

Dropper bottles. Eye drop and dropper bottles for ear and nasal use (see Fig. 26.3) are hexagonal-shaped amber glass containers fluted on three sides. They are fitted with a cap, rubber teat and dropper as the closure. The bottles are

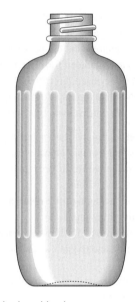

Fig. 9.2 Ribbed oval bottle.

used at a capacity of 10 mL or 20 mL. The label is attached to the plain sides of the bottle.

Jars. Powders and semi-solid preparations are generally packed in wide-mouthed cylindrical jars made of clear or amber glass. The capacity of these jars varies from 15 mL to 500 mL. Ointment jars are used for packing extemporaneously prepared ointments and pastes. They are also used to repackage commercial products where microbial contamination by the patient's fingers is not detrimental to the product.

Containers for parenteral products. Small-volume parenteral products, such as subcutaneous injections, are typically packaged in various containers made of Type I glass. Glass ampoules (Fig. 9.3) are used to package parenteral solutions intended for single use.

Multiple-dose vials (Fig. 9.4) are used to package parenteral formulations that will be used on more than one occasion. Large-volume parenteral fluids have been packaged in 500 mL glass containers but these have been largely superseded by plastic bags.

Plastics

Plastics have been widely used for several years as containers for the product and as secondary packaging in the form of a carton. In more recent times, plastic has been developed for the packaging of parenteral products including infusion fluids and small-volume injections.

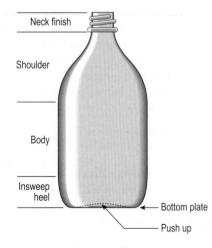

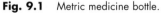

Neck finish

Shoulder

Body

Insweep heel

Bottom plate

Push up

Fig. 9.1 Metric medicine bottle.

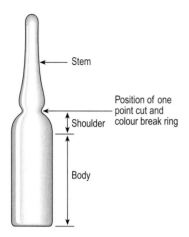

Fig. 9.3 Glass ampoule.

Labels: Stem; Position of one point cut and colour break ring; Shoulder; Body

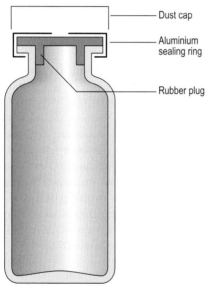

Fig. 9.4 Glass vial.

Labels: Dust cap; Aluminium sealing ring; Rubber plug

Table 9.2 The application of thermoplastic polymers for the packaging of pharmaceutical products

Polymer	Examples of application
High-density polyethylene	Solid dosage form containers
Low-density polyethylene	Flexible eye drop bottles
Linear low-density polyethylene	Heat-sealable containers
Polypropylene	Container closures, intravenous solution bottles
Polyvinyl chloride	Laminate for blister packs, intravenous bags
Polystyrene	Containers for oils and creams and solid dosage forms

Two classes of plastics are used in the packaging of pharmaceutical products. These are known as thermosets and thermoplastics. The thermosets are used for making screw caps for glass and metal containers. Thermoplastic polymers are used in the manufacture of a wide variety of pharmaceutical packages as detailed in Table 9.2.

The advantages of plastics for packaging are that they:

- Release few particles into the product
- Are flexible and not easily broken
- Are of low density and thus light in weight
- Can be heat sealed
- Are easily moulded into various shapes
- Are suitable for use as container, closure and as secondary packaging
- Are cheap.

The disadvantages of plastics are that:

- They are not as chemically inert as Type I glass
- Some plastics undergo stress cracking and distortion from contact with some chemicals
- Some plastics are very heat sensitive
- They are not as impermeable to gas and vapour as glass
- They may possess an electrostatic charge which will attract particles
- Additives in the plastic are easily leached into the product
- Substances such as the active drug and preservatives may be taken up from the product.

Plastic pharmaceutical containers are made of at least one polymer together with additives. The additives used will depend on the composition of the polymer and the production methods used.

Additives used in plastic containers include:

- Plasticizers
- Resins
- Stabilizers

- Lubricants
- Antistatic agents
- Mould-release agents.

Plastic containers

These are used for many types of pack including rigid bottles for tablets and capsules, squeezable bottles for eye drops and nasal sprays, jars, flexible tubes, strip and blister packs. The composition and the physical shape of the containers vary widely to suit the application.

The principal plastic materials used in pharmaceutical packaging

Polyethylene. This is used as high- and low-density polyethylene, both of which are compatible with a wide range of drugs and are extensively used for the packaging of various pharmacy products. Of these two forms of polyethylene, low-density polyethylene (LDPE) is softer, more flexible and more easily stretched than high-density polyethylene (HDPE). Consequently, LDPE is usually the preferred plastic for squeeze bottles. By contrast, HDPE is stronger, stiffer, less clear, less permeable to gases and more resistant to oils, chemicals and solvents. It is commonly pigmented or printed white to block light transmission and improve label clarity. HDPE is widely used in bottles for solid dosage forms.

Disadvantages of LDPE and HDPE for packaging are that they:

- Are softened by flavouring and aromatic oils
- Are unsuitable for packing oxygen-sensitive products owing to high gas permeability
- Adsorb antimicrobial preservative agents
- Crack on contact with organic solvents.

Polyvinyl chloride (PVC). This is extensively used as rigid packaging material and as the main component of intravenous bags.

Polypropylene. This is a strong, stiff plastic polymer with good resistance to cracking when flexed. As a result it is particularly suitable for use in closures with hinges which must resist repeated flexing. In addition, polypropylene has been used as tablet containers and intravenous bottles.

Polystyrene. This is a clear, hard, brittle material with low impact resistance. Its use in drug packaging is limited due to its high permeability to water vapour. However, it has been used for tubes and amber-tinted bottles where clarity

and stiffness are important and high gas permeability is not a drawback. It is also used for jars for ointments and creams with low water content.

CLOSURES

Any closure system should provide an effective seal to retain the container contents and exclude external contaminants. Child-resistant containers (CRCs) commonly consist of a glass or plastic vial or bottle with a specially designed closure. These CRCs are a professional requirement for dispensing of solid and liquid dosage forms in the UK and are ultimately a compromise between child resistance and ease of opening. They are not an absolute barrier to children accessing medicine containers, therefore the containers should be stored in a safe place. Several designs of child-resistant closures are currently used for pharmaceutical packaging, including cap–bottle alignment systems, push down and turn caps and, less commonly, squeeze and turn caps.

The closures in common use with dispensed medicines are the Snap-safe® alignment closure (Fig. 9.5) and the push down and turn Clic-loc® closure (Fig. 9.6). The Clic-loc® child-resistant closures are based on the assumption that young children are unable to coordinate two separate and dissimilar actions. That is, applying pressure and rotating the closure top. The Clic-loc® closure has a two-piece mechanism with springs between the inner and the outer parts. As a result of this design, the closure produces an audible clicking noise when the cap is turned without first being depressed. The inner cap is composed of polypropylene while the outer overcap is made of HDPE.

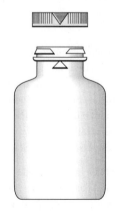

Fig. 9.5 Snap-safe® closure.

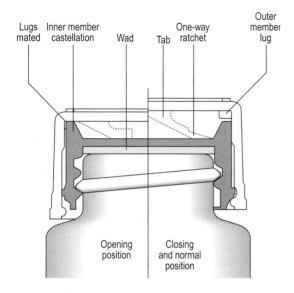

Fig. 9.6 Clic-loc® closure.

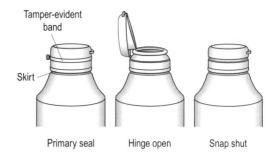

Fig. 9.7 Tamper-evident closure.

Contamination of the screw thread with crystallized sugar arising from syrups can increase the torque necessary to open these Clic-loc® closures. This type of problem can restrict their suitability for use. Owing to opening difficulties experienced by some adults, these closures should not be used on containers supplied to elderly or handicapped patients with poor manual dexterity. They should not be used when a request is made that the product is not dispensed with a child-resistant closure fitted. A Clic-loc® closure must only be dispensed on one occasion as continued use increases the penetration of moisture vapour into the container and decreases the child-resistant properties of the closure.

In recent years greater awareness of the vulnerability of products has led to the development of tamper-evident closures. The closures indicate if unlawful access to the container contents has occurred and are currently available in various designs suitable for different containers and closures. Dispensary stock containers are frequently fitted with a Jaycap® type of tamper-evident closure. These closures are made of either white polypropylene or LDPE. With this closure design the tamper-evident closures snap over a security bead on the neck of the container. The closures cannot be opened until the tamper-evident band connecting the cap to the skirt is torn away (Fig. 9.7). Clic-loc® closures are available with this design whereby an external tamper-evident coloured band must be removed before the closure can be turned. Tamper-evident inner seals are positioned within the closure and are attached to the rim of the opening

to the container isolating its contents. The seal must be torn or removed from the container to gain access to the packaged product. These seals are commonly made of a combination of paper, plastic and foil.

COLLAPSIBLE TUBES

These are flexible containers for the storage and dispensing of creams and ointments. Tubes made of tin are used to package certain sterile formulations. Typically the formulation is aseptically filled into the presterilized tubes. However, the most common metal tubes in current use are made of aluminium with an internal lacquered surface. With this package the tube remains collapsed as the product is removed. These tubes are frequently sealed at both ends and the nozzle must be punctured to access the product. An alternative seal that can be used with these packages is a heat seal band between the closure and the container. This band must be torn to gain access to the container contents.

Metal tubes are being superseded by plastic tubes made from a variety of materials. For example, the tube sleeve may be made of LDPE with either a LDPE or HDPE head or the entire tube may be made of polypropylene.

UNIT-DOSE PACKAGING

This term usually means that a single item such as a tablet or capsule or a specific dose is enclosed within its own disposable packaging. The most commonly used methods for unit-dose packaging are blister packs and strip packs.

Blister packs

These are used for packaging unit doses of tablets and capsules and can act as an aid for patient compliance. The medication is placed in a compartment in a base material made of paper, board, plastic or metal foil or a combination of these. The blister is generally composed of a thermo-formed plastic sheet such as PVC. The protection given by the plastic blister depends on its composition, design and the method used to form it. Perforations in the base material allow individual sections of the package to be broken off. Blister packages are rigid, unlike strip packs that are flexible.

Strip packaging

With strip packaging, two webs of material sandwich various types of medicine such as tablets, capsules, suppos-itories or pessaries. Each of these dosage forms is contained within its own compartment. The composition of the two webs can be selected to meet the necessary protective requirements for the medicine. Aluminium foil is commonly used to manufacture strip packs and provides a good barrier against moisture penetration. The foil is used as a laminate in which the other components add strength to the fragile aluminium foil. They also block small holes which can occur in the thinner foil layer.

PAPER

Paper is used more than any other material in packaging. Although it has an insignificant role in primary packaging it remains the predominant secondary and tertiary pack-aging material. In this role it is used as the carton which contains the primary package and, in the form of board, is the corrugated shipping container which contains both.

PATIENT PACK DISPENSING

A patient pack consists of a course of medication together with a patient information leaflet in a ready to dispense pack. Liquid formulations are supplied in a standard pack. Solid dose forms are supplied as a strip or blister pack. The size of the sealed patient pack is based on a 28, 30 or 56 dose unit appropriate to the medicine. It is supplied in this amount unless a doctor prescribes that a different quantity of medicine is to be dispensed. The patient pack contains an information leaflet as an aid to improving patient compli-ance and to supply information to patients about their medi-cation. Pharmacists should be prepared to respond to enquiries after the patient has read the leaflet. The patient pack is designed as a balance between the need for child resistance and the need for ease of opening by the elderly. If requested by the patient the pack contents can be repack-aged in a more suitable container.

Advantages of patient packs

- They contain product information such as product and manufacturer identification and the batch number.
- More efficient dispensing results in greater opportunity for patient counselling.
- More information is supplied to the patient about the product.

Disadvantages of patient packs

- Increased storage space is required.
- Elderly and debilitated patients may experience difficulty in opening the pack.

Key Points

- Containers should preserve the quality of a medicine for its stated shelf life.
- Glass has both advantages and disadvantages in use, but remains the preferred material in many situations.
- The types of glass have different uses:
  Type I for ampoules and vials
  Type II for eye preparations and dropper bottles
  Type III for metric medical bottles
  Type IV for solid, liquid and semi-solid preparations.
- Fluted bottles are used for preparations not intended to be swallowed.
- Plastics may be thermosets or thermoplastics.
- A variety of additives to plastics may enter medicines with which they are in contact.
- Child-resistant closures (CRCs) may be alignment closures (Snap-safe®) or push and turn (Clic-loc®).
- Use of CRCs is a professional requirement for dispensed medicines unless requested otherwise.
- Tamper-evident closures indicate that there has been no unlawful access to the medicine.
- Aluminium is being replaced by plastics for collapsible tubes.
- Unit dosage packaging may be either blister or strip packaging.
- The main use for paper is for cartons and boxes.
- A patient pack consists of the medicine and patient information leaflet in a ready to dispense outer pack.

10

Storage and stability of medicines

A. J. Winfield

After studying this chapter you will understand about:

The reasons for limited life of medicines
Nature of storage conditions
Expiry dates
Estimating shelf life

Introduction

Medicines do not keep indefinitely. Some can be kept for only a short time. There are many reasons why this is the case. In 1984, Rhodes listed six general causes for the limited time for which medicines can be kept. These are:

- Loss of drug (such as hydrolysis or oxidation)
- Loss of vehicle (such as evaporation of water or other volatile ingredient)
- Loss of uniformity (such as caking of a suspension or creaming of an emulsion)
- Change in bioavailability (particularly with tablets where ageing can reduce availability)
- Change of appearance (such as colour changes)
- Appearance of toxic or irritant products (as a result of chemical change).

To this list may be added changes which arise from microbiological activity.

The underlying physical and chemical processes, together with the formulation steps that can be taken to improve stability, are discussed in *Pharmaceutics: the science of dosage form design* (Aulton 2002).

It is important to recognize and be aware of the potential for instability in both manufactured and extemporaneous products. There is a need to specify storage conditions and a shelf life, to ensure effective stock control and pay attention to the packaging used in dispensing. It is also useful to be able to offer advice to a patient where a medicine has been kept at an incorrect temperature. This chapter will consider these practical implications of product instability in pharmacy practice.

STORAGE CONDITIONS

The *British Pharmacopoeia* (BP) includes storage as a heading in some drug monographs and preparations. These include phrases such as 'protected from moisture' and 'protected from light' which are described as being non-mandatory. Thus they are recommended rather than being required. With commercial products, the manufacturer will specify any special storage requirements on the packaging.

Some products require storage at low temperature. The Royal Pharmaceutical Society of Great Britain (RPSGB) publication *Medicine, Ethics and Practice—a guide for pharmacists* defines the two common requirements. A refrigerator should be between 2 and 8°C and be equipped with a maximum and minimum thermometer. A 'cool place' is between 8 and 15°C. Many pharmacies will not have a room at this temperature, so a refrigerator may be used. It is important that any special storage conditions are complied with, not only in the pharmacy, but also by patients after the medicine has been dispensed. Patients must be given adequate information about the storage of their medicines. The label should state the storage conditions required, and be backed up by a verbal reminder, especially where it is out of the normal. It should also be remembered that there are legal storage requirements in the pharmacy, such as a lockable cabinet for controlled drugs (see Appendix 1).

EXPIRY DATE

The expiry date of a medicine is the date after which it should not be used. Before a shelf life and storage conditions can be specified for a medicine, a range of chemical, physical or microbiological tests are performed. These 'accelerated stability tests' (see Aulton 2002) involve using more extreme conditions to predict behaviour under normal conditions. The results are then confirmed by a series of long-term tests. It is normal to allow the potency of a medicine to fall to 90% of its original. This figure may be varied where toxicity is increased or where an excess is added (such as the addition of a 5% overage above the amount stated on the label). Accelerated testing is time-consuming and costly, but is an important part of the development of a medicine in the pharmaceutical industry.

With extemporaneously dispensed products such methods are impractical, so a more arbitrary method of arriving at a shelf life is used. The BP (and other pharmacopoeia) uses the terms 'freshly prepared' or 'recently prepared' where preparations have a short keeping time. 'Freshly prepared' is defined as having been made no more than 24 hours before issue for use, but there is no indication of when it should be discarded. 'Recently prepared' is used for products which must be discarded 4 weeks after issue when stored at 15–25°C. Whilst the BP does not give a shelf life for 'freshly prepared' medicines an arbitrary 1-week shelf life is often given. Thus there is no indication of a desirable shelf life for an extemporaneous preparation if the monograph does not mention stability. In giving a shelf life, safety for the patient must be paramount. Some aspects of deciding shelf life for extemporaneous mixtures and diluted creams are discussed later in the chapter.

Special storage requirements apply to eye drops (see Ch. 26).

Stock control

For economic reasons, pharmacists do not like to have stock on their shelves for long periods of time. The aim is to keep stock at a level which will just meet demand. Most manufactured medicines have a long storage time so stability is not normally an issue. However, it is essential that there is efficient stock rotation, so that the older stock is used first. It is also good practice to check the expiry date as an integral part of the dispensing process. When short shelf life products are involved, stock levels may have to be modified to prevent items regularly expiring on the shelves.

Packaging

The properties of different types of packaging and containers are discussed in Chapter 9. Containers are designed to afford protection to the medicine which they contain. Part of this may be to protect from light, exclude air and moisture, prevent access of microorganisms or have other more specialized functions.

The official compendia direct to particular containers for some extemporaneous preparations. Manufacturers will have selected the packaging after extensive testing. Any repackaging which takes place during dispensing may remove this protection and reduce the shelf life of the product. Original pack dispensing of manufactured medicines is being introduced. Until it is fully implemented, pharmacists have to repackage dispensed medicines. A number of problems may arise, some of which are summarized in Table 10.1.

The pharmacist should include storage conditions on the label. The expiry date may also require to be changed. The decision about this will be based on a consideration of many factors, including the original expiry date, the specified storage condition, a knowledge of the nature of the instability, the properties of the original container and that to be used for the dispensed product, the duration of the treatment and the likely storage conditions at home or on the hospital ward. Particular care will be required if the medicine is being placed in a compliance aid or monitored dosage system where the level of protection will be much reduced. A shelf life of a few weeks only may be given to products which have a particular susceptibility to chemical, physical or microbiological change. As with any such decision, the

Table 10.1 Some of the stability issues which may arise when redispensing medicines and may cause changes to the expiry date

Change occurring	Effect produced
Access of light	Increased oxidation or photochemical degradation
Access of oxygen	Increased oxidation
Loss of vapour	Loss of water or volatile solvents
Access of microorganisms	Increased contamination, growth, spoilage and possible toxicity
Access of moisture	Hydrolysis, damage to powders, tablets and capsules

safety of the patient is of the greatest importance. The revised shelf life should be clearly indicated on the label and the patient counselled.

EXAMPLES OF STABILITY PROBLEMS

Whilst there are many examples of stability problems, three will be used as illustrations.

Glyceryl trinitrate tablets

The drug glyceryl trinitrate (GTN) is volatile and soluble in some plastics. The vapour pressure of the drug is relatively low at room temperature. This produces a saturated atmosphere within the container. If it remains tightly closed, further loss of drug would be minimal. However, if the vapour is in contact with a material which will dissolve or adsorb the drug, this is likely to occur. Plastic bottles will do this, but so too will some screw cap liners (such as cork or paperboard) and inserts used to reduce movement of the tablets on transport (such as cotton wool or synthetic fibres). In these situations, the loss of drug will be extensive. There are three further complications. One is that, if temperature fluctuates, vaporized drug can condense onto other tablets. This has been shown to cause poor content uniformity. This is most likely to happen shortly after packing and can be minimized by the addition of stabilizers to the tablets, although some of these stabilizers reduce drug stability. Secondly, because patients suffering from angina require to carry the tablets around, many transfer a few tablets to a smaller, more convenient container. These are unlikely to have an effective seal and may contain plastics and other adsorbents. Thirdly, the greatest level of loss occurs at elevated temperatures, such as are encountered when the tablets are carried close to the body.

The recommendation for GTN tablets is to avoid repackaging on dispensing. The tablets must be in glass containers, fitted with a screw cap with an aluminium or tin foil lining and with no other packing materials. They should be protected from light and kept below 25°C. A maximum of 100 tablets per container is specified. The recommended shelf life for dispensed tablets is 8 weeks.

Extemporaneous mixtures

The BP directions on freshly and recently prepared products have been discussed already. However, the actual expiry date will have to be arrived at with an awareness of all the other factors involved. These include chemical stability (such as hydrolysis or oxidation) and physical stability (such as caking of suspensions or precipitation where tinctures are included). Perhaps the main factor is the possibility of microbiological growth which can occur in aqueous medicines. Whilst many contain chloroform water as a preservative, the chloroform is volatile and growth has been observed in such systems when the chloroform has evaporated. Well-filled, well-closed containers appear not to lose much chloroform. However, regular opening of containers, as occurs in normal use, can cause the loss of a third or more of the chloroform over 4 weeks. A loss of about one-fifth would probably allow vegetative organisms to grow. The recommendation for mixtures which are preserved with chloroform is that they should be discarded 2 weeks after dispensing (Lynch et al 1977).

Diluted creams

Creams, being aqueous, are prone to microbial growth. Protecting creams is difficult because of the partitioning of preservatives between the aqueous and oily phases and micelles (see Ch. 20 and Aulton 2002). Dilution of a cream, apart from possibly introducing organisms, can also inactivate the preservative system present through incompatibility, dilution or changes in partition coefficient. The BNF recommends that dilution be avoided. Where it is necessary, only the diluent recommended by the manufacturer should be used. The dilution should be freshly prepared and a 2-week expiry date should be applied.

ESTIMATING SHELF LIFE

Occasionally a product which should have been stored in a refrigerator will have been left at room temperature for a time. It is useful for the pharmacist to be able to advise the patient of a revised expiry date. The manufacturer may be able to give advice. When contact is made, record the query, the advice, the date and the name of the contact in case there is a subsequent problem.

In 1989 the Q_{10} value was recommended as a way of estimating the remaining shelf life. The method is not accurate, but using a 'worse case' approach can give an approximate time if other approaches have failed to give an answer.

Key Points

- Storing in a cool place means 8–15°C and storing in a refrigerator means at 2–8°C.
- Shelf life is normally the time that a medicine can be kept before the potency has fallen to 90% of the original.
- Expiry date is calculated from the shelf life at the time of preparation.
- Extemporaneous preparations often have to be given arbitrary shelf lives.
- 'Freshly prepared' is defined in the BP as prepared no more than 24 hours before issue.
- 'Recently prepared' is defined in the BP as discarded after 4 weeks.

- Dispensing may inadvertently involve shortening the shelf life of a product in view of its susceptibility to chemical, physical or microbiological challenge.
- Glyceryl trinitrate tablets must be dispensed in glass containers with a metal foil cap liner, protected from light, and stored below 25°C with fewer than 100 per container. The shelf life is 8 weeks.
- Preparations made with chloroform water as preservative should normally have a shelf life of 2 weeks.
- Cream dilutions should be avoided, but if prepared a 2-week shelf life is used.
- The Q_{10} value is a method for estimating shelf life following inappropriate storage.

Labelling of dispensed medicines

A. J. Winfield (original author M. M. Moody)

After studying this chapter you will know about:

The reasons for having labels
Requirements for labels:
 Producing labels
 Standard details required on labels
 Additional labels
Specific legal requirements

Introduction

The label on dispensed medicines has two main functions. One is to uniquely identify the contents of the container. The other is to ensure that patients have clear and concise information which will enable them to take or use their medicine in the most effective and appropriate way.

There are both legal (UK and EU) and professional requirements which must be complied with when labelling a dispensed medicine. It is the pharmacist's responsibility to ensure that these requirements are satisfied and that all labelling is accurate and comprehensible. The regulations indicate standard details which must appear on every label. In certain circumstances additional details are also required. Useful sources of information are 'Medicines, Ethics and Practice' and the *British National Formulary* (BNF). It should also be noted that provision of an adequate label does not remove the need to counsel the patient.

STANDARD REQUIREMENTS FOR LABELLING DISPENSED MEDICINES

All labels must be typewritten or computer generated. Most labels are now computer generated. This should mean that the information on the label is legible; however, there have been reports of labels which were unreadable because the printer was not working properly (e.g. worn ribbon). If this type of printer is used check the ribbon regularly to make sure that the print is clear. Equally replace ink or toner cartridges as soon as required. Remember it is easier to read what is on a poorly printed label when you know what is supposed to be there. The patient may not be able to do so!

In summary the details which must appear on the label of a dispensed medicine are:

- The name of the preparation
- The quantity
- Instructions for the patient
- The patient's name
- The date of dispensing
- The name and address of the pharmacy
- 'Keep out of reach of children'.

Additional labelling requirements

- Warning or advisory labels should be attached to the container, where appropriate.
- A batch number should be indicated if the preparation has been prepared extemporaneously.
- An expiry date should be indicated if the preparation has been prepared extemporaneously or the shelf life has been shortened, e.g. a diluted preparation.
- Additional legal requirements, e.g. 'For animal treatment only' on veterinary prescriptions.

The name of the preparation and the quantity

The name which appears on the label must be the same as the one which appears on the prescription. The preparation may be prescribed generically but only be available as a proprietary or branded product; however, the prescribed name must be used. The reason for this is to avoid the patient becoming confused with a variety of names.

The letters NP on a prescription stand for 'nomen proprium'—the proper name of the medicine. Occasionally a prescriber may not wish the name of the preparation to appear on the container. To indicate this they will delete the NP instruction on the prescription. In these cases the type of medicine, i.e. 'the tablets', 'the mixture', should replace the name of the product.

Another occasion when the name may be omitted is when the product contains several active ingredients and has no official or proprietary name and it would be extremely difficult to list all the ingredients on the label. In these instances the pharmaceutical form is used, i.e. 'the ointment', 'the mixture'.

If the preparation is available in more than one strength, the strength must be included on the label.

Normally the quantity which appears on the label will be the quantity which has been prescribed. However, in some cases multiple packs are required to complete a prescription. In these instances, when more than one container of the same medicine is dispensed, the quantity on the label should be the amount in each container.

The instructions

No patient should leave a pharmacy without knowing how much, how often and how to use his or her medication. Although the label should be seen as a back up to the verbal counselling and advice given by the pharmacist, it is still essential to ensure that the wording on the label is clear, concise and comprehensible to the patient. The prescriber's instructions should therefore be translated into an appropriate form. If instructions are missing or incomplete it is the

pharmacist's professional duty to obtain instructions from the prescriber or use professional discretion to interpret BNF statements on dosage.

The way in which instructions are worded is very important and will greatly influence how easily a patient understands the message. Pharmacists should therefore give serious consideration to the wording on medicine labels.

The Royal Pharmaceutical Society Working Party Report (1990) on 'The labelling of dispensed medicines' made several recommendations. The use of active verbs is preferred, i.e. 'take' instead of 'to be taken', 'apply' instead of 'to be applied'. The reason is that research has shown that active verbs are more easily understood and remembered than passive verbs. It is bad practice to have two numbers appearing together in instructions, e.g. 'take two three times daily'. It is easy for a patient to mentally transpose the position of the numbers so that the previous instruction becomes 'three twice daily' in the patient's mind. To avoid this the numbers should *always* be separated by using the formulation name, e.g. 'take two tablets', 'two capsules', 'two powders three times daily'. Other Working Party recommendations can be seen in Table 11.1.

Numbers which are part of an instruction must always be written as words except in the case of 5 mL, when referring to a 5 mL spoonful, or oral syringe quantities, e.g. a 2.5 mL dose using the oral syringe provided.

The patient's name

It is a legal requirement that the name of the patient for whom the medication has been prescribed must appear on the label of all dispensed medicines. If possible, the status

Table 11.1 Recommended wording for directions	
Recommended wording	**Wording to be replaced**
Do not swallow	Not to be taken
Take 'x' times a day, spaced evenly through the day. (This wording was considered preferable for antibiotics. For analgesics it remains desirable to use the previous wording)	Take every 'y' hours
Put two drops in the affected eye	Instil two drops in the affected eye
For creams or ointments:	
Spread thinly	Use sparingly
For pessaries or suppositories:	
Gently put one into the vagina/rectum	Insert one into the vagina/rectum
Patient information leaflets: where appropriate, reference should be made to the patient information leaflet for instructions on how the product should be used	

of the patient, i.e. Mr, Mrs, Miss, Master, Child or Baby should be included in order to clearly differentiate from other members of a household, where there may be persons with the same name. For the same reason a full first name should also be included, if possible, rather than an initial, e.g. Mr James Burnett instead of J. Burnett.

The date and name and address of the pharmacy

The majority of pharmacies use computer systems for prescription labelling and this information will normally appear automatically, with the date being re-set daily.

'Keep out of reach of children'

Virtually all labels for use with typewriters and computer labelling systems come pre-printed with 'Keep out of reach of children' but it is always worth checking that this is the case. Any pharmacist who issues a dispensed medicine without this warning on the label is guilty of contravening the Medicines Act.

ADDITIONAL LABELLING REQUIREMENTS

In addition to the standard details required on all dispensed medicines there are several extra details which are required in certain circumstances.

Additional information specific to a particular type of formulation

Storage

General information for different types of preparation can be found in the relevant chapters in this book. Some formulations require special storage and this information should be attached to the label, e.g. transdermal patches should be stored in a cool place. Any specific pharmaceutical precautions relating to storage should always be indicated. Information on proprietary medicines can be accessed in the Association of British Pharmaceutical Industries (ABPI) *Medicines Compendium.*

Warnings for patients

Ideally, any liquid preparation should state 'Shake the bottle' and 'For external use only' is a legal requirement on external liquid and gel preparations.

Many drugs cause side effects about which the patient should be informed. Information on these can be found in Appendix 9 of the BNF (note: appendix number may change with edition). It is a professional requirement, subject to the pharmacist's discretion, that if indicated, these special warnings should be affixed to the container. Nowadays most computer systems will automatically print these warnings when a label for a particular drug is being produced. However, there are instances when use of this information is inappropriate and professional discretion should be used. For example, the antihistamine chlorphenamine (chlorpheniramine) requires the warning: 'Warning. May cause drowsiness. If affected do not drive or operate machinery. Avoid alcoholic drink.' Young children may be prescribed a drug such as this but this warning would be inappropriate. Obviously it is important to draw attention to the problem of sedation and in this case the more suitable warning 'Warning. May cause drowsiness' could be used. If a doctor does not wish the warning labels to appear, the prescription should be endorsed 'NCL' (no cautionary labels).

Some of the BNF warning labels have been known to cause confusion, such as numbers 5, 6, 7, 11 and 14. All of these may require additional explanation to be given to the patient.

Label number 5: 'Do not take indigestion remedies at the same time of day as this medicine'.

Label number 6: 'Do not take indigestion remedies or medicines containing iron or zinc at the same time of day as this medicine'.

Label number 7: 'Do not take milk, indigestion remedies or medicines containing iron or zinc at the same time of day as this medicine'.

Some patients misunderstand the information on these three labels and think that milk, iron preparations and indigestion remedies must not be taken at all. It should be explained to the patient that as long as there is an interval of approximately 2 hours between taking the medicine and any of the remedies there is not a problem.

Label number 11: 'Avoid exposure of skin to direct sunlight or sun lamps'.

There have been reports of patients who were frightened to venture outside when taking medication which carried this warning. Again an explanation that as long as exposed areas of skin are adequately covered, e.g. a long-sleeved shirt or a sunhat to shade the face, the patient should not suffer any ill effects.

Label number 14: 'This medicine may colour the urine'.

It is useful to give the patient an indication of the colour, e.g. phenolphthalein (pink), levodopa (dark reddish) or rifampicin (red).

A batch number

When a product has been prepared extemporaneously it is good practice to award it a batch number and incorporate this onto the label. This is standard practice in hospital pharmacy. When preparing an extemporaneous product, details of the ingredients used should be recorded. The batch number allows referral back to this information and assists pharmacists in complying with the Consumer Protection Act (see Appendix 1).

Expiry date

It is not normally necessary to put an expiry date on the label of a dispensed medicine, although with the increasing dispensing of manufacturers' original packs this information will be part of the pack labelling. Manufacturers' expiry dates relate to ideal storage conditions but, unfortunately, when a product has been dispensed and given to the patient there is no longer any control over how it is stored. For this reason, under current legislation, when a product is repackaged for dispensing no expiry date is stated. Patients should be encouraged to complete the course of medication or, if for any reason, a supply is not finished and is no longer required, to bring any remainder back to the pharmacy.

There are, however, specific occasions when an expiry date must be added to the label.

- An expiry date should always be put onto any extemporaneously prepared item.
- An expiry date should always be used when a product has been diluted, thereby affecting the stability and shelf life.
- An expiry date should always be indicated when the preparation is sterile, e.g. eye drops. Once opened the product is no longer sterile and if used beyond a certain timescale there is a serious risk of infection. It is therefore recommended that eye drops and eye ointment, unless otherwise specified by the manufacturer, should be discarded 4 weeks after opening. This instruction should be indicated on the label (see Ch. 26 for further details).

- Glyceryl trinitrate tablets lose their efficacy owing to the volatility of the active ingredient and an expiry date must be attached to the container (see Ch. 10). The tablets must be disposed of 8 weeks after the container is first opened.

Although the majority of patients will understand what 'expiry date' means it is important to express the information in a clear and unambiguous way. 'Any unused to be discarded on ... (date)' or 'Do not use after ... (date)' are preferred methods of expressing expiry dates.

LEGAL REQUIREMENTS IN CERTAIN CIRCUMSTANCES

Veterinary dispensed products

The words 'For animal use only' or similar must always be added to the label of a dispensed veterinary product. Instead of the patient's name the name of the animal's owner should appear, along with the owner's address or address where the animal lives.

Emergency supply

When a preparation is dispensed using the emergency supply procedures (see Appendix 1) the words 'Emergency supply' must appear on the label.

Private prescriptions

A label for a medicine dispensed from a private prescription must bear a reference number. This reference number will relate to the entry in the private prescription register and will also be endorsed on the private prescription.

ERRORS

The potential for making errors when producing a label is considerable and it is important that constant checking is carried out. Practice procedures should be such that the chances of errors occurring are minimized (see Ch. 6). One of the commonest ways that errors occur is reading what we think is on a label, not what is actually there. Dispensing is usually carried out in a busy environment with many distractions and it takes considerable effort to maintain the 100% concentration required to ensure that errors do not occur.

Apart from errors in interpreting prescribers' instructions or missing off any of the details already mentioned, the advent of computerized labelling has brought its own problems, two of which will be mentioned.

Patient's name

When using a computer system, if a patient presents a prescription for several items, the patient's name is typed in once and the number of items to be dispensed bearing that patient's name is entered. Occasionally an item may not be dispensed or the number of items may be entered incorrectly. This means that when the next prescription for a different patient is to be dispensed, the name of the first patient will occur on the label even if all the other information is correct.

Transposition of labels

It is not uncommon that two labels have been produced on the pharmacy computer and two medicines have been prepared. At this point the labels could be applied to the incorrect container unless care is taken.

An awareness of how easily these errors can occur is at least one step to ensuring that they do not happen.

Key Points

- A label is used to identify and instruct on the use of a medicine, so simple language should be used.
- All labels must be typewritten or computer generated.
- All labels must state the name and quantity of the preparation, patient's name and instructions, name and address of pharmacy, date of dispensing and 'Keep out of reach of children'.
- Warning labels may also be required.
- Active verbs should be used on the label.
- Adjacent numbers should be separated by the formulation name, e.g. 'take two tablets three ... ' on a label.
- As full a name of the patient as possible should be included on the label.
- The BNF contains details of side effect warnings which should be used unless there is a good reason not to do so.
- Some warning labels may require verbal explanation.
- It is good practice to give an extemporaneous preparation a batch number.
- Expiry dates are required on the label when dispensing diluted, sterile and extemporaneous preparations and for glyceryl trinitrate tablets.
- Computer labelling systems can increase the risk of some types of error.

SELF-ASSESSMENT QUESTIONS

1. The following NHS prescription was received:

   Tabs Ibuprofen 400 mg
   Mitte 60
   one t.i.d.

   The name of the patient was Mrs Marjory Nicol. Comment on the accuracy of the following labels produced for this prescription. (Assume that the name and address of the pharmacy and 'Keep out of the reach of children' are included.)
   a. 60 Tabs Ibuprofen
      Take one tablet three times daily with or after food
      Mrs Marjory Nicol   [12/5/03]
   b. 60 Tabs Ibuprofen 400 mg
      Take one three times daily with or after food
      Mrs Marjory Nicol   [12/5/03]
   c. 60 Tabs Ibuprofen 400 mg
      Take one tablet three times daily with or after food
      M Nicol   [12/5/03]
   d. 60 Tabs Ibuprofen 400 mg
      One to be taken three times daily with or after food
      Mrs Marjory Nicol   [12/5/03]
   e. 60 Tabs Ibuprofen 400 mg
      Take three tablets daily with or after food
      Mrs Marjory Nicol   [12/5/03]

2. The following NHS prescription is received:

   Betnovate Ointment Half Strength
   Mitte 50 g
   Sig. apply to affected area m. et n.
   Mr James Hill   [12/5/03]

   Comment on the following label:

   50 g Betnovate Ointment Half strength
   Apply to affected area morning and night
   Mr James Hill   [12/5/03]

3. You will need to consult Appendix 9 in the BNF to complete this exercise.

   Using the BNF, indicate the cautionary and advisory labels which should appear on the following products. Are there any where you consider additional information may need to be given?
   a. Tildiem Retard tablets
   b. Ledermycin capsules
   c. Solpadol caplets
   d. Madopar capsules.

SELF-ASSESSMENT ANSWERS

1. a. The strength of the drug has been omitted from the label. This will cause problems of identification.
   b. The instructions have been written with the number of tablets and the dose frequency together, i.e. 'Take one three times…'. This is bad practice and may lead to errors in dosing.
   c. The status of the patient and first name have not been included, i.e. M Nicol instead of Mrs Marjory Nicol.
   d. The passive form of the verb has been used, i.e. 'to be taken'. The active form 'take' is the preferred form.
   e. The instructions are not clear. Although the patient has been told the correct number of tablets to take in a 24-hour period, information about frequency is missing. This will lead to loss of efficacy and a possible increase in the incidence of adverse effects.

2. This preparation has been diluted, i.e. Betnovate ointment, 25 g and 25 g of recommended diluent. This has affected the stability and consequently the shelf life so an expiry date should have been indicated on the label. The manufacturer's recommendation is a shelf life of 14 days. This preparation is for external use and the label should have indicated this.

3. a. Tildiem Retard tablets require:

   Label 25: 'Swallowed whole, not chewed'.

   This is a reasonably simple instruction but the patient's attention should be drawn to it and an explanation of why it is necessary given. The modified release of the preparation will be destroyed if the tablets are crushed or chewed.

b. Ledermycin capsules require:

   Label 7: 'Do not take milk, iron preparations or indigestion remedies at the same time of day as this medicine'.
   Label 9: 'Take at regular intervals. Complete the prescribed course unless otherwise directed'.
   Label 11: 'Avoid exposure of skin to direct sunlight or sun lamps'.
   Label 23: 'Take an hour before food or on an empty stomach'.

   The main problem here is the considerable amount of information. The patient's understanding of the information should be checked and further explanation given if necessary.

c. Solpadol caplets require:

   Label 2: 'Warning. May cause drowsiness. If affected do not drive or operate machinery'.
   Label 29: 'Do not take more than 2 at any one time. Do not take more than 8 in 24 hours'.
   Label 30: 'Contains paracetamol'.

   Again there is a considerable amount of information given, all of which is important. The pharmacist should alert the patient to the paracetamol warning and explain that other paracetamol-containing preparations should not be taken.

d. Madopar capsules require:

   Label 14: 'This medicine may colour the urine'.
   Label 21: 'Take with or after food'.

   Reinforcement of dosing in relation to food intake should be given if the pharmacist considers it necessary. If the patient has not received the medication before, an indication that the urine colour will be reddish should be given.

Principles and methods of sterilization

R. M. E. Richards

After studying this chapter you should be able to:

**Define: sterility; sterilization; aseptic
techniques; sterility testing; parametric
release; disinfection; disinfectant; antiseptic**

**Explain: bioburden; death rates; sterility
assurance level/probability of survival
concepts; *D* value; *Z* value; *Q* value**

**Discuss *F* values and the concept of lethality
in relation to heat-sensitive products**

**Discuss sterilization in relation to validation
and monitoring**

Describe factors affecting sterilization

**Explain the moist heat sterilization process
for pharmaceuticals, dressings and
equipment**

**Explain the dry heat sterilization process for
pharmaceuticals and equipment**

**Compare and contrast the advantages and
disadvantages of the two heat sterilization
processes**

**Explain the functioning of the equipment
used in moist and dry heat sterilization**

Describe sterilization by filtration

**Discuss two other methods for sterilizing
pharmaceuticals, dressings and equipment**

GENERAL PRINCIPLES OF STERILIZATION

Introduction

Pharmaceutical products are generally required to be free
from contamination with microorganisms (bacteria, viruses,
yeasts, moulds, etc.). Such organisms may cause spoilage by
adversely affecting the appearance or composition of a
product and may cause serious adverse effects in the patient.
Adverse effects are particularly likely if the preparation is
introduced into the body via a route which bypasses some
of the body's normal defence mechanisms, especially in a
seriously ill or immunocompromised patient.

Dosage forms designed for parenteral, ophthalmic or surgical use, as well as irrigation solutions and topical preparations for application to large open wounds, must be free
from microbial and particulate contamination. These products are required to be prepared and maintained in a sterile
state until used. Some of the terms used in connection with
'sterile pharmaceutical products' are defined below.

Sterility

Sterility may be defined as the total absence of viable
microorganisms and is an absolute state. The production of
sterile pharmaceutical products may be achieved by aseptic
technique (see Ch. 13) or by means of a terminal sterilization process, as described later in this chapter.

Sterilization

This is the subjection of products to a process whereby all
viable life forms are either killed or removed. The sterilization process is usually the final stage in the preparation of the
product. The methods of sterilization in regular use include
exposure to: saturated steam under pressure, dry heat, ionizing radiation, ethylene oxide or passage through a bacteria-
retaining filter. When possible, exposure to saturated steam
under pressure is the sterilization method of choice.

Aseptic technique

This is the preparation of pharmaceutical products from
sterile ingredients by procedures that exclude the access of
viable microorganisms into the products. It is used for those
products that would be adversely affected by being subjected to a sterilization process.

Sterility testing

This is end-product testing for the sterility of pharmaceuticals to reveal the presence or absence of viable microorganisms in a sample number of containers taken from a production batch. From the results of such tests an inference is made as to the sterility of the batch.

Parametric release

This terminology has been used since the mid 1980s. Parametric release is a sterility release procedure which is based on effective control, monitoring and documentation of a completed cycle of a validated sterilization process. It recognizes that such a procedure provides greater assurance of the finished product meeting specification than end product sterility testing. An EC Working Party on Control of Medicines and Inspections (2001) defined parametric release as 'A system of release that gives the assurance that the product is of the intended quality based on information collected during the manufacturing process and on the compliance with specific good manufacturing practice requirements related to parametric release.'

Disinfection

Disinfection is a process which aims to reduce the number of harmful (pathogenic) microorganisms in a particular situation. Disinfection will destroy infective vegetative organisms but not necessarily resistant spores, i.e. it is not an absolute process. It often involves the use of chemicals, although other means of disinfection may be employed, e.g. the pasteurization of milk is a disinfection process that uses heat.

Disinfectant. This is a chemical agent used to destroy harmful microorganisms usually on inanimate objects.

Antiseptic. An antiseptic is a chemical agent usually applied to living tissues in humans or animals in order to destroy harmful microorganisms.

STERILIZATION CRITERIA

The bioburden

In order to select the appropriate parameters for any method intended to kill microorganisms in a given product or associated with a given material, it is necessary to know the initial number of organisms present. That is the 'bioburden' or 'bioload', and the resistance of those organisms to the chosen process. For example, it has been the practice to

choose the time and temperature relationship for steam sterilization to ensure that a large number of the known most resistant pathogens would be killed. This treatment would not necessarily be sufficient to kill a large number of the known most resistant non-pathogenic organisms. However, it is extremely unlikely that such an organism would be present in pharmaceutical solutions immediately before sterilization. The time and temperature chosen for such a steam sterilization process is greatly in excess of the treatment necessary to kill the small number of heat-sensitive contaminants likely to be present in these pharmaceutical solutions.

Establishing microbial death

Death in a microbial population is determined by assessing the reduction in the number of viable microorganisms resulting from contact with a given destructive force. Viable organisms are those which, when transferred to a culture medium, can form a colony. This places the onus on the investigator to provide suitable culture conditions for recovery and growth of any surviving microorganisms.

Death rates

When a population of microorganisms is subjected to a destructive sterilization procedure the order of death is generally logarithmic. That is, a constant proportion of the microbial population is inactivated in any given time interval, approximating to first-order kinetics.

A typical survivor curve is shown in Figure 12.1. It can be represented as follows:

$$\log N_t = \frac{-t}{D + \log N_0}$$

$$\text{i.e. } \log N_0 - \log N_t = \frac{t}{D}$$

where N_0 is the initial number of organisms, N_t is the number of organisms surviving after exposure time t and D is the microbial death rate (the time required for 90% kill).

From Figure 12.1 it can be seen that where $N_0 = 10^6$ and $N_t = 10^2$, then $t = 10$.

Substituting in the equation we have:

$$\log 10^6 - \log 10^2 = \frac{10}{D}$$

$$(6 - 2) \times D = 10$$

$$D = 2.5$$

Since k, the death rate constant, is the reciprocal of D

$$k = 0.4.$$

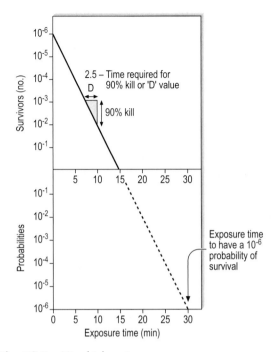

Fig. 12.1 Microbial survivor curve.

The determination of death rate provides the facility to compare the resistance of the same organism at different temperatures or to compare the resistance of different organisms to the same lethal agent, e.g. temperature, ionizing radiation, chemical agent, etc. Death rates may also be used to give a quantitative measure of the effect of environmental factors such as pH, osmolarity and the presence of various chemicals on the sterilization process. Since the same percentage of bacteria dies each minute, it is impossible in theory to reach a point of zero survivors. From Figure 12.1 an extension of the process to 30 minutes would give the assurance that the probability of survival of one member of the original population would be 10^{-6}. This is referred to as a sterility assurance level (SAL) of 10^{-6}. In terms of containers of solution this would mean a probability of not more than one container in a million being contaminated with one microorganism. An SAL of 10^{-6} or better is the aim in terminal sterilization by moist and dry heat and radiations.

The concept of percentage reduction of a bacterial population reinforces the need for as small a bioburden as possible when a product is to be sterilized.

The methods that are used to prepare sterile fluids ensure that the bioburden is very low (see Ch. 25). If containers are filled through a bacteria-proof filter prior to sterilization the bioburden is effectively zero.

D value or decimal reduction time

The death rate can also be expressed as the decimal reduction time or D value. This is the time in minutes at any defined temperature to destroy 90% of viable organisms. In Figure 12.1 this is 2.5 minutes. Numerically it is also the reciprocal of the death rate constant, k. D values are often given a subscript to indicate the temperature at which they were measured, e.g. $D_{121°C}$. From the D value for a particular combination of organism/time/temperature an 'inactivation factor' (IF) can be calculated, e.g. if the D value of an organism exposed to a temperature of 121°C for 15 minutes was 2 minutes the IF would be $10^{15/2}$, i.e. $10^{7.5}$.

Z value or thermal destruction value

This relates the heat resistance of a microorganism to changes in temperature. The Z value is the number of degrees of temperature change required to produce a 10-fold change in D value. Bacterial spores have a Z value in the range 10–15°C, while most non-sporing organisms have Z values of 4–6°C.

Q value or temperature coefficient

This also gives a measure of the relative resistance of different microorganisms and describes the change in the death rate over a 10°C change in temperature.

F values

The F value is a measure of the lethality of the total process of sterilization and equates heat treatment at any particular temperature with the time in minutes at a designated reference temperature that would be required to produce the same lethality in an organism of stated Z value. For a temperature of 121°C and organisms with a Z value of 10°C F becomes F_0. Annex 2 of Appendix XVIII of the *British Pharmacopoeia* (BP 2001) contains the following description of F_0: 'The F_0 value of a saturated steam sterilization process is the lethality expressed in terms of the equivalent time in minutes at a temperature of 121° delivered by the process to the product in its final container with reference to microorganisms possessing a Z value of 10.'

An F unit is equivalent to heating the load for 1 minute at 121°C. Mathematically F is defined as:

$$F_0 = 10^{(Tc-121/Z)}\, dt$$

where Tc = load temperature at time dt and Z = 10°C.

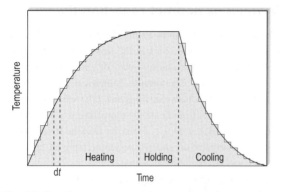

Fig. 12.2 The time–temperature recording of a typical autoclave cycle showing the method of integration by dividing the time axis into a series of segments (d*t*). (From Kirk et al 1982.)

For many years it has been understood that both the heating up and cooling phases of a heat sterilizing cycle contribute to the total lethality of the process. The F principle allows an estimation of the overall lethality by integration of the lethal rates multiplied by the times at discrete temperature intervals (Fig. 12.2).

The total lethality (F_0) for the cycle is equal to the sum of the F_0 values for each individual time/temperature segment. The accuracy of the estimated F_0 is related to the time interval represented by each segment of the profile. Small intervals are conveniently handled by computer. A total F_0 value of not less than 8 applied to every container in the load would be considered satisfactory. Where the product is especially heat sensitive an F_0 of less than 8 is deemed justifiable. Nevertheless it is necessary to demonstrate continually with vigorous microbiological monitoring that for each validated set of conditions the sterilizing process chosen gives a sterility assurance level of not less than 10^{-6}.

STERILIZATION, VALIDATION AND MONITORING

Tests for sterility of the products subjected to a sterilization procedure are discussed in Chapter 14. Whenever possible additional validation and monitoring of the sterilization process is also carried out. This may be done by using indicators other than the product. Biological, chemical and physical indicators have all been used.

Biological indicators

Biological indicators are supplied in one of two main forms, each of which incorporates a viable culture of a stated species of microorganism. One form consists of spores added to a carrier such as a disc or strip of filter paper, glass or plastic, so packaged as to protect the contents before use but to allow the sterilizing agent to reach the spores and exert its effect during use. In the other form the spores are added to representative units of the product to be sterilized or to similar units if it is not practicable to add the spores to selected units of a particular product.

Choice of the biological indicator is critical if the indication given is to be a valid reflection of the efficacy of a sterilization cycle. The viability of the organisms, the storage conditions before use and the incubation and culture conditions after sterilization must be standardized for the result to be meaningful. Gaseous sterilization effectiveness must be checked for each manufacturing batch sterilization cycle using a suitable biological indicator.

Organisms used as biological indicators include:

Bacillus subtilis var. niger—dry heat: ethylene oxide
Bacillus stearothermophilus—steam
Bacillus pumulis—ionizing radiation.

The biological indicator must be so chosen as to provide a greater challenge to the sterilization process than the natural bioburden of the product. The strain must also be non-pathogenic and easy to culture.

Biological indicator for sterilization by filtration

The type of filter chosen must have been shown to be satisfactory by means of a microbial challenge test using a suitable test microorganism. Certain strains of *Pseudomonas diminuta* have been shown to be suitable. The integrity of each assembled sterilizing filter must also be verified in situ before use and confirmed after use (see 'Physical validation and monitoring' below).

Chemical indicators

These are commercially available and are used to indicate whether a particular batch of product has been through a sterilization process; they do not generally indicate whether the process was successful. The indicator chosen undergoes some change in physical or chemical nature when exposed to the conditions of the sterilization process.

Heat-sensitive tape

The Bowie–Dick test is valuable for confirming that steam has displaced all the air from a porous load in a high vacuum autoclave. It consists of using autoclave tape which has heat-sensitive bars, at intervals of about 15 mm, which change colour after contact with steam. The tape is placed suitably wrapped at the centre of a test pack. All the bars on the tape should change colour to demonstrate full penetration of the steam. Duration of exposure or temperature attained is not indicated by this type of indicator.

Chemical dosimeters

These are used to monitor the quantity of the radiation dose in the use of radiation sterilization. Qualitative indicators of exposure to radiation are also available.

Physical validation and monitoring

A master process record (MPR) must be prepared as part of the validation procedure for a particular autoclave (or hot air oven) and for each specified product and load configuration. The MPR is then used as a reference to compare with the process record of each manufacturing batch sterilization cycle, known as the batch process record (BPR). This is automatically recorded on a temperature/time chart or digital printout. The BPR is kept together with the batch manufacturing record to provide evidence that the particular batch has been subjected to the validated sterilization cycle. BPR temperature is sensed from a thermocouple placed in the coolest part of the load.

The MPR should be checked at annual intervals and whenever significant changes occur in the BPR when compared with the MPR. In addition it is also necessary that the equipment is subject to a fully documented programme of planned preventative maintenance (PPM). This is to ensure that the equipment is maintained at the same level of operation as at the time of process validation.

In practice all records associated with the sterilization process are kept. In addition to the aforementioned documents, this includes data on bioburdens and D values, the results obtained with chemical and biological indicators and the F_0 value for each sterilization cycle. Medicines inspectors would expect to be provided with this data for scrutiny.

Microprocessor-controlled sterilization cycles are now a part of modern autoclaves and provide a very tight control and description of sterilization cycles.

Bubble point test for filters

The bubble point of a test filter is the pressure at which the largest pore of a wetted filter is able to pass air. The pressure varies with the surface tension of the liquid with which the filter is wetted. Details for carrying out the test are usually described in the relevant manufacturer's literature.

The generally accepted and widely used methods of sterilization will now be considered.

MOIST HEAT STERILIZATION

The sterilization method of choice for aqueous preparations and for surgical dressings is heating in saturated steam under pressure. A number of time–temperature combinations have been proposed. The BP and EP (2001) recommend 121°C maintained throughout the load for 15 minutes as the preferred combination for this method of terminal sterilization.

Principles of sterilization by steam under pressure

Moderate pressure as used in steam sterilization has no sterilizing power. Steam is used under pressure as a means of achieving an elevated temperature. It is important to ensure that steam of the correct quality is used in order to avoid the problems which follow incorrect removal of air, superheating of the steam, failure of steam penetration into porous loads, etc.

Steam production

This may be achieved in two ways. On a small scale, steam may be generated from water within the sterilizer and because water is present the steam is known as wet saturated steam. For large-scale sterilizers, dry saturated steam may be piped from a separate boiler.

Saturated and supersaturated steam

Steam is described as saturated when it is at a temperature corresponding to the liquid boiling point appropriate to its pressure. Important properties of saturated steam are illustrated by reference to Figure 12.3.

The phase boundary is obtained by joining points representing saturated steam temperatures at different pressures, e.g. 115°C at 172 kPa (1.7 bar), 121°C at 202 kPa (2 bar) and 134°C at 304 kPa (3 bar). In Figure 12.3 if saturated

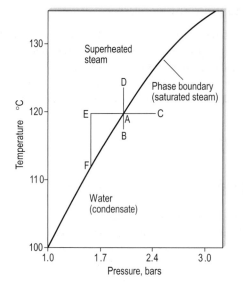

Fig. 12.3 Phase diagram for water and steam.

steam at A is isolated from water and heated without change of pressure from A to D, or the pressure is lowered without change of temperature from A to E, then the steam must become hotter because there is no water from which further evaporation can occur. Therefore it is no longer at the temperature corresponding to the liquid boiling point appropriate to its pressure and it is called superheated steam. Superheat is to be avoided because as steam becomes more superheated it becomes more like hot air and therefore less effective as a sterilizing medium. Very slight cooling will not make superheated steam condense. Before this can occur the temperature must be reduced to the temperature of the corresponding saturated steam point. That is from D to A or from E to F on Figure 12.3. Superheated steam can arise from several sources but sterilizer jacket heat is the predominant source and is caused when the jacket is hotter than

the steam in the chamber. This is a practical consequence of the theory outlined above. In this example the problem arises because the system has, in effect, moved to point D in Figure 12.3. To prevent it, care should be taken to ensure that the jacket and the chamber temperatures are similar.

Now consider again the saturated steam at point A. As soon as the steam is cooled at constant pressure, e.g. from A to B, it will deposit water. (The same would happen if the pressure were raised to point C without alteration of temperature.) The condensation of saturated steam on cooling liberates all of its latent heat immediately. This is a very important property in sterilization.

Heat energy in steam is in the form of 'sensible heat' and 'latent heat'. Sensible heat is the heat required to raise the temperature of water, and latent heat (of vaporization) is the amount of heat required to convert water at its boiling point to steam at the same temperature. Table 12.1 illustrates the high percentage of total heat that is latent heat at various temperatures.

The advantages of saturated steam include:

- *Penetration*. It flows quickly to every article in the load (and into porous articles). This is due to its contraction to a very small volume on condensation creating a low-pressure region into which more steam flows.
- *Rapid heating*. It heats the load rapidly owing to the release of its considerable latent heat.
- *Moist heat*. The condensate produced on cooling contributes to the lethality by coagulating microbial protein.
- *No residual toxicity*. The product is free from toxic contamination.

Presence of air

Air occupies the space in the sterilizer before steam is generated or admitted and air is also present dissolved in water before its conversion to steam. Any air remaining in the

Table 12.1	Heat content of steam at various pressures				
Pressure (lbf/in²(g))	Temperature (°C)		Heat		
		Sensible (kJ/kg)	Latent (kJ/kg)	Latent to total (%)	
10	115–116	483	2216	82	
15	121–123	505	2202	81	
20	126–129	530	2185	80	
'Gauge' (g) = in excess of atmospheric pressure.					

sterilizer forms a thin layer which clings to every surface on which steam condensation occurs. Since air is a poor conductor it provides a barrier to heat penetration. Therefore effective air removal from sterilizers is vital.

Wet steam

Wet steam contains less heat than dry saturated steam and is harmful to dressings.

THE DESIGN AND OPERATION OF AUTOCLAVES

The word autoclave means self-closing. Originally this referred to the closing of the lid by the excess pressure within the vessel. Modern usage of the word is rather wider and it is often used for modern sterilizing equipment which is not necessarily self-closing.

Large sterilizers

The essential features of a large sterilizer are shown diagrammatically in Figure 12.4 and will be used in the following general description. While the basic features are common to all types of sterilizer, the manufacturer's literature should be consulted for details of the features of a particular model.

General procedure

- Load material to be sterilized and close door
- Remove air
- Admit dry saturated steam (venting and condensate removal automatic)
- Allow for heating up and expose for required duration
- Cut off steam supply
- Allow to cool (or spray cool if appropriate).

These steps are now discussed below in turn.

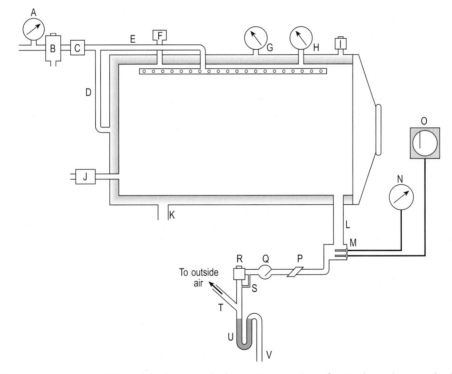

Fig. 12.4 Diagrammatic representation of the features of a large steam sterilizer (for simplicity, the control valves have been omitted). A, Mains pressure gauge; B, separator; C, reducing valve; D, steam supply to jacket; E, steam supply to chambers; F, air filter; G, jacket pressure gauge; H, chamber pressure gauge; I, jacket air vent; J, vacuum pump; K, jacket discharge channel (detail not shown); L, chamber discharge channel; M, thermometer pocket; N, direct-reading thermometer; O, recording thermometer; P, strainer; Q, check valve; R, balanced-pressure thermostatic trap; S, bypass; T, vapour escape line; U, water seal; V, air-break.

Loading

This should be carried out so that heat distribution within the load is optimal and will vary with the type of load, e.g. bottles, plastic containers, dressings, etc.

Remove air

This may be achieved through downward displacement by admitting steam at the top of the sterilizer and allowing air to escape through the discharge channel L in Figure 12.4. An alternative method is to apply a high vacuum (2.5 kPa, 25 mbar) to remove the air before the entry of the steam. This is particularly useful for porous loads since it aids steam penetration.

Admit dry saturated steam

In order to reduce the moisture content of steam delivered from the boiler the steam is passed through a separator (B in Fig. 12.4) which collects suspended condensate. The reducing valve, C, lowers the pressure to the required level and in doing so effects further drying.

Special requirements for plastic containers. For plastic containers there is an additional requirement for an over-pressure inside the autoclave chamber to prevent the containers from bursting during the sterilization cycle. The excess chamber pressure required will depend on the type and design of the container and the amount of air remaining inside the container after filling.

Automatic removal of condensate. Large volumes of condensate are produced, particularly during the heat-up cycle. Condensate runs down to the bottom of the chamber and drains through the same discharge channel as the air (L in Fig. 12.4). A check valve and trap are incorporated to prevent suck-back contamination of the chamber on cooling.

Exposure for required temperature–time cycle

The recommended holding time–temperature relationship is 121°C for 15 minutes. Other possible time–temperature relationships are given in Table 12.2. Whichever is chosen it must be such as to give an SAL of 10^{-6} or better and must be carefully monitored as described under 'Physical validation and monitoring'.

Cut off steam supply

This is done by closing the appropriate control valve.

Allow to cool

The method used for cooling depends on the type of load.

Fluid containers. Fluid containers cool very slowly because of their large heat capacity and the containers may burst if the sterilizer is opened at too high a temperature. Cooling time may be reduced by using a very fine mist of cold water (50–100 micrometres diameter droplets) sprayed over the containers. Table 12.3 shows the time savings with forced cooling. Compressed air is admitted to the bottom of the chamber to compensate for the pressure drop caused by the condensation of steam. For plastic containers spray cooling must take place with an excess pressure outside the bag in order to avoid bursting. Problems may arise if the spray water is contaminated and/or if the closures of the fluid containers are rendered ineffective by the sterilization process.

In Holland autoclaves which are heated by very hot water under pressure and cooled by the same water after it has passed through a suitable heat exchanger have been commissioned. The water is introduced through many small holes at the top of the autoclave and removed from the bottom of the autoclave. The pressure within the autoclave is maintained at a slightly higher pressure than the calcu-

Table 12.2	Possible time/temperature relationships for saturated steam sterilization			
Temperature (°C)	Corresponding nominal pressure (lbf/in²(g))	Minimum holding (min) time	Lethality (F_0)	
115–116	10	30	7.5–15	
121–123	15	15	15–30	
126–129	20	10	32–63	
'Gauge' (g) = in excess of atmospheric pressure.				

Table 12.3 Time for contents to fall from 115°C to 95°C		
Load	Without water cooling	With water cooling
24 × 500 ml bottles	3 h	10 min
200 × 1 litre bottles	22 h	17 min

lated pressure within the glass bottles or plastic containers. It is important with this type of autoclave to monitor the rate of water flow through the autoclave to check that it is maintained within the desired range.

Figure 12.5 represents the autoclave pressure (highest recorded line on the graph), hottest container temperature (second highest line), coldest container temperature (the lowest recorded line), together with the lethality for each of these temperatures. The record is produced in multicoloured graphical form by a linked microcomputer. This graph then forms the batch process record (BPR).

Porous loads. Porous loads are wet at the end of the exposure period due to absorbed condensate and must be dried. This is best achieved by application of high vacuum. A vacuum pump is used to remove the steam and to reduce the pressure to 2.5 kPa (25 mbar) in about 3 minutes. Under these conditions the moisture content of the dressings is only slightly greater than before sterilization.

The air used for breaking the vacuum after drying must be sterile.

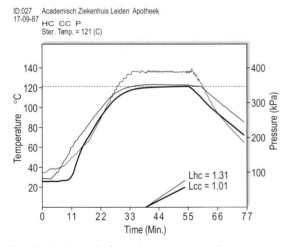

ID:027 Academisch Ziekenhuis Leiden Apotheek
17-09-87
HC CC P
Ster. Temp. = 121 (C)

Lhc = 1.31
Lcc = 1.01

Fig. 12.5 Record of autoclave pressure and container temperature during a sterilization cycle. Lcc, lethality for coldest container; Lhc, lethality for hottest container.

Hydrostatic continuous sterilizers

The need for the production of large batches of sterilized fluids has led to the development of continuous sterilizers. Containers are fed automatically onto an endless conveyor that carries them up and down a series of towers which are 17 m high. The containers are subjected in turn to preheating, sterilizing, water cooling and spray cooling before leaving the sterilizer.

Automatic control of steam sterilizers

Most large sterilizers are operated under automatic control and may offer a series of 'programmes' for different types of load. It is essential that pressure and temperature recordings are checked for each cycle to ensure that no malfunction has occurred and that the selected conditions have been achieved.

DRY HEAT STERILIZATION

This process may be used for heat-stable non-aqueous preparations, powders and certain impregnated dressings. It may also be used for some types of container.

Sterilization by dry heat is usually carried out in a hot-air oven in which heat is transferred from its source to the load by radiation, convection and to a small extent by conduction.

Published evidence on the temperature–time exposures necessary to kill pathogens by dry heat indicates that 90 minutes at 100°C will destroy all vegetative bacteria but that 3 hours at 140°C is needed for resistant spores. Mould spores are of intermediate resistance and are killed by 90 minutes at 115°C. Most viruses have a resistance similar to vegetative bacteria but some viruses are known that are as resistant as bacterial spores, e.g. the virus that causes homologous serum jaundice.

Recommended time–temperature combinations

The *British Pharmacopoeia* (2001) recommends a minimum temperature of 160°C for at least 2 hours. Other combinations of temperature and time are permissible subject to first demonstrating a reproducible level of lethality in routine operation that achieves an SAL of 10^{-6} or better.

Dry heat treatment at greater than 220°C provides a useful method for sterilization and depyrogenation of glassware, in particular containers intended for large-volume parenteral dosage forms. The method chosen should be shown to cause a 3-log reduction in heat-resistant endotoxin.

In each cycle it is important to ensure that the whole of the contents of each container is maintained for an effective combination of time and temperature and especially to allow for temperature variations in hot-air ovens, which may be considerable.

Design and operation of the dry heat sterilizer

Ovens suitable for dry heat sterilization should be specially designed for the purpose and equipped with forced air circulation (Fig. 12.6). It is recommended that the sterilizer be maintained at a positive pressure and all air entering the chamber should be via a bacteria-proof filter. Only a small amount of the heat is transferred from the heat source to the articles in a hot-air oven by conduction, because of the limited pathways and small areas of contact. Convection is responsible for more heat transfer but this is not a very efficient process. Maximum use of the heating capacity of the air is made by circulating it with a fan in order to have the maximum number of air molecules collide with the load and hot chamber surfaces (Fig. 12.7). In addition, pockets of stagnant cool air are prevented.

Radiation is the chief form of heat transfer and this is why the heaters need to be arranged all round the chamber. It is useful to have the oven fitted with the facility for automatic boost heating to give minimum heat-up times. Accurate temperature control by easily set regulators is essential. The loaded oven temperature variation should not exceed 5°C once the sterilizing temperature is reached.

The method of validating sterilization cycles has been given (see p. 127).

It is important to reduce the heating-up time to a minimum, partly for economy, but chiefly to prevent excessive overheating of the outer regions of materials and preparations during the time that heat is penetrating to their centres. The best way is to use small containers through which the heat will be transferred quickly, even if the containers are poor conductors. A wise upper weight limit for substances such as powders and oils is 25 g. It is best to load

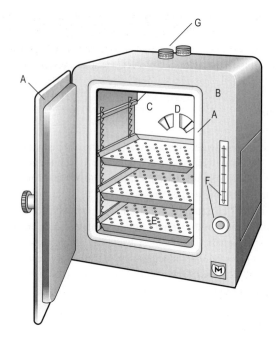

Fig. 12.6 Hot-air oven. A, Asbestos gasket; B, outer case containing glass-fibre insulation, and heaters in chamber wall; C, false wall; D, fan; E, perforated shelf; F, regulator; G, vents.

the oven with only one type of material in one size and type of container. The walls of the container should be as thin as practicable and of good heat-conducting material, e.g. metal rather than glass for powders. Tins should be blackened or dull to absorb and not reflect heat and, as a general rule, all

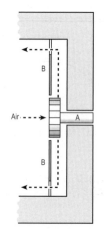

Fig. 12.7 Section of rear of an oven showing forced air circulation produced by a fan. A, Fan; B, false back.

containers should be either both tall and narrow (e.g. a long cylindrical tin) or shallow and very wide (e.g. a Petri dish) so that heat can penetrate rapidly in one direction. Glassware must be cleaned thoroughly because heat transfer will be impaired if the surface is coated with a greasy film.

Because articles sterilized by dry heat are not often used immediately, precautions must be taken to ensure that they are sterile when used. For example, glass pipettes, because they are dipped in sterile liquids, must be externally as well as internally sterile and therefore they are completely wrapped in paper or packed in tubes of card, metal or glass. Items such as glass vessels need protection at the mouth only and this can be given with a metal cap. Containers of products to be sterilized are sealed with a screw cap having a suitable liner.

After suitable packaging the containers are arranged on the oven shelves taking the following into account.

- Spacing to allow air movement, radiation from the oven walls to reach the product and to prevent contact of articles with the sides of the oven.
- Packing of small items in large tins should be avoided. The air inside the tin cannot escape from the tin easily and acts as an efficient insulator of the contents. It is better to wrap such things as Petri dishes in twos or threes.
- Screw caps should be loosened half a turn to prevent distortion of the closure and to prevent the possibility of having the container burst.

The time is noted when the temperature recorder shows that the oven air has reached the required temperature and the appropriate exposure is subsequently given to include lag time and sterilization time. After switching off, the door is left closed until the temperature has fallen to 40°C in order to prevent breakages. The bottle caps are tightened.

A dry heat oven should have a door lock or accidental openings of the door may occur. Automatic control is easy to achieve, consisting of a suitable device to start the timing when the required temperature is reached and to switch off the heating after the appropriate exposure, including lag time, has been given. A record of the temperature and time should be available for each sterilization cycle.

APPLICATIONS OF HEAT STERILIZATION

Moist heat

Dry saturated steam under pressure is used in the sterilization of the following:

- *Aqueous parenteral solutions and suspensions*: 121°C for 15 minutes is recommended.
- *Surgical dressings and fabrics*: 134°C for 3 minutes is recommended.
- *Plastic and rubber closures*: if sterilized separately from the containers.
- *Metal instruments*: immediate drying required to protect against corrosion.
- *Glass apparatus and containers*: if unable to withstand dry heat, e.g. rubber parts.

Dry heat

Dry heat is used to sterilize:

- *Glassware*: prewashing in apyrogenic water is required.
- *Porcelain and metal equipment*.
- *Oils and fats*: including oily injections.
- *Powders*: including natural products, e.g. talc, which may contain resistant spores. Severe heat treatment will destroy pyrogens, e.g. in sodium chloride.

Advantages and disadvantages of moist heat and dry heat sterilization

As a result of reading this chapter so far you should be able to construct a table summarizing the relative advantages and disadvantages of saturated steam and dry heat for sterilization processes.

ALTERNATIVE METHODS FOR THE DESTRUCTION OF MICROORGANISMS

Alternative methods to heat sterilization must be employed for heat-labile materials. Sterilization by filtration, gaseous sterilization and sterilization by ionizing radiations are possible alternatives.

Sterilization by filtration

Sterilization by filtration is a method permitted by the *British Pharmacopoeia* (2001) for solutions or liquids that are not sufficiently stable to withstand the process of heating in an autoclave. Passage through a filter of appropriate pore size (e.g. 0.22 micrometre pore size membrane filter) can remove bacteria and moulds although viruses and mycoplasms may not be retained. After filtration the liquid is aseptically distributed into previously sterilized containers which are then sealed. This method has the disadvantages that specialized facilities and skilled operatives are required and the final preparation cannot be released until the manufacturing batch has passed the appropriate test for sterility. Sterilization by filtration also carries a greater potential risk of failure due to equipment or operator technique than other methods of sterilization.

Membrane filters

These are the preferred type of filter for sterilization. Membrane filters are made from cellulose derivatives or other polymers and there are no loose fibres or particles. The retention of particles larger than the pore size occurs on the filter surface, which also makes this type of filter particularly useful in the detection of small numbers of bacteria in sterility testing (see Ch. 14).

Advantages of membrane filters
- Rigid structure—unaffected by bubbles or pressure surges
- High flow rates—80% of filter surface consists of pores
- Do not shed fibres
- Minimal absorption—concentration unaffected
- Minimal wastage—little retention of solution
- Testable prior to and after filtration.

Although reusable membrane filters are available, the disposable types are generally preferred.

The use of a prefilter. Membrane filters are generally blocked by particles which are near in size to the pore size of the filter. Prefiltration reduces the risk of blockage of the final filter. Since the filtration method of sterilization carries a potentially greater risk of failure than other methods, a second filtration through a sterilized membrane filter provides an additional safeguard.

Gaseous sterilization

Gaseous sterilizing agents are of two main categories, oxidizing and alkylating agents. Vapour phase hydrogen peroxide is an example of the former. Ethylene oxide and formaldehyde are examples of the latter. However, the *British Pharmacopoeia* states that gaseous sterilization is only to be used where there is no suitable alternative. The main advantage of ethylene oxide is that many types of materials, including thermolabile materials, can be sterilized without damage. The gas can diffuse through packaging materials and containers made of paper, fabrics, a range of plastics and rubber and diffuse out again after sterilization.

It has the disadvantages of being toxic and combustible and it requires the correct humidity. In practice the relative humidity in the chamber atmosphere is usually between 40 and 50% with temperatures up to 6°C. An appropriate sample of each manufacturing batch must be tested for sterility.

Low-temperature steam with formaldehyde has been used in northern Europe as an option for sterilizing thermolabile substances.

Both ethylene oxide and formaldehyde have health risks and strict monitoring of personnel exposed to the gases is required to ensure protection from harm. In general it can be concluded that steam sterilization should be used in preference to gaseous sterilization wherever practicable.

Sterilization by radiations

Radiations can be divided into two groups—electromagnetic waves and streams of particulate matter. In the former group are infrared radiation, ultraviolet light, X-rays and gamma rays. In the latter group are alpha and beta radiations. Infrared radiation, ultraviolet light, gamma radiation and high-velocity electrons (a type of beta radiation) are used for sterilization.

Ultraviolet light

Only a narrow range of wavelength (220–280 nm) is effective in killing microorganisms, and wavelengths close to 265 nm are the most effective. This is because wavelengths of 265 nm and adjacent wavelengths are strongly absorbed by nucleoproteins. The most serious disadvantage of ultraviolet light as a sterilizing agent is its poor penetrating power. This is the result of strong absorption by many substances. Applications are therefore limited to treatment of clean air, water in thin layers and hard impermeable surfaces in situations where people are not subjected to either direct or high-intensity reflected radiation. This latter precaution is necessary because bactericidal ultraviolet light damages eyesight and produces erythema of the skin.

Thus in general ultraviolet light should not be relied on for sterilization.

Ionizing radiations

Ionizing radiations suitable for commercial sterilization processes must have good penetrating power, high sterilizing efficiency, little or no damaging effect on irradiated materials and be capable of being produced efficiently. The radiations that best fulfil these four criteria are high-speed electrons from machines and gamma rays from radioactive isotopes. Sterilization by gamma rays is the more common in the UK and is carried out using the radioactive isotope of cobalt, ^{60}Co, as the source of gamma emission at specialized irradiation plants.

Articles for sterilization by radiation are packed in boxes of standard size which are suspended from a monorail and sterilized by a series of slow passages around the gamma ray source. The reference absorbed dose for sterilization is 25 kGy (BP 2001).

Mode of action. Ionizing radiations can cause excitations, ionizations and, where water is present, free radical formation. Free radicals are powerful oxidizing (OH, HO$_2$) and reducing (H) agents which are capable of damaging essential molecules in living cells. Thus all three processes cause disintegration of essential cell constituents such as enzymes and the DNA. This results in cell death.

Undesirable effects. Radiation sterilization appears an attractive method for thermolabile medicaments and equipment because the rise in temperature caused by a sterilizing dose is very small—about 4°C. However, the Association of British Pharmaceutical Industries' (ABPI) investigation on the effects of radiation on pharmaceutical products (Report of a Working Party established by the ABPI 1960) led to the conclusion that in many instances 25 kGy produces changes that may make the preparation unacceptable for administration or presentation.

Undesirable effects include chemical decomposition, immediately or after storage, and alterations in colour, texture and solubility. Potency changes range from nil or almost nil (e.g. certain antibiotics and steroid hormones) to serious loss (e.g. insulin, posterior pituitary hormones and cyanocobalamin). Alterations in colour are common and, although sometimes there is no associated loss in activity, the preparation is less acceptable for sale. Because of the indirect effect of radiation, destruction is often greater when substances are irradiated in solution (e.g. heparin).

Ordinary types of clear glass become brown. Special glasses that are unaffected have been developed but are expensive. Silicone rubber is very resistant but butyl and chlorinated rubbers are degraded.

It is inadvisable to resterilize irradiated articles without careful investigation of possible adverse effects. For example, repeated irradiation of certain dressings and plastics causes degradation, as does autoclaving of cellulosic materials that have been subjected to gamma radiation previously. In addition, some radiation-sterilized products become toxic if exposed to ethylene oxide gas.

Applications of radiation sterilization

Articles regularly sterilized on a commercial scale include plastic syringes and catheters, hypodermic needles and scalpel blades, adhesive dressings, single-application capsules of eye ointment and catgut. Containers made of polythene and packaging materials using aluminium foil and plastic films may also be sterilized by radiation.

Key points

Factors affecting sterilization
- Relating to the bioburden:
  Initial number of organisms
  Their heat resistance
  Recovery and growth requirements.
- Relating to the sterilization process:
  Method chosen
  Sterility assurance level/probability of survival concepts
  Overall lethality
  Validation and monitoring
  Documentation of all sterilization process data.
- Relating to the product:
  Solubility
  pH and nutritive properties
  Heat stability
  Moisture stability.
- Relating to the container:
  Suitability to withstand process chosen
  Suitability to protect/maintain sterility and not interact with the product
  Suitability for transport and storage of product.

Methods of sterilization
- Two major means of sterilization:
  Heat sterilization—consists of moist heat and dry heat sterilization
  Non-heat methods of sterilization—consist of sterilization by filtration, gases and by radiations.
- Moist heat sterilization is method of choice for:
  Heat-stable aqueous preparations
  Surgical dressings.
- Moist heat has the following advantages:
  Penetration—due to contraction on condensing
  Rapid heating—due to the release of latent heat on condensation
  Moisture—the condensate contributes to lethality by coagulation of microbial protein
  No residual toxicity.

- Autoclaves are used to provide the moist heat sterilization conditions.
- The United States Pharmacopoeia, British Pharmacopoeia and European Pharmacopoeia recommend 121°C maintained throughout the load for 15 minutes as the preferred sterilization time–temperature combination. This is the temperature of saturated steam at 15 lb/in^2 (g).
- Dry heat sterilization in the hot air oven is the method of choice for:
  Heat-stable non-aqueous preparations
  Powders
  Certain impregnated dressings
  Glass containers and certain equipment.

- The BP recommended time–temperature combinations for dry heat sterilization are:
  160°C for not less than 2 hours.
- Sterilization by filtration is used for liquids which will not withstand heat sterilization methods. It usually involves:
  0.22 micrometre membrane filters
  Validation of the integrity of the filtration system
  Product validation by sterility testing (see Ch. 14).
- Ethylene oxide is a useful 'non-heat' method of sterilization for thermolabile materials.
- Ionizing radiations are suitable for commercial sterilization of articles which for some reason are not readily sterilized by other methods (plastic containers).

13

Sterile production areas

D. G. Chapman

After studying this chapter you will know about:

The requirements for sterile production
Grades of clean areas
Design and operation of clean areas
Isolators
Environmental monitoring.
Preparation of aseptic products

Introduction

The production of sterile medicinal products has special requirements. These products must be produced in conditions that ensure that they are pure. They must also be free from viable organisms and have limited or ideally no particulate contamination. It is thus important that only carefully regulated and tested procedures are used to manufacture sterile products.

Owing to their special manufacturing requirements, sterile medicinal products are prepared in special facilities known as clean rooms. These rooms are designed to reduce the risk of microbial and particulate contamination at all stages of the manufacturing process.

The clean area used to produce sterile products is commonly designed as a suite of clean rooms. With this system, the operators enter the clean rooms by way of a changing room. Within this area the operators put on clean room clothing before entering into the clean rooms. The changing room has a lower standard of environmental quality. A clean room with a lower environmental standard is also used to prepare solutions. These solutions are then sterilized by filtration before being transferred into the filling room. The clean room used to fill and seal the product containers is the highest quality of clean room. This will reduce the risk of product contamination.

Sterile products that are marketed in the European Union must be produced in conditions which conform with the details in the revised Annex 1 of Volume IV of 'The Rules Governing Medicinal Products in the European Community'. These manufacturing conditions for sterile products in the revised Annex 1 were implemented in January 2002. It contains the standards to which pharmaceutical clean rooms should be built and used.

STERILE PRODUCT PRODUCTION

Production of sterile products should be carried out in a clean environment with a limit for the environmental quality of particulate and microbial contamination. This limit for contamination is necessary to reduce the risk of product contamination. In addition, however, the temperature, humidity and the air pressure of the environment should be regulated to suit the clean room processes and the comfort of the operators.

Clean areas for the production of sterile products are classified into grades A, B, C and D. These grades are categorized by the particulate quality of the environmental air when the clean area is operating in both a 'manned' and 'unmanned' state. In addition, these are graded by the microbial monitoring of the environmental air, surfaces and operators when the area is functioning. The standards are shown in Tables 13.1 and 13.2.

There are two common procedures used to manufacture sterile products. The first method involves the preparation of products that will be terminally sterilized. The second method involves the aseptic filling of containers that are not exposed to terminal sterilization. Aseptic filling requires a higher environmental quality for the preparation of solutions and the filling of containers. The qualities of the clean rooms used for these production procedures are detailed in Tables 13.3 and 13.4.

Table 13.1   Airborne particle contamination for manned and unmanned clean rooms

Grade	Maximum number of particles per cubic metre equal to or above the size indicated			
	Clean room at rest		Clean room operating	
	0.5 μm	5 μm	0.5 μm	5 μm
A	3500	0	3500	0
B	3500	0	350 000	2000
C	350 000	2000	3500 000	20 000
D	3500 000	20 000	Varies with procedure	Varies with procedure

Table 13.2   Limits for microbial contamination of an operating clean room

Grade	Viable organisms per cubic metre of air	90 mm settle plate per 4 hours	55 mm contact plate	Glove print (5 fingers)
A	<1	<1	<1	<1
B	10	5	5	5
C	100	50	25	Not applicable
D	200	100	50	Not applicable

Table 13.3   Conditions for preparing terminally sterilized products

Procedure	Required standard before terminal sterilization
Preparation of solutions for filtration and sterilization	Grade C is used for products which support microbial growth. Grade D acceptable if solutions subsequently filtered
Filling small and large volume parenterals	Grade C. For products with a high risk of contamination such as wide-necked containers a Grade A laminar airflow workstation with Grade C background
Preparation and filling of ointments, creams, suspensions and emulsions	Grade C

Table 13.4   Conditions for the production of aseptically prepared products

Procedure	Required standard
Handling of sterile starting materials	Grade A with Grade B background or Grade C if solution filtered later in production process
Preparation of production solutions	Grade A with Grade B background or Grade C if sterile during filtered production
Filling of aseptically prepared products such as small and large volume parenterals	Grade A with Grade B background
Preparation and filling of ointments, creams, suspensions and emulsions	Grade A with Grade B background

PREMISES

High standards are necessary for the manufacture of sterile medicinal products. The sterile production unit must be separated from the general manufacturing area within the hospital pharmacy or factory. This sterile production unit must not be accessible to unauthorized personnel.

The unit is designed to allow each stage of production to be segregated. It should also ensure a safe and organized workflow and reduce the need for personnel to move around the clean rooms. The unit is built and the equipment positioned to protect the product from contamination. The layout must allow efficient cleaning of the area and avoid the build up of dust. Premises are also arranged to decrease the risk of mix up or contamination of one product or material by another.

The filling room is typically serviced from an adjacent preparation room. This allows supporting personnel to assemble and prepare materials. Staff within the filling room area then use these materials. Figure 13.1 shows the layout of rooms for the production of terminally sterilized medicines such as small or large volume injections.

Design and construction

Access to clean and aseptic filling areas is limited to authorized personnel. Operators enter clean rooms by way of changing rooms. Within the changing room the operators can don and remove their clean room garments.

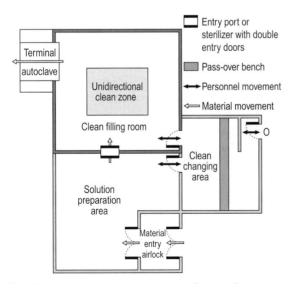

Fig. 13.1 Rooms for the production of terminally sterilized medicines.

A low physical barrier, commonly known as a pass-over (or cross-over) bench, extends across the changing room. It forms a physical barrier that separates the different areas for changing by the operators.

Special precautions are needed to avoid contamination of clean and aseptic filling areas when materials are passed through airlocks or hatchways. Thus, sterilizers and entry ports are fitted with double-sided doors. The doors are interlocked to prevent both doors being opened simultaneously.

Surfacing materials

All clean room surfaces including the floors, walls and ceilings should be smooth, impervious and unbroken. This will decrease the release and build up of contaminating particles and organisms. The surfaces are made of materials that allow the use of cleaning agents and disinfectants. The ceilings are sealed to prevent the entry of contaminants from the space above them. Uncleanable recesses within the clean room should be avoided. This will reduce the collection of contaminating particles. Thus, the junction between the wall and the floor is commonly coved. The presence of shelves, ledges, cupboards and equipment is minimized. Windows should be non-opening and sealed. This will prevent the ingress of contaminants.

Services

Piped liquids and gases should be filtered before entering the clean room. This will ensure that the liquid or gas at the work position will be as clean as the clean room air. The pipes and ducts must be positioned for easy cleaning. All other fittings such as fuse boxes and switch panels should be positioned outside the clean rooms.

Sinks and drains must be excluded from areas where aseptic procedures are performed in clean room areas. They should be avoided in the whole unit wherever possible. In areas where sinks and drains are installed they must be designed, positioned and maintained to decrease the risk of microbial contamination. They are thus often fitted with easily cleanable traps. The traps may contain electrically heated devices for disinfection.

There should be a limited number of entry doors for personnel and ports for materials. Entry doors should be self-closing and allow the easy movement of personnel.

Airlock doors, wall ports, through-the-wall autoclaves and dry heat sterilizers should be fitted with interlocked doors. This will prevent both doors being opened simultaneously. An alarm system should be fitted to all the doors to prevent the opening of more than one door.

Lights in clean rooms are fitted flush with the ceiling to reduce the collection of dust and avoid disturbing the airflow pattern within the room. Similarly, equipment should be positioned in clean rooms to avoid the distribution and the collection of particles and microbial contaminants.

ENVIRONMENTAL CONTROL

Potential sources of particles and microbial contaminants occurring within the clean room are:

- The air supply of the room
- Inflow of external air
- Production of contaminants within the room.

Each of these possible sources can be minimized as described below.

Air supply

The air supply to a Grade A, B or C clean room must be filtered to ensure the removal of particulate and microbial contamination. This is carried out by filtering the air with high-efficiency particulate air (HEPA) filters. The HEPA filter should be positioned at the inlet to the clean room or close to it. A prefilter may be fitted upstream of the HEPA filter. This will prolong the life of the final filter. A fan is required to pump the air through the filter.

The HEPA filters use pleated fibreglass paper as the filter medium. Parallel pleats of this filter material increase the surface area of the filter and increase the airflow through the filter. This structure allows the filter to retain a compact volume. Aluminium foil is used to form spacers in the traditional type of HEPA filter. Spacers are not used in the more modern 'mini-pleat' type of filter design. These mini-pleat filters are now widely used. They have a shallower depth in construction than the traditional HEPA filter. Within the structure of the filter, the filter material is sealed to an aluminium frame (Fig. 13.2). At least one side of the filter is protected with a coated mild steel mesh. HEPA filters exhibit:

- A high flow rate
- High particulate holding capacity
- Low-pressure drop across the filter.

HEPA filters remove larger particles from the air by inertial impaction, the medium-sized particles by direct interception and the small particles by Brownian diffusion. The HEPA filters are least efficient at removing particles of about

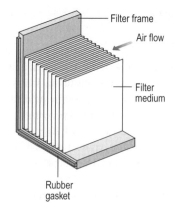

Fig. 13.2 Section through a mini-pleat high-efficiency filter, showing its construction.

0.3 μm. However, the efficiency of removing particles is affected by the air velocity and the filter packing. Larger and smaller particles will be removed more efficiently.

With a new HEPA filter fitted in a clean room, the air exits from the filter face at a rate of about 0.45 m/s and has a 99.997% efficiency at removing 0.3 μm particles. The initial pressure difference across the depth of the filter is about 130 Pascal (Pa). At the end of the effective life of the filter the pressure drop across the filter will increase to about 490 Pa. To retain the operating efficiency of the filter, the fan forcing air through the filter must be able to maintain this pressure difference. Sensors are fitted upstream and downstream of the filters to indicate the pressure differential across the filter. An automatic alarm system should be fitted to indicate failure in the air supply or filter blockage.

The HEPA filters for clean room use must conform with the British Standard 5295 (1989) aerosol test. The filters may have faulty seals and can be damaged during delivery or installation. It is thus important that they are tested in situ before use.

The filter material possesses a uniform resistance and is constructed with a large number of parallel pleats. This results in the air downstream of the filter face flowing uniformly with a unidirectional configuration.

The number of air changes in clean rooms is affected by:

- The room size
- The equipment in use
- The number of operators in the area.

In practice 25–35 air changes per hour are common. The airflow pattern within the clean room must be carefully regulated to avoid generating particles from the clean room floor and from the operators. Various options for ventilating clean rooms may be categorized by the airflow pattern within the room. These are:

- Unidirectional airflow systems
- Non-unidirectional airflow systems
- Combination airflow systems.

Unidirectional airflow systems

Air enters the room through a complete wall or ceiling of high-efficiency filters. This air will sweep contamination in a single direction to the exhaust system on the opposing wall or floor (Fig. 13.3). In the interests of economy, the exhaust grill may be fitted low down on the wall. The velocity of the air is about 0.3 m/s in down-flow air from ceiling filters and 0.45 m/s in cross-flow air. These are highly efficient airflow systems. However, one major disadvantage of these rooms for pharmaceutical use is that they are expensive to construct. They also use much more conditioned air than rooms with non-unidirectional airflow. This greatly increases their operating costs. Owing to these factors, unidirectional airflow clean rooms are not often used for pharmaceutical purposes.

Non-unidirectional airflow systems

Air enters the clean rooms through filters and diffusers that are usually located in the ceiling. It exits through outlet ducts positioned low down on the wall or in the floor at sites remote from the air inlet (Fig. 13.4). With the use of this system, the filtered inlet air mixes with and dilutes the contaminated air within the room. As the clean room air has been previously heated and cleaned it can be recirculated to save energy, a little fresh air being introduced with each air change cycle.

Various designs of diffuser are used with this ventilation system. These affect the air movement and the cleanliness of the rooms. The perforated plate diffuser produces a jet flow of air directly beneath it. This jet of air will carry contamination at its edges. However, it does produce high-quality air directly under the diffuser. It is thus important that production procedures are located directly below the diffuser. By contrast, the air released from the bladed diffuser will mix with the clean room air. This diffuser thus produces a reasonably constant quality of air throughout the room.

Combination systems

In many pharmaceutical clean rooms it is common to find that the background area is ventilated by a non-unidirectional airflow system. Meanwhile, the critical areas are supplied with high-quality air from unidirectional airflow units.

The combination airflow system is often selected for pharmaceutical clean room applications as it:

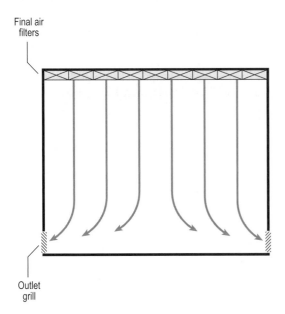

Fig. 13.3 Airflow pattern in a unidirectional airflow clean room.

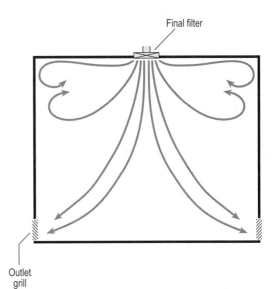

Fig. 13.4 Airflow pattern in a non-unidirectional airflow clean room.

- Produces controlled room pressure
- Separates the manufacturing process from the general clean room
- Is cheaper to use.

Several types of unidirectional flow workstations or benches are used in this combination-type room. Various vertical unidirectional airflow systems are used in combination clean rooms. With one system, the critical area is surrounded by a plastic curtain with vertical unidirectional downflow air 'washing' over the manufacturing process and exiting under the plastic curtains into the general clean room area (Fig. 13.5). An alternative system is often used with the small-scale combination-type clean room in hospital pharmacies. With this system, a horizontal airflow cabinet (Fig. 13.6) is used as the workstation. With these cabinets, a fan forces air through a HEPA filter located at the rear wall of the workstation. The air that exits from the filter firstly washes over the critical work area before washing over the arms and upper body areas of the operator. Contamination arising from the operator is thus kept downstream of the critical procedures. Grade A environmental conditions are achieved at the critical work area. A similar workstation known as a vertical laminar airflow cabinet (Fig. 13.7) could also be used in the combination room. This cabinet passes air vertically downwards from the ceiling of the cabinet over

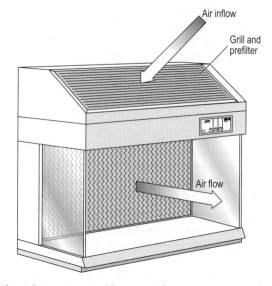

Fig. 13.6 Horizontal laminar airflow unit. (Courtesy of John Bass Ltd.)

the critical working area. It produces a Grade A environmental quality. The air exits from the front of the workstation.

In recent times, there has been a trend towards protecting the critical procedures within combination clean rooms by using isolator cabinets. The isolator cabinet gives a localized

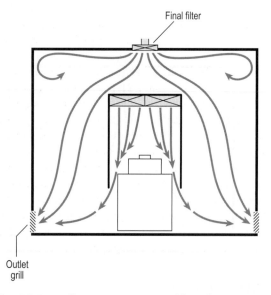

Fig. 13.5 Airflow patterns in a mixed-flow clean room with non-unidirectional airflow background environment and unidirectional airflow protection for a critical area.

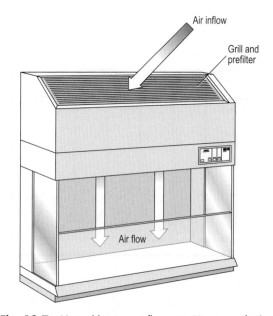

Fig. 13.7 Vertical laminar airflow unit. (Courtesy of John Bass Ltd.)

high-quality environment. Isolators give protection from potential contamination in clean rooms as they are positively pressurized with air supplied through HEPA filters. The operator works outside the confines of the isolator using glove ports to perform procedures within the enclosed chamber. The gloved hands of clean room operators can transfer microbial contamination into critical working areas within the clean room. To indicate that the required clean room standards have been achieved (Table 13.2) the fingertips of a gloved hand are depressed onto the surface of a suitable solid growth medium. This medium is incubated to show any contamination.

There is also a need to avoid contaminated external air passing into the clean room environment. Thus, the clean room air pressure must exceed that of the surrounding areas. The pressure differential between different standards of clean room should be 10–15 Pa. This level should be comparatively easy to monitor and will decrease the unregulated outflow of air. Adjusting grills known as pressure stabilizers located in the walls of rooms regulate the outflow of clean room air and the room pressure. The air moves from an area of high pressure to an area of lower pressure. To maintain the room pressure it is important that the rooms are airtight. However, a small quantity of air will exit from the rooms by way of door spaces.

Temperature and humidity control

The temperature and the humidity are adjusted to suit the procedures being carried out within the clean room and maintain the comfort of the operators. A target temperature of about 20ºC with a relative humidity of about 35–45% is usually preferred.

Personnel

The clean room environment is supplied with high-quality air at positive pressure. The main source of contamination in these areas arises from skin scales that are released by the clean room operators.

To limit clean room contamination by personnel there is a need to:

- Restrict the number of operators working in the clean room
- Restrict operator conversations
- Instruct operators to move slowly
- Minimize general movement throughout the room
- Avoid operators interrupting the airflow between the inlet filter and the work area.

The clean room operator is constantly shedding dead skin scales from the body surface. Not all of these skin particles are contaminated with bacteria. Males shed more particles that are contaminated with bacteria than females. In addition, individual males and females show variable rates of bacterial dispersal. This dispersal from the individual is affected by:

- Personal characteristics
- General health and skin condition.

Body movements of personnel will increase the number of contaminated particles released from the skin surface. Each individual releases more than 10^6 skin scales per minute during normal walking movements. There is a need to contain the dispersion of skin particles from the operators in clean rooms and protect both the environment and the product. Containment of particles is achieved by the operators wearing clean room clothing. This clothing is made from synthetic fabrics that filter out particulate and microbial contamination from the operators without the fabrics releasing contamination. However, this clothing is not absolute and particles can pass through the garments. Operators wearing clean room undergarments reduce this effect. The outer garments are close fitting at the neck, wrists and ankles, but these sites still provide an exit route for particulate matter.

Clean garments should be used for each work session and must provide operator comfort. Disposable single-use garments are available, although most production units employ reusable garments. The clothing is specially laundered in an area with similar standards to those used in the clean room. Garments are laundered by a wet-wash process using particle-free solutions. This is followed by an antibacterial rinse and hot air drying and then the garments are packaged in sealed bags to avoid particulate contamination. This cleaning process fulfils the needs of most pharmaceutical clean room applications, which are a balance between cost and acceptability. For a higher level of sterility assurance the garments are gamma irradiated using ^{60}Co, each garment receiving an approved dose of 25 kGy. This treatment is expensive and decreases the life of the garments. The donning of clean room clothing without contaminating the outer surface of the garments is a rather difficult procedure that is performed in the changing room.

Changing room

Entry of personnel into clean rooms should be through a changing room fitted with interlocking doors. These doors act as an airlock to prevent the influx of external air. This access route is intended for the entry of personnel only. The changing room is subdivided into three areas. Movement through these areas must comply with a strict protocol. They are often colour coded as black, grey and white, black representing the dirtiest area while white represents the cleanest area.

The black area is where jewellery, cosmetics, factory or hospital protective garments and shoes are removed. Long hair may be contained and a mob cap donned to contain the hair completely. The pass-over bench forms a physical separation between the black and the grey areas in the changing room. The operator sits on the pass-over bench, swings his/her legs over the bench and fits clean room covers over their feet before they are placed on the floor of the grey area.

The operator then stands up in the grey area. Wrappings on the various garments are opened to avoid contacting the outer surface of the packaging following the hand-washing procedure. Then the operator washes her hands and forearms using an antiseptic solution. Special attention is paid to cleaning the fingernails. The hands are then dried using an automatic air-blow drier as towels shed particles when used for drying hands.

Clothing garments are donned in sequence from head to foot. Throughout this procedure care must be taken to avoid the hands contacting the outer surface of the clean room clothing. Firstly the head and shoulder hood is fitted, ensuring that all the hair is contained within the head cover. A face mask is fitted to prevent the shedding of droplets. The one-piece coverall or alternatively the two-piece trouser suit is put on. Care must be taken to avoid these garments contacting the floor surface. The shoulder cover of the head and shoulder hood is tucked into the coverall. Then the zip is closed and the studs fastened. Overboots are then fitted over the clean room shoes. The overboots are kept in position with ties that are suitably fastened for operator comfort. For entry into aseptic filling rooms an antiseptic cream is applied to the hands. The clean room powder-free gloves are then donned. Care is needed to avoid contacting the outer surface of the gloves. The cuffs of the coverall are secured within the gloves and the gloved hands disinfected. The operator now enters into the white clean room area and begins work. During the work procedures the gloved hands of the operators are regularly disinfected. Key features of the clothing are given in Table 13.5.

Cleaning

A strict cleaning and disinfection policy is essential to minimize particulate and microbial contamination in the clean

Table 13.5	Clothing for clean room use
Clean room grade	Description of clothing
A/B	Head cover and face mask Single- or two-piece trouser suit Overboots and sterile powder-free rubber or plastic gloves
C	Hair (and beard) cover Single- or two-piece trouser suit Clean room shoes or overshoes
D	Hair (and beard) cover Protective suit Appropriate shoes or overshoes

room. Operators release microbial and particulate contamination within the clean room. These contaminants are mostly deposited onto horizontal surfaces. However, other areas of the clean room can become contaminated due to direct contact with the operators' clothing. It is thus essential that a strict cleaning and disinfection policy is implemented within the clean room to minimize both the particulate and the microbial contamination.

There are two main methods of cleaning. Vacuuming is effective at removing gross particulate contamination of particles greater than 100 μm. However, vacuuming is not very effective at removing smaller particles. Small particles are removed by wet wiping. It is important that the wet wipe is sterile and must not generate particulate contamination. The use of wet wipes involves the use of cleaning agents that will remove particulate contamination and have an antibacterial effect.

The ideal cleaning agent should be:

- Effective in removing undesirable contamination
- Harmless to surfaces
- Fast drying
- Non-flammable
- Non-toxic
- Cost-effective.

Anionic or cationic surfactants are used as cleaning agents within the clean room. The disinfectants of choice for clean room use are generally quaternary ammonium compounds, phenols, alcohols and polymeric biguanides. The disinfectant solutions should be freshly prepared before use.

Different types of disinfectants should be used in rotation to prevent the development of resistant microbial strains. Most surfactants or detergents will dissipate surface static electricity but the most effective and widely used antistatic agents used in clean rooms are cationic surfactants.

Trained personnel regularly clean critical production areas of clean rooms. A less stringent cleaning protocol is required in the general clean room areas. This applies to the walls and floors where contamination cannot directly contaminate the product. As part of the cleaning protocol regular microbiological monitoring should be carried out to determine the effectiveness of the disinfection procedures.

ISOLATORS

Commercial manufacturers are using isolators increasingly for the aseptic filling of products with combination isolators being used. Isolators are also used for sterility testing of products. Robots have been used in isolators for repetitive processes such as sterility testing but they are expensive. Isolators are used in hospital pharmacy departments as an alternative to clean rooms for the small-scale aseptic processing of sterile products. Aseptic procedures performed in the best isolators cannot reach the same levels of sterility assurance achieved by terminal heat sterilisation (Table 13.6). However, when suitably operated they can produce a sterility assurance level better than the conventional clean room. Isolators are often selected for aseptic manipulations of sterile products as they are:

- Relatively inexpensive
- Easily designed for a specific purpose
- Capable of providing operator protection from the product.

Isolators are composed of a chamber that controls the environment surrounding the work procedure (Fig. 13.8). The inlet and exhaust air passes through HEPA filters. The airflow pattern within the isolator chamber may be either unidirectional, non-unidirectional or a combination of both. Vertical unidirectional airflow has the advantage of rapidly purging particles from the isolator chamber. This is an advantage for aseptic processes. The air within the isolator chamber should be frequently changed to maintain the aseptic chamber environment. Particle and microbial contamination of the environment within the isolator chamber must conform with the Grade A standard as detailed in Tables 13.1 and 13.2. The operator remains outside the isolator chamber environment. To perform manual manipulations within the chamber the operator inserts his hands and

arms into the chamber. Entry occurs by way of a glove port using either a one-piece full-arm-length glove or a glove and sleeve system. With the glove and sleeve system, the easily changeable glove is attached to a sleeve that is attached to the wall of the chamber through an airtight seal. Using either of these glove systems the operator is able to perform aseptic manipulations in comfort up to a distance of about 0.5 metres within the chamber. The glove system avoids contamination arising from the operator and maintains the integrity of the isolator chamber environment. As cytotoxic materials can diffuse through the gloves it is important that they are changed regularly. To perform the work procedure within the chamber, materials must be introduced and prepared products removed without compromising the chamber environment. This transfer procedure is a critical factor in the operation of the isolator and is carried out using a transfer system. The transfer system separates the external environment from the controlled isolator environment. It restricts airflow between these areas while allowing the transfer of materials between them. The transfer system is fitted with an interlocked double door entry system. This will provide an airlock that avoids both doors being opened to the external environment simultaneously. A filtered air inlet and exhaust is fitted to the transfer system. However, a risk of microbial contamination during the transfer does exist. This was recorded at the Manchester Children's Hospital in 1994 and detailed below. The isolator must be positioned in a suitable background environment of at least a Grade D classification. This is typically achieved by positioning the isolator in a dedicated room that is only used for the isolator and its related activities.

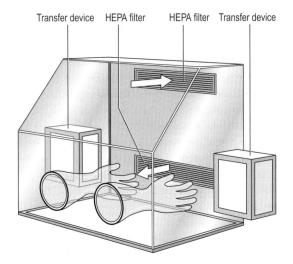

Transfer device   HEPA filter   HEPA filter   Transfer device

Fig. 13.8 Isolator cabinet.

Isolators are divided into positive and negative pressure isolators.

Positive pressure isolator

This isolator operates under positive pressure and protects the product from contamination arising from an external source and from the aseptic process itself. It is used for the aseptic preparation of pharmaceutical products and can be used as a sterility test chamber.

Negative pressure isolator

This isolator will protect the product from contamination arising from an external source and from the aseptic manipulation. In addition, however, this isolator should protect the operator from hazardous materials such as cytotoxic preparations or radiopharmaceuticals in the isolator chamber. This type of isolator operates under negative pressure. The exhaust air is ducted to the outside through at least one HEPA filter and through an adsorption material such as activated carbon. Rigid negative pressure isolators should be used for radiopharmaceutical manipulations. In this situation, the isolator is frequently used with a lead-free vision panel and a lead glass protector around the product. Alternatively, isolators are available with lead acrylic glass windows.

The chambers of isolators are gas sterilized. The ideal sterilant for use in the isolator chamber should have the following properties:

- Non-corrosive to metals and plastics
- Rapidly lethal to all microorganisms
- Good penetration
- Harmless.

The sterilants in most general use for pharmaceutical applications in isolators do not comply with all of these ideal properties. Those used are peracetic acid vapour and hydrogen peroxide vapour. To reduce the risk of chemical contamination of the sterile product, the sterilant contact time should be carefully regulated. The sterilant must be flushed from the isolator before beginning the aseptic manipulations.

Currently marketed isolators are constructed with either a flexible canopy or a rigid containment medium. The rigid type of isolator is often preferred, owing to the reduced risk of the chamber being punctured. This occurs more readily with the flexible canopy design. Rigid isolators are often constructed from a stainless steel frame with a moulded acrylic window. A further isolator known as a half-suit isolator is currently in use. This is a flexible canopy isolator that is made from material such as nylon-lined PVC. It is designed using a half-suit sealed to a wall of the chamber. This system allows the torso of the operator to be introduced into the suit that is located within the chamber of the isolator. To improve visibility, a transparent helmet is sealed to the neck of the suit that is ventilated by a pressurized air supply. This provides operator comfort over prolonged work sessions. The advantage of the half-suit isolator is that the operator can easily access a large area of the chamber and manoeuvre heavier and larger materials. The half-suit isolator is used as dedicated production equipment for the aseptic compounding of products such as total parenteral nutrition (TPN) fluids.

During a 2-week period in September 1992 eight children died from infection after receiving contaminated TPN fluids at four different hospitals in South Africa. These fluids had been prepared in flexible film isolators. The investigation of this incident revealed that the production equipment was suitable for its purpose but inadequate procedures had allowed contamination and subsequent growth of pathogenic bacteria in the TPN fluids. It should therefore be carefully noted that the use of isolators requires trained staff and good manufacturing practices to maintain product quality.

Isolator tests

Isolators must be frequently tested to ensure that they operate as a sealed chamber and conform with the required level of air quality and surface contamination. They are thus subjected to both physical and microbial tests.

Physical tests include:

- *Integrity tests.* These tests will detect leaks that compromise the integrity of the isolator chamber. The procedure is routinely carried out by sealing the chamber and recording changes in the chamber pressure over time.
- *Glove inspection.* The glove and sleeve are visually inspected and leak tested for pin holes.
- *HEPA filter test.* The integrity of the HEPA filter should be tested with an aerosol generator and a detector.
- Airborne particle count. This is carried out in the isolator chamber and the transfer device using a particle counter.

Microbial tests use microbial growth media suitable for the growth of potential contaminants. The tests include:

- *Active air sampling.* This test determines the number of organisms in the air of the isolator chamber. The procedure uses impact and agar impingement samplers.

- *Settle plates*. Settle plates containing growth media are exposed in the chamber for 2–4 hours. Particles and organisms settle by gravity onto the agar surface. The plates are then incubated.
- *Surface tests*. Surfaces are sampled using direct contact plates that are then incubated. Following sampling, it is important to remove materials deposited onto the sampled surfaces during the test. Alternatively, surfaces are sampled using sterile moistened swabs. The swabs are then streaked onto solid growth media and incubated. Soluble swabs may be dissolved in sterile diluent and the viable count determined.
- *Finger dabs*. The fingertips of the gloved hand are pressed onto the surface of solid growth medium. The medium is then incubated.
- *Broth fill test*. This test challenges both the manipulative procedure of the operator and the facilities. The test simulates routine aseptic procedures by using nutrient medium in place of a product to produce broth-filled units. These units are incubated to indicate microbial contamination.

ENVIRONMENTAL MONITORING

Following construction of a clean room, it must be tested to ensure that it is providing the required quality of environment. These verification tests are rigorously performed and are similar to the tests used to monitor the clean room subsequently. The monitoring tests ensure that the clean room continues to provide satisfactory operation.

To ensure that the pharmaceutical clean room is providing the required environmental standards, the following are determined.

Air quality

The air supplied to the clean room must not contribute to particulate or microbial contamination within the room. The HEPA filters for the inlet air must be tested to ensure that neither the filter fabric nor the filter seals are leaking. This is done by introducing a smoke with a known particle size upstream of the filter. The clean room surface of the filter is then scanned for smoke penetration using a photometer or a particle counter.

Air movement

Adequate ventilation throughout the clean room can be determined by air movement tests. These are carried out at the time of clean room validation. Air movement within the clean room is determined by measuring the decay profile of smoke particles released into the clean room. Smoke particle release is also used to ensure that a clean area within a unidirectional workstation is not being contaminated with air from the clean room environment.

The outflow of air from a clean room with a higher standard of cleanliness to an area with a lower standard is indicated by the pressure differential between the rooms. This is determined using a manometer or magnahelic gauge.

Air velocity

The velocity of the air at several points in a clean room area of critical importance should be determined. This is done both at validation of the clean room and at timed intervals. The procedure involves the use of an anemometer.

Airborne particulate and microbial contamination

The particle count and the microbial bioburden of the clean room provide the basis for the air classification system for grading a clean room as detailed in Table 13.1. The points for sampling and the number of samples taken at each position are determined by the size and the grade of the clean room. Airborne particles are normally sized and counted by optical particle counters.

Microbial monitoring

There should be very few viable organisms present in the clean room air. However, operators within the clean room disperse large numbers of skin particles. Many of these particles are contaminated with bacteria. The dispersal of contaminated particles by the clean room operator is greatly decreased by the wearing of occlusive clothing together with appropriate air ventilation. Sampling for microbial contamination is necessary when people are present in the clean room during production. Monitoring of the microbial contamination during production will ensure that both the use of clean room clothing by the operators and the air ventilation system are producing the required environmental standards. Air sampling is carried out by volumetric sampling or by the use of settle plates. With volumetric sampling a measured volume of air is drawn from the environment and contaminants are impinged onto a suitable microbial growth medium. The medium is then incubated and the colonies of microbial growth counted. Settle plates rely on bacteria-carrying particles being deposited onto the exposed solid surface of sterile microbial growth media contained in a 90 or 140 mm diameter Petri dish. When positioning the plates, care is needed to avoid accidental contamination. Owing to the small number of microbial contaminants in the clean room the settle plates are preferably exposed for about 4 hours.

The surfaces of the clean room should also be tested for microbial contamination, notably in areas that may be contacted by the clothing of the operators. This is achieved by using contact plates or by using sterile moistened swabs. The contact plates allow a sterile agar surface to be pressed onto the clean room surface. These plates are then incubated to reveal microbial growth. Swabbing procedures are carried out as previously detailed in isolator tests.

ASEPTIC PREPARATION

Parenteral products such as injections, infusions and eye products must be sterile for administration to the patient (see Chs 25 and 26). The preferred method of manufacturing parenteral medicines is to place the product in its final container and then seal this package. The product is then protected from further contamination and is terminally sterilized (see Ch. 12). At worst this achieves the risk of one product in a million being contaminated following terminal sterilization by dry or moist heat or by irradiation. Some products cannot withstand this sterilization process. An alternative approach known as aseptic preparation must then

be used to prepare these medicines. This procedure is carried out in industry with selected products but is extensively used in hospital pharmacy where products are specially compounded to meet the specific needs of patients (see Chs 27 and 28).

As shown in Table 13.6, aseptic preparation of parenteral products provides the lowest level of assurance of sterility of all the methods currently used to produce these formulations. In the pharmaceutical industry presterilized medicines are aseptically filled into sterile containers. The filling process must avoid recontamination of the sterile medicine and its container during this process. A sterility assurance level of 10^{-6} is achieved but in order to achieve this requires highly sophisticated industrial production procedures. In hospital pharmacy presterilized product components are aseptically compounded using sterile apparatus and then aseptically added to appropriate packaging for subsequent patient administration. It is critical that the sterile product components and the packaging are not recontaminated with organisms or particulate matter during these aseptic procedures. In order to achieve this, the sterile product components and the sterile package must be manipulated in a high-quality environment. The aseptic preparation and filling of products is performed in a localized Grade A zone that is achieved by a laminar airflow cabinet with a Grade B background. The Grade A environment within an isolator cabinet is also suitable for the compounding of aseptic preparations. It is important that this quality environment is continuous throughout the aseptic preparation process. Great reliance is not only placed on the facility and equipment used to

Table 13.6 Microbial contamination of batch-produced sterile products	
Place of production	**Microbial contamination**
Industrial production	
Terminal sterilization by dry or moist heat or irradiation	1 in at least 10^6 containers
Aseptic preparation in sealed, gassed isolator using sophisticated transfer system	1 in 10^6
Aseptic preparation in conventional clean room using sophisticated laminar airflow system	1 in 10^5
Aseptic preparation in conventional clean room	1 in 10^4
Aseptic complex preparation of large-volume TPN fluids	1 in 10^3
Production in hospital pharmacy	
Terminal sterilization by dry or moist heat containers	1 in at least 10^6
Aseptic preparation in an isolator with surfaces cleaned and wiped with sterile alcohol. Extensively used in many pharmacies	1 in 10^3
Aseptic preparation in a well-managed clean room	1 in 10^3 (or less)

produce the product, but also on the ability of the trained operators to avoid product contamination. It achieves a sterility assurance level of about one in a thousand. The manufacture of aseptic products also needs a stringent quality assurance system to ensure production of a quality product that is fit for its intended purpose. The quality assurance system should have documented, validated and audited procedures with in-process monitoring and standard operating procedures defining each step of the production process (see Ch. 27).

There is a need for awareness of the potential risk of infection that can occur during the aseptic preparation of pharmacy products. This has been shown by the tragic outcome of the supply of contaminated parenteral nutrition fluids to children at the Royal Manchester Children's Hospital in 1994. These fluids were aseptically compounded in an isolator. Microorganisms were unknowingly transferred from a sink into the isolator chamber on components used to prepare the feeds. The contaminating organisms grew in fluid remaining in assembled tubing used to prepare the feeds in the isolator. Reuse of this tubing resulted in contamination of the feeds that infected the patients. During these events it was shown that the equipment was not faulty, only the manner in which it had been used. This demonstrates the importance of adequately disinfecting the components being transferred into the isolator and for a total quality system for the manufacture of aseptic products.

Chapters 27 and 28 deal with the aseptic preparation of a range of commonly used sterile products.

In order to aseptically prepare a parenteral medicine, it is critical that validated procedures are stringently followed. This must go hand in hand with the other components of the quality assurance system for the preparation of aseptically prepared products of quality that are right first time and every time.

Key Points

- Particulate and microbial contamination of sterile products is minimized by preparation in a clean environment.
- Quality of clean areas is graded A, B, C, D in decreasing stringency for particulate and microbial content.
- Premises must allow segregation of stages of production and protect products from contamination by all possible means of design and operation.
- Access to clean areas is restricted and special clothing must be worn.
- Environmental control, particularly of the air supply to the room, is required to ensure a minimal contamination hazard.
- HEPA filters have a 99.997% efficiency at removing 0.3 μm particles, the size at which their efficiency is lowest.
- Airflow may be designed as unidirectional, non-unidirectional or as a combination system.
- In addition to general air quality, localized areas of higher quality can be produced either by airflow design in enclosed areas, or by isolator cabinets.
- The main source of contamination in clean rooms is the skin scales from operators.
- Clean room clothing, made from synthetic fabrics, is designed to minimize release of operator contaminants.
- Changing areas are designed and used to minimize the entry of contamination on personnel.
- During cleaning, vacuuming and wet wiping are used to remove large and small particles respectively.
- Isolators give protection to both the product and the operator at relatively low cost.
- Type II isolators protect the operator from hazardous materials in addition to providing the Type I facilities of protection of the product from contamination.
- Isolator interiors are sterilized using a gas sterilant.
- Isolator integrity is tested using physical and microbial tests.
- A range of environmental tests is used in clean rooms to monitor air quality, movement and velocity, airborne particles and microbial contamination.
- Aseptic preparation is involved with repackaging sterile products for patient use without terminal sterilization.
- Aseptic preparation is performed in laminar airflow cabinets in clean rooms or in isolator cabinets to avoid product contamination.
- A stringent quality assurance system is required for aseptic production to ensure a quality product is prepared.

14

Sterility testing

R. M. E. Richards

After studying this chapter you should be able to:

Discuss the role and the limitations of the sterility test

Explain the factors affecting the growth of bacteria

Explain the factors affecting the growth of moulds

Explain the reasons for the various media used in sterility testing

Discuss the properties required of a medium used in sterility testing

Describe the two test methods—membrane filtration and direct inoculation

Discuss the interpretation of the results of the test for sterility of the *British Pharmacopoeia* and the *European Pharmacopoeia*

Discuss the issues involved in the selection of samples for sterility testing

LIMITATIONS OF THE TEST

Sterility testing of pharmaceutical preparations purporting to be sterile is a procedure that has limitations both inherent (technical and biological) and imposed (numerical and economical), which means that it can only provide partial answers to the state of sterility of the product batch under test.

The test for sterility discussed and explained in this chapter relates especially to the test of the *British Pharmacopoeia* (BP 2001) which meets the standards of the *European Pharmacopoeia* (EP 2001). These are now also very similar to those recommended by the *United States Pharmacopoeia* (USP 25).

It is acknowledged that sterility testing is inadequate as an assurance of sterility for a terminally sterilized product. This is because the level of probability of an accidental microbial contaminant in an aseptic process can be as high as one in a thousand (10^{-3}) but the probability of a microbial survivor in a terminal sterilization process is at worst only one in a million (10^{-6}) (see Ch. 13). Nevertheless, the test is still a regulatory test in most countries. However, there has been a move towards exempting from the sterility test products which have been prepared by manufacturers who provide evidence of good manufacturing practice combined with properly validated and controlled sterilization cycles. This has been referred to as 'parametric release' (see Ch. 12). The parameters for release are the initial validation data and physical and biological data routinely collected in process. However, sterility testing still has valuable application for products prepared using aseptic processes, where it is the only analytical test available. It is also the only analytical method available to regulatory authorities who have to examine a specimen of a product for sterility.

Stated very simply, sterility testing attempts to reveal the presence or absence of viable microorganisms in a sample number of containers taken from a batch of product. Based on the results obtained from testing the sample a decision is made as to the sterility of the batch. Great care is taken to try to eliminate false positives which might arise from operator error. This has led to some major pharmaceutical companies introducing robotics. Experience has shown that robotic sterility testing can reduce false-positive rates quite markedly.

In addition to operator technique other factors of importance in sterility testing include: the environment in which the test is conducted; the quality of the culture conditions provided; the test method; the sample size and sampling procedure.

STERILITY TEST CONDITIONS

Environmental conditions required for the test

The basic requirement of the facility used for carrying out sterility testing is that it should be designed to provide conditions which avoid accidental contamination of the product during the test, that is conditions equivalent to those for the aseptic preparation of pharmaceutical products. A suitable environment is a class A laminar airflow cabinet located in a class B clean room or an isolator (see Ch. 13). Regular microbiological monitoring of the working area with contact swabs, settle plates, etc. should be carried out.

Chemical antimicrobial agents should be used with care. There must be no possibility of such an agent adversely affecting either microorganisms which may be present in the sample under test or the culture medium subsequently inoculated with the test sample.

Culture conditions

Sterility testing involves testing for viable microorganisms which are likely to have been damaged by the sterilization process. Consequently it follows that appropriate conditions for growth of any surviving organisms should be provided by the culture media selected.

The following account of factors affecting the growth of microorganisms indicates the importance of selecting the most appropriate culture conditions for sterility testing.

FACTORS AFFECTING GROWTH OF BACTERIA

Nutrition, moisture, air, temperature, pH, light, osmotic pressure and the presence of growth inhibitors are all important factors which affect the growth of bacteria.

Nutrition

To produce vigorous growth of bacteria, suitable and adequate sources of carbon, nitrogen, mineral salts and growth factors must be present in the culture medium.

Moisture

Bacteria require moisture in order to utilize the aforementioned food substances. Usually a medium for the growth of

bacteria must contain at least 20% of water. In the absence of moisture, bacteria cease to multiply but spore-bearing forms may continue to exist in spore form for many years.

Air

Many bacteria will grow in the presence of air and are called 'aerobes', e.g. *Pseudomonas aeruginosa*; others can multiply only in the absence of oxygen and are known as 'anaerobes', e.g. *Clostridium tetani*. A third group, 'facultative anaerobes', are able to grow with or without air, e.g. *Escherichia coli*.

Anaerobic bacteria may be cultivated successfully either by providing an oxygen-free atmosphere or by adding reducing substances to the growth media. The state of oxidation or reduction of a medium can be measured and is known as the oxidation-reduction potential.

Temperature

Most pathogenic bacteria multiply best at normal human body temperature, i.e. approximately 37°C. However, some common and serious contaminants of wounds, eye drops and injections (e.g. *Pseudomonas* spp.) have an optimum growth temperature of about 30°C and may not be detected at 37°C.

Some saprophytes have an optimum range of 55–80°C and are known as 'thermophiles'. The spores of some species, e.g. *Bacillus stearothermophilus*, are extremely heat resistant and are used to test the efficiency of heat sterilization processes.

At temperatures approaching 0°C and below most organisms stop multiplying, but they remain alive, and this behaviour is utilized in the preservation of cultures of microorganisms by freeze drying.

Temperatures above 50°C are harmful, particularly if moisture is present. All vegetative cells are killed by exposure to dry heat at 100°C for 1.5 hours or moist heat at 80°C for 1 hour. Spores are more resistant.

pH

The optimum pH for growth is about 7.4, although this varies with different organisms. Growth is less rapid as the liquid is made more acid or more alkaline. Solutions that are strongly acid or alkaline are bactericidal.

Light

Exposure to sunlight in the presence of air has a harmful action on bacteria and may inhibit growth or destroy the organism. It is for this reason that the incubators used for growing bacteria have no windows. The damage is caused chiefly by light waves from the ultraviolet region. This explains the occasional use of ultraviolet lamps for reducing the contamination of atmospheres and surfaces (see Ch. 12).

Osmotic pressure

Bacteria respond rather slowly to changes in osmotic pressure, but they are plasmolysed by strongly hypertonic solutions and they swell and may burst when placed in hypotonic medium. Suspensions of bacteria used for test purposes should be suspended in diluents of optimum osmotic pressure. When used in sterility testing the inhibitory effect of strongly hypertonic solutions must be allowed for.

Growth inhibitors

Many substances can inhibit the growth of bacteria. Substances that prevent the growth of bacteria without destroying them are called 'bacteriostats', while substances that kill bacteria are called 'bactericides'. However, substances can be bacteriostatic at low concentrations and bactericidal at high concentrations and bacteria may die if subjected to prolonged contact with bacteriostatic concentrations. Bactericides are extensively used in injections as preservatives.

Application to sterility testing

Consideration of the foregoing factors is necessary to establish the most suitable conditions for the growth of bacteria. Thus to produce the rapid and luxuriant growth required in the preparation of bacterial cultures, or testing for sterility, it is necessary to provide ample nutrients, sufficient water and a suitable hydrogen ion concentration. The temperature will also need to be maintained in the optimum region by using an incubator which will exclude light. For anaerobes precautions must be taken to ensure a low oxidation-reduction potential. In all cases the presence of excessive quantities of substances having bacteriostatic or bactericidal action must be avoided.

FACTORS AFFECTING GROWTH OF FUNGI

Although there is an overlap in the growth requirements of moulds and yeasts with those required by bacteria, there are

also some differences. The similarities and differences are pointed out in the following comments on the factors affecting the growth of moulds and yeasts.

Nutrition

Moulds and yeasts require the same classes of nutrients as bacteria but the carbohydrate and nitrogen sources are particularly important. A supplementary source of carbohydrate must be added to most media because a high concentration is essential; examples are 2% dextrose, 3% sucrose and 4% maltose.

Extracts are used as nitrogen sources and are often obtained from vegetable materials, such as malt and potato extracts. However, the pathogenic fungi grow better in media containing extracts from animal sources. Thus the soya bean casein digest medium used in the fungal sterility test of the USP, EP and BP contains tryptone (a pancreatic digest of casein) as well as the vegetable extract (soya peptone). Peptones are often used to supplement or replace extracts.

Air

The common saprophytic moulds are strongly aerobic but yeasts can grow both aerobically and anaerobically. For example, anaerobic growth can occur deep in large containers of unpreserved syrups, or syrupy preparations, producing alcohol and carbon dioxide, which may eventually expel the stopper or burst the container. However, special anaerobic media are unnecessary.

Temperature

The optimum temperatures for the growth of most moulds and yeasts lie between 20 and 25°C. As many moulds grow rather slowly, tests should be incubated for at least 14 days.

pH

Moulds and yeasts prefer a pH well on the acid side of neutrality. Test media are usually adjusted to between pH 5 and 6. A pH of less than 5 is avoided when the medium contains agar because this is hydrolysed, with consequent loss of gel strength, if autoclaved at low pH. If a higher acidity is essential it is obtained by adding sterile acid after sterilization.

Light

Most moulds and yeasts grow equally well in the light and dark. Since incubators are not made with windows it is more convenient to incubate in the dark.

Osmotic pressure

Moulds and yeasts are more tolerant of high osmotic pressure than bacteria and are often found as contaminants of unpreserved syrups, semisolid creams and ointments. Additional sodium chloride is unnecessary in mould media.

Growth inhibitors

Substances used to prevent the growth of moulds and yeasts are known as 'fungistats' while substances used to kill them are called 'fungicides'. These must be neutralized or 'diluted out' in sterility testing.

CULTURE MEDIA FOR STERILITY TESTING

Culture media suitable for sterility testing must be capable of initiating and maintaining the vigorous growth of a small number of organisms. These organisms may consist of aerobic and anaerobic bacteria and the lower fungi.

The BP (2001) suggests the use of two dual-purpose or joint media. These are fluid thioglycollate medium and soya bean casein digest medium.

Fluid thioglycollate medium

The fluid thioglycollate medium is intended primarily for the culture of anaerobic bacteria but will also sustain the growth of aerobic bacteria. Resazurin is included as an oxidation-reduction indicator and agar is present to increase the viscosity and thus reduce the inward diffusion of oxygen into the medium.

The nutrients include sodium chloride, glucose and pancreatic digest of casein. Yeast extract is present as a growth factor and the amino acid L-cystine is included to encourage the growth of certain clostridia.

The formulation is suitable for the detection of anaerobes if not more than the upper third of the medium in the container, such as a 100 mL bottle, has been oxygenated. This is indicated by a green coloration of the medium. If necessary, reducing conditions can be restored immediately

before using by heating the medium in a water-bath, until the green colour disappears, and then cooling rapidly. However, repeated reheating can give rise to toxic degradation products.

A medium with the top 10% oxygenated is very suitable for use because aerobic growth will be more quickly initiated under such conditions and anaerobic growth will also take place.

Soya bean casein digest medium

The soya bean casein digest medium is intended primarily for the growth of aerobic bacteria but also supports the growth of fungi. Owing to the inclusion of tryptone (from casein) and soya peptone, this medium is particularly supportive to injured or fastidious aerobic bacteria that grow slowly in fluid thioglycollate medium (especially if trapped in the anaerobic region), because of the low oxidation-reduction potential. In addition, it has given good results in the membrane filtration method of sterility testing.

Certain tests must be carried out either previous to, or in parallel with, the sterility test on the product being examined. The tests should be designed to demonstrate the sterility of the medium, its nutritive properties and its effectiveness in the presence and absence of the preparation being examined.

Sterility of the media

Assurance that the media to be used in the sterility test are sterile is necessary in order to eliminate the possibility of false positives arising from contaminated media. This assurance is obtained by incubating portions of the media at appropriate temperatures for 14 days. Media intended for detection of bacteria are incubated at 30–35°C and media intended for detection of fungi are incubated at 20–25°C. Sterility is confirmed by the absence of microbial growth.

Nutritive properties of the media— growth promotion test

Tubes of the chosen media are individually inoculated with 10–100 viable microorganisms of one of a selection of culture types. These organisms are representative of the various types of contaminant that the test is seeking to detect. The BP (2001) suggests the use of the following aerobes: *Staphylococcus aureus*, (e.g. NCTC 10788), *Pseudomonas aeruginosa* (e.g. ATCC 6633) and the spore-forming *Bacillus subtilis* (e.g. NCIMB 8054). The recommended anaerobe is *Clostridium sporogenes* (e.g. ATCC 19404) and the fungi *Candida albicans* (e.g. ATCC 10231) and *Aspergillus niger* (e.g. ATCC 16404). For the fluid thioglycollate a minimum of one anaerobic and one aerobic bacteria are used and for the soyabean casein digest a minimum of one fungi and one aerobic bacteria.

Incubation at the appropriate temperature for bacteria and fungi is for not more than 3 and 5 days respectively. Early and copious growth of the microorganism confirms the suitability of that medium.

Effectiveness of media under test conditions—validation test

This test is to demonstrate whether or not culture conditions are satisfactory in the presence of the product being examined or a membrane filter, where applicable. It is performed for culture media for aerobic bacteria, anaerobic bacteria and fungi. A control set of cultures is included to provide a means of comparing the rate of onset and the density of growth in the presence and absence of the material being examined. The inoculations should be carried out in a separate laboratory from the test for sterility.

Aerobic bacterial test

An appropriate sample, as used in the test for sterility, of the preparation being examined is added to at least two containers of selected medium. Each container is then inoculated with 10–100 viable organisms of a suitable aerobic organism, such as *Staphylococcus aureus*. It should be noted that if the preparation being examined is an antibiotic then the organism used must be sensitive to that antibiotic.

A control set of containers is prepared without the addition of the product being examined. All containers are incubated at 30–35°C for not more than 3 days.

Anaerobic bacterial test

This is performed in a similar manner to the aerobic bacterial test, except that a suitable strain of anaerobic organism (such as *Clostridium sporogenes*) and a suitable medium for anaerobic organisms is used.

Fungal test

The test is carried out similarly to the aerobic bacterial test, except that a suitable strain of a fungus (such as *Candida*

albicans) and a suitable medium for fungi is used. Incubation is at 20–25°C for not more than 5 days.

If cultures containing the preparation being examined show equivalent growth to the cultures in the absence of the preparation, it indicates that the preparation has no antimicrobial action under the conditions of the test. Then the test for sterility of the preparation may be carried out without modification. If weaker growth, delayed growth or no growth occurs in the presence of the preparation compared with the control cultures, then the material being examined has antimicrobial action. This must be eliminated before or during the test for sterility of the preparation. Suitable methods include neutralization, dilution or filtration. Whichever way is chosen its effectiveness must be demonstrated by repeating the foregoing test procedure.

TEST METHODS FOR TESTING THE STERILITY OF THE PRODUCT

The BP (2001) states:

> *The test may be carried out using the technique of membrane filtration or by direct inoculation of the culture media with the product being examined. Appropriate negative controls are included in either case using preparations known to be sterile.*

The negative control may be an ampoule or ampoules of sterile medium or media. However, the negative control may be samples of the product being tested, e.g. antibiotic powder which has been terminally sterilized. The negative control is of assistance in interpreting false positives and provides a check on operator technique.

Membrane filtration is used for the following:

- Filterable aqueous preparations
- Alcoholic or oily preparations
- Preparations miscible with or soluble in aqueous or oily solvents which do not possess antimicrobial activity under the conditions of the test.

Membrane filtration

Membrane filters having a nominal pore size of not greater than 0.45 μm and whose effectiveness in retaining microorganisms has been established are recommended for this method. Filters of the appropriate composition for filtering the various solvents are available; e.g. cellulose nitrate filters for aqueous, oily or weakly alcoholic solutions and cellulose acetate for strongly alcoholic solutions. Filter discs commonly used are about 50 mm in diameter. For filters of different diameter, the volumes of dilutions used may have to be adjusted.

The filtration system and membrane are first sterilized by appropriate means. They should be so designed that solutions to be examined are introduced and filtered under aseptic conditions. One of two procedures may then be followed. The membrane can be removed intact (or divided into two) and aseptically transferred to one (or two) containers of appropriate culture medium. Alternatively, culture medium is passed through the closed system to the membrane which is then incubated in situ in the filtration apparatus. The latter technique may be conveniently performed with one of the commercially available systems, for example the Sartorius system which consists of a multiple suction filtration device. The system is capable of being sterilized by autoclaving at 121°C for 30 minutes (a deliberate excess) prior to use.

Millipore produce a transparent blister-packed system which has been sterilized by ethylene oxide. The system known as Steritest uses a peristaltic pump to provide pressure filtration. After completion of the test the plastic test system is disposed of suitably. Various fully automatic systems have also been developed.

Aqueous solutions

Each membrane is prepared by moistening with a small quantity of suitable sterile diluent such as 0.1% w/v neutral solution of meat or casein peptone. This renders the membrane less liable to damage in use and reduces the retention of inhibitors. The diluent may contain suitable neutralizing and/or acceptable inactivating substances.

The quantity of the preparation to be examined depends on the end-use of the product. Tables 14.1 and 14.2 summarize the BP (and EP) requirements.

The appropriate quantity is transferred from the container or containers to be tested to the membrane or membranes. If necessary, dilution is made to about 100 mL with a suitable sterile diluent (as used in the validation test) and filtration is carried out immediately. For those solutions being

Table 14.1   Minimum samples to be used in each culture medium in the test for sterility of parenterals (based on the BP 2001)

Culture medium properties	Volume/weight		
Liquids			
Volume in container (mL)	<1	≥1	
Sample volume	All	Half the contents up to 20 mL	
Solids			
Weight in container (mg)	<50	50–<300	300 or more
Solids			
Sample weight	All	Half	150 mg

Table 14.2   Quantities to be used in the test for sterility of ophthalmic and other non-injectable preparations. (Based on the BP 2001)

Type of preparation	Quantity to be used for each culture medium
Aqueous solutions	Whole contents of 1 or more containers to provide not less than 2.5 mL
Preparations soluble in water or isopropyl myristate	Whole contents of 1 or more containers to provide not less than 0.25 g
Insoluble preparations, creams and ointments (suspend or emulsify)	Whole contents of 1 or more containers to provide not less than 0.25 g

tested that have antimicrobial properties, the membrane is immediately washed with three successive 100 mL quantities of the chosen diluent. Where necessary, a suitable antimicrobial inactivating substance is added to the diluent or to the medium (Table 14.3).

A membrane is transferred to the same volume of each of the culture media as used in the validation test. Alternatively each medium is transferred onto a separate membrane in the sealed apparatus. The media are incubated for not less than 14 days at 30–35°C for the detection of bacteria and 20–25°C for the detection of fungi.

Another option is that the combined quantity of the material being examined for both media is transferred to the membrane—diluting, filtering and washing as previously described. The membrane is then aseptically cut into two equal parts. One part is transferred to each medium. Incubation is then carried out for not less than 14 days at the appropriate temperatures as just described.

Soluble solids

For each medium the appropriate quantity (indicated in Tables 14.1 and 14.2) is dissolved in a suitable solvent such as 0.1% w/v neutral solution of meat or casein peptone. The

test is then followed as described for aqueous solutions. If non-aqueous solvent is used it may be necessary to use membranes made of a material other than cellulose nitrate.

Oils and oily solutions

At least the quantities indicated in Tables 14.1 and 14.2 are used for each medium. Using a dry membrane, oils and oily solutions may be filtered without dilution. Heat-sterilized isopropyl myristate is used to dilute viscous oils. After the oil has been in contact with the membrane and has penetrated the membrane by gravity, filtration should be commenced by applying either pressure or suction gradually. The membrane is then washed at least three times with 100 mL quantities of sterile solution containing a suitable surface-active agent. Neutral meat or casein peptone 0.1% w/v containing either 1% w/v polysorbate 80 or 1% w/v (4-tert-octylphenoxy)-polyethoxyethanol are suitable washing fluids. The divided membrane segments, or whole membranes, are then transferred to the appropriate culture media. Alternatively the culture media are transferred to the membranes as described for the aqueous solutions. Incubation is also as described in the procedure for aqueous solutions.

Table 14.3   Inactivating agents for selected antimicrobials

Antimicrobial	Inactivating agent
Alcohols	None (dilution 1 to 50)
Arsenic compounds	Thioglycollate (<0.5%)
Cefalosporins	Cefalosporinase
Cefaloridine	
Cefalotin	
Hydroxybenzoates	Polysorbate 80 (1%) or (dilution 1 to 50)
Mercury compounds	Cystine (0.1%) or thioglycollate (0.05%) + polysorbate 80 (3%)
Penicillins	Penicillinase
Ampicillin	
Carbenicillin	
Penicillin G	
Penicillin V	
Pheneticillin	
Propicillin	
Phenols, cresols	Polysorbate 80 (1%) or (dilution 1 to 50)
Quaternary ammonium compounds	Polysorbate 80 (3%) + lecithin (0.3%)
Sulfonamides	p-aminobenzoic acid (25 mg will neutralize up to 5 g sulfanilamide)

Ointments and creams

The minimum quantities for each medium are shown in Table 14.2. Again isopropyl myristate forms a suitable diluent and it can be used to dilute ointments in a fatty base or water-in-oil emulsions to 1%. If necessary gentle heat may be used up to a maximum of 40°C, followed immediately by filtration, as described under oils and oily solutions. The BP (2001) and EP (2001) permit heating to not more than 44°C in exceptional cases.

Any antimicrobial activity in the product to be tested must be neutralized by inactivation or by dilution in a suitable quantity of culture medium before incubation. After filtration, washing and incubation procedures are carried out similar to those described for the oils and oily solutions.

Advantages of the filtration method

- Wide application. It can be used for:
  solutions with or without inhibitory properties
  soluble solids with or without inhibitory properties
  insoluble solids without inhibitory properties
  oils
  ointments, provided a non-inhibitory solvent or dispersing medium can be found
  articles, such as syringes, that can be rinsed with a sterile fluid.
- A large volume can be tested with one filter. Therefore the method is applicable to the testing of poorly soluble solids.
- A much smaller volume of broth is required than for testing by direct inoculation into culture media.
- It is applicable to substances for which no satisfactory inactivators are known, e.g. certain antibiotics.
- Some strongly adsorbed antibacterial agents, such as the mercurials and quaternary ammonium compounds, can be inactivated on the filter by treatment with the appropriate neutralizing solution.
- Subculturing—which could be required in the case of oils and oily preparations and substances that like the barbiturates give precipitates mimicking growth in broth—is usually unnecessary.

Disadvantage of the filtration method

An expensive facility, highly trained staff and a consistently high level of operation are required. However, there is no easy alternative.

Direct inoculation of the culture medium

The quantity of the preparation to be examined (as shown in either Table 14.1 or 14.2) is transferred directly into the appropriate culture medium. Antimicrobial properties are neutralized as described under 'Membrane filtration' above.

To ensure that the sample does not excessively dilute the ingredients and so impair the growth-promoting properties of the medium, the volume of culture medium must be at least 10 times the liquid sample volume. For solids it is recommended that the proportion of medium to sample is 100 to 1 in order to negate any effect of the dissolved solid on the nutritive properties of the medium. However, when the volume of sample is large, it is difficult for bacteria and yeasts to produce a detectable turbidity in the correspondingly large volume of medium within the incubation period of the test. Therefore in such circumstances it is better to use a concentrated medium which when diluted with sample gives the correct strength of medium. Where appropriate the concentrated medium may be added directly to the preparation in its container.

Oily liquids

When oily liquids are being examined it is necessary to add to the media used an appropriate emulsifying agent which has no antimicrobial activity under the conditions of the test. The two agents described under the membrane filtration test are suitable, i.e. 1% w/v polysorbate 80 or 0.1% w/v (4-tert-octylphenoxy)-polyethoxyethanol.

Ointments and creams

The sample is diluted to about 1 in 10 in a suitable sterile diluent (0.1% w/v neutral solution of meat or casein peptone) containing the chosen emulsifying agent. The emulsified diluted product is transferred to medium not containing an emulsifying agent.

Incubation for the direct inoculation method is for not less than 14 days at 30–35°C (mainly for the detection of bacteria) and 20–25°C (mainly for the detection of fungi). The cultures are observed periodically throughout the incubation period, preferably every day. This is because some bacteria produce a detectable turbidity at first which later settles as an insignificant deposit at the bottom of the tube or medium above. Therefore it is advisable to swirl containers gently before examination to stir up any sediment. It is also necessary to gently shake media containing oily products daily. However, great care must be taken with the thioglycollate medium not to destroy the anaerobic conditions at the base of the medium.

Daily examination of the medium also means that a repeat test (where permitted) can be commenced immediately contamination is detected.

Observation and interpretation of results

The batch passes the test for sterility if there is no sign of growth in any of the test media. When microbial growth is present then the sample fails the test for sterility. In such a situation the media showing growth are kept to one side and the identity of the contaminants determined. If it can be demonstrated that there was a breakdown in the aseptic technique, then the test is declared invalid and the initial test may be repeated. The following may invalidate the test:

* The monitoring of the sterility of the test facility indicates a fault
* Review of the test procedure indicates a fault
* The negative controls show growth
* The identity of the microorganisms isolated implies contamination during the performance of the test for sterility, i.e. a false positive (see below).

No evidence of microbial growth on subsequent retest indicates the product complies with the test for sterility. Microbial growth in the repeat test indicates that the product examined does not comply with the test for sterility.

A false positive might be due to the growth of *Staphylococcus epidermis*, which was found to be killed by the preservative used in the product being tested. It would then be reasonable to conclude that the contaminant did not originate from the product under test but rather from a breakdown in the testing procedure. That is it could have originated from the skin of a test operator. However, the growth of *Escherichia coli*, should it occur, would not be attributed to a breakdown in the testing procedure because this organism would not be expected to be present in a sterility testing environment.

Applications of the test

The BP (2001) contains advice on how to apply the test to injectables, ophthalmic products and other non-injectables.

Injectables

With the membrane filtration method it is best to use the whole contents of the container whenever possible; otherwise the quantities indicated in Table 14.1 are used. Where it is necessary to dilute the sample, it is diluted to about 100 mL with a suitable sterile solution (e.g. 0.1% w/v neutral meat of casein peptone). With the direct inoculation method the quantities shown in Table 14.1 are used.

The tests to detect bacterial and fungal contamination are carried out on the same sample of the product being examined. In the situation where the amount contained in a single container is insufficient to carry out the test, then the contents of two or more containers are used to inoculate the different media. In those cases where the contents of the container exceed 100 mL the membrane filtration method is the procedure of choice. The total volume to be filtered through one membrane filter should not normally exceed 1000 mL.

Ophthalmic and other non-injectable preparations

For these products the contents of an appropriate number of containers are combined to provide not less than the minimum quantities shown under 'Quantity to be used for each culture medium' in Table 14.2.

Sampling

The selection of samples and the number of samples to be taken from any given batch of sterile product or materials is obviously an important aspect of testing for sterility.

Selection of the samples

Samples must be representative of the whole of the bulk material and each batch of final containers. For the bulk, the material must be thoroughly mixed before the sample is taken. For the final containers, the sample must be selected at random, but:

* When a load from a heat sterilization process is being tested, samples should be taken from every shelf and from any parts of the sterilizer in which less satisfactory conditions are believed to exist.
* For aseptically processed preparations, samples must be taken throughout the filling operation. This may be considered as a period not exceeding 24 consecutive hours during which no interruptions or changes affecting the

integrity of the filling assembly have occurred and in which an identical group of containers has been filled with the same product from the same bulk lot.

- For articles sterilized by a continuous process, such as radiation sterilization, samples are selected from the total number of similar items subjected to uniform sterilization during an appropriate period which should not exceed 24 consecutive hours.

Sample size

There has been much debate on sample size. This has involved statistically based arguments related to the lack of assurance that the test for sterility will detect low levels of contamination. The present situation, however, has changed to where the test is seen as part of a total process aimed at providing assurance of sterility. This has reduced the reasons for criticism of the test. It has already been stated (see Ch. 12) that in the case of terminally sterilized products full documentation of a completed validated sterilization cycle provides greater assurance than the sterility test. Nevertheless, as stated at the beginning of this chapter, the sterility test provides an independent analyst the only means

of confirming that a particular product complies with pharmacopoeial standards for sterility. Thus for this purpose, in addition to the situation where the product has been prepared by an aseptic process, the test is indispensable.

The BP (2001) suggests minimal sample sizes for various products. These are summarized in Table 14.4. This is by way of guidance to manufacturers who have to include in their decisions on the size of samples such factors as: the environmental conditions of the manufacture, the volume of preparation per container and any other special considerations applying to the preparation concerned. The suggestions summarized in Table 14.4 assume that the preparation has been manufactured under conditions designed to exclude contamination.

Sterility test record

An example of the type of records that need to be kept on each test for sterility that is carried out is given in Figure 14.1. In situations where the material being tested produces turbidity in the test medium, samples are removed after 14 days' incubation and inoculated into fresh medium, which is then incubated for a further 7 days.

Table 14.4 Minimum sample size related to batch size. (Based on the BP 2001)	
Number of items in the batch*	**Minimum number containers/packages to be tested for each medium†**
Injectables	
≤100	10% or 4 whichever is the greater
>100 but ≤500	10
>500	2% or 20 whichever is the lesser
Ophthalmics and other non-injectables	
≤200	5% or 2 whichever is the greater
>200	10
If the product is presented in the form of single-dose containers apply the scheme for injectables	
Bulk solids	
<4	Every one
4 to ≤50	20% or 4 whichever is the greater
>50	2% or 10 whichever is the greater
*Batch = homogeneous collection of sealed containers so prepared that the possibility of microbial contamination is uniform.	
† If the contents of one container are enough to inoculate the two media, this column gives the number of containers needed for both media together.	

Sterility test record Direct inoculation method

Date test commenced	First test	Retest	
Product	Batch no.	Method of sterilization	
Vol/wt. in each container	Vol/wt. of sample	No. tested	
Antimicrobial and conc.	Inactivator/diluent		

Results of incubation. Day number 1,2,3,4,5,6,7,14

		Thyoglycollate medium 31°C		Soya bean casein digest medium 25°C	
		Anaerobic	Aerobic	Aerobic	Fungal
Test organisms		*Cl. sporog.*	*S. aureus*	*S. aureus*	*C. albicans*
Density of growth Scale 1–3	'Growth promotion test'				
	'Validation test'				
Controls	'Negative'				

Conclusion:			
	Sample passed	Batch passed	
	Sample failed	Retest allowed	
	Sample failed	Batch failed	
Signed		Date completed	

Fig 14.1 Sterility test record: direct inoculation method. 'Growth promotion test' = media + organism; 'Validation test' = media + organism + product and for the membrane filtration method + membrane; 'Negative control' = sterile media, or terminally sterilized product + media. This latter control is to check the operator technique and should be negative. *Note*: The same sterility test record format can be used for the 'Filter membrane method' noting the difference in the 'Validation test'.

Key Points

- The sterility test has limitations related to:
  Sample size—cannot guarantee to detect a small level of contamination
  The possibility of false positives—due to the fallibility of the test conditions and/or operator technique.
- Sterility test conditions need to be controlled and these include:
  Environmental conditions of the test laboratory
  General culture conditions for the microorganisms
  Species and strains of the test microorganisms.
- Bacteria and moulds have different specific culture requirements and need their own specific culture media, incubation temperature and length of incubation. Examples of sterility test media are:
  Fluid thioglycollate medium—primarily for anaerobic bacteria but also sustains growth of aerobic bacteria
  Soyabean casein digest medium—primarily for aerobic bacteria but will also support the growth of fungi.
- There are two methods recommended in the BP, EP and USP for testing the sterility of the product. The methods have to be followed in exact detail if they are to have the possibility of success. The two methods are:
  Membrane filtration—the method of choice where applicable
  Direct inoculation.
- The tests specify:
  The use of inactivating agents and/or neutralizing procedures which are effective for the antibacterial agents contained in the product
  Sample sizes to be tested in relation to the original manufacturing batch size of the product
  How the results obtained are to be interpreted with regard to passing or failing the test or whether a retest is allowed.

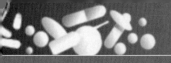

PART 3

PHARMACEUTICAL PRODUCTS

The prescription

J. A. Rees

After studying this chapter you will know about:

The place of the prescription in the prescribing process
The types of prescription forms and prescribers
Writing a prescription
The information required on a prescription
The routine procedure for checking and dispensing prescriptions
Information sources required for prescription writing and dispensing
Record keeping and standard operating procedures

Introduction

The access to medicines by the general public varies dependent on the laws of each country. In the UK, the Medicines Act 1968 classifies medicines into three categories, namely,

- General Sales List (GSL)
- Pharmacy medicine (P)
- Prescription Only Medicine (POM).

GSL medicines are available to the public through many retail outlets. These medicines are for the treatment of minor ailments/conditions and have a history of being safe and effective. P medicines are available only from pharmacies and are sold under the supervision of a pharmacist. Some P medicines are those that have recently been 'deregulated' from the POM classification, others may have potential for abuse or require the supervision of a pharmacist in the sale. POMs are only available on a prescription from an authorized prescriber. The Medicines Act defines an authorized prescriber. Medicines for use in animals (veterinary medicines) follow a similar pattern of regulation.

At the present time, a prescription is a paper document written, typed or computer generated detailing the medicine(s) to be dispensed for an individually named patient and issued by an authorized prescriber. The medicine can be any of the above three legal categories. A prescription item is one named medicine on a prescription, e.g. aspirin tablets. A prescription may contain more than one prescription item, e.g. aqueous cream, pholcodeine linctus and aspirin tablets (three prescription items), in which case the prescription may be referred to as a multiple item prescription. In addition to medicines, a prescription may contain other items required by the patient for their treatment, e.g. wound dressings, elastic hosiery, blood glucose monitoring equipment, needles and syringes, nutritionally complete feeds and gluten-free foods.

In the UK, a state-funded National Health Service (NHS) and a private system of health care run alongside each other. Prescriptions can be provided to patients by prescribers in both systems. In the NHS system, access to some medicines is limited in an attempt to reduce costs (see below).

Traditionally in the UK and according to the Medicines Act, prescribers have been doctors, dentists and veterinary surgeons, who can prescribe all categories of medicines (with chiropodists and ophthalmic opticians being allowed to prescribe a few specified medicines). A recent review of the prescribing, supply and administration of medicines (the Crown report published in 1998) recommended radical changes to the system. As a result, nurse prescribing was piloted and then introduced throughout England from 1998. Nurses allowed to prescribe have to hold appropriate qualifications and have to successfully complete prescribing training courses. The range of medicines available for nurse prescribing is limited to all GSL and P medicines currently available for NHS prescribing by GPs and a list of POMs to enable them to manage a range of specified medical conditions (the latter only prescribable by 'extended formulary nurse prescribers'). More recently, the second Crown report

(1999) proposed two new classifications of prescribers, namely, independent and dependent prescribers.

- Independent prescribers would assess patients, make diagnoses and prescribe.
- Dependent prescribers would be responsible for continuing the care of patients previously diagnosed by independent prescribers.

Specialist pharmacists and pharmacists carrying out reviews of patients on multiple therapy were cited as possible dependent prescribers. The latter group of pharmacists would have some discretion to amend various aspects of the prescription in terms of dose, frequency, presentation or active ingredient, within an individual treatment plan.

Another recent advance in the supply of medicines is the introduction of Patient Group Directions (PGDs). PGDs are used for the supply of POM and P medicines by designated health professionals to individual patients, subject to any exclusions stated in the PGD. PGDs are written directions signed by a doctor or dentist and by a pharmacist relating to the supply and administration, or administration only, of certain POMs and P medicines. The particulars to be included in a PGD are detailed in Box 15.1. A medicine supplied under a PGD does not require the patient to obtain a prescription and so medicines supplied via a PGD are dispensed without a prescription. However, records of supply to individual patients are required within a PGD. PGDs have

been used successfully for the supply of emergency hormonal contraception and head lice lotions.

The NHS Plan 2000 stated that by 2004, electronic prescriptions would be routine in both community and hospital. Electronic prescriptions will have the same legal force as prescriptions signed in writing and will replace paper prescriptions. The benefits of electronic prescriptions include patient convenience, easier ordering of repeat prescriptions and more complete information about prescribing. In addition, it will mean an end to incomplete and illegible prescriptions. Although electronic prescriptions will become the norm in the NHS, private prescriptions will, for the foreseeable future, remain as paper documents. This chapter will concentrate on paper prescriptions in use at the time of writing. The information contained on both paper and electronic prescriptions and the method of dispensing and recording is essentially the same.

WRITING A PRESCRIPTION

Writing a prescription is part of the prescribing process. The stages in the prescribing process are:

- Define the patient's problem (diagnosis)
- Specify the therapeutic objectives
- Verify the suitability of the medicinal treatment
- Write a prescription for the medicinal treatment
- Monitor the progress of the patient.

Thus the contents of the prescription are dependent on previous actions of the prescriber. However, appropriate prescribing is not a simple process and relevant factors need to be considered before 'putting pen to paper'. The National Prescribing Centre developed seven principles of good prescribing for the training of nurse prescribers. These seven principles are outlined below with appropriate explanations.

Examine the holistic needs of the patient

Before prescribing, the patient's social and medical history should be taken and considered with regard to possible treatment. Such an investigation may show that the needs of the patient would be better met by non-drug therapy, or such an approach complementary to the prescription. The WWHAM approach (see Ch 37) may be a useful way of obtaining the required information. Over-the-counter (OTC) medicines and alternative therapies taken by the patient and any allergies need to be taken into account before prescribing. Any new information should be recorded in the patient's notes.

Box 15.1   Particulars to be included on a patient group direction

Time period the PGD is in force
Class of medicine
Restriction on quantity to be supplied
Clinical situation
Clinical criteria
Class of persons excluded
Circumstances when advice from a doctor is required
Pharmaceutical form
Strength or maximum strength
Applicable or maximum dosage
Route of administration
Frequency of administration
Minimum or maximum period of administration
Relevant warnings
Details of follow-up action
Arrangements for referral for medical advice
Records to be kept

Consider the appropriate strategy

At this stage it is important to consider whether a prescription is really necessary or is it just an expectation of the patient? Should alternative non-drug treatment be considered? Are you sure that the diagnosis is correct and prescribing is an appropriate measure or should the patient be referred to their GP?

Consider the choice of product

Four points (forming the mnemonic EASE) need to be considered to enable a correct and appropriate choice of product.

E—How **E**ffective is the product? Is there sufficient evidence to show that the product will be effective for this condition of this patient?

A—Is the potential choice of product **A**ppropriate for this patient? Could the formulation be changed to accommodate the needs of the patient, e.g. would a tablet be more convenient to the patient than a liquid dosage form? Is the dose appropriate for the patient taking into account their age, liver and kidney function etc?

S—How **S**afe is the chosen product for the patient? Adverse drug reactions are more serious for some patients, e.g. those with impaired liver and kidneys, children or the very old. Will the chosen product react with other concurrently administered drugs, including OTC medicines? Has the patient any known allergies, sensitivities to drugs?

E—Is the proposed choice of product cost **E**ffective? Are the costs of using this drug outweighed by the effectiveness and the benefits? Is there a cheaper alternative that is just as effective?

Negotiate a 'contract' and achieve concordance with the patient

Is the patient going to use or take the prescribed medicines? Many patients fail to take their medicines for a variety of reasons (see Ch. 40). Would the patient be more likely to take the medicine if a different medicine, formulation, dosage regimen was chosen? Perhaps a once-a-day dosage would be preferable for a very busy person or one who can be a little forgetful. Perhaps the person has difficulty with taking tablets or doesn't like the taste of a medicine. If the patient has any doubts about the medicine then it is better to address them at this stage. Prescribing a medicine that will not be used by a patient is both wasteful and non-effective.

In addition it does not address the needs of the patient. Concordance is about sharing the decisions on medicines with the patient, i.e. negotiating a 'contract' with the patient. This process involves good communication skills.

Review the patient on a regular basis

There must be some follow up after writing a prescription. The follow up will involve seeing the patient to ensure that the treatment is effective and acceptable to the patient. Also it is important to ensure that the patient is not experiencing any side effects due to the medicine. In addition it is important to establish if the patient is using the medicine, as non-compliance will result in ineffective and wasteful treatment.

Ensure record keeping is both accurate and up to date

Responsible prescribing must include good record keeping that is up to date. All legal and professional records must be completed and maintained on a regular basis.

Reflect on your prescribing

As with all processes, it is important that we reflect on our actions. Look back over the prescribing process to see how you could improve in the future. In this way your prescribing becomes more efficient and more effective for the patients.

INFORMATION REQUIRED ON A PRESCRIPTION

When writing a prescription, the prescriber is giving information and instructions to the dispenser. The information and instructions that are required as a minimum are detailed below:-

Name, address and telephone number of the prescriber. This identifies the prescriber and where to contact him.

Date of the prescription. This identifies when the prescription was written. Some legal requirements require prescriptions to be dispensed within a certain time from the date on the prescription, e.g. Controlled Drugs in the UK.

Name of the medicine with strength and dosage form, if this is relevant. The name of the medicine can be written as either the generic or proprietary name.

Dose and dosage regimen, if relevant. Topical products, e.g. creams and ointments, are unlikely to have a specific dose.

Total amount to be dispensed or length of treatment time.

Directions for use. The directions for use can include how to use (spread thinly, dissolve in water) and where to use (in the eye, in the ear, on the scalp).

Name, address and age of the patient. This identifies the patient and whether they are a child or adult.

Prescriber's signature. This is usually a legal requirement of prescriptions.

The above details are not totally inclusive depending on the prescription type and the legal requirements of the country. For example, all NHS prescriptions would require the NHS registration number of the GP and veterinary prescriptions may require the type of animal to be stated.

A number of specific terms, e.g. dose, dosage regimen, etc., are used in the above list and are often confused. These are explained below and Example 15.1 demonstrates these terms using an extract from a prescription.

Dosage form. The term dosage form refers to the type of formulated product. These include, as examples, tablets, capsules, creams, ointments, ear/eye/nasal drops, aerosols, suppositories, vaginal pessaries and creams, mixtures, linctuses and patches. Each dosage form may also be presented in a number of specialist forms. For example, tablets are available as modified-release, enteric-coated, dispersible, buccal, soluble, chewable. The dosage form should be stated on the prescription if there is more than one form available. For example, glyceryl trinitrate is available as tablets, modified-release tablets, a pump spray, an aerosol spray, an injection, ointment and patches, thus, the prescriber will need to state the form, if the prescription is to be complete.

Strength. The strength refers to the amount of drug in the dosage form or a unit of the dosage form (e.g. a capsule, a tablet, a patch). The strength of a dosage form can be expressed in a number of ways. For example, the strength of oral liquids is usually expressed as the amount of drug per usual dose volume (e.g. ampicillin suspension is available as 125 mg/5 mL and 500 mg/5 mL) or the strength may be expressed in units (e.g. nystatin suspension is available as 100 000 units/mL). External liquids, topical preparations and injections are usually expressed as an amount per millilitre or gram (e.g. naloxone hydrochloride injection 400 micrograms/mL, nystatin cream 100 000 units/g, terbutaline sulphate nebulizer solution 25 mg/mL) or as a concentration (e.g. chloramphenicol eye drops 0.5%, ketoconazole cream 2%, benzyl benzoate application 25%, lidocaine (lignocaine) injection 0.5%). Single-dose forms, e.g. suppositories, are usually expressed as the amount of drug in one suppository (e.g. diclofenac sodium suppositories are available in 25 mg, 50 mg and 100 mg strengths).

Dose. This is the amount of drug taken at any one time. This can be expressed as the weight of drug (e.g. 500 mg) or volume of drug solution (e.g. 5 mL, 2 drops) or as the number of dose forms (2 capsules, $^{1}/_{2}$ a tablet, 1 sachet, 1 patch) or some other quantity (2 puffs, 1–2 inches of ointment).

Dosage regimen. Dosage regimen refers to the frequency of administration or the number of times the dose is to be taken in a period of time. Examples include 5 mL twice a day, use the cream night and day, one injection every 4 weeks, 3 tablets three times a week.

Total daily dose. The total daily dose can be calculated from the dose and the number of times per day that the dose is taken. Some maximum doses of drugs are expressed in terms of per day rather than each separate dose (e.g. the dose for digitoxin in the BNF is 100 micrograms daily).

Total amount. This refers to the total amount of the medicine to be supplied to the patient. This can be expressed as a number of units (e.g. 21 tablets, 12 suppositories) as a volume (e.g. 100 mL of mixture, 5 mL of eye drops) or as a weight (e.g. 30 g of cream) or as a single pack size or multiple thereof (e.g. 1 tube of ointment, 2 inhalers).

Proprietary name. This can also be referred to as the brand name or trade name. The company that first produces and markets a drug will give it a proprietary name. The company will apply for a trademark in respect of the proprietary name. The granting of a trademark means that no other company can use that name. Usually trademarks are short, distinct and easy to remember and write. Sometimes trademarks reflect the name of the company. After expiry of the patent (in the UK 20 years from first date of discovery or, under a certificate of Supplementary Protection, 15 years from the date of first marketing) the drug may be produced by other companies using the approved (or generic) name (see below). Drugs may be prescribed by their proprietary name.

Generic name. The generic name is also known as the approved name. All drugs are given an approved name, which is adopted by the World Health Organization and is known as the recommended International Non-proprietary Name (rINN). In the UK these names are usually co-opted as a British Approved Name (BAN). A recent directive 92/27/EEC requires that only the rINN be used and at the present time there is a 5-year transitional period in the UK.

During this period the rINN name of some drugs will be adopted for use in the UK because the rINN and BAN are very similar, e.g. amoxycillin (BAN) and amoxicillin (rINN), sulphasalazine (BAN) and sulfasalazine (rINN), whilst for some drugs both the rINN and BAN will be used alongside each other e.g. adrenaline/epinephrine, lignocaine/lidocaine, bendrofluazide/bendroflumethiazide. The use of generic names is commonly used on prescriptions, particularly hospital prescriptions. Prescribers in the UK are encouraged to use generic names for cost-saving reasons.

Length of treatment. The length of treatment may be stated on the prescription (e.g. use for 1 week) or it may be possible to calculate the length of time for which the treatment is prescribed (e.g. 21 capsules to be taken 'one three times a day' will be sufficient for 7 days' treatment).

EXAMPLE 15.1

The following details have been abstracted from a prescription.

Brufen® tablets 200 mg
Two tablets to be taken three times a day
Send 84 tablets

Using the above prescription as an example the terms dosage form, strength, dose, dosage regimen, total daily dose, proprietary name and generic name are described.

Term	Example
Dosage form	Tablets
Strength	200 mg
Dose	400 mg (2 tablets of 200 mg)
Dosage regimen	400 mg three times a day
Total daily dose	1200 mg
Total amount	84 tablets
Proprietary name	Brufen®
Generic name	Ibuprofen
Length of treatment	14 days

TYPES OF PRESCRIPTION FORMS

As stated previously, in the UK there are two providers of health care: the private sector and the NHS. Concomitantly there are two categories of prescriptions, namely private prescriptions and NHS prescriptions. Additionally, prescriptions may be provided in both the primary care sector (e.g. community) and the secondary care sector (e.g. hospitals). The format of prescriptions in these two sectors will be different.

Mr I Drillem BDS
Dental Surgeon
Mediton Dental Practice
Mediton

℞

Sodium fluoride tablets 500 microgram

Take one tablet daily

Send 56

I Drillem
14.2.03

Miss Isabel Featherstone
Molesworth Manor
Mediton

Fig. 15.1 A typical private prescription, in this case issued by a dental practitioner.

Private prescription forms

Private prescriptions are normally written on a form that includes the name, address and qualifications of the prescriber. The symbol ℞ is often used on private prescription forms to indicate that the form is a prescription. Figure 15.1 shows a typical private prescription for a human patient. All veterinary prescriptions are private prescription and Figure 15.2 shows a veterinary prescription.

Mr R Cowes MRCVS
Mediton Veterinary Practice
Animal Lane
Mediton

℞

Betsolan eye drops

Use four times a day

Supply 5 mL
For an animal under my care and attention

R Cowes
31.3.03

Fluffy the cat
Miss Kate Riley
The Crescent
Mediton

Fig. 15.2 A typical private veterinary prescription.

NHS prescription forms

NHS prescriptions are only issued for NHS patients. There are nine types of NHS prescription forms available in England and Wales that may be dispensed at any community pharmacy. Similar NHS prescription forms are available in other parts of the UK. Each type of prescription form is given a different number depending on either the prescriber or the source of the prescription. These nine forms are:

FP10.   This form is the usual form used by general practitioners to prescribe for their patients.

FP10 NC.   This form is the same as FP10 but is available in pads.

FP10 C.   This form is used by GPs for computer-generated prescriptions and is thus designed for use in computer printers.

FP10 MDA.   This form is used for the prescribing on an instalment basis of methadone and other drugs for community-based registered drug addicts. The prescriber is community based.

FP10 (HP) Ad.   This form is used for the instalment prescribing of methadone but is distinct from FP10 MDA as the prescriber is hospital based, although the patient will be community based.

FP10 P.   This form is used by all nurse prescribers in England.

FP10 CN.   This form is used by community-based nurse prescribers and extended formulary nurse prescribers in Wales.

FP10 PN.   This form is used by practice-based nurse prescribers and extended formulary nurse prescribers in Wales.

FP10 (HP).   This form is used by hospital prescribers for prescription item(s), which are to be dispensed in the community. This form may be used for outpatients and discharge patients if dispensing services are not available in the hospital.

FP10 D.   This form is used for prescribing by dentists.

FP10 L.   This form is a loose-leaf prescription to be used by deputizing services, or where the normal prescriptions are unavailable for any reason, personalized by the health authority.

All NHS prescription forms except FP10 L are personalized for use by one prescriber. Figure 15.3 shows a typical NHS form.

Hospital prescription forms

There is no standard form for hospital prescribing for inpatients, and the actual format and design will depend on the

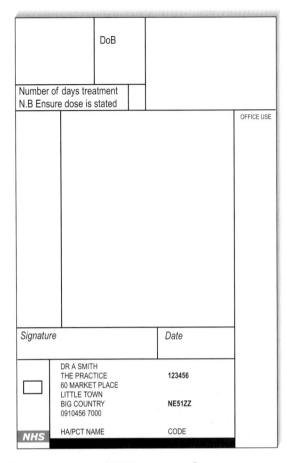

Fig. 15.3   A typical NHS prescription form.

individual hospital trust. However, the forms usually have space for the prescription details as well as space for confirmation of administration of the medicine by nursing or other staff. For convenience most hospital forms are divided into three separate areas, namely medicines to be administered on a regular basis, medicines to be administered once only and medicines to be administered on an 'as required' basis. Some forms may also have an area for listed medicines that can be administered by nursing staff at their discretion. Such medicines may be simple analgesics, sore throat lozenges, laxatives, etc. In addition all hospital prescription forms will require space for identification and important details about the patient, e.g. allergies. Figure 15.4 illustrates a typical hospital prescription and administration form.

MEDITON HEALTH TRUST

REGULAR PRESCRIPTIONS

Date Commenced	DRUG (Block Letters)	DOSE	MEDICINE ROUNDS								OTHER TIMES & DIRECTIONS	METHOD OF ADMIN	SIGNATURE	DISCONTINUED Date and Initials	PHARMACIST
			6	10	12	14	18	22	24						
A															
B															
C															
D															
E															
F															
G															
H															
I															
J															
K															
L															
M															

ONCE ONLY PRESCRIBING

DATE GIVEN	DRUG (Block Letters)	DOSE	TIME OF ADMIN	METHOD OF ADMIN	SIGNATURE	GIVEN BY

AS REQUIRED PRESCRIPTIONS

DATE COMMENCED	DRUG (Block Letters)	DOSE	Max No of Doses per Day	Min. Interval Between doses	METHOD OF ADMIN	SIGNATURE
N						
M						
O						
P						
Q						
R						
S						
T						
U						

TAKE HOME PRESCRIPTIONS

When this sheet is full please transfer all current treatments to a new sheet

DRUG SENSITIVITY

DRUG SENSITIVITY

NAME OF PATIENT	AGE	UNIT NUMBER	BODY WT. KG	CONSULTANT
WARD				

Fig. 15.4 A typical hospital prescription and administration form.

INFORMATION SOURCES

Both writing prescriptions and the dispensing will necessitate consulting some information source. Drugs are continually being introduced to the market and the indications for some drugs change, as well as doses and formulations. In addition, some drugs are removed from the market for a variety of reasons. Prescribers will need independent, accessible and unambiguous reviews of effective treatments, whilst dispensers will require similar information in addition to information on products and their availability, drug interactions, legal aspects and costs, etc. Some of the most useful information sources in the UK are listed below:

British National Formulary (BNF)
ABPI Summary of Product Characteristics
Medicines , Ethics and Practice Guide
Drug and Therapeutics Bulletin
MeReC Bulletin
Effective Health Care
Prescribers' Journal
Pharmaceutical Codex
Current Problems in Pharmacovigilance
Martindale: the Extra Pharmacopoeia

The BNF is published and updated every 6 months and lists the products available for dispensing in the UK. It is sent to all doctors, pharmacists and prescribing nurses in the NHS. The *Nurse Prescribers' Formulary* and the *Dental Practitioners' Formulary* are included in the BNF and published as separate booklets. The BNF is the major source of easily available information on the characteristics of individual medicines, including proprietary and generic formulations, strengths, dose and dosage regimens, drug side effects and drug interactions. The most recent copy should always be used.

If you cannot find the information that you require, then it is always possible to contact the local medicines information department. See also Chapter 33 for more on information sources.

ROUTINE PROCEDURE FOR DISPENSING PRESCRIPTIONS

The dispensing of prescriptions requires a logical and very thorough approach, but in addition it requires knowledge and ability in order to:

- Interpret the prescriber's instructions
- Check the appropriateness of the prescription for the patient
- Check the legal requirements
- Dispense the correct product
- Label correctly the dispensed medicines
- Complete the legal records
- Provide patient advice, information and counselling.

Some of the above stages are covered elsewhere in this book (see Chs 11 and 38 and Appendix 1). Some prescribers may use Latin abbreviations in their prescription writing. Appendix 4 details some of the abbreviations in common use. In order to accomplish the first three of the above tasks a series of checks needs to be thoroughly made as follows:

Check the patient details

It is essential that the details of the patient are known so that:

- The appropriateness of the prescription for that patient can be assessed.
- Any required records can be completed correctly.
- The product can be labelled for that patient.
- If necessary the prescription can be delivered to the correct patient at the correct address.
- The patient can be contacted, if necessary, after the medicine has been dispensed and supplied to the patient.

Thus, the full name of the patient is required. This information will indicate the sex of the patient, if it is not given elsewhere on the prescription. The sex of the patient may be necessary in the assessment of the appropriateness of the medicine for the patient (see Example 15.2).

The full address of the patient is required. It may be possible that two patients have the same name and so the address will identify the patient. If two patients have the same address and name, then it is helpful if the age or date of birth of the patient is stated. The age/date of birth is required on NHS prescriptions, but is not a legal requirement in the UK for private prescriptions. However, it is usual practice to state the age for children under 12 years old. The age of the patient may be essential in order to calculate the appropriate dose for children and for some elderly patients. On private prescriptions, the age of very young children may be expressed as a fraction. If the age is expressed in days, weeks or months, then the denominator is 7, 52 and 12, respectively. For example, an age of 3 days may be abbreviated to 3/7, an age of 3 weeks may be abbreviated to 3/52 and an age of 3 months to 3/12.

EXAMPLE 15.2

A prescription contains the following details.

Mrs Joyce Hind
2 High Street
Mediton

Hytrin BPH 2 mg tablets
1 at night
Send 28

Hytrin is the proprietary name for terazosin, an alpha-blocker drug which is used for the treatment of urinary retention in benign prostatic hyperplasia and for the treatment of mild to moderate hypertension. It is available as two named products, Hytrin and Hytrin BPH, in a number of strengths. The product Hytrin BPH is marketed for benign prostatic hyperplasia. In the above prescription the patient is female and the drug is most likely to be prescribed for the treatment of hypertension. Thus an indication of the sex of the patient is useful to the pharmacist in this case, since the drug may be incorrectly named. However, it is important to check with the prescriber that this is the case.

If the prescription is for an animal, then the name of the animal is not required but the name and address of the owner should be stated on the prescription. However, all veterinary prescriptions should include the type of animal and, ideally, the weight of the animal. This information will allow the dispenser to check if the medicine is appropriate for that type of animal and to calculate the appropriate dose.

Check the legal requirements

The legal requirements will be dependent on the legislation in place in the individual country at the time of writing the prescription. Legal aspects are outlined in Appendix 1, but detailed information is beyond the scope of this book and the reader should seek current legislation details elsewhere. For example, the 'Medicines, Ethics and Practice' guide covers the legislation relating to prescriptions generated in the UK adequately for most purposes. However the legal requirements are likely to require the prescription, at the very least, to be signed and dated by the prescriber. Clearly it is the responsibility of the pharmacist to check that the signature is genuine and the date correct.

Check the product details

Checking the product details will include checking the name of the product, its pharmaceutical form, strength and total amount to be dispensed and its availability. At this stage it is important to consult reference material, if at all in doubt. The name of the product can be either the generic or proprietary name. It is important to check if the product is available in the generic and/or proprietary form and also if it is legal or within the payer's 'formulary' (see later) and hence permissible or cost effective to swap the generic for the proprietary or vice versa. Names of medicines can be very similar and it is essential to make sure that you are dealing with the correct product. Mistakes can be made by incorrectly choosing the wrong product because the name is similar. Also manufacturers' packs of different drugs can be of a very similar design. Box 15.2 shows a list of a few products with similar names. A much more complete list can be obtained from the National Pharmaceutical Association (NPA).

Some drugs are available in many different formulations and it is essential to check that the product on the prescription is available in the correct formulation and to correctly choose the formulation. Again confusion and mistakes can be made if the name of the formulation is similar to another formulation, e.g. tablet formulations of the drug Voltarol are available as Voltarol tablets 25 mg and 50 mg, dispersible tablets, Voltarol Rapid tablets, Voltarol 75 mg SR and Voltarol Retard tablets. Clearly there is the potential for errors in the writing of prescriptions, the checking and interpretation of prescriptions and in the picking of the product with so many different tablet formulations of the same drug all with similar names.

Box 15.2	A few products with similar names
Aldactide	Aldactone
Betaloc	Berotec
Betnesol	Betnelan
Co-amilofruse	Co-amilozide
	Co-amocyclav
Cardene	Codeine
Daonil	Danol
Fucidin	Fulcin
Gliclazide	Glipizide
Migril	Mictral
Nicardipine	Nifedipine
Promazine	Promethazine
Zocor	Zoton

If more than one strength of the product is available, then it is important to check that the strength is stated on the prescription and that the strength is appropriate for the patient. If no strength is stated on the prescription then it may be necessary to contact the prescriber for confirmation of the appropriate strength. If only one strength of a product is available, then clearly it does not need to be entered on the prescription.

The prescription will need to indicate the total amount to be supplied to the patient. This amount should be checked to confirm that the amount is appropriate for the patient and that the product can be supplied in such an amount. Clearly if an ointment is available in a 25 g tube, it would be unprofessional to squeeze out 2.5 g if the prescriber had requested 22.5 g. The pharmacist would either make a professional decision to supply 25 g or seek to arrange for the prescription to be altered. Nowadays many products are available in a complete patient pack (original pack) and so the whole pack would be given to the patient. In such cases the prescription may indicate a complete (original) pack by the abbreviation OP (see Example 15.3).

EXAMPLE 15.3

Co-amoxiclav 250/125 tablets
1 tablet every 8 hours
Send 1 OP

Co-amoxiclav tablets are available only in 21 tablet patient packs and with the instruction on the prescription as 'send 1 OP' the patient would be given a 21 tablet patient pack.

Some prescriptions are written to indicate that a number of days' supply should be dispensed rather than a total amount stated (see Example 15.4). NHS prescription forms have a box in which the prescriber can state the number of days treatment that should be dispensed, rather than state the total amount.

EXAMPLE 15.4

Paracetamol tablets
Two tablets to be taken four times a day
Send 10 days' supply

In the above, the dispenser would need to calculate the total number of tablets to be dispensed, which in this case would be 80 tablets.

Some prescribers may abbreviate the amount to be dispensed in a similar way to the abbreviations used for age. For example, send 3/7 and 3/52 would indicate that an amount of medicine suitable for the treatment of the patient for 3 days and 3 weeks, respectively, should be dispensed (see Example 15.5).

EXAMPLE 15.5

Simple linctus
5 mL four times a day
Send 1/52

Amoxicillin 250 mg capsules
1 to be taken three times a day
Send 5/7

From the above prescription it can be seen that the prescriber requires 1 week's supply (1/52) of the simple linctus. This can be calculated: 5 mL four times a day is 20 mL per day. Therefore 7 days is 7 × 20 mL = 140 mL.

5 days' supply (5/7) of amoxicillin capsules is required. If 1 capsule is to be taken three times a day for 5 days, then 15 capsules should be dispensed.

With much of the above checking procedure, pharmacists should use their professional decision-making skills as to whether the prescriber needs to be contacted for some incomplete prescriptions or whether the pharmacist can deal with the problem. For NHS prescriptions there are two endorsements which can be used by pharmacists. If a prescriber can be contacted by phone regarding any aspects of quantity, strength and dose, then the pharmacist is allowed to amend the prescription provided the prescription is endorsed 'pc' (prescriber contacted) and initialled and dated by the pharmacist. If the prescriber cannot be contacted and the pharmacist has sufficient information to make a professional judgment, then the product may be dispensed. If the total quantity is missing then up to 5 days' supply can be provided. In all cases the prescription must be endorsed with 'pnc' (prescriber not contacted) and initialled and dated by the pharmacist. If the pharmacist has any doubts about exercising discretion, an incomplete prescription should be referred back to the prescriber.

Some products and their details may be correctly written on the prescription form, available on the market but not available in the 'formulary' used by the payer. An example of this, in the UK, is products that are 'blacklisted' by the NHS (Parts XV111A/B/C of the Drug Tariff). Such products cannot be dispensed against an NHS prescription. This method is used to reduce or rationalize costs. Similar schemes are used in private health systems, in which instances the payer develops a 'formulary'. Only those drugs in the 'formulary' can be dispensed. If the patient wants the non-formulary drug then she will have to pay the full market price. It is important that the pharmacist checks each prescription to confirm that he will be recompensed for dispensing.

Check the dosage and directions for use.

Are these present and do they need to be? If appropriate to the product, the dose should always be checked taking into account the patient's age, if a child or elderly (see Ch. 8). Maximum doses and dosage regimens are published in the BNF. These can be expressed in a number of ways.

A specific dose per day, e.g. 200 mg per day

A specific dose per day for a specific time, e.g. 200 mg per day for 7 days

A specific dose for a specific number of times per day, e.g. 200 mg three times daily

A combination of the above, e.g. 200 mg per day, in divided doses, for 15 days

An initial dose, e.g. 200 mg initially, then …

A dose per kg of body weight, e.g. 250 micrograms per kg

A dose per square metre of body surface, e.g. 25 mg per metre squared

A maximum dose, e.g. Do not take more than 2 tablets at any one time. Do not take more than 8 in 24 hours.

The pharmacist should always check that the dose, dosage regimen and any directions for use are appropriate for the patient and the drug (see Example 15.6). Any suspected drug overdoses should always be referred to the prescriber.

EXAMPLE 15.6

The following details are written on a prescription.

Elizabeth Riley
2 Black Avenue
Mediton

Furosemide (frusemide) tablets 40 mg
1 tablet to be taken at night
Send 28 tablets

On the above prescription there is no indication of the age of the patient. It cannot be assumed that the patient is an adult. If the patient is not an adult, then the dose will be inappropriate and possibly the dosage form (young children are usually given liquid formulations).

Furosemide (frusemide) is usually taken in the morning not at night, but night workers may take the tablets at night. In this case it is essential to check with the patient and the prescriber for the correctness of the prescription.

In the case of a veterinary prescription, the dose and dosage regimen can be checked using the *Veterinary Pharmacopoeia* and the *Summary of Product Characteristics for Veterinary Medicines*.

Check for drug interactions

Many drugs are known to interact with other drugs. Appendix 1 in the BNF is a good, up-to-date source for drug interactions. All multiple-item prescriptions should be checked for drug interactions. In addition, if patient medication records are available and current, these should be checked for interactions with concurrent medication. If a prescribed item is known to interact with many drugs or to interact with OTC medicines then it is imperative that the pharmacist checks with the patient which other drugs the patient is taking in order to eliminate possible drug interactions. All potential drug interactions should be referred to the prescriber.

Repeat prescriptions

Pharmacists should check if the prescription is repeatable or being dispensed on a repeat basis. Repeats are stated on the prescription as defined time intervals (e.g. repeat every month) or a defined number of occasions (e.g. repeat twice). NHS prescriptions are nonrepeatable, although NHS forms FP10 MDA and FP10 (HP) Ad allow a total amount of medicine to be supplied on an instalment basis. If a repeatable prescription is dispensed then records need to be made and the prescription should be returned to the patient. If the final repeat is being dispensed then the pharmacist should retain the prescription.

All the above checks should be made on every prescription before the prescription item(s) is assembled, dispensed and labelled (see Ch. 11).

After the dispensing and labelling, the dispensed product and the label should be checked against the prescription to ensure that the right product has the right label. The dispensed product should be handed to the patient (making sure it is the right patient) with appropriate counselling and advice (see Ch. 38).

There are a few other tasks after the dispensing and labelling stages that should be carried out for completion. These tasks are described below.

Records

Pharmacists should complete any legally and professionally required records. Records of prescriptions dispensed can be of two types.

1. Patient medication records. These are maintained for individual patients (see Ch. 31).
2. Legal records. The extent and content of legal records will depend on the legislation in the country of dispensing. In the UK, legal records are only maintained for private prescriptions and prescriptions written for Controlled Drugs.

Endorsement

Depending on the type of prescription, the prescription may need to be stamped with the place and date of dispensing. Additionally if it is an NHS prescription, it will need to be endorsed with exactly what was supplied to the patient so that the Prescription Pricing Authority can reimburse the pharmacist. Similarly private prescriptions will need to be priced for payment by the patient or third party payer.

Fate of prescription

All NHS prescriptions are submitted to the Prescription Pricing Authority for reimbursement. Similarly copies of private prescriptions may be forwarded to a third party payer for payment. Private prescriptions will normally be stored in the pharmacy after dispensing.

STANDARD OPERATING PROCEDURES

In order to support clinical governance, the Royal Pharmaceutical Society is to introduce the requirement for pharmacists to put into place written Standard Operating Procedures (SOP) within individual pharmacies to cover the dispensing process and the transfer of prescribed items to patients. This will apply to both community and hospital pharmacies from 1 January 2005. SOPs will be pharmacy specific, dependent on the competence of the staff working in the pharmacy and applicable at all times. The guidance

document recommends that for each procedure covered by the SOP, pharmacists should consider the following:

- Objectives—what is the procedure trying to achieve?
- Scope—what areas of work are to be covered by the procedure?
- Stages of the process—describe how the task is to be carried out.
- Responsibility—who is responsible for carrying out each stage of the process under normal working conditions and during staff holidays/sickness/maternity leave, etc?
- Other useful information—could anything else be included in the SOP? Is there a mechanism for audit?
- Review—how are you going to ensure that the procedure continues to be useful, relevant and up to date?

Additionally, the guidance document suggests the SOP is set out under the following headings:

- Receipt of prescription
- Assessment of the prescription for validity, safety and clinical appropriateness
- Making interventions and problem solving
- Assembly and labelling of required medicine or product
- Checking procedure
- Transfer of the medicine or product to the patient
- Record keeping and completion of documentation.

Clearly all of the above will need considerable input from pharmacists in the near future. For more details of SOP requirements consult the Royal Pharmaceutical Society.

Key Points

- Prescriptions are paper or electronic documents issued by an authorized prescriber for an individual patient.
- Prescriptions detail the medicinal treatment required for the treatment of the patient.
- Prescription writing is part of the prescribing process.
- The prescribing process should follow a logical sequence.
- Prescriptions can contain more than one prescription item.
- All prescriptions should be checked for clinical and patient appropriateness before assembly and dispensing.
- Standard Operating Procedures should be used in the dispensing process.

Routes of administration and dosage forms

A. J. Winfield (original author M. M. Moody)

> After studying this chapter you will know about:
>
> **The different routes of administration of drugs**
> **The advantages and disadvantages of each route**
> **The types and uses of dosage forms**

Introduction

Following the administration of a medicine, the drug has to reach its site of action or receptor in order to produce an effect. How this is achieved is often a complex process affected by many factors. The first stage will be the release of the drug from the dosage form, to be followed by absorption into the body (unless it is for a surface effect at the site of administration). There is then a distribution process, usually in the blood, which will take the drug to the site of action. As soon as it is in the body metabolic processes, especially in the liver, will start to change the drug and the elimination process will also commence. A detailed discussion of these processes is outside the scope of this book, although it does have a significant impact on the choice of both the route of administration and the actual dosage form. There is a growing awareness that the correct choices can have an important impact on therapeutic outcomes for the patient. Further details about biopharmacy can be found in Aulton (2002) and on pharmacokinetics in Walker and Edwards (1999). This chapter will review the various routes of administration used for drug delivery and discuss some of their advantages and disadvantages. Brief details of a variety of dosage forms are also given. Figure 16.1 illustrates the principle routes of administration.

1 Buccal (inside mouth)
2 Oral (swallow)
3 Sublingual (under tongue)
4 Nasal
5 Rectal
6 Vaginal
7 Inhalation (to lungs)
8 Eye
9 Ear

10 Parenteral
  a Intravenous
  b Subcutaneous
  c Intramuscular
  d Intraspinal
Topical-skin (any site)

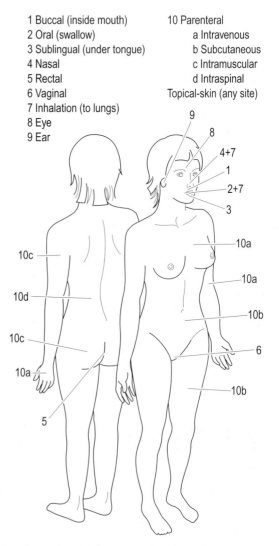

Fig. 16.1 Diagrammatic representation of the main routes of administration.

THE ORAL ROUTE

The oral route can produce either a systemic or local effect. For a systemic effect the drug, formulated in either a solid or a liquid form, is absorbed from the gastrointestinal tract (GIT) and is the most commonly used route for drug administration. There are several reasons for this.

- From a patient's point of view it is the simplest route.
- Self-administration of drugs can be carried out.
- If used properly, it is also the safest route.

However, there are disadvantages which should be borne in mind:

- The onset of action is relatively slow.
- Absorption from the GIT may be irregular.
- Some drugs are destroyed by enzymes and other secretions found in the GIT.
- Because the blood supply from the GIT passes through the liver via the hepatic portal system, it is subject to hepatic metabolism before it enters the systemic circulation. This is called first pass or presystemic metabolism.
- Drug solubility may be altered by the presence of other substances in the GIT, e.g. calcium.
- Gastric emptying is very variable and can be influenced by factors such as food, drugs, disease state and posture. Not only does it affect the onset of action, but if it is extended it may cause a drug to be inactivated by gastric juices owing to prolonged contact.
- It is an unsuitable route of administration in unconscious or vomiting patients and for immediate pre- or postoperative use.

THE BUCCAL ROUTES

A drug is administered by these routes by being formulated as a tablet or spray and is absorbed from the buccal cavity. The highly vascular nature of the tongue and buccal cavity, and the presence of saliva which facilitates the dissolution of the drug, make this a highly effective and useful route for drug administration. It can also be used for a local action.

Two sites are used for absorption from the buccal cavity.

- For sublingual absorption, the area under the tongue is used. This gives a very fast onset of action of the drug but duration is usually short.
- For buccal absorption, the buccal sulcus is used. This is the area between the upper lip and the gum. Tablets formulated for absorption from the buccal sulcus give a quick onset of action but will also give a longer duration of action than the sublingual route. This route can also administer drugs with a longer half-life for an extended duration of action.

It is important that patients are made aware of the difference between the two sites and they should be given full instructions on how to administer their tablets, to ensure maximum benefit. For details of suitable patient instructions see Chapter 23.

The advantages of the buccal route are:

- There is a relatively quick onset of action.
- Drugs are absorbed into the systemic circulation, thereby avoiding the 'first pass' effect.
- Drugs can be administered to unconscious patients.
- Because the tablet is not swallowed, antiemetic drugs can be given by this route.

THE RECTAL ROUTE

For administration by this route drugs are formulated as liquids, solid dosage forms, and semi-solids (see Ch. 21). The chosen preparation is inserted into the rectum from where the drug is released to give a local effect or it may be absorbed to give a systemic effect.

The rectum is supplied by three veins, namely the middle and inferior (lower) rectal veins which drain directly into the systemic circulation and the upper rectal vein which drains into the portal system which flows into the liver. This means that, depending on the position within the rectum, only some of the drug absorbed from the rectum will be subject to the first pass effect. Bioavailability therefore, may be less than 100% but may be better than obtained from other parts of the GIT.

The amount of fluid present in the rectum is small, estimated at approximately 3 mL of mucus. This affects the rate of dissolution of the drug released from the suppository. However, there is also muscular movement which spreads the drug over a large area and promotes absorption.

The advantages and disadvantages of this route of administration are as follows.

Advantages

- Can be used when the oral route is unsuitable, e.g. severe vomiting, unconscious patient, with uncooperative patients such as children, elderly or mentally disturbed and patients with dysphagia.

- Useful when the drug causes GIT irritation.
- Can be used for local action.

Disadvantages

- Absorption can be irregular and unpredictable, giving rise to a variable effect.
- Less convenient than the oral route.
- There is low patient acceptability of this route in the UK. A wider acceptance is found in other parts of the world.

THE VAGINAL ROUTE

For administration by this route, drugs may be formulated as pessaries, tablets, capsules, solutions, sprays, creams, ointments and foams which are inserted into the vagina. Most often this route is used for a local effect. However, drugs absorbed from the vagina are not subject to the first pass effect and can give systemic bioavailability better than with the oral route.

THE INHALATION ROUTE

Drugs are administered, usually by inhalation through the nose or mouth to produce either local or systemic effects. This route is used predominantly for local administration to treat respiratory conditions such as asthma. For this, drugs are delivered directly to the site of action, i.e. the lungs. A variety of dosage forms are used, from simple inhalations consisting of volatile ingredients such as menthol to sophisticated inhaler devices (see Ch. 24). A major benefit of the inhaled route is that the drug dose required to produce the desired effect is much smaller than for the oral route, with a consequent reduction in side-effects. Because of the high blood flow to the lungs and their large surface area, drug absorption by this route is extremely rapid and can be used to give systemic action.

THE NASAL ROUTE

The nasal cavity has been traditionally used for producing local effects using solutions as drops or sprays. More recently it has been used for systemic action because of its good vascular supply which avoids first pass metabolism, although it does have local enzymic activity.

THE TOPICAL ROUTE

In the topical route the skin is used as the site of administration. This route is most commonly used for local effects using liquid and powder dosage forms in addition to the traditional ointments, creams and pastes (see Ch. 20). The skin has a natural barrier function, but specialized dosage forms have been developed which, when applied to the skin, allow the drug to pass through and produce a systemic effect. This avoids first pass effects and can produce close to zero-order kinetics over prolonged time intervals. A more detailed discussion of this route of administration can be found in Chapter 20.

THE PARENTERAL ROUTE

This is the term used to describe when drugs are given by injection. Within this general term there are a variety of different routes. The main ones are:

- *Intravenous route*, where drugs are injected directly into the systemic circulation. This produces a very fast onset of action.
- *Subcutaneous route*, where drugs are injected into the subcutaneous layer of the skin. This is the easiest and least painful type of injection to administer.
- *Intramuscular route*, where drugs are injected into muscle layers. This method can be used to produce a fairly fast onset of action when the drug is formulated as an aqueous solution. A slower and more prolonged action will occur when the drug is presented as a suspension or in an oily vehicle.

These and other specialized types of injection are discussed more fully in the chapter on parenteral products (see Ch. 25).

DOSAGE FORMS

Drugs are presented in a wide variety of dosage forms. How a drug is formulated is dependent on a variety of factors and the same drugs may be presented in several different dosage forms. It is important for pharmacists to appreciate the different properties of the varying dosage forms in order that the most appropriate or most acceptable formulation is given to the patient. This section gives brief information on the different types of dosage forms. Additional, more detailed, information is found in the chapters dealing with specific formulations (see Chs 17–26) and in Aulton (2002).

Aerosols

These consist of pressurized packs which contain the drug in solution or suspension and a suitable propellant. They are most commonly used for their local effect in the treatment of asthma. These devices are fitted with a metering valve which allows a known dose of drug to be delivered each time the device is fired. Some aerosols are for topical use, particularly in the treatment of muscle sprains and injuries. These may contain substances such as non-steroidal anti-inflammatory drugs or counterirritants.

Applications

This is the name given to solutions, suspensions or emulsions which are for topical use. They contain substances such as ascaricides or antiseptics.

Capsules

These are solid dosage forms, generally for oral use. Some drugs formulated as capsules are intended to be inhaled. It is therefore important to inform the patient on their appropriate use. For both types of capsule the drug is contained in a gelatin shell, usually as a powder or a liquid. Modified-release preparations are available where the drug is presented in the gelatin container as small pellets with different coatings.

Collodions

These are liquid preparations for external use. The liquid is painted on the skin, where it forms a flexible film. They contain substances such as salicylic acid which is useful in the treatment of corns.

Creams

These are semisolid emulsions for external use. Because of the water content they are susceptible to microbial contamination and either include a preservative or are given a short shelf life. Creams are easier to apply and are less greasy than ointments, so patients often prefer them.

Dusting powders

These are finely divided powders for external use. Their main uses are as lubricants to prevent friction between skin surfaces and for disinfection and antisepsis in minor wounds.

Ear drops

These are used topically to treat a variety of ear problems. The drug, or mixture of drugs, is presented as a solution or suspension in a suitable vehicle such as water, glycerol, propylene glycol or alcohol. The drops are inserted into the ear, using a dropper. Some vehicles, such as alcohol, may cause a degree of stinging when applied to the ear. Ensure that the patient is aware of this and is assured that it is a normal sensation. If patients find the degree of stinging unacceptable they may have to be given ear drops with an aqueous vehicle. Oils such as almond or olive are often recommended for the alleviation of impacted earwax. It is usually suggested that such oils, before being dropped into the ear, should be warmed. This must be done very carefully and only minimal heat applied, i.e. the oil placed on a warm spoon. Excessive heat will have serious consequences for the integrity of the ear.

Elixirs

An elixir is a solution of one or more drugs for oral use. The vehicle generally contains a high proportion of sucrose or, increasingly nowadays, a 'sugar-free' vehicle such as sorbitol solution, which is less likely to cause dental caries. The therapeutic action of drugs presented as elixirs varies widely and includes antihistamines, antibiotics and decongestants.

Emulsions

These are mixtures of two immiscible liquids, usually oil and water. When the term 'emulsion' is used this refers to a preparation for oral use.

Enemas

An enema is an oily or aqueous solution which is administered rectally. A variety of drugs are formulated as enemas and are used to treat conditions such as constipation or ulcerative colitis. They are also used in X-ray examination of the lower bowel and for systemic effects, such as the use of diazepam in status epilepticus and febrile convulsions.

Eye drops

These are sterile preparations used to administer drugs to the eye.

Gargles

Gargles are aqueous solutions used to treat infections of the throat. They are often presented in a concentrated form with instructions to the patient for dilution. Gargles should not be swallowed but held in the throat while exhaling through the liquid. After a suitable time period, usually a minute or so, the patient should spit out the gargle.

Gels

Gels are semisolid dosage forms for topical or other local use. They are usually transparent or translucent and have a variety of uses. Spermicides and lubricants are often presented in a gel form. Preparations containing coal tar or other drugs used in the treatment of psoriasis and eczema are also presented in this form. Many patients prefer this formulation because it is non-greasy.

The term 'gel' is also used to describe colloidal suspensions of drugs such as aluminium and magnesium hydroxides.

Granules

This term is used to describe a drug which is presented in small irregularly shaped particles. Granules may be packed in individual sachets containing a unit dose of medicament or may be provided in a bulk format where the dose is measured using a 5 mL spoon. Some laxatives are among the drugs currently presented as granules.

Implants

This term refers to solid dosage forms which are inserted under the skin by a small surgical incision. They are most commonly used for hormone replacement therapy or as a contraceptive. Release of the drug from implants is generally slow and long-term therapy is achieved. In the case of the contraceptive implant the effect continues for up to 3 years. A testosterone implant used in the treatment of male hypogonadism will maintain adequate hormone levels in the patient for 4–5 months. Implants must be sterile.

Inhalations

These are preparations which contain volatile medicaments which may have a beneficial effect in upper respiratory tract disorders such as nasal congestion. Some inhalations contain substances which are volatile at room temperature and the patient can obtain a degree of relief by adding a few drops to a handkerchief or a pillowcase and breathing in the vapour. Other inhalations are added to hot water and the impregnated steam is then inhaled. Many users of the latter type of inhalation use boiling water. Pharmacists should advise against this, as the steam produced is too hot and can damage the delicate mucous membranes of the upper respiratory tract. Overuse of this type of preparation should also be avoided as it may cause a chronic condition to develop. The use of these strong aromatic decongestants is contraindicated in children under 3 months owing to the risk of apnoea.

Injections

These are used parenterally and are sterile (see Ch. 25).

Insufflations

This term is used to describe drugs presented in a dry powder form, usually in a capsule, which is inserted into a specially designed device where the capsule is broken, the contents released and the patient inhales the powder. Today, the most common use being made of insufflations is in the treatment of asthma. Some patients find these 'breath-actuated' devices easier to use than aerosol devices.

Irrigations

These are sterile solutions most commonly used in the treatment of infected bladders. Sterile solutions of sodium chloride 0.9% (physiological saline) are used to treat a wide range of common urinary tract pathogens. Antifungal drugs such as amphotericin and locally acting cytotoxics, e.g. doxorubicin and epirubicin, are introduced into the bladder, as irrigations, to treat mycotic infections and bladder tumours, respectively.

Linctuses

A linctus is a viscous liquid for oral use, the majority being for the relief of cough. The viscous nature of the preparation coats the throat and helps to alleviate the irritation which is causing the problem. Previously, many linctuses contained a high level of sucrose; however, many have been reformulated as 'sugar-free' products to reduce the risk of dental caries. Because the viscous nature of linctuses is beneficial they should not be diluted prior to administration.

Liniments

These are liquids for external use. They are used to alleviate the discomfort of muscle strains and injuries. Because of the rubefacient nature of some of the ingredients some sportsmen will use them prior to starting a sporting activity in an attempt to avoid any muscle damage. Examples of active ingredients found in liniments are turpentine oil and methyl salicylate.

Lotions

These are liquids for external use and may be solutions, suspensions or emulsions. They have a variety of uses which include antiseptic, parasiticidal and soothing. Care should be taken when recommending lotions for the treatment of head lice. Those which have an alcohol base should be avoided in asthmatics and young children, as the alcoholic fumes may cause breathing difficulties. Aqueous-based products should be advised.

Lozenges

These are large tablets designed to be sucked and remain in the mouth for up to 15 minutes. They do not contain a disintegrant and the active ingredient is normally incorporated into a sugar base, such as sucrose or glucose. The main use of lozenges is in the treatment of mouth and throat infections.

Mixtures

This is a generic term which is used for many liquid preparations for oral use.

Mouthwashes

These are similar to gargles but are used specifically to treat conditions of the mouth. The active ingredients are usually antiseptics or bactericidal agents.

Nasal drops and sprays

These are isotonic solutions used to treat conditions of the nose. Locally acting decongestants are commonly presented as nose drops. The container includes a dropper device to allow the patient to deliver the appropriate dose into the affected nostril(s). Overuse of nose drops is common as patients find it difficult to judge the number of drops being delivered. Other preparations for both local and systemic use are presented as sprays (metered or pump).

Ointments

Ointments are semisolids for topical use.

Paints

Paints are solutions for application to the skin or mucous membranes. Those used on the skin are often formulated with a volatile vehicle. This evaporates on application and leaves a film of active ingredient on the skin surface. Paints to be used on the throat and mucous surfaces normally include a viscous vehicle such as glycerol, which enables the preparation to remain in contact with the affected area. Paints are used for their antiseptic, analgesic, caustic or astringent properties, and should be supplied with a brush to assist application.

Pastes

These are semisolids for external use. They differ from creams and ointments in that they contain a high proportion of fine powder, such as starch. This makes them very stiff and means they do not spread readily over the skin's surface. Corrosive drugs such as dithranol are often formulated as pastes so that paste applied to the psoriatic lesion will not spread onto healthy skin and cause irritation.

Pastilles

Pastilles are for oral use and, like lozenges, are designed to be sucked. They contain locally acting antiseptics, astringents or anaesthetics and are used to treat, or give symptomatic relief of, conditions affecting the mouth and throat. They are jelly like in consistency produced by their basis of gelatin or acacia.

Pessaries

Pessaries are solid dosage forms for insertion into the vagina. They are used for both local and systemic action.

Pills

Pills are a moulded oral dosage form which has been superseded by tablets and capsules. The term is still used, incorrectly, to describe any solid oral dose form.

Powders (oral)

These occur as both bulk and divided powders. Bulk powders usually contain non-potent active ingredients such as antacids. The dose is measured using a 5 mL spoon.

Individual powders are used for more potent drugs where accuracy of dosage is more important. An individual dose is packaged separately, either in a sheet of paper or in a sachet.

Suppositories

These are solid dosage forms for insertion into the rectum. They are used for both local and systemic actions.

Suspensions

Suspensions are liquid dose forms where the active ingredient is insoluble. Suspensions are available for both oral and external use.

Syrups

These are concentrated aqueous solutions of sugars such as sucrose. The term 'syrup' is frequently, but incorrectly, applied to certain sweetened liquids intended for oral use. The term 'syrup' should nowadays only be used to refer to flavouring vehicles. Sucrose is being replaced by sorbitol as the sweetening agent in many preparations to give 'sugar-free' syrups to reduce the risk of dental caries.

Tablets

This is the term used to describe compressed solid dosage forms generally intended for oral use, although some pessaries are tablets for vaginal use. As well as the standard tablet made by compression, there are many different types of tablet designed for specific uses, e.g. dispersible, enteric-coated, modified release or buccal.

Transdermal delivery systems

This term is used to describe the adhesive patches which, when applied to the skin, deliver a controlled dose of drug over a specified time period to produce a systemic effect.

Key Points

- The route can be chosen to give local or systemic effects, fast or slow onset and is influenced by biopharmacy and pharmacokinetics.
- The oral route is the most commonly used route.
- Gastric emptying, stability and other materials present in the GIT may limit availability of drug from the oral route.
- Sublingual absorption gives a short, fast-onset activity.
- Buccal absorption takes place between the gum and lip.
- Buccal routes of administration can be used with unconscious patients and avoid first pass metabolism.
- Rectal absorption partially avoids first pass metabolism.
- Rectal administration is useful for nil-by-mouth patients and in cases of gastric irritation. However, it is poorly accepted in the UK.
- Vaginal administration can give systemic effects avoiding first pass metabolism.
- Inhalation requires a much lower dose than the oral route, with a rapid onset.
- Administration to the skin may be used for both local and systemic effects.
- Injections can give the fastest onset of action but prolonged action is also possible using oily intramuscular injections.
- A wide range of different dosage forms have been devised which have different properties and uses.
- The same drug may usefully be used in different formulations to assist different types of patients.

Solutions

A. J. Winfield (original author E. J. Kennedy)

After studying this chapter you will know about:

Definitions of solutions and expressions of solubility

Advantages and disadvantages of using solutions

Methods of controlling solubility

Selection of vehicles

Use of preservatives and other ingredients in solutions

Principles of dispensing:
Solutions for oral use
Mouthwashes
Nasal, oral and aural solutions
Enemas

Use of oral syringes

Introduction

Solutions are homogeneous mixtures of two or more components. They contain one or more solutes dissolved in one or more solvents, usually solids dissolved in liquids. The solvent is often aqueous but can be oily or alcoholic.

There are many types of pharmaceutical solutions, based on their composition or medical use. Solutions as oral dosage forms may be used, mouthwashes, gargles, nasal drops, ear drops and externally as lotions, liniments, paints, etc. Solutions may also be used in injections and ophthalmic preparations, which are discussed in Chapters 25 and 26 respectively.

SOLUTIONS FOR ORAL DOSAGE

Oral solutions are usually formulated so that the patient receives the usual dose of the medicament in a conveniently administered volume, usually a multiple of 5 mL, given to the patient using a 5 mL medicine spoon. The term 'teaspoon' and 'tablespoon' should not be used as expressions of a dose for an oral liquid because they are not accurate measures.

Advantages of solutions for oral use over a solid dosage form are that liquids are much easier to swallow than tablets or capsules and the medicament is readily absorbed from the gastrointestinal tract. Ease of taking is especially useful for children, elderly patients or those with chronic conditions such as Parkinson's disease, who may have difficulty swallowing a solid oral dosage form. An advantage of solutions over suspensions is that the medicament is dispersed homogeneously throughout the preparation, without the need to shake the bottle. This makes the preparation easier for the patient to use and should ensure more even dosage. Sometimes substances with a low aqueous solubility may be made into solution by the addition of another solvent rather than formulate the medicine as a suspension.

Disadvantages of solutions are that they are bulky and not as convenient to carry around as a solid dosage forms. They are also less microbiologically and chemically stable than their solid counterparts. Drugs that have an unpleasant taste may not be suitable for administration as an oral solution. The accuracy of oral dosage is dependent on the patient measuring the dose carefully.

The different forms of oral solutions are:

- *Syrups*, which are aqueous solutions that contain sugar. An example is Epilim syrup (sodium valproate).
- *Elixirs*, which are clear, flavoured liquids containing a high proportion of sucrose or a suitable polyhydric alcohol and sometimes ethanol. Examples are phenobarbital elixir and chloral elixir (see Example 17.5).
- *Linctuses*, which are viscous liquids used in the treatment of cough. They should be sipped and swallowed slowly and usually contain a high proportion of sucrose, other sugars or a suitable polyhydric alcohol or alcohols. Examples are Simple Linctus BP and diamorphine linctus (see Example 17.4).

- *Mixtures* is a term often used to describe pharmaceutical oral solutions and suspensions. Examples are chloral hydrate mixture and ammonia and ipecacuanha mixture BP (see Example 17.3).
- *Oral drops* are oral solutions or suspensions which are administered in small volumes, using a suitable measuring device. A proprietary example is Abidec vitamin drops.

Containers for dispensed solutions for oral use

Plain, amber medicine bottles should be used, with a reclosable child-resistant closure. Exceptions to this are if the medicine is in an original pack or patient pack, if there are no suitable child-resistant containers for a particular liquid preparation or if the patient requests it, e.g. if they have severe arthritis in their hands. Advice to store away from children should then be given. A 5 mL measuring spoon or an appropriate oral syringe should be supplied to the patient.

Special labels and advice for dispensed oral solutions

An expiry date should appear on the label for extemporaneously prepared solutions. Most 'official' mixtures and some oral solutions are freshly or recently prepared (see Ch. 10). 'Official' elixirs and linctuses and manufactured products are generally more stable, unless diluted. Diluted products generally have a shorter shelf life than the undiluted preparation. Linctuses should be sipped and swallowed slowly, without the addition of water.

SOLUTIONS FOR OTHER PHARMACEUTICAL USES

Topical solutions for external use are considered in Chapter 20. Some topical solutions are designed for use in body cavities, such as the nose, mouth and ear.

Mouthwashes and gargles

Gargles are used to relieve or treat sore throats and mouthwashes are used on the mucous membranes of the oral cavity, rather than the throat, to refresh and mechanically clean the mouth. Both are concentrated solutions, although gargles tend to contain higher concentrations of active

ingredients than mouthwashes. Both are usually diluted with warm water before use. They may contain antiseptics, analgesics or weak astringents. The liquid is usually not intended for swallowing. Examples are Phenol Gargle BPC and Compound Sodium Chloride Mouthwash BP (see Example 17.7). Proprietary examples are chlorhexidine (Corsodyl) mouthwash and povidone-iodine (Betadine) mouthwash.

Containers for mouthwashes and gargles

An amber, ribbed bottle should be used for extemporaneously prepared solutions. Medicine bottles may be used for products which are intended to be swallowed. Manufactured mouthwashes and gargles are usually packed in plain bottles.

Special labels and advice for mouthwashes and gargles

Directions for diluting the preparations should be given to the patient. If the preparation is not intended for swallowing, the following label is appropriate: 'Not to be swallowed in large amounts'.

Nasal solutions

Most nasal preparations are solutions, administered as nose drops or sprays. They are isotonic to nasal secretions (equivalent to 0.9% normal saline) and buffered to the normal pH range of nasal fluids (pH 5.5–6.5) to prevent damage to ciliary transport in the nose. The most frequent use of nose drops is as a decongestant for the common cold or to administer local steroids for the treatment of allergic rhinitis. Examples are normal saline nose drops and ephedrine nose drops, 0.5% or 1%. Overuse of topical decongestants can lead to oedema of the nasal mucosa and they should only be used for short periods of time (about 4 days) to avoid rebound congestion, called rhinitis medicamentosa. The nasal route may also be useful for new biologically active peptides and polypeptides which need to avoid the first pass metabolism and destruction by the gastrointestinal fluids. The nasal mucosa rapidly absorbs medicaments applied there to give a systemic effect. There are some products utilizing nasal delivery currently available on the market, e.g. desmopressin (Desmospray, DDAVP), used in the treatment of pituitary diabetes insipidus. Accurate dosage is achieved using metered spray devices.

Ear drops

Ear drops are solutions of one or more active ingredient which exert a local effect in the ear, e.g. by softening earwax or treating infection or inflammation. They may also be referred to as otic or aural preparations. Propylene glycol, glycerol (to increase viscosity) and water may be used as vehicles. Examples are aluminium acetate ear drops, almond oil ear drops and Sodium Bicarbonate Ear Drops BP (see Example 17.8).

Containers for nasal and aural preparations

Nose and ear drops that are prepared extemporaneously should be packed in an amber, ribbed hexagonal glass bottle which is fitted with a teat and dropper. Manufactured nasal solutions may be packed in flexible plastic bottles which deliver a fine spray to the nose when squeezed, or in a plain glass bottle with a pump spray or dropper. Manufactured ear drops are usually packed in small glass or plastic containers with a dropper.

Special labels and advice for nasal and aural preparations

Patients should be advised not to share nasal sprays or nose and ear drops in order to minimize contamination and infection. Manufactured nasal sprays and nose and ear drops will usually contain instructions for administration. Patients should be given advice on how to administer extemporaneously prepared nose and ear drops, accompanied by written information if possible (Fig. 17.1). For nose drops it may be easier if the patient is lying flat with the head tilted back as far as comfortable, preferably over the edge of a bed. The patient should remain in this position for a few minutes after the drops have been administered to allow the medication to spread in the nose.

For ear drops, it may be easier for someone other than the patient to administer the drops. If desired the drops can be warmed by holding the bottle in the hands before putting them in, but they must not be overheated. The ear lobe should be held up and back in adults, down and back in children, to allow the medication to run in deeper. They may cause some transient stinging. If the drops are intended to soften earwax, then the ears should be syringed after use.

Extemporaneous preparations should be labelled with the appropriate expiry date following the official monographs. 'For external use' is not an appropriate label and so 'Not to be taken' is advised.

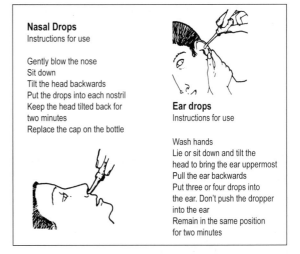

Nasal Drops
Instructions for use

Gently blow the nose
Sit down
Tilt the head backwards
Put the drops into each nostril
Keep the head tilted back for two minutes
Replace the cap on the bottle

Ear drops
Instructions for use

Wash hands
Lie or sit down and tilt the head to bring the ear uppermost
Pull the ear backwards
Put three or four drops into the ear. Don't push the dropper into the ear
Remain in the same position for two minutes

Fig. 17.1 Patient instruction leaflets for use of nose and ear drops.

Enemas

Enemas are oily or aqueous solutions that are administered rectally. They are usually anti-inflammatory, purgative, sedative or given to allow X-ray examination of the lower bowel. Examples are arachis oil enema and magnesium sulphate enema. Retention enemas are administered to give either a local action of the drug, e.g. prednisolone, or for systemic absorption, e.g. diazepam. They are used after defecation. The patient lies on one side during administration and remains there for 30 minutes to allow distribution of the medicament. Microenemas are single-dose, small-volume solutions. Examples are solutions of sodium phosphate, sodium citrate or docusate sodium. They are packaged in plastic containers with a nozzle for insertion into the rectum. Large-volume (0.5–1 litre) enemas should be warmed to body temperature before administration.

Containers for enemas

If extemporaneously produced, enemas are packed in amber, fluted glass bottles. Manufactured enemas will usually be packed in disposable polythene or polyvinyl chloride bags sealed to a rectal nozzle.

Special labels and advice for enemas

Patients should be advised on how to use the enema if they are self-administering and the time that the product will take to work. The label 'For rectal use only' should be used.

EXPRESSION OF CONCENTRATION

Strengths of pharmaceutical solutions can be expressed in a number of ways. The two most commonly used are in terms of amount of drug contained in 5 mL of vehicle or percentage strength. Thus for example a 100 mg/5 mL solution contains 100 mg of drug in each 5 mL. The volume 5 mL is used because it is the usual oral dose administered. A percent weight in volume (% w/v) describes the number of grams of a constituent in 100 mL of preparation. For example, a 2% w/v preparation contains 2 g of a constituent in 100 mL of preparation. A percent volume in volume (% v/v) describes the number of millilitres of a constituent in 100 mL of preparation. For example, a 1% v/v preparation contains 1 mL of a constituent in 100 mL of preparation (see also Ch. 8).

FORMULATION OF SOLUTIONS

Solutions comprise the medicinal agent in a solvent as well as any additional agents. These additional agents are usually included to provide colour, flavour, sweetness or stability to the formulation. Most solutions are now manufactured on a large scale although it may be occasionally required to make up a solution extemporaneously. When compounding a solution, information on solubility and stability of each of the solutes must be taken into account.

Chemical and physical interactions that may take place between constituents must also be taken into account, as these will affect the preparation's stability or potency. For example, esters of *p*-hydroxybenzoic acid, which can be used as preservatives in oral solutions, have a tendency to partition into certain flavouring oils. This could reduce the effective concentration of the preservative agent in the aqueous vehicle of the preparation to a level lower than that required for preservative action.

Solubility

The saturation solubility of a chemical in a solvent is the maximum concentration of a solution which may be prepared at a given temperature. For convenience, this is usually simply called solubility. Solubilities for medicinal agents in a given solvent are given in the *British Pharmacopoeia* (BP) and 'Martindale' and other reference sources. Solubilities are usually stated as the number of parts of solvent (by volume) that will dissolve one part (by weight or volume) of the substance. In other situations, words are used to describe the solubility (see Example 17.2). Using this information it is often possible to calculate whether a solution can be prepared. Most solutions for pharmaceutical use are not saturated with solute.

EXAMPLE 17.1

Potassium chloride is soluble in 2.8–3 parts of water.

This means that 1 g of potassium chloride will dissolve in 2.8–3 mL of water at a temperature of 20°C (taken as normal room temperature).

EXAMPLE 17.2

Diazepam is described as being 'very slightly soluble' in water (which means 1 in 1000 to 1 in 10 000), 'soluble' in alcohol (which means 1 in 10 to 1 in 30) and 'freely soluble' in chloroform (which means 1 in 1 to 1 in 10).

This means that 1 g of diazepam will dissolve in between 10 and 30 mL of alcohol, but would need 1000–10 000 mL of water to dissolve, at a temperature of 20°C.

Vehicles

In pharmacy the medium which contains the ingredients of a medicine is called the vehicle. In solutions this is the solvent. The choice of a vehicle depends on the intended use of the preparation and on the nature and physicochemical properties of the active ingredients.

Water as a vehicle

Water is the vehicle used for most pharmaceutical preparations. It is widely available, relatively inexpensive, palatable and non-toxic for oral use and non-irritant for external use. It is also a good solvent for many ionizable drugs. Different types of water are available as outlined below.

- *Potable water* is drinking water, drawn freshly from a mains supply. It should be palatable and safe for drinking. Its chemical composition may include mineral impurities which could react with drugs, e.g. the presence of calcium carbonate in hard water.
- *Purified water* is prepared from suitable potable water by distillation, by treatment with ion-exchange materials or by any other suitable treatment method such as reverse osmosis. Distilled water is purified water that has been prepared by distillation.

- *Water for preparations* is potable or freshly boiled and cooled purified water, which can be used in oral or external preparations which are not intended to be sterile. The boiling removes dissolved oxygen and carbon dioxide from solution in the water. Any stored water, for example drawn from a local storage tank, should not be used because of the risk of contamination with microorganisms.
- *Water for injections* is pyrogen-free distilled water, sterilized immediately after collection and used for parenteral products (for further details see Ch. 25).
- *Aromatic waters* are near-saturated aqueous solutions of volatile oils or other aromatic or volatile substances, and are often used as a vehicle in oral solutions. Some have a mild carminative action, e.g. dill. Aromatic waters are usually prepared from a concentrated ethanolic solution, in a dilution of 1 part of concentrated water to 39 parts with water. Chloroform water is used as an antimicrobial preservative and also adds sweetness to preparations (see also Ch. 7).

Other vehicles used in pharmaceutical solutions

- *Syrup BP* is a solution of 66.7% sucrose in water. It will promote dental decay and is unsuitable for diabetic patients. Hydrogenated glucose syrup, mannitol, sorbitol, xylitol, etc. can replace the sucrose to give 'sugar-free' solvents.
- *Alcohol (ethyl alcohol, ethanol)*. This is rarely used for internal preparations but is a useful solvent for external preparations.
- *Glycerol (glycerin)* may be used alone as a vehicle in some external preparations. It is viscous and miscible both with water and alcohol. It may be added as a stabilizer and sweetener in internal preparations. In concentrations above 20% v/v it acts as a preservative.
- *Propylene glycol* is a less viscous liquid and a better solvent than glycerol.
- *Oils*. Bland oils such as fractionated coconut oil and arachis oil may be used for fat-soluble compounds, e.g. Calciferol Oral Solution BP. Care is required when using nut oils due to hypersensitivity reactions.
- *Acetone* is used as a cosolvent in external preparations.
- *Solvent ether* can be used as a cosolvent in external preparations for preoperative skin preparation. The extreme volatility of ether and risk of fire and explosion limit its usefulness.

Factors affecting solubility

Compounds that are predominantly non-polar tend to be more soluble in non-polar solvents, such as chloroform or a vegetable oil. Polar compounds tend to be more soluble in polar solvents, such as water and ethanol. The pH will also affect solubility, as many drugs are weak acids or bases. The ionized form of a compound will be the most water soluble, therefore a weakly basic drug will be most soluble in an aqueous solution that is acidic. Acid or alkali may therefore be added to manipulate solubility. Most compounds are more soluble at higher temperatures. Particle size reduction will increase the rate of solution.

Increasing the solution of compounds with low solubility

Cosolvency

The addition of cosolvents, such as ethanol, glycerol, propylene glycol or sorbitol can increase the solubility of weak electrolytes and non-polar molecules in water. They are discussed in more detail in Aulton (2002).

Solubilization

Surfactants may be used as solubilizing agents. Above the critical micelle concentration (CMC) they form micelles which are used to help dissolve poorly soluble compounds. The dissolved compound may be in the centre of the micelle, adsorbed onto the micelle surface or sit at some intermediate point depending on the polarity of the compound. Examples of surfactants used in oral solutions are polysorbates, whilst soaps are used to solubilize phenolic disinfectants for external use.

Preservation of solutions

Most water-containing pharmaceutical solutions will support microbial growth unless this is prevented. Contamination may come from raw materials or be introduced during extemporaneous dispensing.

Preservatives may be added to the formulation to reduce or prevent microbial growth. Chloroform is the most widely used in oral extemporaneous preparations although there are disadvantages to its use, including its high volatility and reported carcinogenicity in animals. Use in the UK is limited to a chloroform content of 0.5% (w/w or w/v). For oral solutions, chloroform at a strength of 0.25% v/v will usually be incorporated as Chloroform Water BP. Alternatively, double strength chloroform water may be included in pharmaceutical formulae as half the total volume of the solution, to effectively give single strength chloroform water in the finished medicine (see Example 17.3). Benzoic acid at a strength of 0.1% w/v is also suitable for oral administration, as are ethanol, sorbic acid, the hydroxybenzoate esters and syrup. Some of the alternative preservatives have pH-dependent activity.

Syrups can be preserved by the maintenance of a high concentration of sucrose as part of the formulation. Concentrations of sucrose greater than 65% w/w will usually protect an oral liquid from growth of most microorganisms by its osmotic effects. A problem with their use occurs when other ingredients are added to the syrup, as this decreases the sucrose concentration. This may cause a loss in the preservative action of the sucrose. Accidental dilution by, for example, using a damp bottle, may have a similar effect.

Preservatives used in external solutions include chlorocresol (0.1% w/v), chlorbutanol (0.5% w/v) and the para-hydroxybenzoates (parabens).

Additional ingredients

Solutions that are intended for oral use may contain excipients such as flavouring, sweetening and, sometimes, colouring agents. These are added to improve the palatability and appearance of a solution for the patient. Stabilizing and viscosity enhancing agents may also be used.

Flavouring agents

Flavours added to solutions can make a medicine more acceptable to take, especially if the drug has an unpleasant taste. Selection of flavours is a complex process in the pharmaceutical industry. Flavours should be chosen to mask particular taste types, e.g. a fruit flavour helps to disguise an acid taste. The age of the patient should be taken into account when selecting a flavour, as children will tend to enjoy fruit or sweet flavours. Some flavours are associated with particular uses, e.g. peppermint is associated with antacid preparations. The flavour and colour should also complement each other. Extemporaneous medicines tend to use natural flavours added as juices (raspberry), extracts (liquorice), spirits (lemon and orange), syrups (blackcurrant), tinctures (ginger) and aromatic waters (anise and cinnamon). Some synthetic flavours are used in manufactured medicines.

Sweetening agents

Many oral solutions are sweetened with sugars, including glucose and sucrose. Sucrose enhances the viscosity of liquids and also gives a pleasant texture in the mouth. Prolonged use of liquid medicines containing sugar will lead to an increased incidence of dental caries, particularly in children. Attempts should be made to formulate oral solutions without sugar as a sweetening agent, using sorbitol, mannitol, xylitol, saccharin and aspartame as alternatives. Oral liquid preparations that do not contain fructose, glucose or sucrose are labelled 'sugar free' in the *British National Formulary* (BNF). These alternatives should be used where possible.

Colouring agents

Colouring agents are added to pharmaceutical preparations to enhance the appearance of a preparation or to increase the acceptability of a preparation to the patient. Colours are often matched to the flavour of a preparation, e.g. a yellow colour for a banana-flavoured preparation. Colour is also useful to give a consistent appearance where there is natural variation between batches. Colours can give distinctive appearances to some medicines, e.g. the green colour of the Drug Tariff formula of methadone mixture.

Colouring agents should be non-toxic and free of any therapeutic activity themselves. Natural colourants are most likely to meet this criterion and include materials derived from plants and animals, e.g. carotenoids, chlorophylls, saffron, red beetroot extract, caramel and cochineal. As with all natural agents, the disadvantage is that batches may vary in quality. Mineral pigments such as iron oxides are not often used in solutions because of their low solubility in water. Synthetic organic dyes such as the azo compounds are alternatives for colouring pharmaceutical solutions as they give a wide range of bright, stable colours. Colours appear in pharmaceutical formulae less often now, especially in children's medicines. Some consumers see their use as unnecessary and some colouring agents, e.g. tartrazine, have been implicated in allergic reactions and hyperactivity of children. Additionally, coloured dyes in medicines can lead to confusion when diagnosing diseases, e.g. a red dye appearing in vomit could be wrongly assumed to be blood. In the European Union, colours are selected from a list permitted for medicinal products, with designated 'E' numbers between 100 and 180.

Stabilizers

Antioxidants may be used where ingredients are liable to degradation by oxidation, e.g. in oils. Those which are added to oral preparations include ascorbic acid, citric acid, sodium metabisulphite and sodium sulphite. These are odourless, tasteless and non-toxic.

Viscosity-enhancing agents

Syrups may be added to increase the viscosity of an oral liquid. They also improve palatability and ease pourability. Other thickening agents may also be used (see Ch. 18).

SHELF LIFE OF SOLUTIONS

There may be individual variations, but most solutions which are prepared extemporaneously should be freshly or recently prepared. The data sheets should be consulted for information about particular manufactured solutions and for storage conditions.

ORAL SYRINGES

If fractional doses are prescribed for oral liquids, they should not be diluted, but an oral syringe should be supplied with the dispensed oral liquid. The standard oral syringe is marked in 0.5 mL divisions from 1 to 5 mL to measure doses of less than 5 mL. An adapter fits into the neck of all common sizes of the medicine bottle. Instructions should be supplied with the oral syringe. Shake the bottle and then remove the lid and insert the adapter firmly into the top of the bottle. Push the tip of the oral syringe into the hole in the adapter and turn the bottle upside down. Pull the syringe plunger to draw liquid to the appropriate volume. It may be desirable to indicate this on the syringe. Turn the bottle right way up and carefully remove the syringe, holding the barrel. Gently put the tip into the child's mouth to be inside the cheek. Slowly and gently push the plunger in and allow the child to swallow the medicine before removing the syringe. Do not squirt the liquid or direct it towards the throat. After completing the process, remove the adapter and replace the cap on the bottle. The adapter and syringe should be rinsed and left to dry. Patient information leaflets are available to accompany the oral syringe (Fig. 17.2).

INFORMATION ABOUT THE *Exacta-Med*® ORAL MEDICINE SYRINGE

Baxa *Exacta-Med*® Oral Medicine Syringes are intended for the accurate measurement, and giving by mouth, of liquid medicines in doses prescribed by a Pharmacist or Doctor. The Syringes cannot be used with an injection needle. They are made from material which allows them to be cleaned and re-used. The Syringes comply with BS.3221/7:86 and the 5ml Syringe Pack complies with BNF No.23 and is available on prescription under the Drug Tariff, Pt.IV.

Two types of **Bottle Adaptor** are available. They are designed to make it easier to fill the Syringe. The **Universal Bottle Adaptor**, illustrated below, fits a number of bottle neck sizes. It must be removed and the bottle re-capped after use. The **Press-in Adaptor** (normally only supplied by the Hospital Pharmacist) fits snugly into the neck of certain bottle sizes. After use the **Press-in Adaptor** is left in position and the bottle cap replaced over it.

INSTRUCTIONS FOR USE

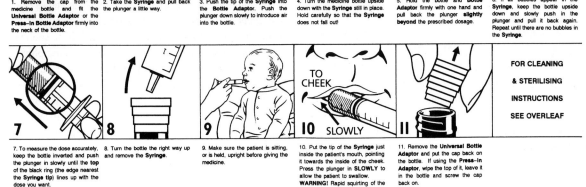

1. Remove the cap from the medicine bottle and fit the **Universal Bottle Adaptor** or the **Press-in Bottle Adaptor** firmly into the neck of the bottle.

2. Take the **Syringe** and pull back the plunger a little way.

3. Push the tip of the **Syringe** into the **Bottle Adaptor**. Push the plunger down slowly to introduce air into the bottle.

4. Turn the medicine bottle upside down with the **Syringe** still in place. Hold carefully so that the **Syringe** does not fall out!

5. Hold the bottle and **Bottle Adaptor** firmly with one hand and pull back the plunger **slightly beyond** the prescribed dosage.

6. If air bubbles appear in the **Syringe**, keep the bottle upside down and slowly push in the plunger and pull it back again. Repeat until there are no bubbles in the **Syringe**.

7. To measure the dose accurately, keep the bottle inverted and push the plunger in slowly until the **top** of the black ring (the edge nearest the **Syringe tip**) lines up with the dose you want.

8. Turn the bottle the right way up and remove the **Syringe**.

9. Make sure the patient is sitting, or is held, upright before giving the medicine.

10. Put the tip of the **Syringe** just inside the patient's mouth, pointing it towards the inside of the cheek. Press the plunger in **SLOWLY** to allow the patient to swallow. **WARNING!** Rapid squirting of the medicine may cause choking.

11. Remove the **Universal Bottle Adaptor** and put the cap back on the bottle. If using the **Press-in Adaptor**, wipe the top of it, leave it in the bottle and screw the cap back on.

FOR CLEANING
& STERILISING
INSTRUCTIONS
SEE OVERLEAF

Fig. 17.2 Patient information leaflet with instructions for the use of an oral syringe. (Reproduced by permission of Baxa Corporation. An updated version will be available from Baxa during 2003.)

DILUENTS

If a prescriber insists that a manufactured solution is diluted, then a suitable diluent must be selected. Information sources to obtain this information are the *Medicines Compendium* or the National Pharmaceutical Association (NPA) *Diluent Directory*. An indication of the expiry date for the diluted preparation is also given in these references. The dilution should be freshly prepared.

A short shelf life for a diluted solution may require patients to return to the pharmacy to collect the balance of their medication. This may happen, for instance, where an oral sodium chloride solution has been prescribed for 1 month. The solution has a 2-week expiry, and must therefore be supplied in two instalments. The patient, or their representative, should be issued with an owing slip, or some similar documentation. This should state the name of the patient, the pharmacy, the item and quantity of medicine owed and the date of issue. A record should also be kept in the pharmacy. Most computer labelling systems have the facility to handle 'owings'.

EXAMPLE 17.3

℞ Ammonium and Ipecacuanha Mixture BP. Mitte 100 mL.

	Master formula	For 100 mL
Ammonium bicarbonate	200 mg	2 g
Liquorice liquid extract	0.5 mL	5 mL
Ipecacuanha tincture	0.3 mL	3 mL
Concentrated camphor water	0.1 mL	1 mL
Concentrated anise water	0.05 mL	0.5 mL
Double strength chloroform water	5 mL	50 mL
Water	to 10 mL	to 100 mL

Action and uses. Expectorant cough preparation. The benefit of expectorant mixtures is doubtful, but they may be useful as a placebo and they are inexpensive.

Formulation notes. Ammonium bicarbonate, ipecacuanha and camphor water are mild expectorants. Anise water acts as a mild expectorant and a flavouring agent. Liquid liquorice extract is used as a mild expectorant, flavouring and sweetening agent. Chloroform water acts as a sweetener and a preservative. Ammonium bicarbonate is

soluble 1 in 5 of water, so will dissolve to give a solution. All other ingredients are liquids.

Method of preparation. The ammonium bicarbonate should be weighed on a suitable balance and dissolved in approximately 15 mL water, in a 100 mL conical measure. The double strength chloroform water should be added to this solution. The other liquid ingredients should be measured and added to the solution. The mixture should then be made up to volume in the conical measure. It should be packed into an amber medicine bottle with a child-resistant closure. The bottle should be polished and labelled, and a 5 mL spoon should be given with the medicine.

Shelf life and storage. Store in a cool, dry place. It is recently prepared, therefore a shelf life of 2–3 weeks is applicable.

Advice and labelling. 'Shake well before use'. Whilst this is not strictly required, it is good practice to include it.

EXAMPLE 17.4

℞ 200 mL of Diamorphine linctus.

	Master formula	For 200 mL
Diamorphine hydrochloride	3 mg	120 mg
Oxymel	1.25 mL	50 mL
Glycerol	1.25 mL	50 mL
Compound tartrazine solution	0.06 mL	2.4 mL
Syrup	to 5 mL	to 200 mL

Action and uses. A cough suppressant in terminal care.

Formulation notes. Oxymel is a solution of acetic acid, water and purified honey, used as a demulcent and sweetening agent in linctuses. Glycerol is also a demulcent and sweetener. Compound tartrazine solution is a colouring agent and syrup is a demulcent vehicle. Diamorphine is soluble 1 in 1.6 of water and 1 in 12 of alcohol, so a solution will be produced.

Method of preparation. Weigh 120 mg diamorphine on an appropriate balance. Transfer to a 200 mL measuring cylinder. Dissolve the diamorphine in the oxymel and glycerol. Add about 50 mL of syrup, then add the compound tartrazine solution. Transfer to a previously tared amber medicine bottle (see Ch. 7). Make up to volume with the syrup in the tared bottle in order to overcome difficulties in draining all the viscous mixture from a measure. Close with a child-resistant closure, polish and label the bottle and give a 5 mL medicine spoon or oral syringe with the medicine (depending on the dosage prescribed).

Shelf life and storage. Store in a cool, dry place. It is recently prepared, therefore a shelf life of 2–3 weeks is applicable.

Advice and labelling. 'Shake well before use'. The linctus should be sipped and swallowed slowly, undiluted. 'The medicine may cause drowsiness. Avoid alcoholic drink' (BNF Label 2). Since this patient is terminally ill, they are unlikely to be driving or operating machinery so this part of the advisory label can be omitted. Alcohol should be avoided as this will increase the sedative effect.

EXAMPLE 17.5

℞ 50 mL Chloral elixir, paediatric. For an 8-month-old baby.

	Master formula	For 50 mL
Chloral hydrate	200 mg	2 g
Water	0.1 mL	1 mL
Blackcurrant syrup	1 mL	10 mL
Syrup	to 5 mL	to 50 mL

Action and uses. For short-term use in insomnia.

Formulation notes. Chloral hydrate is soluble 1 in 0.3 of water and has an unpleasant taste. Blackcurrant syrup is used as a flavouring agent to mask this.

Method of preparation. Weigh 2 g chloral hydrate on a suitable balance. Transfer it to a 50 mL measuring cylinder and dissolve it in water. Add the blackcurrant syrup. Add some of the syrup (rinsing the measure used for the blackcurrant syrup). Transfer the mixture to a tared, 50 mL amber medicine bottle and make up to volume, to avoid loss of the viscous product in the measures. Polish and label the bottle and give a 5 mL medicine spoon or oral syringe with the medicine.

Shelf life and storage. Store in a cool, dry place. Chloral hydrate is volatile and sensitive to light. It is recently prepared and a shelf life of 2–3 weeks is appropriate.

Advice and labelling. 'Shake well before use' and BNF Labels 1 and 27. An appropriate dose for a child up to 1 year is one 5 mL spoonful to be given, well diluted with water, at bedtime. The parent should be advised that this might make the child drowsy.

EXAMPLE 17.6

℞ 200 mL Potassium Citrate Mixture BP.

	Master formula	For 200 mL
Potassium citrate	3 g	60 g
Citric acid monohydrate	500 mg	10 g
Syrup	2.5 mL	50 mL
Quillaia tincture	0.1 mL	2 mL
Lemon spirit	0.05 mL	1 mL
Double strength chloroform water	3 mL	60 mL
Water	to 10 mL	to 200 mL

Action and uses. Alkalinization of urine to relieve discomfort in mild urinary tract infections or cystitis.

Formulation notes. Citric acid and potassium citrate are the active ingredients, both are soluble 1 in 1 of water. Lemon spirit, which is lemon oil in alcoholic solution, is a flavouring agent. The oil tends to be displaced from solution in an aqueous medium, especially in the presence of a high concentration of salts. The quillaia tincture is a surfactant used to emulsify any displaced lemon oil. Syrup is a sweetening agent.

Method of preparation. The solids should be size reduced, weighed and dissolved in the double strength chloroform water and syrup. The quillaia tincture should be added before the lemon spirit is added with stirring, so that immediate emulsification of the oil will be achieved if required. Make up to volume with water. Pack in an amber medicine bottle with a child-resistant closure. Polish and label the bottle and give a 5 mL medicine spoon with the medicine.

Shelf life and storage. Store in a cool, dry place. It is recently prepared, therefore a shelf life of 2–3 weeks is applicable.

Advice and labelling. 'Shake well before use'. The medicine should be diluted with plenty of water (BNF Label 27).

EXAMPLE 17.7

℞ Compound Sodium Chloride Mouthwash BP. Mitte 500 mL.

	Master Formula	For 500 mL
Sodium chloride	1.5 g	7.5 g
Sodium bicarbonate	1 g	5 g
Concentrated peppermint emulsion	2.5 mL	12.5 mL
Double strength chloroform water	50 mL	250 mL
Water	to 100 mL	to 500 mL

Action and uses. Mechanically cleans and freshens the mouth.

Formulation notes. Concentrated peppermint emulsion is used as a flavouring and the chloroform water is a sweetener and preservative. Sodium chloride is soluble 1 in 3 of water and sodium bicarbonate is soluble 1 in 11 of water.

Method of preparation. The solids are weighed on a suitable balance and dissolved in a 500 mL conical measure in approximately 100 mL of water. Add the double strength chloroform water and the concentrated peppermint emulsion. Make up to volume with water. Pack in an amber ribbed bottle with a child-resistant closure. Polish and label the bottle.

Shelf life and storage. Store in a cool, dry place. It is recently prepared, therefore a shelf life of 2–3 weeks is applicable.

Advice and labelling. 'Shake well before use'. The patient should be directed to use about 15 mL diluted in an equal volume of warm water, usually morning and night, unless otherwise directed. The solution should be used as a mouthwash and should not be swallowed, although reassure the patient that it is not harmful to swallow small amounts of the mouthwash.

EXAMPLE 17.8

℞ 10 mL Sodium Bicarbonate Ear Drops BP.

	Master formula	For 10 mL
Sodium bicarbonate	5 g	500 mg
Glycerol	30 mL	3 mL
Water	to 100 mL	to 10 mL

Action and uses. For the softening and removal of earwax (usually prior to syringing with warm water).

Formulation notes. Sodium bicarbonate is soluble 1 in 11 of water. Glycerol is a viscous liquid used to thicken the drops, but presents problems in measuring the volume accurately.

Method of preparation. Weigh 500 mg sodium bicarbonate and dissolve in 6 mL of water, using a 10 mL conical measure. Carefully make up to 7 mL using water. Carefully add glycerol up to the 10 mL mark (this will result in 3 mL of glycerol being added to the solution). Pack in a 10 mL hexagonal, amber, ribbed bottle with a dropper. Polish and label the bottle on the three smooth sides.

Shelf life and storage. Store in a cool, dry place. The drops are recently prepared, therefore a shelf life of 2–3 weeks is applicable.

Advice and labelling. 'Shake well before use' and 'Not to be taken'. The bottle may be warmed in the hands before placing drops in the ears. A patient information leaflet should be used to describe how to use the drops (Fig. 17.1).

Key Points

- Pharmaceutical solutions are given different names depending on their nature and use.
- There are both advantages and disadvantages in the use of oral solutions.
- Most oral solutions would be freshly or recently prepared.
- Solutions may also be used for mouthwashes, gargles, nasal drops and sprays, ear drops and enemas.
- Many different vehicles may be used in pharmaceutical solutions, but water is the most common.
- Water is available in different forms for different uses.
- Saturation solubility of a drug in a solvent is affected by polarity of both drug and solvent.
- Saturation solubility can be increased by techniques such as cosolvency and solubilization.
- Antimicrobial preservation is required for most aqueous solutions.
- Various additives such as flavours, sweeteners and colours may be added to improve the palatability of oral solutions.
- Oral syringes will be required for doses of less than 5 mL and its use explained.

Suspensions

A. J. Winfield (original author E. J. Kennedy)

After studying this chapter you will know about:

The nature of suspensions
The pharmaceutical uses of suspensions
The properties of an ideal suspension
Matters which need to be considered in formulating a suspension
Ingredients which may be added to suspensions
The dispensing of suspensions for internal and external use

Introduction

Suspensions contain one or more insoluble medicaments in a vehicle, with other additives such as preservatives, flavours, colours, buffers and stabilizers. Most pharmaceutical suspensions are aqueous, but an oily vehicle is sometimes used. Suspensions may be used for oral administration, inhalation, topical application, as ophthalmic preparations, for parenteral administration and as aerosols.

A definition of a pharmaceutical suspension is a disperse system in which one substance (the disperse phase) is distributed in particulate form throughout another (the continuous phase). Most are classified as a coarse suspension which is a dispersion of particles with a mean diameter greater than 1 μm. A colloidal suspension is a dispersion of particles with a mean diameter less than 1 μm. Suspended solids slowly separate on standing, but redispersion may be difficult if they form a compacted sediment.

PHARMACEUTICAL APPLICATIONS OF SUSPENSIONS

Suspensions may be used pharmaceutically for a number of reasons. Some are given below:

- Drugs that have very low solubility are usefully formulated as suspensions.
- If people have difficulty swallowing solid dosage forms, the drug may need to be dispersed into a liquid form.
- Drugs that have an unpleasant taste in their soluble form can be made into insoluble derivatives, and formulated as a suspension, which will be more palatable. For example chloramphenicol (soluble) → chloramphenicol palmitate (insoluble).
- In oral suspensions the drug is delivered in finely divided form, therefore optimal dissolution occurs immediately in the gastrointestinal (GI) fluids. The rate of absorption of a drug from a suspension is usually faster than when delivered as a solid oral dosage form, but slower than the rate from solution. The rate of availability of drug from a suspension is also dependent on the viscosity; the more viscous the product, the slower the release of drug.
- Insoluble forms of drugs may prolong the action of a drug by preventing rapid degradation of the drug in the presence of water.

Oxytetracycline
in aqueous solution

Hydrochloride (soluble,   Calcium salt (insoluble):
tablet form): hydrolyses rapidly   stable

- If the drug is unstable when in contact with the vehicle, suspensions should be prepared immediately prior to handing out to the patient in order to reduce the amount of time that the drug particles are in contact with the dispersion medium. For example with ampicillin suspension, water is added to powder or granules prior to giving out to the patient. A 14-day expiry date is given, if kept in the fridge.
- Drugs which degrade in aqueous solution may be suspended in a non-aqueous phase, for example tetracycline hydrochloride is suspended in a fractionated coconut oil for ophthalmic use.

- Bulky, insoluble powders can be formulated as a suspension so that they are easier to take, for example kaolin or chalk (see Example 18.2). Examples of suspensions for oral use are Kaolin Mixture Paediatric BP, kaolin and morphine mixture (see Example 18.1) and antacids such as Magnesium Trisilicate Mixture BP.
- Intramuscular, intra-articular or subcutaneous injections are often formulated as suspensions to prolong the release of the drug.
- Lotions containing insoluble solids are formulated to leave a thin coating of medicament on the skin. As the vehicle evaporates, it gives a cooling effect and leaves the solid behind. Examples are Calamine Lotion BP (see Example 18.5) and Sulphur Lotion Compound BPC (see Ch. 20).

PROPERTIES OF A GOOD PHARMACEUTICAL SUSPENSION

In preparing a pharmaceutically elegant product, several desirable properties are sought:

- There is ready redispersion of any sediment which accumulates on storage.
- After gentle shaking, the medicament stays in suspension long enough for a dose to be accurately measured.
- The suspension is pourable.
- Particles in suspension are small and relatively uniform in size, so that the product is free from a gritty texture.

FORMULATION OF SUSPENSIONS

The three steps that can be taken to ensure formulation of an elegant pharmaceutical suspension are:

1. Control particle size. On a small scale, this can be done using a mortar and pestle, to grind down ingredients to a fine powder.
2. Use a thickening agent to increase viscosity of vehicle, by using suspending or viscosity-increasing agents.
3. Use a wetting agent.

Some of the theoretical and practical aspects of these will be considered in the context of extemporaneous dispensing. Further details about the industrial aspects are given in Aulton (2002).

The insoluble medicament may be a diffusible solid or an indiffusible solid:

Diffusible solids (dispersible solids). These are insoluble solids that are light and easily wetted by water. They mix readily with water, and stay dispersed long enough for an adequate dose to be measured. After settling they redisperse easily. Examples include magnesium trisilicate, light magnesium carbonate, bismuth carbonate and light kaolin (see Example 18.1).

Indiffusible solids. Most insoluble solids are not easily wetted, and may form large porous clumps in the liquid. These solids will not remain evenly distributed in the vehicle long enough for an adequate dose to be measured. They may not redisperse easily. Examples for internal use include aspirin, phenobarbital, sulfadimidine and chalk (see Example 18.2) and for external use calamine, hydrocortisone, sulphur and zinc oxide.

Problems encountered when formulating insoluble solids into a suspension

Various factors need to be considered when formulating insoluble solids into a suspension.

Sedimentation

The factors affecting the rate of sedimentation of a particle are described in Stokes' equation:

$$v = \frac{2r^2(\sigma - \rho)g}{9\eta}$$

where v = velocity of a spherical particle of radius r, and density σ, in a liquid of density ρ, and viscosity η, and where g is the acceleration due to gravity.

The basic consequences of this equation are that the rate of fall of a suspended particle in a vehicle of a given density is greater for larger particles than it is for smaller particles. Also, the greater the difference in density between the particles and vehicle, the greater will be the rate of descent. Increasing the viscosity of the dispersion medium, within limits so that the suspension is still pourable, will reduce the rate of sedimentation of a solid drug. Thus a decrease in settling rate in a suspension may be achieved by reducing the size of the particles and by increasing the density and the viscosity of the continuous phase.

Flocculation

The natural tendency of particles towards aggregation will determine the properties of a suspension. In a deflocculated suspension, the dispersed solid particles remain separate and settle slowly. However, the sediment that eventually forms is hard to redisperse and is described as a 'cake' or clay. In a flocculated suspension, individual particles aggregate into clumps or floccules in suspension. Because these flocs are larger than individual particles, sedimentation is more rapid, but the sediment is loose and easily redispersible. Excess flocculation may prevent 'pourability' due to its effect on rheological properties.

The ideal is to use either a deflocculated system with a sufficiently high viscosity to prevent sedimentation, or controlled flocculation with a suitable combination of rate of sedimentation, type of sediment and pourability.

Wetting

Air may be trapped in the particles of poorly wetted solids which causes them to float to the surface of the preparation and prevents them from being readily dispersed throughout the vehicle. Wetting of the particles can be encouraged by reducing the interfacial tension between the solid and the vehicle, so that adsorbed air is displaced from solid surfaces by liquid. Suitable wetting agents have this effect, but decrease interparticular forces thereby affecting flocculation.

Hydrophilic colloids such as acacia and tragacanth can act as wetting agents. However, care should be taken when using these agents as they can promote deflocculation. Intermediate HLB (hydrophilic–lipophilic balance) surfactants such as polysorbates and sorbitan esters are used for internal preparations. Solvents such as ethanol, glycerol and the glycols also facilitate wetting. Sodium lauryl sulphate and quillaia tincture are used in external preparations.

Suspending agents

Suspending agents increase the viscosity of the vehicle, thereby slowing down sedimentation. Most agents can form thixotropic gels which are semisolid on standing, but flow readily after shaking. Care must be taken when selecting a suspending agent for oral preparations, as the acid environment of the stomach may alter the physical characteristics of the suspension, and therefore the rate of release of the drug from suspension. Some suspending agents may also bind to certain medicaments, making them less bioavailable.

Suspending agents can be divided into five broad categories: natural polysaccharides, semisynthetic polysaccharides, clays, synthetic agents and miscellaneous compounds. Brief information on these classes of suspending agents is

given below, with more detailed information available from the *Pharmaceutical Codex* or Aulton (2002).

Natural polysaccharides

The main problem with these agents is their natural variability between batches and microbial contamination. Tragacanth is a widely used suspending agent and is less viscous at pH 4–7.5. As a rule of thumb, 0.2 g tragacanth powder is added per 100 mL suspension or 2 g compound tragacanth powder per 100 mL suspension. Tragacanth powder requires to be dispersed with the insoluble powders before water is added to prevent clumping (see Example 18.2). Compound Tragacanth Powder BP 1980 contains tragacanth, acacia, starch and sucrose and so is easier to use. Other examples include acacia gum, starch, agar, guar gum, carrageenan and sodium alginate. These materials should not be used externally as they leave a sticky feel on the skin.

Semisynthetic polysaccharides

These are derived from the naturally occurring polysaccharide, cellulose. Examples include methylcellulose (Cologel, Celacol), hydroxyethylcellulose (Natrosol 250), sodium carboxymethylcellulose (Carmellose sodium) and microcrystalline cellulose (Avicel).

Clays

These are naturally occurring inorganic materials which are mainly hydrated silicates. Examples include bentonite and magnesium aluminium silicate (Veegum).

Synthetic thickeners

These were introduced to overcome the variable quality of natural products. Examples include carbomer (Carboxyvinyl polymer, Carbopol), colloidal silicon dioxide (Aerosil, Cabo-sil) and polyvinyl alcohol.

Miscellaneous compounds

Gelatin is used as a suspending and viscosity-increasing agent.

Preservation of suspensions

All pharmaceutical preparations that contain water are therefore susceptible to microbial growth. Water is the most common source of microbial contamination. Also the naturally occurring additives such as acacia and tragacanth may be sources of microbes and spores. Preservative action may be diminished because of adsorption of the preservative onto solid particles of drug, or interaction with suspending agents. Useful preservatives in extemporaneous preparations include chloroform water, benzoic acid and hydroxybenzoates.

THE DISPENSING OF SUSPENSIONS

The method of dispensing suspensions is the same for most, with some differences for specific ingredients.

1. Crystalline and granular solids are finely powdered in the mortar. The suspending agent should then be added and mixed thoroughly in the mortar. Do not apply too much pressure, otherwise gumming or caking of the suspending agent will occur and heat of friction will make it sticky.
2. Add a little of the liquid vehicle to make a paste and mix well until smooth and free of lumps. Continue with gradual additions until the mixture can be poured into a tared bottle. Further liquid is used to rinse all the powder into the bottle, where it is made up to volume.

Variations

- If wetting agents are included in the formulation, add them before forming the paste.
- If syrup and/or glycerol are in the formulation, use this rather than water to form the initial paste.
- If soluble solids are being used, dissolve them in the vehicle before or after making the paste.
- Leave addition of volatile components, colourings or concentrated flavouring tinctures such as chloroform spirit, liquid liquorice extract and compound tartrazine solution until near the end.

Most 'official' suspensions will be prepared from the constituent ingredients. There may be some occasions where an oral solid dosage form, such as a tablet or capsule, will have to be reformulated by the pharmacist into an oral suspension, e.g. where the medicine is for a child (see Example 18.3). It is important to obtain as much information (physical, chemical and microbiological) as possible about the manufactured drug and its excipients. This can usually be obtained from the manufacturer. Typically, the tablet will be crushed or capsule contents emptied into the mortar and a

suspending agent added. A paste is formed with the vehicle and then diluted to a suitable volume, with the addition of any other desired ingredients such as preservative or flavour. A short expiry of no more than 2 weeks (more likely to be 7 days) should be given owing to the lack of knowledge about the stability of the formulation.

Preparation of suspensions from dry powders and granules for reconstitution

Suspensions may have to be prepared from previously manufactured dry powders or granules if the liquid preparation has a limited shelf life because of chemical or physical instability. Powders should firstly be loosened from the bottom of the container by lightly tapping against a hard surface. The specified amount of cold, purified water should then be added, sometimes in two or more portions, with shaking, until all the dry powder is suspended. The container is usually over-sized in order to allow adequate shaking for reconstitution. The patient may prepare some suspensions immediately before taking from individually packed sachets of powder or from bulk solids. This is considered in more detail in Chapter 22.

Containers for suspensions

Suspensions should be packed in amber bottles, plain for internal use and ribbed for external use. There should be adequate air space above the liquid to allow shaking and ease of pouring. A 5 mL medicine spoon or oral syringe should be given when the suspension is for oral use.

Special labels and advice for suspensions

The most important additional label for suspensions is 'Shake well before use', as some sedimentation of medicament would normally be expected. Shaking the bottle will redisperse the medicament and ensure that the patient can measure an accurate dose.

'Store in a cool place'. Stability of suspensions may be adversely affected by both extremes and variations of temperature. Some suspensions, such as those made from reconstituting dry powders, may need to be stored in a refrigerator.

Extemporaneously prepared and reconstituted suspensions will have a relatively short shelf life. They are usually required to be recently or freshly prepared, with a 1–4-week expiry date. Some official formulae state an expiry date, but many do not. The pharmacist may have to make judgments about the expiry date for a particular preparation, based on its constituents and likely storage conditions. The manufacturer's literature for reconstituted products will give recommended storage conditions.

Inhalations

Suspensions are useful formulations for inhalations. The volatile components are adsorbed onto the surface of a diffusible solid to ensure uniform dispersion throughout the liquid. When hot water is added the oils vaporize. Where quantities are not stated, 1 g of light magnesium carbonate is used for each 2 mL of oil (such as eucalyptus oil) or 2 g of volatile solid (such as menthol). An example of an inhalation is menthol and eucalyptus inhalation (see Example 18.4).

EXAMPLE 18.1

℞ 150 mL Kaolin and Morphine Mixture BP.

	Master formula	For 150 mL
Light kaolin	2 g	30 g
Sodium bicarbonate	500 mg	7.5 g
Chloroform and		
morphine tincture	0.4 mL	6 mL
Water	to 10 mL	to 150 mL

Action and uses.   As an adjunct to fluid replacement in treatment of acute diarrhoea.

Formulation notes.   Light kaolin is a diffusible solid, therefore no suspending agent is required.

Method of preparation.   Weigh the light kaolin and place in the mortar. Dissolve the sodium bicarbonate in about 100 mL of water. Gradually add this to the light kaolin in the mortar with mixing to disperse the solid. Add the chloroform and morphine tincture. Wash the mixture into a tared, amber medicine bottle, and make up to volume with water. Seal with a child-resistant closure. Polish and label the bottle and give a 5 mL medicine spoon with the medicine.

Shelf life and storage.   Store in a cool, dry place. It is recently prepared (unless the kaolin has been sterilized), therefore a shelf life of 2–3 weeks is applicable.

Advice and labelling.   'Shake well before use'. The usual dose is 10 mL every 4 hours in water. The importance of rehydration therapy should be stressed to the patient.

EXAMPLE 18.2

℞ Chalk Mixture, Paediatric BP. Mitte 100 mL.

	Master formula	For 100 mL
Chalk	100mg	2 g
Tragacanth	10 mg	200 mg
Syrup	0.5 mL	10 mL
Concentrated cinnamon		
water	0.02 mL	0.4 mL
Double strength chloroform		
water	2.5 mL	50 mL
Water	to 5 mL	to 100 mL

Action and uses.   As an antidiarrhoeal mixture for children, in addition to fluid replacement.

Formulation notes.   Chalk is practically insoluble in water and is an indiffusible solid which requires a suspending agent. Tragacanth powder is used in this formulation. The concentrated cinnamon water is a flavouring agent and the syrup increases the viscosity as well as acting as a sweetener. Chloroform water is the preservative.

Method of preparation.   The chalk and tragacanth should be weighed and lightly mixed in a mortar and pestle. Add the syrup and mix to make a paste. The double strength chloroform water should be gradually added, with mixing, followed by the concentrated cinnamon water. The mixture should be rinsed into a previously tared 100 mL amber medicine bottle and made up to volume with water. Shake the suspension well and seal with a child-resistant closure. Polish and label the bottle and give a 5 mL medicine spoon with the medicine.

Shelf life and storage.   Store in a cool, dry place. It is freshly prepared, therefore a shelf life of 1 week is applicable.

Advice and labelling.   'Shake well before use'. A dose of 5 mL every 4 hours is normally used. Advice on the importance of fluid replacement, using oral rehydration sachets should be given if necessary.

EXAMPLE 18.3

℞ Spironolactone suspension 15 mg/5 mL. Sig. 5 mL t.d.s. Mitte 100 mL. For a 4-year-old child.

	Master formula	For 100 mL
Spironolactone	q.s.*	300 mg
Compound orange spirit	0.2%	0.2 mL
Cologel	20%	20 mL
Water	to 100%	100 mL

* q.s. means sufficient (see Appendix 4).

Action and uses. A potassium-sparing diuretic used in oedema of heart failure and nephrotic syndrome.

Formulation notes. Spironolactone is practically insoluble in water. Cologel (methylcellulose) acts as the suspending agent. Compound orange spirit is a flavouring agent.

Method of preparation. Tablets may be used, and sufficient crushed in a mortar and pestle to give 300 mg spironolactone (e.g. 6 × 50 mg tablets). Alternatively, weigh the powder and transfer to a mortar and pestle. Add the Cologel and mix to a paste. Gradually add some of the water. Add the compound orange spirit. Rinse the suspension into a tared, amber medicine bottle and make up to volume with water. Shake the bottle well and seal with a child-resistant closure. Polish and label the bottle and give a 5 mL medicine spoon with the medicine.

Shelf life and storage. It is recently prepared with a shelf life of 4 weeks when stored in a refrigerator. Spironolactone should be protected from light.

Advice and labelling. 'Shake well before use' and 'Give one 5 mL spoonful three times a day'. Reinforce the storage conditions.

EXAMPLE 18.4

℞ Menthol and Eucalyptus Inhalation BP 1980. Mitte 100 mL.

	Master formula
Menthol	2 g
Eucalyptus oil	10 mL
Light magnesium carbonate	7 g
Water	to 100 mL

Action and uses. For relief of nasal congestion.

Formulation notes. Light magnesium carbonate has a large surface area and is used to adsorb the volatile ingredients which helps to ensure a uniform dispersion. Menthol is freely soluble in fixed and volatile oils, so will dissolve in the eucalyptus oil.

Method of preparation. Grind the menthol to a fine powder in a glass mortar and add the eucalyptus oil, which will dissolve the menthol. Gradually add the light magnesium carbonate to the mortar and mix well. Add the water gradually to produce a pourable suspension; this may take a while to achieve. Rinse into a tared, amber ribbed bottle and make up to volume. Seal with a child-resistant closure.

Shelf life and storage. Store in a cool, dry place. It is recently prepared, therefore a shelf life of 2–3 weeks is applicable.

Advice and labelling. 'Shake well before use' and 'Not to be taken'. The patient should be told to add 1 teaspoonful to 1 pint of hot, not boiling, water. A towel should be placed over the head and bowl and the vapour inhaled for 5–10 minutes. Patients should be aware of the potential danger of scalding to themselves and others, particularly small children.

EXAMPLE 18.5

℞ 200 mL Calamine Lotion BP.

	Master formula	For 200 mL
Calamine	15 g	30 g
Zinc oxide	5 g	10 g
Bentonite	3 g	6 g
Sodium citrate	500 mg	1 g
Liquefied phenol	0.5 mL	1 mL
Glycerol	5 mL	10 mL
Water	to 100 mL	to 200 mL

Action and uses. As a cooling lotion for sunburn or skin irritation and pruritis.

Formulation notes. Calamine is a coloured zinc carbonate and is practically insoluble in water, as is zinc oxide. Both are indiffusible solids. Sodium citrate is added to control the flocculation of calamine. Bentonite is a thickening agent, glycerol will thicken the product and help powder adherence to the skin. Liquefied phenol acts as a preservative and antiseptic.

Method of preparation. The dry powders should be weighed and mixed in a mortar so that the bentonite is well distributed. Add the glycerol to the powders and mix. The sodium citrate is dissolved in about 140 mL of water, and gradually added to the mixture in the mortar, so that a smooth paste is produced. Add the liquefied phenol, taking care not to splash, as it is caustic. Transfer the mixture to a tared, amber ribbed glass bottle, adding washings from the mortar, and make up to volume. Seal with a child-resistant closure.

Shelf life and storage. Store in a cool, dry place. It is recently prepared, therefore a shelf life of 2–3 weeks is applicable.

Advice and labelling. 'For external use only', 'Shake well before use' and 'Do not apply to broken skin'. The lotion should be applied to the affected areas when required and allowed to dry.

Key Points

- Suspensions can be used to administer an insoluble solid by the oral route.
- Suspensions may be used to replace tablets, to improve dissolution rate, to prolong action and to mask a bad taste.
- Solids may be diffusible or indiffusible and require different dispensing techniques.
- Stokes' equation can be applied when formulating a suspension to help ensure accurate dosage of the drug.
- Flocculated particles settle quickly and redisperse easily, whilst deflocculated particles settle slowly but tend to cake.

- Hydrophobic solids may require wetting agents.
- Suspending agents are added to slow down the rate of settling of the solid.
- Suspending agents may be natural polysaccharides, semisynthetic polysaccharides, clays or synthetic polymers.
- Some suspensions are made by adding water to reconstitute manufactured powders when stability is a problem.
- 'Shake well before use' and 'Store in a cool place' should be part of the labels on a suspension.
- Inhalations are suspensions of a volatile material adsorbed onto a diffusible solid.

Emulsions

A. J. Winfield (original author E. J. Kennedy)

After studying this chapter you will know about:

The uses of pharmaceutical emulsions
The different types of emulsion and their identification
Considerations during the formulation of emulsions
Selection of emulsifying agents and other ingredients
The dispensing processes for emulsions

Introduction

An emulsion consists of two immiscible liquids, one of which is uniformly dispersed throughout the other as fine droplets normally of diameter 0.1–100 μm. To prepare a stable emulsion a third ingredient, an emulsifying agent, is required. Oral emulsions are stabilized oil-in-water dispersions that may contain one or more active ingredients. They are a useful way of presenting oils and fats in a palatable form. Emulsions for external use are known as lotions, applications or liniments if liquid, or creams if semisolid in nature. Some parenteral products may also be formulated as emulsions. Most important of these is total parenteral nutrition (TPN), which is discussed in detail in Chapter 28. Pharmaceutically the term 'emulsion' when no other qualification is used is taken to mean an oil-in-water preparation for internal use. Information about other types of emulsion, together with some of the science of emulsions, can be found in Aulton (2002).

PHARMACEUTICAL APPLICATIONS OF EMULSIONS

Emulsions have a wide range of uses, including:

- Oral, rectal and topical administration of oils and oil-soluble drugs.

- Formulation of oil- and water-soluble drugs together.
- To enhance palatability of oils when given orally by disguising both taste and oiliness.
- Increasing absorption of oils and oil-soluble drugs through intestinal walls. An example is griseofulvin suspended in oil in an oil-in-water emulsion.
- Intramuscular injections of some water-soluble vaccines provide slow release and therefore a greater antibody response and longer-lasting immunity.
- Total parenteral nutrition makes use of a sterile oil-in-water emulsion to deliver oily nutrients intravenously to patients, using non-toxic emulsifying agents, such as lecithin (see Ch. 28).

Examples of emulsions for oral use are cod liver oil emulsion (see Example 19.3), liquid paraffin oral emulsion (see Example 19.4) and castor oil emulsion. Examples of emulsions for external use are Turpentine Liniment BP (see Example 20.3) and Oily Calamine Lotion BP (see Example 19.5).

Emulsion types

Emulsions may be oil-in-water emulsions (o/w), where oil is the disperse phase in a continuous phase of water, or water-in-oil emulsions (w/o), where water is the disperse phase in a continuous phase of oil. It is also possible to form a multiple emulsion, e.g. a water droplet enclosed in an oil droplet, which is itself dispersed in water—a w/o/w emulsion. These may be used for delayed-action drug delivery systems.

If the emulsion is for oral or intravenous administration it will always be oil-in-water. Intramuscular injections may be water-in-oil for depot therapy. When selecting emulsion type for preparations for external use, the therapeutic use, texture and patient acceptability will be taken into account. Oil-in-water emulsions are less greasy, easily washed off the skin and more cosmetically acceptable than water-in-oil emulsions. They have an occlusive effect, which hydrates upper layers of skin (called an emollient, see Ch. 20). Water-in-oil emulsions rub in more easily.

Identification of emulsion type

There is a range of tests available to identify the emulsion type. Some of the tests that can be used are outlined below.

Miscibility test. An emulsion will only mix with a liquid that is miscible with its continuous phase. Therefore an o/w emulsion is miscible with water, a w/o emulsion with an oil.

Conductivity measurement. Systems with an aqueous continuous phase will conduct electricity, whilst systems with an oily continuous phase will not.

Staining test. A dry filter paper impregnated with cobalt chloride turns from blue to pink on exposure to stable o/w emulsions.

Dye test. If an oil-soluble dye is used, o/w emulsions are paler in colour than w/o emulsions and vice versa. If examined microscopically, an o/w emulsion will appear as coloured globules on a colourless background whilst a w/o emulsion will appear as colourless globules against a coloured background.

FORMULATION OF EMULSIONS

An ideal emulsion has globules of disperse phase that retain their initial character, that is the mean size does not change and the globules remain evenly distributed. The formulation of emulsions involves the prevention of coalescence of the disperse phase (often called 'cracking') and reducing the rate of creaming.

Emulsifying agents

Emulsifying agents help the production of a stable emulsion by reducing interfacial tension and then maintaining the separation of the droplets by forming a barrier at the interface. Most emulsifying agents are surface-active agents. Emulsion type is determined by the solubility of the emulsifying agent. If the emulsifying agent is more soluble in water (i.e. hydrophilic) then water will be the continuous phase and an o/w emulsion will be formed. If the emulsifying agent is more soluble in oil (i.e. lipophilic), oil will be the continuous phase and a w/o emulsion will be formed. If a substance is added which alters the solubility of the emulsifying agent, this balance may be altered and the emulsion

may change type. This is called phase inversion. The ideal emulsifying agent is colourless, odourless, tasteless, non-toxic, non-irritant and able to produce stable emulsions at low concentrations.

Emulsifying agents can be classed into three groups: naturally occurring, synthetic surfactants and finely divided solids.

Naturally occurring emulsifying agents

These agents come from vegetable or animal sources. Therefore the quality may vary from batch to batch and they are susceptible to microbial contamination and degradation.

Polysaccharides. Acacia is the best emulsifying agent for extemporaneously prepared oral emulsions as it forms a thick film at the oil–water interface to act as a barrier to coalescence. It is too sticky for external use. Tragacanth is used to increase the viscosity of an emulsion and prevent creaming. Other polysaccharides, such as starch, pectin and carrageenan, are used to stabilize an emulsion.

Semisynthetic polysaccharides. Low-viscosity grades of methylcellulose (see Example 19.4) and carboxymethyl-cellulose will form o/w emulsions.

Sterol-containing substances. These agents act as water-in-oil emulsifying agents. Examples include beeswax, wool fat and wool alcohols (see Ch. 20).

Synthetic surfactants

These agents are classified according to their ionic characteristics as anionic, cationic, non-ionic and ampholytic. The latter are used in detergents and soaps but are not widely used in pharmacy.

Anionic surfactants. These are organic salts which, in water, have a surface-active anion. They are incompatible with some organic and inorganic cations and with large organic cations such as cetrimide. They are widely used in external preparations as o/w emulsifying agents. They must be in their ionized form to be effective and emulsions made with anionic surfactants are generally stable at more alkaline pH.

Many different ones are used pharmaceutically. Some examples include:

- Alkali metal and ammonium soaps such as sodium stearate (o/w).
- Soaps of divalent and trivalent metals such as calcium oleate (w/o) (see Example 19.5).
- Amine soaps such as triethanolamine oleate (o/w).
- Alkyl sulphates such as sodium lauryl sulphate (o/w).

Cationic surfactants. These are usually quaternary ammonium compounds which have a surface-active cation and so are sensitive to anionic surfactants and drugs. They are used in the preparation of o/w emulsions for external use and must be in their ionized form to be effective. Emulsions formed by a cationic surfactant are generally stable at acidic pH. The cationic surfactants also have antimicrobial activity. Examples include cetrimide and benzalkonium chloride.

Non-ionic surfactants. These are synthetic materials and make up the largest group of surfactants. They are used to produce either o/w or w/o emulsions for both external and internal use. The non-ionic surfactants are compatible with both anionic and cationic substances and are highly resistant to pH change. The type of emulsion formed depends on the balance between hydrophilic and lipophilic groups which is given by the HLB (hydrophilic–lipophilic balance) number (see below). Examples of the main types include glycol and glycerol esters, macrogol ethers and esters, sorbitan esters and polysorbates.

The HLB (hydrophilic–lipophilic balance) system. An HLB number, usually between 1 and 20, is allocated to an emulsifying agent and represents the relative proportions of the lipophilic and hydrophilic parts of the molecule. High numbers (8–18) indicate a hydrophilic molecule, and produce an o/w emulsion. Low numbers (3–6) indicate a lipophilic molecule and produce a w/o emulsion. Oils and waxy materials have a 'required HLB number' which helps in the selection of appropriate emulsifying agents when formulating emulsions. Liquid paraffin, for example, has a required HLB value of 4 to obtain a w/o emulsion and 12 for an o/w emulsion. Two or more surfactants can be combined to achieve a suitable HLB value and often give better results than one surfactant alone. (See Aulton (2002) or the *Pharmaceutical Codex* for more details.) HLB values of some commonly used emulsifying agents are given in Table 19.1.

Table 19.1 HLB values of emulsifying agents	
Emulsifying agent	**HLB value**
Acacia	8.0
Sorbitan laurate (Span 20)	8.6
Sorbitan stearate (Span 60)	4.7
Polysorbate 20 (Tween 20)	16.7
Polysorbate 80 (Tween 80)	15.0
Sodium lauryl sulphate	40.0
Sodium oleate	18.0
Tragacanth	13.2
Triethanolamine oleate	12.0

Finely divided solids

Finely divided solids can be adsorbed at the oil–water interface to form a coherent film that prevents coalescence of the dispersed globules. If the particles are preferentially wetted by oil, a w/o emulsion is formed. Conversely, if the particles are preferentially wetted by water, an o/w emulsion is formed. They form emulsions with good stability which are less prone to microbial contamination than those formed with other naturally derived agents. Examples are bentonite, aluminium magnesium silicate and colloidal silicon dioxide. Colloidal aluminium and magnesium hydroxides are used for internal preparations. For example Liquid Paraffin and Magnesium Hydroxide Oral Emulsion is stabilized by the magnesium hydroxide.

Choosing an emulsifying agent

The active ingredients that are to be emulsified and the intended use of the product will determine the choice of emulsifying agent. Because they are non-toxic and non-irritant the natural polysaccharides (acacia) and non-ionic emulsifying agents are useful for internal emulsions. Quillaia can be used in low concentrations, but soap emulsions irritate the gastrointestinal tract and have a laxative effect. The taste should be bland and palatable, again suggesting the natural polysaccharides. Polysorbates have a disagreeable taste, therefore flavouring ingredients are necessary. Only certain non-ionic emulsifying agents are suitable for parenteral use including lecithin, polysorbate 80, methylcellulose, gelatin and serum albumin. A wider range of emulsifying agents can be used externally, although the polysaccharides are normally considered too sticky.

Antioxidants

Some oils are liable to degradation by oxidation and therefore antioxidants may be added to the formulation. They should be preferentially soluble in the oily phase.

Antimicrobial preservatives

Emulsions contain water, which will support microbial growth. Microbes produce unpleasant odours, colour changes and gases and may affect the emulsifying agent, possibly causing breakdown of the emulsion. Other ingredients of emulsions can provide a growth medium for microbes. Examples include arachis oil which supports *Aspergillus* species and liquid paraffin which supports

Penicillium species. Contamination may be introduced from a variety of sources including:

- Natural emulsifying agents, e.g. starch and acacia
- Water, if not properly stored
- Carelessly cleaned equipment
- Poor closures on containers.

Antimicrobial preservative agents should be free from toxic effects, odour, taste (for internal use) and colour. They should be bactericidal rather than bacteriostatic, have a rapid action and wide antibacterial spectrum over a range of temperatures and pH. Additionally emulsion ingredients should not affect their activity and they should be resistant to attack by microorganisms. The effect of the partition coefficient is also important. Microbial growth normally occurs in the aqueous phase of an emulsion, therefore it is important that a sufficient concentration of preservative is present in the aqueous phase. A preservative with a low oil/water partition coefficient will have a higher concentration in the aqueous phase. A combination of preservatives may give the best preservative cover for an emulsion system. The ratio of the disperse phase volume to the total volume is known as the phase volume or phase volume ratio. If a preservative is soluble in the oil and if the proportion of oil is increased, the concentration of preservative in the aqueous phase decreases, and vice versa.

Some preservatives in use are listed below:

- Benzoic acid: effective at a concentration of 0.1% at a pH below 5
- Esters of parahydroxybenzoic acid such as methyl paraben (0.01–0.3%)
- Chloroform, as chloroform water (0.25% v/v)
- Chlorocresol (0.05–0.2%)
- Phenoxyethanol (0.5–1.0%)
- Benzyl alcohol (0.1–3%)
- Quaternary ammonium compounds, e.g. cetrimide, which can be used as a primary emulsifying agent but can also be used as a preservative
- Organic mercurial compounds such as phenyl mercuric nitrate and acetate (0.001–0.002%).

Colours and flavourings

Colour is rarely needed in an emulsion, as most have an elegant white colour and thick texture. Emulsions for oral use will usually contain some flavouring agent.

Stability of emulsions

Phase inversion

This is the process in which an emulsion changes from one type to another, say o/w to w/o. The most stable range of disperse phase concentration is 30–60%. If the amount of disperse phase approaches or exceeds a theoretical maximum of 74% of the total volume, then phase inversion may occur. Addition of substances which alter the solubility of an emulsifying agent may also cause phase inversion. The process is irreversible.

Creaming

The term 'creaming' is used to describe the aggregation of globules of the disperse phase at the top or bottom of the emulsion, similar to cream on milk. The process is reversible and gentle shaking redistributes the droplets throughout the continuous phase. Creaming is undesirable because it is inelegant and inaccurate dosing is possible if shaking is not thorough. Additionally, creaming increases the likelihood of coalescence of globules and therefore break down of the emulsion due to cracking.

Cracking

Cracking is the coalescence of dispersed globules and separation of the disperse phase as a separate layer. It is an irreversible process and redispersion cannot be achieved by shaking.

Causes and prevention of cracking or creaming

- *Globule size*. Stable emulsions require a maximal number of small sized (1–3 μm) globules and as few as possible larger (>15 μm) diameter globules. A homogenizer will efficiently reduce droplet size and may additionally increase the viscosity if more than 30% of disperse phase is present. Homogenizers force the emulsion through a small aperture to reduce the size of the globules.
- *Storage temperature*. Extremes of temperature can lead to an emulsion cracking. When water freezes it expands, so undue pressure is exerted on dispersed globules and the emulsifying agent film, which may lead to cracking. Conversely, an increased temperature decreases the viscosity of the continuous phase and disrupts the integrity of the interfacial film. An increasing number of collisions between droplets will also occur, leading to increased creaming and cracking.

- *Potential for globule coalescence.* Increasing the viscosity of the continuous phase will reduce the potential for globule coalescence as this reduces the movement of globules. Emulsion stabilizers, which increase the viscosity of the continuous phase, may be used in o/w emulsions, e.g tragacanth, sodium alginate and methylcellulose.
- *Changes which affect the interfacial film.* These may be chemical, physical or biological effects:

  microbiological contamination may destroy the emulsifying agent, especially if a polysaccharide emulsifying agent is being used

  addition of a common solvent

  addition of an emulsifying agent of opposite charge, for instance cationic to anionic.
- *Incorporation of excess disperse phase*, as discussed above.

DISPENSING EMULSIONS

Emulsions can be extemporaneously prepared on a small scale using a mortar and pestle. Electric mixers can also be used, although incorporation of excess air may be a problem. All equipment used must be thoroughly clean and dry. All oil-soluble and water-soluble components of the emulsion are separately dissolved in the appropriate phase. A suitable emulsifying agent must then be chosen.

Emulsions for oral use

Acacia gum is usually used when making extemporaneous o/w emulsions for oral use, unless otherwise specified. A primary emulsion should be prepared first. This is a thick, stable emulsion prepared using optimal proportions of the ingredients. These vary with the nature of the oil.

Calculating quantities for primary emulsions

Proportions or 'parts' for preparation of primary emulsions are given in Table 19.2. These refer to parts by volume for the different types of oil and water and weight for the acacia gum. If more than one oil is to be incorporated, the quantity of acacia for each is calculated separately and the sum of the quantities used.

EXAMPLE 19.1

Calculate the quantities for a primary emulsion for the following:

Cod liver oil	30 mL
Water	to 100 mL

Primary emulsion quantities

Cod liver oil is a fixed oil, therefore the primary emulsion proportions are 4 : 2 : 1. Hence:

Cod liver oil	30 mL	4
Water	15 mL	2
Powdered acacia gum	7.5 g	1

Variations to primary emulsion calculations

If the proportion of oil is too small, modifications must be made. Acacia emulsions containing less than 20% oil tend to cream readily. A bland, inert oil, such as arachis, sesame, cottonseed or maize oil, should be added to increase the amount of oil and so prevent this from happening. Care should be taken in selection of the bulking oil because of the increasing incidence of nut allergy. It is often, therefore, advisable to avoid oils such as arachis, especially for children.

EXAMPLE 19.2

Calciferol solution, 0.15 mL per 5 mL dose.

The percentage of oil in each dose is 3%. The oil content must be made up to at least 20% to produce a stable emulsion.

Since 20% of 5 mL = 1 mL the volume of bland oil required is 1–0.15 = 0.85 mL.

Table 19.2	Quantities for primary emulsions			
Type of oil	**Examples**	**Oil**	**Water**	**Gum**
Fixed	Almond, arachis, cod liver, castor	4	2	1
Mineral (hydrocarbon)	Liquid paraffin	3	2	1
Volatile	Turpentine, cinnamon, peppermint	2	2	1
Oleo-resin	Male fern extract	1	2	1

Formula for primary emulsion (for 50 mL)		
Calciferol solution	1.5 mL	4
Cottonseed oil	8.5 mL	
Water	5 mL	2
Acacia	2.5 g	1

METHODS OF PREPARATION OF EXTEMPORANEOUS EMULSIONS

There are two possible methods, the dry gum method being the most popular.

Dry gum method of preparation

1. Measure the oil accurately in a dry measure. It is important that the measure is dry.
2. Allow measure to drain into a dry mortar with a large, flat, bottom.
3. Weigh acacia gum.
4. Measure the water for the primary emulsion in a clean measure.
5. Add acacia to the oil and mix lightly to disperse lumps. Do not over-mix, and keep the suspension in the bottom of the mortar.
6. Immediately add all of the water (aim to do this within 10–15 seconds of adding the acacia to the oil) and stir continuously and vigorously until the mixture thickens and the primary emulsion is formed. The mixture thickening, becoming white and producing a 'clicking' sound, characterizes this.
7. Continue mixing for a further 2–3 minutes to produce the white stable emulsion. The whiter the product, the smaller the globules.
8. Gradually dilute the primary emulsion with small volumes of the vehicle, ensuring complete mixing between additions.
9. Gradually add any other ingredients, transfer to a measure and make up to final volume with vehicle.

Wet gum method of preparation

Water is added to the acacia gum and quickly triturated until the gum has dissolved, to make a mucilage. Oil is added to this mucilage in small portions, triturating the mixture thoroughly after each addition until a thick primary emulsion is obtained. The primary emulsion should be stabilized by mixing for several minutes and then completed in the same way as for the dry gum method.

Problems when producing the primary emulsion

The primary emulsion may not form and a thin oily liquid is formed instead. Possible causes are:

- Phase inversion has occurred
- Incorrect quantities of oil or water were used
- There was cross-contamination of water and oil
- A wet mortar was used
- The mortar was too small and curved, or the pestle head was too round, giving insufficient shear
- Excessive mixing of oil and gum (dry gum method)
- Diluting the primary emulsion too soon
- Too rapid dilution of primary emulsion
- Poor quality acacia.

EMULSIONS FOR EXTERNAL USE

Liquid or semiliquid emulsions may be used as applications, liniments and lotions (see Ch. 20). The extemporaneous preparation of emulsions for external use does not require the preparation of a primary emulsion. Soaps are commonly used as the emulsifying agent and some are prepared 'in situ' by mixing the oily phase containing a fatty acid and the aqueous phase containing the alkali. Alternatively the emulsifying agent can be dissolved in the oily or aqueous phase and the disperse phase added to the continuous phase, either gradually or in one portion.

Creams are semisolid emulsions which may be o/w (e.g. aqueous cream) or w/o (e.g. oily cream). These are considered in more detail in Chapter 20.

SHELF LIFE AND STORAGE

Emulsions should be stored at room temperature and will either be recently or freshly prepared. Some official preparations will have specific expiry dates. They should not be frozen.

CONTAINERS

An amber medicine bottle is used, plain for internal use and ribbed for external use, with an airtight child-resistant closure. Containers with a wide mouth are useful for very viscous preparations.

SPECIAL LABELLING AND ADVICE FOR EMULSIONS

- 'Shake well before use'.
- 'Store in a cool place'. This is to protect the emulsion against extremes of temperature which will adversely affect its stability.
- Expiry date.
- 'For external use only', for external emulsions.

EXAMPLE 19.3

℞ Prepare 200 mL cod liver oil emulsion to the following formula:

Cod liver oil	60 mL
Chloroform	0.4 mL
Cinnamon water	to 200 mL

Action and uses
A rich source of vitamins A and D.

Formulation notes. Cod liver oil is a fixed oil that requires the addition of acacia gum as an emulsifying agent. The proportions are 4 oil : 2 water : 1 gum. Therefore 60 mL cod liver oil, 30 mL of cinnamon water and 15 g of acacia gum will be used to prepare the primary emulsion. Cinnamon water acts as a flavouring agent and vehicle. It may need to be prepared from concentrated cinnamon water, at a dilution of 1 part to 39 parts of water. Since 60 mL of the emulsion is the cod liver oil, it is not necessary to prepare 200 mL, 160 mL is adequate. Therefore, 4 mL of concentrated cinnamon water will be diluted to 160 mL with water. Chloroform is dense and only slowly soluble and acts as a preservative.

Method of preparation. Use the dry gum method. Weigh 15 g of acacia, measure 60 mL of cod liver oil and 30 mL of cinnamon water, which will be used to create the primary emulsion. Place the cod liver oil in a dry, flat-bottomed mortar. Add the acacia and mix very lightly and briefly. Immediately add the cinnamon water, mixing vigorously until a clicking sound is heard and a white primary emulsion is formed. Continue mixing for a few minutes to stabilize the primary emulsion. Scrape the mortar and pestle with a spatula to ensure that all the oil is incorporated. Add the chloroform by pipette and mix thoroughly. Gradually add

most of the remainder of the cinnamon water to the emulsion in the mortar, stirring well between additions. Transfer the emulsion to a 200 mL measure, rinsing the mortar adding these washings to the measure. Make up to volume with cinnamon water and pack in an amber medicine bottle with a child-resistant closure. Polish and label the bottle and give a 5 mL medicine spoon with the medicine.

Shelf life and storage. Store in a cool, dry place. It is recently prepared, therefore a shelf life of 2–3 weeks is applicable.

Advice and labelling. This is an unofficial formula, and should be labelled 'Cod liver oil 30% v/v emulsion'. 'Shake well before use.' A normal dose is 10 mL three times a day, with or after food.

EXAMPLE 19.4

℞ 100 mL Liquid Paraffin Oral Emulsion BP 1968.

Liquid paraffin	50 mL
Vanillin	50 mg
Chloroform	0.25 mL
Benzoic acid solution	2 mL
Methylcellulose 20	2 g
Saccharin sodium	5 mg
Water	to 100 mL

Action and uses. A lubricant laxative for chronic constipation.

Formulation notes. Methylcellulose 20 at a concentration of 2% acts as an emulsifying agent for the mineral oil, liquid paraffin. A primary emulsion is not required. Benzoic acid and chloroform act as preservatives and vanillin and saccharin sodium act as flavouring and sweetening agent respectively. The amount of saccharin sodium is not weighable on a Class B dispensing balance and will be obtained by trituration using water as the diluent (since this is the vehicle for the emulsion).

Trituration for saccharin sodium:

Saccharin sodium	100 mg
Water to	100 mL

5 mL of water will contain 5 mg of saccharin sodium.

Method of preparation. Firstly, prepare a mucilage by mixing the methylcellulose 20 with about six times its weight of boiling water and allow to stand for 30 minutes to hydrate. Add an equal weight (about 15 g) of ice and stir mechanically until the mucilage is homogeneous. Dissolve the vanillin in the benzoic acid solution and chloroform. Add this mixture to the mucilage and stir for 5 minutes.

Make up the saccharin sodium trituration and stir in the appropriate volume of solution to the mucilage. Make the volume of the mucilage up to 50 mL, taking care to ensure that there is no entrapped air in the mucilage. Make the emulsion by mixing together 50 mL of liquid paraffin and 50 mL of prepared mucilage with constant stirring. The emulsion is more stable if passed through a hand homogenizer. Pack in an amber medicine bottle with a child-resistant closure. Shake well to ensure that the emulsion is thoroughly mixed. Polish and label the bottle and give a 5 mL medicine spoon with the medicine.

Shelf life and storage. Store in a cool, dry place. This is an official preparation and should remain stable on storage, however a 4-week expiry date is recommended.

Advice and labelling. 'Shake well before use'. The emulsion should not be taken within 30 minutes of meal times and preferably on an empty stomach. The importance of fibre and fluid intake in the diet should be emphasized.

EXAMPLE 19.5

℞ 100 mL Oily Calamine Lotion BP 1980.

Calamine	5 g
Wool fat	1 g
Oleic acid	0.5 mL
Arachis oil	50 mL
Calcium hydroxide solution	to 100 mL

Action and uses. Soothing lotion for the treatment of eczema, sunburn and other inflammatory conditions.

Formulation notes. The emulsifying agent for the arachis oil is the soap calcium oleate produced from the calcium hydroxide and oleic acid when they are shaken together. Wool fat is included as an emulsion stabilizer. This is a w/o emulsion.

Method of preparation. The wool fat, oleic acid and arachis oil should be warmed together in an evaporating basin (using a water-bath or heating block) until melted. Mix them thoroughly. The calamine should be sieved and weighed and placed on a warm ointment tile. Add a little of the oily mixture and rub in with a large spatula until smooth. Gradually add more of the oily mixture until it is fluid.

Transfer back to the evaporating basin and stir to evenly distribute the calamine powder. Pour into a previously tared, amber ribbed bottle and add the calcium hydroxide solution to the bottle in small amounts, shaking well between additions. Make up to volume and seal with a child-resistant closure. Polish and label the bottle.

Shelf life and storage. Store in a cool, dry place. It is unpreserved, therefore a shelf life of 2–3 weeks is applicable.

Advice and labelling. 'Shake well before use' and 'For external use only'.

Key Points

- Emulsions may be oil-in-water (o/w) or water-in-oil (w/o).
- Emulsions may be used orally, externally or by intramuscular and intravenous injection.
- Oral emulsions are always o/w.
- The type of emulsion may be determined by miscibility, conductivity, staining and dye tests.
- Emulsifying agents are required to reduce the interfacial tension and act as a barrier between the oil and water phases.
- Naturally occurring emulsifying agents include polysaccharides (acacia), semisynthetic polysaccharides (methylcellulose) and sterols (wool fat).
- Synthetic surfactants can be used and are selected using the HLB number.
- Care is required to avoid anion–cation incompatibilities.
- Some finely divided solids will stabilize emulsions.
- Emulsions require antimicrobial preservation.
- Phase inversion, creaming and cracking are instabilities of emulsions which must be avoided.
- A primary emulsion is prepared when making an emulsion using acacia as the emulsifying agent using either the 'dry gum' or 'wet gum' method.
- The ratio of oil : water : acacia used for the primary emulsion will vary with the type of oil in the formulation.
- Liquid emulsions should have 'Shake well before use' and 'Store in a cool place' labels and should not be frozen.

20

External preparations

A. J. Winfield

After studying this chapter you will know about:

Skin structure and sites of action of drugs
The types and function of solid, liquid and
**   semisolid skin preparations**
The ingredients used in skin preparations
Dispensing preparations for use on the skin
Transdermal drug delivery for systemic
**   activity**

Introduction

Skin is the largest organ in the body and has three distinct regions. The hypodermis is the innermost and is often called subcutaneous fat. The dermis is the bulk of the thickness of the skin and contains blood vessels, nerve fibres, sweat glands and hair follicles. The outermost region is the epidermis, which is made up of several layers. Cells divide in the stratum basale, and as they move towards the surface change appearance and function. The outermost layer, the stratum corneum, acts as the skin barrier. It is made up of about 20 layers of dead keratinized cells. The hair follicles and sweat ducts pass through the stratum corneum to reach the surface. A simplified diagram showing the main skin structures is given in Figure 20.1.

There are a large number of diseases which may affect different regions of the skin. Any drug used will require to reach the site of the disease in order to act. Unless it is for a surface effect only, the drug must either pass through the stratum corneum or go through hair follicles or sweat glands. Examples of drugs applied to the skin and their sites of action are shown in Figure 20.1. Once in the skin, a lipid-soluble drug will tend to accumulate in lipid regions,

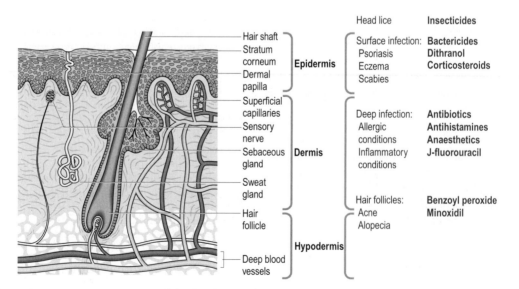

Fig. 20.1 Diagrammatic representation of the skin showing the main structures, location of diseases and the sites of action of drugs.

whilst more water-soluble drugs will tend to enter the blood capillaries and be removed from the skin. There are also many metabolic enzymes in the skin which can deactivate drugs. A more detailed discussion of these factors and the physicochemical principles involved is given in Aulton (2002, see Chapter 33).

Pharmacokinetics is seldom applied to skin administration and dosage is often imprecise. However, by effective formulation it is possible to achieve adequate and reproducible percutaneous absorption. The main advantage is that close to zero order kinetics can be produced. This also carries an inherent warning because traditionally it has been assumed that absorption from the skin is minimal. As a consequence, the skin is seen as 'safe' even if quite toxic materials are applied. This is not true and great care is required.

There are an increasing number of drugs that are effective against skin diseases, but drugs are not the only way of treating skin conditions. Creating physiological change in the skin can bring about beneficial changes. The main one is to control the moisture content of the skin. Normal skin has 10–25% moisture in the stratum corneum. This level may be reduced in, for example, eczema, or increased, as in skin maceration between the toes. By using an occlusive product (that is an oily product), water leaving the body through the skin will be trapped and moisture content will increase. These products are called emollients. An excess of moisture may be removed using an astringent, a hygroscopic material or, to a lesser extent, a dusting powder. Where an oily vehicle is needed, but moisture must not increase, adding solid particles to the vehicle will allow water to escape. Lubrication of sensitive skin is achieved by using finely divided solids, applied either as a powder or, more efficiently, as a suspension. Cooling the skin relieves inflammation and eases discomfort. It is achieved by evaporating a solvent, usually water or a water and alcohol mixture. Volatile solvents sprayed on the skin give intense cooling.

TYPES OF SKIN PREPARATION

There are a large number of different types of external medicine, ranging from dry powders through semisolids to liquids. The names are often traditional. Figure 20.2 illustrates the formulation of the main types of preparation used on the skin.

Solids

Dusting powders are applied to the skin for a surface effect such as drying or lubricating, or an antibacterial action. They are made of a fine-particle-size powder which may be a drug alone or together with excipients.

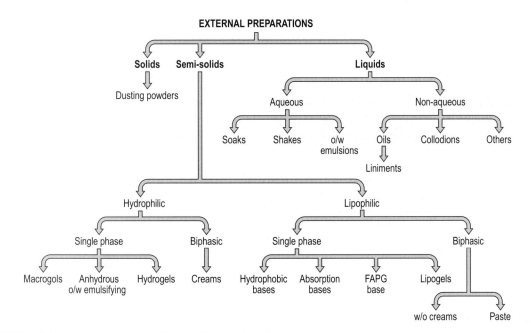

Fig. 20.2 Schematic representation of types of external medicines.

Liquids

Soaks have an active ingredient dissolved in an aqueous solvent and are often used as astringents, for cooling or to leave a film of solid on the skin. Oily vehicles can be used in bath additives to leave an emollient film on the skin surface.

Applications are solutions or emulsions that frequently contain parasiticides (see Example 20.4).

Liniments are alcoholic or oily solutions or emulsions (see Example 20.3) designed to be rubbed into the skin. The medicament is usually a rubefacient.

Lotions are aqueous solutions, suspensions (see Example 20.1) or emulsions that cool inflamed skin and deposit a protective layer of solid.

Paints and *tinctures* are concentrated aqueous or alcoholic antimicrobial solutions.

Collodions are organic solvents containing a polymer and keratolytic agent for treating corns and calluses.

There are also many other liquid products including shampoos, pomades, foot washes.

Semi-solids

Ointments are usually oily vehicles that may contain a surfactant to allow them to be washed off easily (barrier creams). They are used as emollients, or for drug delivery either to the surface or for deeper penetration.

Creams are traditionally o/w emulsions whilst *oily creams* are w/o emulsions. However, there are also 'creams' that are not emulsions. Emulsified creams usually give cooling, are less greasy than ointments and can be used for drug delivery onto or into the skin. They require antimicrobial preservatives.

Pastes are vehicles (aqueous or oily) with a high concentration of added solid. This makes them thick so they do not spread and so localizes drug delivery (e.g. Dithranol in Lassar's Paste, see Example 20.11). They can also be used for sun blocks.

Gels (jellies) are usually aqueous gels used for lubrication or applying a drug to the skin. Oily gels are also available where occlusion is required.

INGREDIENTS USED IN SKIN PREPARATIONS

Water-miscible vehicles

These include water, alcohol and the macrogols. Alcohol is often added to water to increase the rate of evaporation and produce a more intense cooling effect. Industrial methylated spirit (IMS) is normally used for external preparations because it is exempt from excise duty. The macrogols (polyethylene glycols) are available with a range of molecular weight. As chain length increases, so the properties change from liquid, through semisolid to waxy solid. They have good solvent properties for a wide range of drugs and can be blended to produce intermediate consistencies. They tend to dry the skin, inactivate some antimicrobials, interact with some plastics and can give poor release of drugs.

Oily vehicles

Oils used in external preparations come from one of three sources.

Mineral oils (paraffins) are the most widely used. They are complex mixtures of mainly saturated hydrocarbons which are available in different fractions. Different names are used in different pharmacopoeias (Table 20.1).

Light liquid paraffin is not normally used in external medicines. Soft paraffin is the main ingredient in many products, with liquid or hard paraffin being used to thin or thicken them respectively. There are two forms of soft paraffin—yellow and white. The latter has been bleached, residues of which may remain. As a rule, white is used in white or pale coloured products, whilst yellow is used for darker products. The paraffins are occlusive and chemically inert, but do not give good skin penetration.

Table 20.1 Paraffins used in external preparations: the names used are different in the UK, USA and European pharmacopoeias

UK	USA	European
Light liquid paraffin	Light mineral oil	Paraffinium perliquidum
Liquid paraffin	Mineral oil	Paraffinium liquidum
Soft paraffin	Petrolatum	Paraffinium molle
Hard paraffin	Paraffin	Paraffinium durum

Table 20.2 Materials based on wool fat: different names are used in the UK, USA and European pharmacopoeias		
UK	**USA**	**European**
Wool fat	Lanolin	Adeps lanae
Wool alcohols	Lanolin alcohols	Alcoholes adipis lanae
Hydrous wool fat	Hydrous lanolin	Adeps lanae cum aqua

Vegetable oils come from many plant sources such as peanut, castor, olive and coconut. They may be used as a mobile solvent (as in a liniment, see Example 20.2) or as part of an ointment or cream. If they require thickening, a high melting point material such as cetostearyl alcohol can be used. They are occlusive and give good skin penetration, but may go rancid. Sufficient skin penetration may occur to cause severe reactions in patients with nut allergies.

Synthetic oils, such as the silicone oils (Dimeticone BP), are used as water repellents and occlusives because they are very hydrophobic. The semisynthetic isopropylmyristate is similar to vegetable oil in properties and use.

Emulsifying agents

Liquid and semisolid emulsions, both o/w and w/o, are used externally and require the addition of emulsifying agents. The latter may also be added to an oil without water as in Emulsifying Ointment BP. The presence of a surfactant usually increases the skin penetration of any drug. A wide range of materials can be used as surfactants, either alone or in combinations. Selection is made in view of the type of emulsion required (o/w or w/o) and the charge on the other ingredients (anionic, cationic or non-ionic).

Emulsifiers—w/o

Wool fat, obtained from sheep wool, is a pale yellow sticky material. It is a complex mixture of fatty acid esters of cholesterol and other sterols and alcohols. Whilst it is similar to human sebum, it has been implicated in sensitization in some people. Where this is a problem there are an increasing number of hypoallergenic commercial products available. Wool alcohols, a solid, is richer in cholesterol and lanesterol and freer from impurities. Both it and wool fat increase the 'water-holding' capacity of greasy bases. Hydrous wool fat is 7 parts wool fat and 3 parts water and is a softer material. Different names are used as shown in Table 20.2. Beeswax is a traditional w/o emulsifier which is occasionally used.

Emulsifiers—o/w

The main group of materials used extemporaneously are the emulsifying waxes. Each one has two ingredients—cetostearyl alcohol and a surface-active agent as shown in Table 20.3. All three are waxy solids that mix with oily materials. Addition of water produces an o/w emulsion—a cream. Both the non-aqueous blends and the creams are easily washed off the skin. Varying the amount of bodying agent, usually cetostearyl alcohol, can control consistency. The ratio of oil to water will also alter the consistency of a cream.

Other emulsifiers

The gums, used in oral emulsions (see Ch. 19), are too sticky for external use, but a number of other emulsifying agents are used.

Table 20.3 The ingredients used in the emulsifying waxes described in the *British Pharmacopoeia* (BP) and *British Pharmaceutical Codex* (BPC)			
Charge	**Surfactant**	**CSA : SAA ratio**	**Name**
Anionic	Sodium lauryl sulphate	9 : 1	Emulsifying Wax BP
Cationic	Cetrimide	9 : 1	Cetrimide Emulsifying Wax BPC
Non-ionic	Cetomacrogol 1000	8 : 2	Cetomacrogol Emulsifying Wax BPC
CSA, cetostearyl alcohol; SAA, surface active agent.			

Calcium soaps are produced by mixing a fatty acid with lime water (calcium hydroxide solution) to form a soap in situ (see Example 19.5). They form w/o emulsions. Soft soap is a sticky green material that can be used to make o/w emulsions (see Example 20.3).

Synthetic surface-active agents can also be used. Low HLB (hydrophilic–lipophilic balance) materials will produce w/o emulsions, whilst higher HLB surfactants give o/w emulsions.

Suspending agents

These materials can be used for suspending solids in shake lotions, or to produce gels, depending on the concentration used. Those used in oral suspensions (see Ch. 18) are too sticky for use in external liquid suspensions. The main group of materials used for this purpose are the clays, of which there are many forms including bentonite, attapulgite, mont-morrilonite and Veegum (aluminium magnesium silicate). They leave a lubricant layer of powder on the skin. They are unsuitable for use below pH 3.5 and their consistency may be affected by alcohol and electrolytes (see Example 18.5).

Gelling agents can be used to produce a wide range of consistency from slightly thickened (as in artificial tears), through lubricants and semisolids for the delivery of drugs to very thick bases used to immobilize the skin. For aqueous gels the materials used include tragacanth, alginates, pectin, gelatin, methylcelluloses, carbomer, polyvinyl alcohol and clays. Oils may be thickened using cetostearyl alcohol, hard paraffin, beeswax (see Example 20.7), wool alcohols and polyvalent soaps such as magnesium stearate. The latter, when heated with an oil, produces a clear 'lipogel'.

Other ingredients

Wetting agents are required for hydrophobic solids. Tincture of quillaia is the traditional material (see Example 20.1), but alcohol alone may be effective. Synthetic materials, such as Manoxol OT, can also be used.

Humectants are materials added to reduce the rate of water loss from creams and gels. They are all hygroscopic materials and include glycerol, propylene glycol, PEG 300 and sorbitol syrup, typically used at concentrations of 5–15%.

Solids may be added to semisolid occlusive bases. They provide channels for the migration of water from the skin surface and so reduce the occlusiveness. Solids used include zinc oxide, talc, starch and Aerosil. Some, such as talc, must be sterilized to kill bacterial spores (see Ch. 22).

Whenever there is a danger of microbial growth, anti-microbial preservation is required.

DISPENSING OF EXTERNAL PREPARATIONS

A wide range of dispensing techniques are used in compounding external medicines some of which have been reviewed in other chapters (see Chs 7, 17, 18, 19 and 22). In the section which follows, only those types of product which require different dispensing techniques are described in detail.

Dusting powders

A simple mixing in a mortar and pestle using 'doubling-up' is used (see Ch. 22). Sieving may be necessary to disperse aggregates of cohesive powders. A 180 μm sieve should be used. Powders such as starch, which contains a lot of moisture, may need drying to ensure optimum flow properties. With coloured materials, considerable working with the pestle is required before proceeding to 'doubling-up' otherwise a speckled product may result. A liquid may be added by pipette to a small quantity of the powder and be worked in before further mixing. A worked example of a dusting powder is given in Example 22.3.

Liquid preparations

These include solutions, suspensions and emulsions. The same basic dispensing techniques employed in making the corresponding oral systems are used (see Chs 17, 18 and 19). Most liquid preparations are used unsterilized, but if they are intended for application to broken skin, eyes or body cavities, they should be sterilized. They should be packed in ribbed bottles, labelled 'For external use only' and carry a 'Shake the bottle' label if they are emulsions or suspensions. Worked examples are given of a lotion in Example 18.5 and of an oily lotion in Example 19.5.

EXAMPLE 20.1

℞ Compound Sulphur Lotion BPC
Send 100 mL Compound Sulphur Lotion BPC.

	Master Formula	For 100 mL
Precipitated sulphur	40 g	4 g
Quillaia tincture	5 mL	0.5 mL
Glycerol	20 mL	2 mL
Industrial methylated spirit	60 mL	6 mL
Calcium hydroxide solution	to 1000 mL	to 100 mL

Action and uses. This is used as a treatment for acne, scabies and as a mild antiseptic.

Formulation notes. This an example of a shake lotion, an aqueous suspension prepared without a suspending agent, but including a wetting agent for the hydrophobic sulphur.

Method of preparation. Sieve the precipitated sulphur. Weigh out 4 g and place in a glass mortar. Using a 1 mL pipette add 0.5 mL quillaia tincture and work well into the sulphur using a pestle. Add 6 mL of industrial methylated spirits followed by 2 mL glycerol working in after each addition (thus achieving maximum wetting before water is added). Add 20–30 mL calcium hydroxide solution to produce a pourable suspension. Transfer to a tared bottle. Rinse the mortar with calcium hydroxide solution, adding it to the bottle, before making up to volume.

Shelf life and storage. There are no special requirements for storage. An expiry date of 4 weeks is suitable.

EXAMPLE 20.2

℞ Methyl Salicylate Liniment BP
Prepare 100 mL methyl salicylate liniment.

	Master Formula	For 100 mL
Methyl salicylate	250 mL	25 mL
Arachis oil	to 1000 mL	to 100 mL

Action and uses. Methyl salicylate is a rubefacient, used to treat muscular aches and pains.

Formulation notes. The methyl salicylate requires to enter the skin. The vegetable oil, arachis oil, is used as the solvent to assist in this process. Other similar fixed oils can be used.

Method of preparation. Measure 25 mL of methyl salicylate in a 100 mL measure and add arachis oil to make up to volume. Transfer to a dry 100 mL amber ribbed bottle.

Shelf life and storage. This liniment should be kept in a well-closed container in a cool place. An expiry date of 4 weeks is appropriate.

EXAMPLE 20.3

℞ Turpentine Liniment BP
Send 100 mL of turpentine liniment.

	Master Formula	To send 100 mL (120 units)
Turpentine oil	650 mL	78 mL
Racemic camphor	50 g	6 g
Soft soap	75 g	9 g
Purified water, freshly boiled and cooled	225 mL	27 mL

Action and uses. Both turpentine oil and camphor are rubefacients which are rubbed into the skin to relieve muscular aches and pains.

Formulation notes. The BP formula adds up to 1000. However, this is a mixture of weights and volumes so the final volume is not known. It is usual to calculate in the ratio 120 'units' per 100 mL.

This is an emulsion made using an alkali soap. When using soft soap, it is usual to use it at 10% by weight of an oil (as in this example), or 20% by weight of a fat.

Method of preparation. Weigh the camphor and place in a porcelain mortar. Grind it to a small particle size. Choose the softer, greener parts of the soap. Weigh (on a piece of paper) and mix thoroughly with the camphor. Measure the turpentine oil and add small aliquots (5–10 mL at first) to the soap and camphor followed by thorough mixing. When an even, pourable dispersion is obtained, transfer this to a 250 mL stoppered measuring cylinder. Use the remaining oil to rinse the mortar and add to the cylinder. Measure the water and add it, as quickly as possible, to the measure, stopper and shake it vigorously until a creamy white emulsion is formed. Allow it to stand for a few minutes (for air bubbles to separate) before transferring 100 mL to a tared bottle. Avoid plastic containers because turpentine reacts with some plastics.

Shelf life and storage. There are no special storage requirements. An expiry date of 4 weeks is appropriate.

EXAMPLE 20.4

℞ Benzyl Benzoate Application BP
Prepare 100 mL of benzyl benzoate application.

	Master Formula	For 100 mL
Benzyl benzoate	250 g	25 g
Emulsifying wax	20 g	2 g
Purified water, freshly boiled and cooled	to 1000 mL	to 100 mL

Action and uses. Benzyl benzoate is a liquid insecticide used for treating scabies and lice. It is usually applied with a brush over the whole body below the neck for scabies. It should not be applied to broken or inflamed skin.

Formulation notes. Benzyl benzoate is water immiscible and is being emulsified using the anionic Emulsifying Wax BP. The application is an o/w emulsion.

Method of preparation. Weigh the emulsifying wax and place it in an evaporating basin on a water-bath or hot plate to melt. Add the benzyl benzoate and mix and warm. Warm about 75 mL of the water to the same temperature. Add about half of this to the evaporating basin and mix very gently. Transfer the mixture, again very gently to avoid frothing, to a tared bottle. Add warmed water to volume. Close the bottle and shake vigorously. Care is required to avoid frothing when water is present, because it will be very difficult to make up to the tare mark when froth has formed. Shake frequently during cooling.

Shelf life and storage. The application should be kept in a cool place, but not be allowed to freeze. An expiry date of 4 weeks is appropriate.

Semisolid preparations

Mixing by fusion

The compounding of many semisolid preparations includes the blending together of oily materials, some of which are solids at room temperature. The process called 'mixing by fusion' achieves this. As the name implies, it involves melting the ingredients together (see Example 20.5). The process is carried out in an evaporating basin on a water-bath or hot plate. It should be noted that a high temperature is not required so 60–70°C is usually adequate. Waxy solids should be grated before weighing and should be added first, so that melting can start whilst other ingredients are being measured. When all the ingredients are melted, remove the basin from the water-bath and gently stir until cold. Mixing, which should be gentle to avoid air bubbles, is necessary to avoid lumps forming. This could happen because the higher melting point ingredients in the eutectic system may precipitate out. Any medicament may be added at different stages of preparation depending on its properties. If soluble and stable, it can be added when the base is molten. If it is less stable, or insoluble but easy to disperse, it can be added during cooling. However, if it is unstable or if dispersion is difficult, it should be added when cold using mixing by trituration.

When evaporating basins are being used recovery of all the product is not possible. Thus, in order to be able to pack the prescribed amount, it is necessary to make an excess of about 10%.

EXAMPLE 20.5

℞ Simple Ointment BP
Send 50 g simple ointment.

	Master Formula	For 60 g
Wool fat	50 g	3 g
Hard paraffin	50 g	3 g
Cetostearyl alcohol	50 g	3 g
Yellow or white soft paraffin	850 g	51 g

Action and uses. Simple ointment is used as an emollient, or for making other ointments.

Formulation notes. This is a simple blend of solid and semisolid oily ingredients made by fusion. Yellow or white soft paraffin is chosen according to the colour of the finished product. In this case, since there is nothing else to be added, white soft paraffin should be used; 60 g is made to allow 50 g to be dispensed.

Method of preparation. Grate the hard paraffin and cetostearyl alcohol. Weigh 3 g of each and place in an evaporating basin on a water-bath or hot plate. Weigh the wool fat, using a piece of paper to allow full recovery of the material, and add it to the evaporating basin, followed by the soft paraffin (also weighed on paper). Stir gently until fully melted. Remove from the heat and continue to stir gently until cold. Weigh 50 g of base into a tared ointment jar or pack into a collapsible tube (see Example 20.10). If an ointment jar is used, a greaseproof paper disc should be placed on the surface of the ointment to protect the liner of the lid from the greasiness.

Shelf life and storage. Store in a cool place. An expiry date of 4 weeks is appropriate.

Mixing by trituration

Insoluble solids or liquids are incorporated into bases using the technique called 'mixing by trituration'. Any powders should be passed through a 180 µm sieve before weighing to avoid grittiness. Mixing by trituration is carried out on an ointment slab or tile, which may be made of glass or glazed porcelain. A flexible spatula is used to work the materials together. Powders are placed on the tile and incorporated into the base using 'doubling-up' as it is worked in. However, it is usually necessary to have two to three times the volume of base to powder, otherwise it will 'crumble'. Liquids, if present, are usually present in small amounts. To incorporate a liquid a portion of the base is placed on the slab and a recess made to hold the liquid which is then worked in gently. Larger quantities of liquid should be added a little at a time using the same method. In theory it is possible to recover all material from the slab, but it is normal to allow up to 10% excess for losses. These processes can be carried out in a mortar with a flat base using a pestle with a flat head. However, because recovery of the product is difficult, this is usually reserved for larger-scale batches.

EXAMPLE 20.6

℞ Sulphur Ointment BP
Send 50 g sulphur ointment.

	Master Formula	For 50 g	For 55 g
Precipitated sulphur, finely sifted	100 g	5 g	5.5 g
Simple ointment	900 g	45 g	49.5 g

Action and uses. The ointment is used to treat acne and scabies.

Formulation notes. The BP directs that the simple ointment be prepared with white soft paraffin. If simple ointment is available, the trituration can be carried out on a slab and all the product recovered. However, if simple ointment is also being made, 50 g should be adequate to ensure that 45 g is available. Precipitated sulphur, whilst of smaller particle size than sublimed sulphur, can give a gritty feel unless it is passed through a 180 μm sieve.

Method of preparation. Sieve and then weigh out the precipitated sulphur and place it on the slab. Weigh out the simple ointment (using a piece of paper to prevent it sticking to the balance), and place it on a different part of the slab. Take a portion of the sulphur and a portion of the base of about three times the volume of the sulphur and work them together vigorously until there is no sign of any particles of sulphur. Spreading a thin layer on the slab can check this. Gradually add the remaining sulphur and base. Collect the ointment together on the slab using the spatula and pack 50 g.

Shelf life and storage. Store in a cool place. An expiry date of 4 weeks is appropriate.

EXAMPLE 20.7

℞ Methyl Salicylate Ointment BP
Send 30 g methyl salicylate ointment.

	Master Formula	For 35 g
Methyl salicylate	500 g	17.5 g
White beeswax	250 g	8.75 g
Hydrous wool fat	250 g	8.75 g

Action and uses. Methyl salicylate is a volatile material used as a rubefacient.

Formulation notes. Methyl salicylate is a liquid. With the high proportion present, the product would be runny without the addition of the beeswax as a thickening agent. The base ingredients require to be blended by fusion.

Method of preparation. Grate and weigh the beeswax. Melt it with the hydrous wool fat (weighed on a piece of paper) in an evaporating basin on a water-bath or hot plate. Remove from the heat and stir until almost cold before adding the methyl salicylate (it is volatile). Continue stirring until cold. Pack 30 g in a glass ointment jar (plastic should be avoided with methyl salicylate).

Shelf life and storage. Store in a cool place. An expiry date of 4 weeks is appropriate.

Creams

Creams are emulsified preparations containing water. They are susceptible to microbial growth which may cause spoilage of the cream or disease in the patient. Whilst preservatives are included, they are usually inadequate to cope with a heavy microbial contamination (see Ch. 12) and so the possibility of microbial contamination during preparation should be minimized. Ideally aseptic techniques should be used, but this is not normally possible in extemporaneous dispensing and so thorough cleanliness is employed. As a minimum, all apparatus and final containers should be thoroughly cleaned and rinsed with freshly boiled and cooled purified water, then dried just prior to use. Swabbing of working surfaces, spatulas and other equipment with ethanol will also reduce the possibility of microbial contamination.

The basic method of making an emulsified cream is to warm the oily phase and aqueous phase to a temperature of about 60°C, mix the phases and stir until cold. It is important that the temperatures of the two phases are within a few degrees the same and it is advisable to use a thermometer to check this. Rapid cooling will cause the separation of high melting point materials, and excessive aeration as a result of vigorous stirring will produce a granular appearance in the product. Medicaments may, if they are stable, be dissolved in the appropriate phase before emulsification, or can be added by trituration when cold.

EXAMPLE 20.8

℞ Aqueous Cream BP
Send 50 g aqueous cream.

	Master Formula	For 55 g
Emulsifying ointment	300 g	16.5 g
Phenoxyethanol	10 g	0.55 g
Purified water, freshly boiled and cooled	690 g	37.95 g

Action and uses. Aqueous cream is an emollient and can be used as a base for drugs.

Formulation notes. This is an o/w cream made using an anionic emulsifying agent. To reduce the risk of microbial contamination all equipment should be washed before use. Phenoxyethanol is present as an antimicrobial preservative. It is a liquid, so has to be weighed, or, if its density is obtained, it could be measured by pipette. If the emulsifying ointment has to made, exactly 16.5 g can be made because the emulsification can be carried out in the same evaporating basin.

Method of preparation. The phenoxyethanol is dissolved in the water warmed to 60°C. Weigh the emulsifying ointment (using a piece of paper to prevent it sticking) and melt it in an evaporating basin on a water-bath or hot plate. Ensure that both phases are close to 60°C, then add the aqueous phase to the melted ointment. Remove from the heat and stir continuously until cold, taking care not to incorporate too much air. Weigh 50 g and pack in an ointment jar or collapsible tube.

Shelf life and storage. The preparation should be stored in a cool place, but not allowed to freeze. A shelf life of 2–3 weeks is appropriate because the preparation has not been made in the cleanest conditions.

EXAMPLE 20.9

℞ Hydrous Ointment BP (also known as Oily Cream)
Send 50 g oily cream.

	Master Formula	For 60 g
Wool alcohols ointment	500 g	30 g
Phenoxyethanol	10 g	0.6 g
Dried magnesium sulphate	5 g	0.3 g
Purified water, freshly		
boiled and cooled	485 g	29.1 g

Actions and uses. Oily cream is used as an emollient in treating dry skin conditions.

Formulation notes. This is a w/o cream prepared using wool alcohols as the emulsifying agent. Phenoxyethanol is present as preservative, but all equipment should be washed before use. Phenoxyethanol is a liquid and so must be weighed, or, if its density is obtained, it can be measured by pipette. Quantities for 55 g produce amounts that cannot be weighed on a Class B balance, so 60 g is made. If the wool alcohols ointment is also to be made, exactly 30 g is adequate, because it does not have to be removed from the evaporating basin.

Method of preparation. All equipment should be thoroughly cleaned before use. Dissolve the magnesium sul-

phate and phenoxyethanol in the water and warm to 60°C on a water-bath or hot plate. Weigh the wool alcohols ointment, using a piece of paper, and melt it in an evaporating basin at 60°C. Check that the two temperatures are the same. Add the water, little by little, to the ointment, stirring constantly until a smooth creamy mixture is produced, whilst maintaining the temperature at 60°C. When all the water is added, stir gently until the cream is at room temperature. Pack 50 g in an ointment jar or collapsible tube.

Shelf life and storage. Store in a cool place but do not allow to freeze. If liquid separates on storage stirring may reincorporate it. An expiry date of 4 weeks is appropriate.

Dilution of creams

It is sometimes necessary to prepare a dilution of a commercially produced cream, although the practice is undesirable. Choice of diluent is crucial, since the diluent may impair the preservative system in the cream, may affect the bioavailability of the medicament, or be incompatible with other ingredients. The process of dilution also increases the risk of microbial contamination. Thus, dilutions should only be made with the diluent(s) specified in the manufacturer's data sheet. All diluted creams should be freshly prepared and be given a 2-week shelf life.

EXAMPLE 20.10

A method for filling a collapsible tube extemporaneously.

1. Cut a piece of greaseproof paper about 5 cm longer than the tube and of a width that will go round the tube about twice. Place this on a clean slab, and fold up about 1 cm on one long edge (Fig. 20.3).

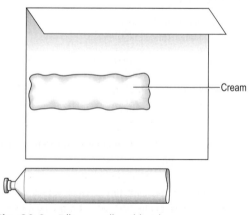

Fig. 20.3 Filling a collapsible tube.

---

2. Place the cream on the paper, parallel to the fold, so that the length is about the same as that of the tube. Then fold the loose edge of the paper into the fold, so covering the cream (This stage is rather like wrapping a powder—see Fig 22.1.) Roll the paper from the fold, so that the cream is held in a cylinder of paper which will slide inside the tube.

3. Push the paper and cream right down the tube. Then, using a spatula or fingers, close the paper at the open end and gently pull it out, leaving the cream behind in the tube.

4. When fully withdrawn hold a spatula blade firmly down on the open end of the tube, about 2.5 mm in from the end and raise the cap end to produce a fold. Use the spatula, or a crimping tool if one is available, to complete the fold. Repeat this to produce a second fold.

Pastes

Pastes are dispersions of high concentrations of solid in either an aqueous or oily vehicle. They can be used to treat infections by making use of their high osmotic pressure, or as very thick materials to prevent irritant drugs spreading over the skin surface. Incorporation of the solid is by mixing on an ointment slab.

EXAMPLE 20.11

℞ Dithranol Paste BP
Send 100 g of weak dithranol paste.

	Master Formula	For 100 g
Dithranol	1 g	0.1 g
Lassar's paste	999 g	99.9 g

Lassar's Paste

	Master Formula	For 110 g
Zinc oxide	240 g	26.4 g
Salicylic acid	20 g	2.2 g
Starch	240 g	26.4 g
White soft paraffin	500 g	55 g

Action and uses. Dithranol is used to treat psoriasis. There are two strengths of dithranol paste, 'weak' is 0.1% and 'strong' is 1%, although a range of intermediate strengths are prescribed by dermatologists.

Formulation notes. The Lassar's paste has to be made first before incorporating the dithranol. Dithranol is prone to oxidation, so contact with metal should be avoided.

Method of preparation. Sieve the zinc oxide and salicylic acid through a 180 μm sieve before weighing. Weigh the soft paraffin (on a piece of paper) and melt in an evaporating basin on a water-bath. Take some of the powder and stir into the melted base. Continue until all the powder is added, then stir gently until cold. Weigh out the Lassar's paste (using paper to avoid sticking). Only when the Lassar's paste has been completed, weigh out the dithranol. Care is required because it is very irritant to skin. Place it on a slab and incorporate it in a small portion of the paste using a plastic spatula, ensuring that a smooth, even product is produced. Dilute gradually with the remainder of the paste. Pack in a 120 g (4 ounces) brown ointment jar, with a circle of greaseproof paper and a tight-fitting closure, or a collapsible tube. The label should include the words 'To be spread thinly … ' (BNF Label 28).

Shelf life and storage. The product should be kept in a cool place, protected from light. An expiry date of 2 weeks is appropriate because of chemical instability.

TRANSDERMAL DELIVERY SYSTEMS

Transdermal drug delivery aims to provide continuous drug release over a period of time which can be from a few hours 1 to 7 days.

The principle of this dosage form is that, by optimization of physicochemical factors the drug is absorbed through the skin into the systemic circulation. Absorption through the skin is variable so the rate of release of the drug must be controlled to a slower rate than the skin can absorb it. This may be achieved either by using a matrix system or a rate-limiting membrane. These devices are known as 'patches'. Further details about the pharmaceutics of the patches are given in Aulton (see Ch. 33). There is also a glyceryl trinitrate cream which gives systemic activity.

Drugs available as transdermal therapeutic systems include:

- Glyceryl trinitrate for the treatment of angina. These patches are designed to deliver the drug over a 24-hour period, although it is recommended that a drug-free period is allowed each day to prevent tolerance. These patches are normally applied to the chest area.
- Estradiol for the alleviation of menopausal symptoms and the prevention of osteoporosis. These patches are applied once or twice weekly to skin below the waist (away from the breasts). They can be used alone or in combination with progestogens.

- Nicotine, in the alleviation of withdrawal symptoms in smoking cessation provides an alternative route of administration to the gums, sprays etc. Patches are used for 16–24-hour periods and are available in a range of 'strengths'—that is rate of delivery of nicotine. By providing a steady delivery of nicotine, they avoid the high plasma levels obtained during smoking. They may also have beneficial effects in other disease states. They are applied to the trunk.
- Hyoscine is available for the prevention of symptoms of travel sickness for up to 72 hours. It is applied behind the ear.
- Testosterone is used for hormone replacement and is applied to the trunk.
- Fentanyl patches can treat chronic intractable pain over a 72-hour period. They are applied to the torso.

The main advantages of this type of dosage form are:

- Continuous drug delivery, producing steady-state plasma levels
- No drug deactivation by digestive juices
- No first pass effect, as the liver is bypassed (although there is metabolism in the skin)
- Cessation of treatment by removing the patch. (This is not immediate because of a reservoir effect which will continue to deliver drug from the skin for several hours.)

Although these are benefits, various problems are associated with this type of dosage form. For these reasons few drugs so far have been formulated in this way.

Disadvantages

- Only potent drugs, i.e. those with a small therapeutic dose, are suitable to be incorporated into a patch. Skin permeability is inadequate to allow larger doses from an acceptable size of patch.
- Because the drug is being absorbed through the skin, lipid-soluble drugs are most likely to be effective.
- Drugs with long half-lives are not suitable for this type of formulation.

- There have been reports of local skin reactions due to irritancy of drugs. Clonidine was withdrawn for this reason. To minimize possible skin reactions, new patches should be placed on fresh skin each time.
- In some instances the steady-state blood levels have produced tolerance, e.g. glyceryl trinitrate. This has led to the practice of patients being given a 'nitrate-free' period which prevents tolerance occurring. A patch is applied and remains in place for 16 hours and is then removed. A period of 8 hours is allowed to elapse before a new patch is applied.
- Steady-state blood levels of nicotine have caused central nervous system disturbance, in particular, patients have reported suffering nightmares. Normally nicotine levels in a smoker will fall during the hours of sleep as no cigarette smoking occurs. No such fall will occur when 24-hour nicotine patches are used. For this reason one manufacturer has developed a patch which is applied for 16 hours then removed. A new one is applied 8 hours later.

Method of use

It is important that patients are informed how to use patches correctly. All patients who purchase or are prescribed patches should be given the following information about their use.

- To ensure adequate adhesion the patch must be applied to a clean, dry area of skin.
- The old patch must always be removed before applying a new one.
- When a patch is replaced with a new one it must be applied to a different area of skin. The area of skin from which a patch has just been removed will be soft and possibly moist. This alters the permeability of the skin. In order to maintain the same level of drug absorption a different, intact area of skin must be used.
- The patch must be disposed of carefully. It should be folded together to prevent it being stuck onto another person's skin. Particular care should be taken to keep patches away from children.

Key Points

- Drugs applied to the skin are usually for a local effect, although systemic action is possible.
- Skin preparations may be solids, liquids or semisolids.
- For liquids and semisolids, the vehicles may be water based, water miscible, oily or emulsified.
- A wide range of emulsifying agents may be used to produce either o/w or w/o emulsions.
- Suspending agents used on the skin are usually clays.
- Other ingredients include wetting agents, humectants and finely divided solids.
- Powders should normally be passed through a 180 μm sieve before use.
- Containers for liquid preparations should be brown and ribbed.
- All skin preparations should carry the label 'For external use only'.

- Dusting powders are simple mixtures made by 'doubling-up'.
- Lotions are aqueous solutions, suspensions or emulsions.
- Liniments are oily solutions or emulsions.
- Mixing by fusion is the process of melting together the ingredients of ointment bases followed by stirring until cold.
- Mixing by trituration is the incorporation of solids or liquids into semisolid vehicles on an ointment slab.
- Cleanliness is essential when making creams to avoid excessive microbial contamination.
- Transdermal delivery systems (skin patches) are used to give prolonged constant plasma concentrations for a number of drugs.
- Patients must be carefully counselled on the use of skin patches.

Suppositories and pessaries

A. J. Winfield (original author M. M. Moody)

After studying this chapter you will understand about:

Ideal suppository bases
Types of base
Suppository moulds and mould calibration
Displacement values
Methods of preparation of suppositories and pessaries
Containers, labelling and patient advice for suppositories and pessaries

Introduction

Drug administration by the rectum can be used for local or systemic action. Dosage forms used include suppositories, tablets, capsules, ointments and enemas. Vaginal administration can also be for both local or systemic action using dosage forms which include pessaries, tablets, capsules, solutions, sprays, creams, ointments and foams. This chapter gives details of how suppositories and pessaries are prepared extemporaneously, the substances and equipment used in their preparation, the calculations involved and patient advice. Details about the formulation, manufacture and biopharmacy can be found in Aulton (2002).

Suppositories and pessaries are drug delivery systems where the drug is incorporated into an inert vehicle. This vehicle is referred to as the base. They are formed by melting the base, incorporating the drug and then allowing them to set in a suitable mould (metal or plastic).

SUPPOSITORY BASES

A range of materials is available for use as bases. A number of criteria can be identified as desirable in an ideal base, including:

- Melt at, or just below body temperature or dissolve in body fluids
- Solidify quickly after melting
- Be easily moulded and removed from the mould
- Be chemically stable even when molten
- Release the active ingredient readily
- Be easy to handle
- Be bland, i.e. non-toxic and non-irritant.

No base meets all these requirements, so a compromise is usually required. There are two groups, the fatty bases and the water-soluble or water-miscible bases.

The fatty bases

These bases, which melt around body temperature, are the naturally occurring theobroma oil and synthetic fats.

Theobroma oil, which has been used as a suppository base for over 200 years, has a melting point range of 30–36°C and so readily melts in the body. It liquefies easily on heating but also sets rapidly when cooled. It is also bland, therefore no irritation occurs. However, for a number of reasons the newer synthetic bases have now largely superseded it. The main technical difficulty is the ease with which lower melting point polymorphic forms of theobroma oil are formed. The stable β-form has a melting point of 34.5°C and forms after melting at 36°C and slowly cooling. However, if it is overheated, the unstable α-form (melting point 23°C) and γ-form (melting point 19°C) are produced. These forms will eventually return to the stable form but this may take several days. The melting point is also a problem in hot climates and when it is reduced by the addition of a soluble drug. The latter can be counteracted by adding beeswax (up to 10%), but care must be taken not to raise the melting point too high, as the suppository would then not melt in the rectum. In addition theobroma oil is prone to oxidation and in common with many naturally occurring substances, may vary from batch to batch. Theobroma oil shrinks only slightly on cooling and therefore tends to stick to the suppository mould. For this reason the mould must be lubricated before use.

Synthetic fats

These are prepared by hydrogenating suitable vegetable oils. They have many of the advantages of theobroma oil but fewer disadvantages. However, there are a few potential problems.

- The viscosity of the melted fats is lower than that of theobroma oil. As a result there is a greater risk of drug particles sedimenting during preparation leading to a lack of uniform drug distribution which can give localized irritancy. This problem is partly compensated for in that these bases set very quickly.
- These bases become brittle if cooled too rapidly, so should not be refrigerated during preparation.
- Most manufacturers produce a series of grades of synthetic fatty bases, each with different hardness and melting point ranges. These can be used to compensate for melting point reduction. However, release and absorption of the drug in the body may vary depending on the base being used.

Further information on these bases can be found in the *Pharmaceutical Codex* (1994).

Water-soluble and water-miscible bases

Glycerol-gelatin bases

These bases are a mixture of glycerol and water stiffened with gelatin. The commonest is Glycerol Suppositories Base BP, which has 14% w/w gelatin, and 70% w/w glycerol. In hot climates the gelatin content can be increased to 18% w/w. Gelatin is a purified protein produced by the hydrolysis of the collagenous tissue, such as skins and bones, of animals. Grades of gelatin for pharmaceutical use must be heat treated during their preparation to ensure that the product is pathogen free. Some people may have ethical problems with the use of material from an animal source.

Two types of gelatin are used for pharmaceutical purposes, Type A, which is prepared by acid hydrolysis and is cationic, and Type B, which is prepared by alkaline hydrolysis and is anionic. Type A is compatible with substances such as boric acid and lactic acid while Type B is compati-

ble with substances like ichthammol and zinc oxide. The 'jelly strength' or 'Bloom strength' of gelatin is important, particularly when it is used in the preparation of suppositories or pessaries.

Glycerol-gelatin bases have a physiological effect which can cause rectal irritation because of the small amount of liquid present. As they dissolve in the mucous secretions of the rectum, osmosis occurs producing a laxative effect. They are also hygroscopic and therefore require careful storage. They are much more difficult to prepare and handle than other bases and the solution time depends on the content and quality of the gelatin and also the age of the suppository. Because of the water content, microbial contamination is more likely than with the fatty bases. Preservatives may be added to the product, but can lead to problems of incompatibilities. As a consequence, this type of base is used for pessaries rather than suppositories.

Macrogols

These polyethylene glycols can be blended together to produce suppository bases with varying melting points, dissolution rates and physical characteristics. Drug release depends on the base dissolving rather than melting (the melting point is often around 50°C). Higher proportions of high molecular weight polymers produce preparations which release the drug slowly and are also brittle. Less brittle products which release the drug more readily can be prepared by mixing high polymers with medium and low polymers. Details of combinations which are used are found in the *Pharmaceutical Codex* (1994, p. 172). Macrogols have several properties which make them useful as suppository bases including that they have no physiological effect, are not prone to microbial contamination and have a high water-absorbing capacity. As they dissolve, a viscous solution is produced which means there is less likelihood of leakage from the body.

There are, however, a number of disadvantages. They are hygroscopic which means they must be carefully stored and this could lead to irritation of the rectal mucosa. This latter disadvantage can be alleviated by dipping the suppository in water prior to insertion. They become brittle if cooled too quickly and also may become brittle on storage. Incompatibility with several drugs and packaging materials, e.g. benzocaine, penicillin and plastic, may limit their use. In addition crystal growth occurs with some drugs causing irritation to the rectal mucosa and, if the crystals are large, prolonged dissolution times.

PREPARATION OF SUPPOSITORIES

Suppositories are made using a suppository mould which may be made of metal or plastic. Traditional metal moulds (Fig. 21.1) are in two halves which are clamped together with a screw. The internal surface is normally plated to ensure that the suppositories have a smooth surface.

Before use it is important to ensure that the mould is completely clean and it should be washed carefully in warm, soapy water and thoroughly dried taking care not to scratch the internal surface. The exact shape can vary slightly from one mould to another.

Preparation of suppositories containing an active ingredient which is insoluble in the base

The bases used most commonly for extemporaneous preparation of suppositories and pessaries are the synthetic fats and glycerol-gelatin base.

1. It is always advisable when calculating the quantity of ingredients to calculate for an excess of 2 to allow for unavoidable wastage, e.g. if required to prepare 12 suppositories, calculate for 14.
2. The mould should be carefully washed and dried.
3. Ensure that the two halves fit together correctly. This is necessary to ensure that there is no leakage of material. They usually have code letters and/or numbers which should match.
4. For some bases the mould will need to be lubricated. The lubricants are given in Table 21.1.
5. If lubricant is necessary, apply it carefully to the two halves of the mould using gauze or other non-fibrous material. Do not use cotton wool as fibres may be left on the mould surface and become incorporated into the suppositories.

Table 21.1   Lubricants for use with suppository bases

Base	Lubricant
Theobroma oil	Soap spirit
Glycerol-gelatin base	Almond or arachis oil, liquid paraffin
Synthetic fats	No lubricant required
Macrogols	No lubricant required

6. Invert the mould to allow any excess lubricant to drain off.
7. Accurately weigh the required amount of base. If large lumps are present the material should be grated.
8. Place in a porcelain basin and warm gently using a water-bath or hot plate. Allow approximately two-thirds of the base to melt and remove from the heat. The residual heat will be sufficient to melt the rest of the base.
9. Reduce the particle size of the active ingredient, if necessary. Either grinding in a mortar and pestle or sieving will do this.
10. Weigh the correct amount of medicament and place on a glass tile (ointment slab).
11. Add about half of the molten base to the powdered drug and rub together with a spatula.
12. Scrape the dispersion off the tile using the spatula and place it back in the basin.
13. If necessary, put the basin back over the water-bath to remelt the ingredients.
14. Remove from the heat and stir constantly until almost on the point of setting. If the mixture is not stirred at this stage the active ingredient will sediment and uniform distribution of the drug will not be achieved.
15. Quickly pour into the mould, slightly overfilling each cavity to allow for contraction on cooling. Do not start pouring the suppositories while the mixture is still very molten. If this is done, the drug sediments to the bottom of the mould and the base shrinks excessively so that the tops become concave.
16. Leave the mould and its contents to cool for about 5 minutes and then, using a spatula, trim the tops of the suppositories. Do not leave the suppositories too long before trimming as they will be too hard and trimming becomes very difficult.
17. Allow cooling for another 10–15 minutes until the suppositories are completely firm and set. Do not try to speed up the cooling process by putting the mould in a

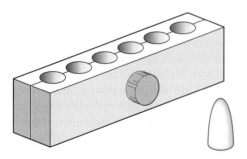

Fig. 21.1   Dispensing suppository mould.

refrigerator. Synthetic fats in particular are inclined to become brittle and break if cooled too quickly.

18. Unscrew the mould and remove the suppositories
19. Each perfect suppository should then be wrapped in greaseproof paper and packed in an appropriate container and labelled.

When preparing suppositories where the active ingredient is a semisolid, is soluble in the base or is a liquid which is miscible with the base, the melting point of the base will be lowered. In these situations a base with a higher than normal melting point should to be used if available. The base is melted as normal and the active ingredient is added directly to the base and incorporated by stirring.

Moulds are made in four sizes, 1 g, 2 g, 4 g and 8 g. Unless otherwise stated, the 1 g size is used for suppositories. The same moulds are used to prepare pessaries, when the two larger sizes are generally used. A suppository mould is filled by volume, but the suppository is formulated by weight. The capacity of a suppository mould is nominal and each mould will have minor variations. Therefore the weight of material contained in different moulds may be different and will also depend on the base being used. It is therefore essential that each mould be calibrated for each different base.

Mould calibration

The capacity of the mould is confirmed by filling the mould with the chosen base. The total weight of the perfect suppositories is taken and a mean weight calculated. This value is the calibration value of the mould for that particular base.

EXAMPLE 21.1

A 1 g suppository mould is to be used to prepare a batch of suppositories. The base to be used is a synthetic fat. Some base is melted in an evaporating basin over a water-bath or hot plate. When about two-thirds of the base has melted the basin is removed from the heat. The contents of the basin are stirred and the remaining base melts with the residual heat. Continue stirring the base until it is almost on the point of setting (it starts to thicken, becomes slightly cloudy and small crystals occur on the surface). The base is then poured into the mould cavities, slightly overfilling to allow for shrinkage. They are trimmed after about 5 minutes and left to set for a further 10–15 minutes. The mould is then opened and the suppositories removed. Only the perfect products should be weighed. Any which are chipped or damaged should be discarded.

From the above exercise five perfect suppositories were obtained. The total weight was 5.05 g. The mould calibration figure is therefore 5.05/5 = 1.01 g. This is the value which should be used for that particular combination of mould and base.

Displacement values

The volume of a suppository from a particular mould is uniform but its weight can vary when a drug is present because the density of the drug may be different from that of the base. For example a drug which has twice the density of the base will occupy half the volume which the same weight of base occupies, and a drug whose density is four times that of the base will occupy a quarter the volume which the same weight of base occupies. Allowance must be made for this by using displacement values (DVs).

The displacement value of a drug is the number of parts by weight of drug which displaces 1 part by weight of the base.

Displacement values for a variety of medicaments are given in Table 21.2. Other reference sources such as the *Pharmaceutical Handbook* (Wade 1980) and the *Pharmaceutical Codex* also give information on displacement values. Minor variations may occur in the values quoted so it is always advisable to indicate the source of your information.

Table 21.2   Displacement values with respect to fatty bases

Medicament	Displacement value
Aspirin	1.1
Bismuth subgallate	2.7
Chloral hydrate	1.4
Cinchocaine hydrochloride	1.0
Codeine phosphate	1.1
Hamamelis dry extract	1.5
Hydrocortisone	1.5
Ichthammol	1.0
Liquids	1.0
Metronidazole	1.7
Morphine hydrochloride	1.6
Paracetamol	1.5
Pethidine hydrochloride	1.6
Phenobarbital	1.1
Zinc oxide	4.7

Displacement values in the literature normally refer to values for theobroma oil. These values can also be used for other fatty bases. With glycerol-gelatin suppository base, approximately 1.2 g occupies the same volume as 1 g of theobroma oil. Using this information the relevant displacement values can be calculated.

EXAMPLE 21.2

Prepare six suppositories each containing 250 mg bismuth subgallate.

Not all material can be removed from the evaporating basin, so quantities are calculated for an excess of two suppositories. Therefore calculate for eight suppositories.

DV of bismuth subgallate = 2.7 (*Pharmaceutical Codex*), i.e. 2.7 g of bismuth subgallate displaces 1 g of base.

A 1 g mould will be used with mould calibration = 0.94.

To calculate the amount of base required, a simple equation is used:

$$\text{Amount of base} = (N \times y) - N \times D/DV$$

where N is the number of suppositories to be made, y is the mould calibration, D is the dose in one suppository, DV is the displacement value.

Using the terms in the equation for this example:

$$N = 8$$
$$Y = 0.94$$
$$D = 250 \text{ mg} = 0.25 \text{ g}$$
$$DV = 2.7$$

Using the equation:

Amount of base required
$$= (8 \times 0.94) - 8 \times 0.25/2.7 = 7.52 - 0.741$$
$$= 6.779 \text{ g} = 6.78 \text{ g}$$

There may be occasions when information on the DV of a drug is not available. In these situations the DV must be determined.

EXAMPLE 21.3

To calculate the DV of a drug. A batch of unmedicated suppositories is prepared and the products weighed.

A batch of suppositories containing a known concentration of the required drug is prepared and the products are weighed.

Weight of six unmedicated suppositories = 6 g.

Weight of six suppositories containing 40% drug = 8.8 g.
Weight of base is then =
  60% = 60/100 × 8.8 = 5.28 g.
Weight of drug in suppositories
  = 40% = 40/100 × 8.8 = 3.52 .
Weight of base displaced by drug = 6 × 5.28 = 0.72 g.

If 0.72 g of drug is displaced by 3.52 g of base, then 1 g of base will be displaced by 3.52/0.72 g = 4.88 g. Therefore displacement value of drug = 4.9 (rounded to one decimal place).

Calculation of quantities when the active ingredient is stated as a percentage

A displacement value is not required when calculating quantities stated as percentages.

EXAMPLE 21.4

Prepare eight suppositories containing 18% zinc oxide.
  Calculate for 10 suppositories (2 excess).

Mould calibration = 1
Weight of base required to fill mould = 10 × 1 = 10 g.
Zinc oxide is 18% of total = 1.8 g
Weight of base required = 10 − 1.8 = 8.2 g.

When there is more than one active ingredient present the quantity of each medicament is calculated and the amount of base is calculated using the displacement value for each ingredient.

EXAMPLE 21.5

Calculate the quantities required to make 15 suppositories each containing 150 mg hamamelis dry extract and 560 mg of zinc oxide. A 2 g mould, with mould calibration of 2.04, will be used.
  Calculate for 17 suppositories (2 excess).

DV of hamamelis dry extract = 1.5 (*Pharmaceutical Codex*).
DV of zinc oxide = 4.7 (*Pharmaceutical Codex*).
Weight of hamamelis dry extract = 17 × 0.15 = 2.55 g.
Weight of zinc oxide = 17 × 0.56 = 9.52 g.
Weight of base = 17 × 2.04 − (2.55/1.5 + 9.52/4.7)
  = 34.68 − (1.7 + 2.03) = 30.95 g.

Preparation of suppositories using a glycerol-gelatin base

The formula for Glycerol Suppository Base BP is:

Gelatin   14%
Glycerol   70%
Water   to 100%

1. The gelatin strip is cut into small pieces, approximately 1 cm square, trimming off any hard outer edges.
2. The required amount of gelatin is weighed and placed in a previously weighed, porcelain evaporating basin.
3. Sufficient water to just cover the gelatin is added and the contents left for about 5 minutes.
4. When the gelatin has softened (hydrated) any excess water is drained off. This step is not necessary if powdered gelatin is being used.
5. The exact amount of glycerol is then weighed into the basin.
6. The basin is heated gently on a water-bath or hot plate and the mixture gently stirred until the gelatin has melted. Do not stir vigorously as this will create air bubbles which are very difficult to remove. At this stage the base may need to be heat treated as noted below.
7. When the gelatin is dissolved the basin is removed from the heat and weighed. If the weight is less than the required total (basin plus ingredients), water is added to give the correct weight. If the contents of the basin are too heavy it must be heated further to evaporate the excess water.
8. When the correct weight is achieved the active ingredient is added, with careful stirring.
9. The mixture is then poured into the prepared mould, lubricated with an oil such as arachis or almond oil or liquid paraffin. The mould must not be overfilled because glycerol-gelatin base cannot be trimmed.
10. The preparation is left to set. After unmoulding, each suppository should then be smeared with liquid paraffin before being wrapped in greaseproof paper.

Note: Gelatin which is of a grade suitable for pharmaceutical use should not contain any pathogens but as a precaution, the base may be heat treated. This is done by heating the base for 1 hour at 100°C in an electric steamer. This should be done before the base is adjusted to weight (at Stage 7 above).

This base is commonly used for the preparation of pessaries, as described in the following example.

EXAMPLE 21.6

Prepare 12 pessaries containing 10% ichthammol. A 4 g mould (calibration value 4.0) is used.

Calculate for 14 pessaries to allow for wastage. Additional base is required because it is more dense than the oily bases. The density factor is 1.2

Mould calibration for glycerol-gelatin base is $4.0 \times 1.2 = 4.8$ g

A displacement value is not required because the ichthammol is expressed as a percentage.

Formula for the base:

Gelatin 14 g
Glycerol 70 g
Water to 100 g

Formula for the pessaries:

Ichthammol 10% w/w
Glycerol-gelatin base 90% w/w

The total weight required to prepare the pessaries is 14×4.8 g = 67.2 g. For ease of calculation prepare 70 g. Quantities are therefore:

Ichthammol 7 g
Base 63 g

It is advisable to make a small excess of base, taking care to choose quantities which give easily weighable amounts, i.e. do not try to weigh to several decimal points. In this case 65 g can be prepared.

Using the method described above, prepare 65 g of the base, taking care that the correct type of gelatin is chosen. Because the active ingredient is ichthammol, Type B should be used. When the 65 g of base has been prepared 2 g should be removed from the basin, leaving the required 63 g. The base is removed from the heat, allowed to cool a little before 7 g of ichthammol is added with careful stirring. The mixture is then poured into the lubricated mould and left to set.

CONTAINERS FOR SUPPOSITORIES

Glass or plastic screw-topped jars are possibly the best choice of container for extemporaneously prepared suppositories and pessaries. Cardboard cartons may be used but these offer little protection from moisture or heat. They are therefore not suitable for hygroscopic materials.

SHELF LIFE

Provided they are well packaged and the storage temperature is low, suppositories and pessaries are relatively stable preparations. Unless other information is available, an expiry date of 1 month is appropriate.

LABELLING FOR SUPPOSITORIES

Adequate information should appear on the label so that the patient knows how to use the product. In addition the following information should appear:

'Store in a cool place' and *'For rectal use only'* or *'For vaginal use only'*, whichever is appropriate.

'Do not swallow' can be put on the label but do not use 'For external use only'. The preparation is being inserted into a body cavity and this instruction is therefore incorrect.

PATIENT ADVICE

In addition to what appears on the label, patients should be told to unwrap the suppository or pessary (this may appear to be unnecessary advice but there is sufficient evidence to show that it is not always done) and insert it as high as possible into the rectum or vagina. It may be helpful to provide the patient with a diagram and instruction leaflet, such as that produced by the National Pharmaceutical Association.

When suppositories are for use with children it is likely that an adult will have to carry out the insertion.

Key Points

- Both rectal and vaginal administration can be used for local or systemic drug action.
- Bases may be fatty or water miscible.
- Synthetic bases, made from hydrogenated vegetable oils, are easier to use than theobroma oil.
- Glycerol-gelatin base produces a laxative effect.
- Type A (anionic) or Type B (cationic) gelatin can be used to avoid incompatibilities.
- Macrogol bases are blends of high and low molecular weight polymers which dissolve in rectal contents.
- Suppository moulds have nominal capacities of 1, 2, 4 and 8 g and must be calibrated with the base to be used.
- When using theobroma oil and glycerol-gelatin base the mould has to be lubricated.
- To allow for contraction on cooling, overfilling with oily bases is required.
- Each mould should be calibrated for each base.
- Because glycerol-gelatin base has a higher density than fatty bases, moulds hold approximately 1.2 times the nominal weight.
- The displacement value is the number of parts by weight of drug which displaces one part by weight of base.
- Unless the density of the drug and base are the same, a displacement value is required to calculate the amount of base displaced by the drug.
- Labels should include either 'For rectal use only' or 'For vaginal use only' and 'Store in a cool place'.

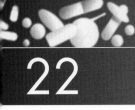

22

Powders and granules

A. J. Winfield (original author E. J. Kennedy)

After studying this chapter you will know about:

The pharmaceutical uses of powders
Bulk and divided powders
The mixing of powders
Diluents used with powders
Calculations required when preparing powders
How to dispense powders
The folding of powders

Introduction

A powder may be defined as a solid material in a finely divided state. Granules are powders agglomerated to produce larger free-flowing particles. Powders and granules can be used to prepare other formulations, such as solutions, suspensions and tablets. A powdered drug on its own can be a dosage form for taking orally (called a simple powder), when they are usually mixed with water first, or for external application as a dusting powder. Alternatively the drug may be blended with other ingredients (called a compound powder).

POWDERS FOR INTERNAL USE

Powders for oral administration will comprise the active ingredients with excipients such as diluents, sweeteners and dispersing agents. These may be presented as undivided powders (bulk powders) or divided powders (individually wrapped doses).

Magnesium Trisilicate Powder, Compound BP (see Example 22.4) and Compound Kaolin Powder BP are examples of bulk powders for internal use. Proprietary powders and granules include Dioralyte, Rehidrat (oral rehydration salts), Normacol (sterculia) and Fybogel

(ispaghula husk). Individually wrapped powders tend not to be official formulae (see Examples 22.1 and 22.2).

Bulk powders

Supplying as an undivided powder is useful for non-potent, bulky drugs with a large dose, e.g. antacids, or when the dry powder is more stable than its liquid-containing counterpart. A bulk powder can be supplied to the patient although this is rarely seen nowadays because the dosage form is inconvenient to carry and there are possible inaccuracies in measuring the dose. Some liquid mixtures may be prepared in the pharmacy from a bulk powder by the addition of a specific volume of water, e.g. Magnesium Trisilicate Mixture BP. This reduces transport and packaging costs.

Individually wrapped powders

Individually wrapped powders are used to supply some potent drugs, where accuracy of dose is important. Extemporaneously produced powders are wrapped separately in paper. They are convenient dosage forms for children's doses of drugs which are not commercially available at the strength required, such as levothyroxine (thyroxine) or ibuprofen (see Example 22.2). Sealed sachets of powders are available commercially, e.g. Paramax (paracetamol and metoclopramide), Stemetil (prochlorperazine) and oral rehydration sachets. They are mixed with water prior to taking and are useful for patients who have difficulty swallowing or where rapid absorption of the drug is required.

Granules for internal use

Some preparations are supplied to the pharmacy as granules, for reconstitution immediately before dispensing, e.g. antibiotic suspensions. This protects drugs which are susceptible to hydrolysis, or other degradation, in the presence of water until the time of dispensing in order to give an adequate shelf life (see Ch. 18).

Particle size

The particle size of a powder is described using standard descriptions given in the *British Pharmacopoeia* (BP). These refer to either the standardized sieve size that they are capable of passing through in a specified time under shaking, or to the microscopically determined particle size. Thus powders for oral use would normally be a 'moderately fine' or a 'fine' powder. The former is able to pass through a sieve of nominal mesh aperture 355 μm and the latter one of 180 μm. Comminution is the process of particle size reduction. On a small scale, this can be achieved using a mortar and pestle when it is often called trituration. This is a common first step in extemporaneous dispensing, after which the powder should be passed through the appropriate sieve before weighing.

Mixing the powder

Ingredients of powders should be mixed thoroughly, using the technique of 'doubling-up' to ensure an even distribution (sometimes called geometric dilution). This process involves starting with the ingredient which has the smallest bulk. In Example 22.1 this is hyoscine hydrobromide. The other ingredient(s) are added progressively in approximately equal parts by volume. In this way the amount in the mortar is approximately doubled at each addition. Mixing in between additions continues until all the ingredients are incorporated. The powder can then be packed.

PREPARING INDIVIDUALLY WRAPPED POWDERS

The minimum weight of an individually wrapped powder is 120 mg. Dilution of a drug with a diluent, usually lactose, is often necessary to produce this weight.

Occasionally manufactured tablets or capsules may be used to prepare oral powders (see Example 22.2). This involves either crushing the tablet in a mortar and pestle, or emptying the contents of the capsule and adding a suitable diluent. Lactose is the most commonly used diluent because it is colourless, odourless, soluble, is generally harmless and has good flow properties. Some patients may be unable to tolerate lactose and a suitable inert alternative diluent, for instance light kaolin, would then be used.

Powder calculations

Quantities should be calculated to allow for loss of powder during manipulation. It is usual to allow for at least one extra powder. If the total amount of active ingredient required is less than the minimum weighable quantity, dilutions will be necessary. In this process, also called trituration, the minimum quantity of the active ingredient(s) is weighed and diluted, over several steps if necessary, in order to obtain the dose(s) required. Example 22.1 illustrates the process where two dilution steps are required (see also Ch. 8).

EXAMPLE 22.1

{R} Hyoscine hydrobromide 300 micrograms Mitte 4 powders
Label 'One to be given 30 minutes before the journey'.

Action and uses. Antimuscarinic drug used in the prevention of motion sickness.

Calculation and method of preparation. Calculate for five powders. Use lactose as the diluent, each powder to weigh 120 mg.

Hyoscine hydrobromide (5 × 300) = 1.5 mg
   (1500 micrograms)
Lactose (5 × 120 mg)   to 600 mg

The minimum weighable quantity (using a Class B balance) is 100 mg.

Step A
Hyoscine hydrobromide   100 mg
Lactose   900 mg

Mix, by doubling-up and remove 100 mg (triturate A).
100 mg of triturate A contains 100/1000 × 100
      = 10 mg hyoscine hydrobromide.

Step B
Triturate A   100 mg
Lactose   900 mg

Mix, by doubling-up and remove 150 mg (triturate B).
150 mg of triturate B contains 10/1000 × 150
      = 1.5 mg hyoscine hydrobromide.

Step C
Triturate B   150 mg
Lactose ((5 × 120 mg) – 150 mg) = 450 mg

Mix, by doubling-up. 120 mg portions of this final powder will contain 300 micrograms of hyoscine hydrobromide. Weigh 120 mg aliquots and wrap in a powder paper.

Folding papers

White glazed paper, called demy paper, is used for wrapping powders. A suitable size is 120 mm × 100 mm. The wrapping should be carried out on a clean tile or larger sheet of demy to protect the product. The papers should be folded with their long edges parallel to the front of the bench. Follow the steps illustrated in Figure 22.1 in order to fold the paper:

- The long edge, furthest away from the dispenser, should be turned over to about one-seventh of the paper width (step A).
- The powder should be weighed accurately and placed on the paper towards the folded edge of the centre of the paper (step B).
- The unfolded long edge (nearest the dispenser) should then be brought over the powder to meet the crease of the folded edge and the flap closed over it (step C).
- The folded edge should then be folded over (towards the dispenser) so that it covers about half the powder packet (step D).
- The short edges of the powder packet should be folded over, using a powder cradle if available, so that the flaps are of equal lengths and the folded powder fits neatly into

a box or jar (step E and F). Before making these folds, ensure that there is no powder in the ends to be folded, otherwise it may fall out and be lost.

The creases can be sharpened with a spatula, taking care not to tear the paper or use excessive pressure which would compress the powder inside the pack.

The powders can be packed in pairs, back to back, or in one bundle, with the final powder placed back to back. They should be held together with an elastic band. In a well-wrapped product, there will be no powder in the fold or flaps, so that all the powder is available for easy administration when unwrapped.

Manufactured powders are subject to a uniformity of weight test, or uniformity of content test if each dose contains less than 2 mg of active ingredient or the content of active ingredient represents less than 2% of the total weight.

Shelf life and storage of internal powders

Extemporaneously prepared powders should have an expiry of between 2 and 4 weeks. Proprietary powders often have a longer shelf life because of the protective packaging. Some powders may be hygroscopic, deliquescent or volatile and will need to be protected from decomposition. Storage for these powders should be moisture proof and airtight.

Containers for internal powders

Extemporaneously prepared individually wrapped powders are often dispensed in a paperboard box. However, it is preferable to use a screw-top glass or plastic container which provides an airtight seal and protection against moisture. Proprietary powders in individual sachets, which are moisture proof, may be dispensed in a paperboard box. Bulk powders are packed in an airtight glass or plastic jar. A 5 mL spoon should also be supplied.

Special labels and advice for internal powders

Powders are usually mixed with water or another suitable liquid before taking, depending on their solubility. Powders for babies or young children can be placed directly into the mouth on the back of the tongue, followed by a drink to wash down the powder. Bulk powders should be shaken and measured carefully before dissolving or dispersing in a little water and taking.

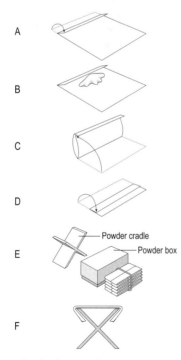

Fig. 22.1 Steps for the folding of individually wrapped powders.

POWDERS FOR EXTERNAL USE

Powders, with or without medicament, are frequently applied to the skin. Dusting powders contain one or more substances in fine powder and may be dispensed as single dose or multi-dose preparations (see Example 22.3). They are used to treat a variety of skin conditions or to soothe skin. Examples are antifungal powders for athlete's foot or talc dusting powder for the prevention of chafing and skin irritation. Zinc oxide and starch are added to formulations to absorb moisture and talc is used for lubricant properties. Talc, kaolin and other natural mineral materials are liable to contamination with bacteria such as *Clostridium tetani*, *C. perfringens* and *Bacillus anthracis*. These ingredients should be sterilized by dry heat or the final product should be sterilized. Dusting powders should be sterile if they may be applied to large areas of open skin or wounds. They should not be used where there is a likelihood of large volumes of exudate, as hard crusts will form.

Preparing powders for external use

A sieve size of 180 μm should be used to obtain the finely divided powder. The constituents should be mixed using the doubling-up method, as described previously.

Shelf life and storage for powders for external use

Dry powders should remain stable over a long period of time if packaged and protected from the atmosphere. For extemporaneously prepared products, an expiry of 4 weeks is appropriate.

Containers for powders for external use

Powders for external use may be packed in glass, metal or plastic containers with a sifter-type cap. Some are also available commercially in pressurized containers, containing other excipients such as a propellant and lubricants.

Special labels and advice for powders for external use

'For external use only' and 'Store in a cool, dry place'.

Examples of official powders for external use include Zinc Oxide Dusting Powder Compound BPC, Chlorhexidine Dusting Powder BP and Talc Dusting Powder BP. Proprietary examples of powders for external use include

Daktarin (miconazole), Cicatrin (neomycin sulphate, bacitracin zinc, cysteine, glycine and threonine) and Ster-zac powder (hexachlorophene, zinc oxide, talc and starch).

EXAMPLE 22.2

Send 18 ibuprofen powders for a child of 3 years to provide 20 mg/kg daily. Take 1 twice daily (child's weight is 14 kg).
 The dose required = 20 × 14 = 280 mg daily. Therefore each powder to contain 140 mg.

	For 1 powder	For 20 powders (2 excess)
Ibuprofen	140 mg	2.8 g

Action and uses. Non-steroidal anti-inflammatory drug, used to treat juvenile arthritis at a dose of up to 40 mg/kg daily.

Formulation notes. A diluent is not required, since the weight of each powder will be above the minimum 120 mg required. Pure ibuprofen powder can be used. However if it is not available, manufactured 200 μg ibuprofen tablets (not modified release) can be used to prepare these powders.

Method of preparation. Take 14 × 200 mg ibuprofen tablets (contain 2.8 g ibuprofen) and weigh them. This is necessary to allow for the weight of the tablet excipients. Grind to a fine powder in a mortar and pestle. Pass the resulting powder through a 250 μm sieve and lightly remix. Divide the original weight of tablets by 20, and weigh aliquots of the resulting amount of powder. Pack into individual powder papers. Fasten the 18 powders together with an elastic band and pack in an amber glass jar or plastic container with a screw cap.

Shelf life and storage. Store in a cool, dry place. A shelf life of 2–3 weeks is appropriate.

Advice and special labels. The powders should be given after food, in water (or directly into the child's mouth, followed by a drink of water).

EXAMPLE 22.3

℞ Zinc, Starch and Talc Dusting Powder BPC. Mitte 100 g.

	Master formula	For 100 g
Zinc oxide	25%	25 g
Starch	25%	25 g
Sterilized purified talc	50%	50 g

Action and uses. A soothing preparation to absorb moisture and act as a lubricant, preventing friction in skin folds.

Method of preparation. Sieve the powders, using a 180 μm sieve, weigh and mix them by doubling-up in a mortar and pestle. Pack in an amber glass jar or plastic container with a screw cap (with a perforated, reclosable lid if possible).

Shelf life and storage. Store in a dry place. An expiry date of 4 weeks is advisable.

Advice and special labels. 'For external use only'. Lightly dust the powder onto the affected area. The area should not be too wet as the powder will cake and abrade the skin. It should not be applied to broken skin or large raw areas.

EXAMPLE 22.4

{℞} Compound Magnesium Trisilicate Oral Powder BP 1988. Mitte 200 g.

	Master formula	For 200 g
Magnesium trisilicate	250 mg	50 g
Chalk	250 mg	50 g
Heavy magnesium carbonate	250 mg	50 g
Sodium bicarbonate	250 mg	50 g

Action and uses. Antacid preparation for dyspepsia.

Method of preparation. Sieve the powders, using a 250 μm sieve, weigh and mix them by doubling-up, using a mortar and pestle. Pack in an amber glass jar or plastic container with a screw cap.

Shelf life and storage. Store in a dry place. A 4-week expiry date is reasonable if kept dry.

Advice and special labels. 'Dissolve or mix with water before taking' (BNF Label 13). A normal dose is 1–5 g of the powder taken in liquid, when required. Antacids are usually taken between meals and at bedtime.

Key Points

- Powders may be prepared as bulk powders, divided powders or granules.
- Powders may be used internally or externally.
- The particle size of a fine powder should be less than 180 μm.
- The minimum weight of a divided powder is 120 mg.
- Lactose is a good diluent for internal powders.
- Trituration is the process used to obtain small doses which are below the minimum weighable quantity.
- Ideally powders should be packed in a glass or plastic container.
- A 5 mL spoon should be provided with bulk powders for oral use.
- When dispensing divided powders, an excess of one or two should be prepared to allow for losses during processing.

Oral unit dosage forms

A. J. Winfield (original author E. J. Kennedy)

After studying this chapter you will know about:

Different types of tablets
Excipients used in tablets and capsules
Dispensing commercially produced tablets and capsules
Extemporaneous dispensing of capsules and cachets

Introduction

Tablets and capsules are the most popular way of delivering a drug for oral use. They are convenient for the patient and are usually easy to handle and identify. They are mass produced on a commercial scale at a relatively low manufacturing cost. Because they are manufactured by the pharmaceutical industry where quality assurance is in place, a high accuracy of dosage is achievable with oral unit dosage forms and they are free from the problems of stability found in aqueous mixtures and suspensions. Packaging in blister packs can also enhance the stability of these dosage forms (see Ch. 9). Their main disadvantages are that there is a slower onset of action relative to liquids and some people have difficulty swallowing solid oral dosage forms, e.g. the very young or very old.

TABLETS

Tablets are solid preparations each containing a single dose of one or more active ingredient(s). They are normally prepared by compressing uniform volumes of particles, although some tablets are prepared by moulding. The process of tablet production is outside the scope of this book, but can be found in Aulton (2002) or the *Pharmaceutical Codex*.

Many different types of tablet are available, which may also be in a variety of shapes and sizes. The types include dispersible or effervescent, chewable, sublingual and buccal tablets, lozenges, tablets for rectal or vaginal administration and solution tablets. Some tablets are designed to release the drug after a time lag, or slowly for a prolonged drug release or sustained drug action (see Ch. 16). The design of these modified-release tablets uses formulation techniques to control the biopharmaceutical behaviour of the drug. These issues are discussed in Aulton (2002).

In addition to the drug(s), several excipients must be added. These will aid the process of tableting and ensure that the active ingredient will be released as intended. Excipients include:

- *Diluents*. These add bulk to make the tablet easier to handle. Examples include lactose, mannitol, sorbitol and calcium carbonate.
- *Binders*. These enable granules to be prepared which improves flow properties of the mixture during manufacture. Examples include acacia mucilage, polyvinylpyrrolidone and microcrystalline cellulose.
- *Disintegrants*. These encourage the tablet to break into smaller particles after ingestion. Examples include modified cellulose and modified starch.
- *Lubricants, glidants, antiadherents*. These are essential for flow of the tablet material into the tablet dies and preventing sticking of the compressed tablet in the punch and die. Examples of lubricants are magnesium and calcium stearate, sodium lauryl sulphate and sodium stearyl fumarate. Colloidal silica is usually the glidant of choice. Talc and magnesium stearate are effective antiadherents.
- *Miscellaneous agents* may be added, such as colours and flavours in chewable tablets.

Some tablets have coatings, such as sugar coating or film coating. Coatings can protect the tablet from environmental damage, mask an unpleasant flavour, aid identification of the tablet and enhance its appearance. Enteric coatings on tablets resist dissolution or disruption of the tablet in the stomach, but not in the intestine. This is useful when a drug is destroyed by gastric acid, is irritating to the gastric mucosa, or when bypassing the stomach aids drug absorption. See Aulton (2002) for details about coatings and other specialized formulation and manufacturing techniques.

Dispensing of tablets

The majority of tablets in the UK are packaged by the manufacturer into patient packs suitable for issue to the patient without repacking by the pharmacist. Patient information leaflets are also contained in these patient packs. When dispensing these packs to patients, the pharmacist must ensure that they are labelled correctly, according to the prescriber's instructions (see Ch. 11) and that the patient is counselled on the use of the medication (see Ch. 38). For some controlled-release tablets, variations in bioavailability may occur with different brands. It is important that patients are given the brand that they are stabilized on to maintain therapeutic outcome. Examples where this is important include theophylline, lithium and phenytoin.

Tablets are also supplied in a bulk container. The required number of tablets needs to be counted out (see Ch. 7) and placed in a suitable container for dispensing to the patient (see Ch. 9). It is important to minimize errors by ensuring that the correct bulk container has been selected and the correct drug dispensed. The pharmacist should verify this by checking the label of the bulk container and by examining the shape, size and markings on the dispensed tablets where appropriate, with the prescription.

Some tablets are supplied in a strip-packed form where each tablet has its own blister. A development of this is the calendar pack where the day or date on which the tablet is to be taken is indicated on the pack.

Shelf life and storage

Most tablets should be stored in airtight packaging, protected from light and extremes of temperature. When stored properly they generally have a long shelf life. The expiry date will be printed on the package or the individual strip packs. Some tablets need to be stored in a cool place, e.g. Ketovite and Leukeran (chlorambucil) (store between 2 and 8°C). Some tablets contain volatile drugs, e.g. glyceryl trinitrate, and must be packed in glass containers with tightly fitting metal screw caps (see Ch. 10). An additional warning must be placed on these tablets, when dispensed to patients, to advise them to throw away the tablets 8 weeks after opening, as they lose potency.

Containers

Strip or blister packs are dispensed in a paperboard box and tablets counted from bulk containers are placed in amber glass or plastic containers with airtight, child-resistant closures.

Special labels and advice on tablets

Most tablets should be swallowed with a glass or 'draught' of water. A draught of water refers to a volume of water of about 50 mL. This prevents the dosage form becoming lodged in the oesophagus, which can cause problems such as ulceration. Tablets may be coated and shaped to aid swallowing.

Some tablets should be dissolved or dispersed in water before taking, e.g. effervescent analgesic tablets. Other tablets, particularly those with coatings or modified-release properties, should be swallowed whole. There are also some tablets which should be chewed or sucked before swallowing, e.g. antacid tablets. Appropriate labels should be placed on the container (see Ch. 10).

Coated tablets, e.g. enteric coatings, require specific advice on avoiding indigestion remedies at the same time of day, as these will affect the pH of the stomach, and therefore cause premature breakdown of the enteric coating on the tablet.

Buccal and sublingual tablets are not swallowed whole and it is important that patients know how to use them. If these formulations are swallowed then they will not have their intended therapeutic effect. Figure 23.1 illustrates the positioning for buccal tablets. Sublingual tablets are placed under the tongue.

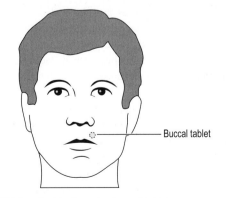

Fig. 23.1   Positioning of a buccal tablet.

CAPSULES

Capsules are solid preparations intended for oral administration made with a hard or soft gelatin shell. One (or more) medicament is enclosed within this gelatin container. Most capsules are swallowed whole, but some contain granules which provide a useful premeasured dose for administering in a similar way to a powder, e.g. formulations of pancreatin. Some capsules enclose enteric-coated pellets, e.g. Erymax (erythromycin). Capsules are elegant, easy to swallow and can be useful in masking unpleasant tastes. Capsules may also be used to hold powder or oils for inhalation, e.g. Intal capsules (sodium cromoglicate) or Karvol (see Ch. 24), or for rectal and vaginal administration (see Ch. 21).

Soft shell capsules

A soft gelatin capsule consists of a flexible solid shell containing powders, non-aqueous liquids, solutions, emulsions, suspensions or pastes. Such capsules allow liquids to be given as solid dosage forms, e.g. cod liver oil. They also offer accurate dosage, improved stability and overcome some of the problems of dealing with powders. They are formed, filled and sealed in one manufacturing process.

Hard shell capsules

Empty capsule shells are made from gelatin and are clear, colourless and essentially tasteless. Colourings and markings can be easily added for light protection and easy identification. The shells are used in the preparation of most manufactured capsules and for the extemporaneous compounding of capsules. The shell comprises two sections, the body and the cap, both being cylindrical and sealed at one end. Powder or particulate solid, such as granules and pellets, can be placed in the body and the capsule closed by bringing the body and cap together (Fig. 23.2). Some capsules have small indentations on the body and cap which 'lock' together. If not, they must be sealed by moistening the outside top of the

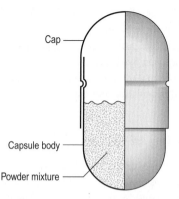

Fig. 23.2 Hard gelatin capsule shell: body and cap.

body before putting the top in place. Technical aspects of capsule manufacture are given in Aulton (2002).

Compounding of capsules

Occasionally hand filling of capsules may be required, particularly in a hospital pharmacy or when preparing materials for clinical trials. A suitable size of capsule shell should be selected so that the finished capsule looks reasonably full. Hard shell capsules are available in eight sizes. These are listed in Table 23.1, with the corresponding approximate capacity (based on lactose). The bulk density of a powder mixture will also affect the choice of capsule size.

Calculations for compounding capsules

The recommended minimum weight for filling a capsule is 100 mg. If the required weight of the drug is smaller than this a diluent should be added by trituration (see Ch. 22). If the quantity of the drug for a batch of capsules is smaller than the minimum weighable amount, 100 mg on a Class B balance, then trituration will also be required. Lactose, magnesium carbonate, starch, kaolin and calcium phosphate are commonly used diluents. To allow for small losses of powder, a small excess should be calculated for, e.g. two extra capsules. Example 23.1 gives a worked example.

Table 23.1	Sizes of hard gelatin capsules and their approximate capacities							
				Capsule no.				
	000	**00**	**0**	**1**	**2**	**3**	**4**	**5**
Content (mg)	950	650	450	300	250	200	150	100

EXAMPLE 23.1

{℞} Caps atropine sulphate 600 micrograms. Mitte 4. Calculate for six capsules.

Atropine sulphate (6 × 600)	3.6 mg (3600 micrograms)
Lactose (6 × 100 mg)	to 600 mg

Step A

Atropine sulphate	100 mg
Lactose	900 mg

Mix, by doubling-up, in a small mortar and pestle. Weigh 100 mg of this mixture (triturate A). Triturate A contains 10 mg of atropine sulphate.

Step B

Triturate A	100 mg
Lactose	900 mg

Mix, by doubling-up, in a small mortar and pestle. Weigh 360 mg of this mixture (triturate B) which contains 3.6 mg of atropine sulphate.

Step C

Add sufficient lactose to triturate B to make the final weight up to 600 mg.
The powder mixture is now ready to be placed into capsules.

Filling capsules

The number of capsules to be filled should first be taken and set aside. This avoids the danger of contaminating empty capsules. The powder to be encapsulated should be finely sifted (180 μm sieve) and prepared. Magnesium stearate (up to 1% w/w) and silica may be added as a lubricant and glidant respectively, to aid filling of the capsule. Various methods of filling capsules on a small scale are possible.

Filling from a powder mass

The prepared powder can be placed on a clean tile or piece of demy paper and powder pushed into the capsule body with the aid of a spatula until the required weight has been enclosed. The empty capsule body could also be 'punched' into a heap of powder until filled. Alternatively create a small funnel from demy paper and fill the capsule body with the required weight. Gloves or rubber finger cots should be worn to protect the capsules from handling with bare fingers.

Filling with weighed aliquots

Weighed aliquots of powder may be placed on paper and channelled into the empty capsule shell. A sharp fold in the paper helps direct the powder. Alternatively, simple apparatus is useful for small-scale manufacture of larger numbers of capsules. A plastic plate with rows of cavities to hold the empty capsule bodies is used, different rows holding different sizes of capsules. A plastic bridge containing a row of holes corresponding to the position of the capsule cavities can then be used to support a long-stemmed funnel. The end of the funnel passes into the mouth of the capsule below. The stem of the funnel should be as wide as possible for the size of the capsule. A weighed aliquot of powder can then be poured into the capsule via the funnel. A thin glass or plastic rod or wire may be used to 'tamp' the powder to break blockages or to lightly compress the material inside the capsule. After filling the capsule, the top can be fitted loosely and the weight checked before sealing.

Capsules are subject to tests for uniformity of weight and content of active ingredient and uniformity of content where the content of active ingredient is less than 2 mg or less than 2% by weight of the total capsule fill.

Shelf life and storage

If stability data are not available for extemporaneously filled capsules, then a short expiry date, up to 4 weeks, should be given. Manufactured capsules will generally be very stable and will be assigned expiry dates on the container or on the packed strips or blister packs. Most capsules need to be stored in a cool, dry place. Some capsules need to be stored in a cool place, e.g. Restandol (testosterone), which needs to be stored in the refrigerator at 2–8°C until it is dispensed to the patient, when it can be stored at room temperature for 3 months.

Containers

Containers used are similar to those for tablets. Some capsules are susceptible to moisture absorption, and desiccants may be included in the packaging, either integrally (e.g. in the cap of the container for Losec capsules) or as separate sachets. These capsules have a limited shelf life once dispensed to a patient. Desiccant sachets should not be dispensed to patients, in case they are mistaken for a capsule and ingested.

Special labels and advice on capsules

Capsules should be swallowed whole with a glass of water or other liquid. Advice may be sought from the pharmacist about whether it is acceptable to empty the contents of a capsule onto food or into water for ease of swallowing. In giving this advice, the release characteristics of the dosage form should be considered; for instance, whether it is an enteric-coated or prolonged-release formulation. Additional labels and advice may be required for capsules, depending on the drug contained.

OTHER ORAL UNIT DOSAGE FORMS

Pastilles

These contain a glycerol and gelatin base. They are sweetened, flavoured and medicated and are popular over-the-counter remedies for soothing coughs and sore throats.

Cachets

These are very rarely used in practice today. They are made from rice flour and each cachet comes in two halves ready to be filled with powder. They are available as dry seal or wet seal. They are dipped in water then swallowed whole with water and prevent the patient from tasting the powder. Filled cachets are packed in cardboard boxes.

EXAMPLE 23.2

{℞} Droperidol 10 mg capsules, with 1% w/w magnesium stearate. Mitte 8 caps.

	For 1 capsule	For 10 capsules
Droperidol	10 mg	100 mg
Magnesium stearate	1 mg	10 mg
Lactose	89 mg	890 mg

Action and uses. Antipsychotic drug, used for tranquillization and control in mania.

Formulation notes. Magnesium stearate is added to act as a lubricant to aid flow of the powder into the capsule. 10 mg is not weighable, so a trituration must be carried out. Lactose acts as a diluent to bring the weight of each capsule fill to 100 mg.

Trituration for magnesium stearate
Magnesium stearate	100 mg
Lactose	900 mg

Take a 100 mg portion of this mixture, which will contain 10 mg of magnesium stearate and 90 mg of lactose.

Method of preparation. Sieve the powders using a 180 μm sieve. Prepare the magnesium stearate triturate. Weigh 100 mg of droperidol, and mix this with the magnesium stearate triturate in a mortar and pestle. Gradually add 800 mg of lactose to this mixture, by doubling-up. This gives a total powder quantity of 1000 mg (equivalent to 10 × 100 mg capsules). Fill the capsule shells (size 4 or 5) with 100 mg aliquots, checking the weight of each capsule before sealing. Pack eight capsules in an amber glass or plastic tablet container with a child-resistant closure.

Storage and shelf life. Store in a cool dry place and protect from light. Expiry date of 2 weeks, since stability in capsule form is unknown.

Advice and labelling. 'Warning. May cause drowsiness. If affected do not drive or operate machinery. Avoid alcoholic drink' (BNF Label 2).

Key Points

- Tablets and capsules are the most common dosage forms.
- Excipients are added to improve manufacture, handling and release of the drug.
- Bioavailability of some tablets may vary between manufacturers.
- Checking of labels and contents of bulk containers is essential in minimizing errors.
- Tablets should be swallowed with about 50 ml of water.
- Ensure that the patient knows how to take the tablet—chew, dissolve, swallow whole, buccal or sublingual.
- Indigestion remedies should be avoided with enteric-coated tablets and capsules.
- Tablets cannot be made extemporaneously, but capsules are filled, especially in hospitals and when preparing for clinical trials.
- Capsule size is selected so that they look reasonably full.
- The minimum weight of contents in an extemporaneous capsule is 100 mg.
- Manufactured tablets and capsules are subject to uniformity of weight and drug content tests.
- Medicated glycerol-gelatin based pastilles are popular for coughs and sore throats.
- Rice flour cachets are little used today.

Inhaled route

P. M. Richards

After studying this chapter you will know about:

The rationale for using the inhaled route
The condition for which the inhaled route is most frequently used—asthma
The appropriate use of the most widely prescribed inhaled medicines
The key role of the peak flow meter in the management of asthma
The different types of inhaler, and inhaler technique
Nebulized therapy

Introduction

Inhaled products are specialized dosage forms, which are designed to deliver medicines directly to the lung. A variety of inhaler devices are in use, all of which require the user of the inhaler to adopt an appropriate inhaler technique. Failure to use the correct inhaler technique will result in treatment failure. The pharmacist, who is usually the person who gives (dispenses) the inhaler to the patient, is clearly ideally placed to demonstrate the appropriate inhalation technique for that inhaler. Using an inhaler is a skill subject to the development of 'bad habits' which can lead to poor technique. Inhaler technique should therefore be regularly checked to ensure that the technique is optimal; again the pharmacist is ideally placed to perform this function. This chapter describes the most frequently prescribed inhaler devices and outlines how to use them correctly.

Many patients on inhaled therapy will be using more than one inhaler and may also have been prescribed a peak flow meter to aid them in monitoring their condition. In order for pharmacists to be able to provide useful education and advice to these patients they will need to understand the condition being treated and the role of the medicines and devices prescribed. This chapter will provide that understanding in the context of asthma and its treatment because by far the widest use of inhaler therapy is in the treatment of asthma. Pharmacists can also be assured that the advice that they give patients is likely to be consistent with that given by other health care professionals, as there are national treatment guidelines for asthma, part of which is reproduced in this chapter, and are widely available e.g. in the British National Formulary (BNF).

Asthma is a very common condition in the UK, affecting at least 5% of adults and up to 20% of children. It is therefore likely that 1 in 5 of the population will experience symptoms attributable to asthma at some time in their life.

The prevalence of asthma and related conditions mean that pharmacists will not only frequently be encountering patients on inhaled therapy during dispensing, but will also encounter patients on inhaled therapy when giving advice on the sale of over-the-counter medicines. This chapter not only provides pharmacists with the knowledge to deal confidently with patients on inhaled therapy but also to be able to spot symptoms that may be associated with poorly controlled or undiagnosed asthma and symptoms that may be due to unwanted effects of inhaled medicines.

Some pharmacists choose to take a more pro-active role in dealing with patients on inhaled therapy. A multidisciplinary approach is likely to be of most benefit to the patient. The pharmacist may then receive requests from the doctor, e.g. to check or demonstrate inhaler technique, and likewise be able to refer patients to a nurse-run asthma clinic or to the doctor. For agreed asthmatics the pharmacist may also be able to perform a review of inhaler technique, peak expiratory flow and asthma control to re-authorize a repeat prescription. Consistency of patient education and information can also be achieved by the multidisciplinary approach. This multidisciplinary approach is facilitated by asthmatics having a written asthma self-management plan.

There are a number of pharmacist-run asthma clinics in general practitioners' surgeries. This number is likely to increase due to government proposals to allow supplementary prescribing by pharmacists by 2003. Pharmacist supplementary prescribing is thought to be of most value for patients with specific non-acute medical conditions such as asthma.

Pharmacists wishing to become involved in asthma management require a range of skills in addition to knowledge. A course such as that run by the National Respiratory Training Centre (Warwick) provides a good grounding for pharmacists (and doctors and nurses) who run asthma clinics.

THE INHALED ROUTE

The inhaled route delivers medicines to the lungs. Inhaled medicines may have a local effect on the lungs, or may be absorbed to give a systemic effect. The inhaled route is generally used when the lung is the target organ, e.g.:

- The antibiotic colistin is nebulized to treat lung infections associated with cystic fibrosis.
- The antiviral zanamivir is presented as a dry-powder inhaler for treating influenza.

Using the inhaled route when the lung is the target organ has a number of advantages:

- A smaller dose can be used. The normal adult oral dose of salbutamol is 4 mg, the normal inhaled dose of salbutamol is 200 micrograms (0.2 mg).
- The risk of unwanted systemic effects is reduced.
- A faster onset of action may be achieved with some drugs, e.g. salbutamol.
- Topically active drugs with poor oral bioavailability can be used.

The main disadvantage of the inhaled route is that inhaling a drug is more difficult than swallowing a tablet. Also some drugs are ineffective by the inhaled route, e.g. theophylline.

Using the inhaled route does not result in all the drug reaching the lung. Even if an inhaler device is used perfectly it is unlikely that any more than 20% of the drug reaches the lung. The majority of the rest of the drug remains in the oropharynx and is normally swallowed.

The lungs are designed to prevent the inhalation of anything other than gas. However particles with a diameter of approximately 5 μm can be inhaled and have sufficient mass to settle in the lung. Particles larger than 10 μm remain in

the oropharynx. Particles smaller than 1 μm are inhaled, but are then exhaled. Decreasing particle size increases the chance of penetration further down the tracheobronchial tree. It may be that a particle needs to be less than 3 μm to reach the 8th to 23rd branch generation.

For inhaled steroids, reaching the entire lung may be of benefit, as the inflammatory process in asthma is thought to be present throughout the lung. Beta$_2$ agonists however will only exert their bronchodilatory effects in those areas of the lung that contain smooth muscle.

Medicines to be inhaled are presented as:

- Aerosol inhalers
- Dry-powder inhalers
- Liquids to be nebulized.

Inhaled therapy is most commonly used in asthma and chronic obstructive pulmonary disease (COPD). In this chapter inhaled therapy is dealt with primarily in the context of treating asthma.

ASTHMA

Asthma can be defined as generalized airways obstruction that is reversible, either spontaneously over time, or on treatment. It is an inflammatory condition. This causes airways obstruction, through swelling of the walls of airways and increased mucus production. Inflammation also causes hyperresponsiveness of the smooth muscle of the airways resulting in airways obstruction due to bronchospasm (see also Walker and Edwards 2003). Airways obstruction in asthma is illustrated in Figure 24.1.

Symptoms

The symptoms of asthma include breathlessness, cough, wheeze and chest tightness. In asthmatics the normal diurnal (circadian) variation in lung function is often increased resulting in symptoms at night, causing nocturnal and early morning waking.

Trigger factors

Asthma symptoms can be triggered by numerous factors including exercise, cold air, allergens, smoke, emotion, stress, anxiety and the common cold. COPD produces symptoms similar to asthma but is a generalized airways obstruction or restriction that is predominantly irreversible. COPD includes conditions such as emphysema and chronic

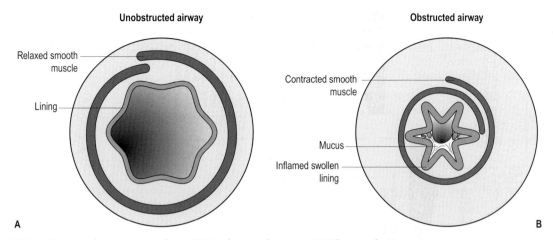

Fig. 24.1 Airways obstruction in asthma. (**A**) Unobstructed airway. (**B**) Obstructed airway.

bronchitis. Smoking is almost always the sole cause of COPD. COPD often presents in combination with asthma, resulting in airways obstruction which is partly reversible.

The British Thoracic Society publishes guidelines on COPD management.

It should be remembered that cancer, inhaled foreign body and congenital malformation of the bronchus can all cause localized airways obstruction, causing symptoms similar to COPD and asthma. Heart failure also causes shortness of breath. The lungs become congested due to back pressure of blood caused by the inadequate pumping of the heart. Shortness of breath due to heart failure was formerly known as cardiac asthma.

ASTHMA TREATMENT GUIDELINES

The British Thoracic Society (BTS) first published British guidelines on asthma management in 1990. The latest revision of the guidelines was published in 1997. The guidelines cover both chronic and acute severe asthma. The BNF contains a summary of the guidelines. Figure 24.2 is a chart outlining the management of chronic asthma reproduced from the BTS guidelines. Local asthma management guidelines exist in some areas. Individual GP practices may have treatment guidelines as part of their practice formulary.

Asthma management is based on a stepwise approach to treatment. Treatment should be started at the step most likely to achieve control of symptoms. If control of symptoms is not achieved then treatment should be stepped up. However treatment should not be stepped up until inhaler technique and compliance with treatment has been checked.

The most common reasons for poor control of asthma are:

- Incorrect technique in using inhaler(s)
- Lack of understanding of the role of different inhalers leading to inappropriate use
- Not using inhaled steroid because of lack of perceived benefit or fear of side-effects.

Once control of asthma is achieved and maintained for 3–6 months, treatment may be stepped down.

The treatment of asthma is primarily via the inhaled route, but it should be remembered that oral therapy is sometimes appropriate (Fig. 24.2). The most important oral treatment is the use of oral steroids. A short course of oral steroids can be life saving when prescribed for severe acute asthma. A typical short course of oral steroids is 30–60 mg of prednisolone daily, taken as a single dose in the morning for 2 weeks, then stopped. Inhaled steroids should be continued (or started) and used concomitantly with oral steroids so that the prophylactic cover provided by the inhaled steroids is in place when the oral steroids are stopped. Asthma control should be actively monitored during a course of oral steroids and for several weeks afterwards.

GOALS OF ASTHMA MANAGEMENT

- To recognize asthma
- To abolish symptoms
- To restore/maintain normal lung function
- To enable normal school/work attendance and participation in sports/social/leisure activities.

Management of chronic asthma in adults and schoolchildren

- Avoidance of provoking factors where possible
- Patient's involvement and education
- Selection of best inhaler device
- Treatment stepped up as necessary to achieve good control
- Treatment stepped down if control of asthma good

Notes

- Patients should start treatment at the step most appropriate to the initial severity. A rescue course of prednisolone may be needed at any time and at any step. The aim is to achieve early control of the condition and then to reduce treatment.
- Until growth is complete any child requiring beclomethasone or budesonide > 800 µg daily or fluticasone > 500 µg daily should be referred to a paediatrician with an interest in asthma.

Prescribe a peak flow meter and monitor response to treatment

Stepping down:

Review treatment every three to six months. If control is achieved a stepwise reduction in treatment may be possible. In patients whose treatment was recently started at step 4 or 5 or included steroid tablets for gaining control of asthma this reduction may take place after a short interval. In other patients with chronic asthma a three to six month period of stability should be shown before slow stepwise reduction is undertaken.

Step 1:

Occasional use of relief bronchodilators

Inhaled short acting β agonists "as required" for symptom relief are acceptable. If they are needed more than once daily move to step 2. Before altering a treatment step ensure that the patient is having the treatment and has a good inhaler technique. Address any fears.

Step 2:

Regular inhaled anti-inflammatory agents

Inhaled short acting β agonists as required
plus
beclomethasone or budesonide 100–400 µg twice daily or fluticasone 50–200 µg twice daily. Alternatively, use cromoglycate or nedocromil sodium, but if control is not achieved start inhaled steroids

Step 3:

High dose inhaled steroids or low dose inhaled steroids plus long acting inhaled β agonist bronchodilator

Inhaled short acting β agonists as required
plus either
beclomethasone or budesonide increased to 800–2000 µg daily or fluticasone 400–1000 µg daily via a large volume spacer
or
beclomethasone or budesonide 100–400 µg twice daily or fluticasone 50–200 µg twice daily plus salmeterol 50 µg twice daily. In a very small number of patients who experience side effects with high dose inhaled steroids, either the long acting inhaled β agonist option is used or a sustained release theophylline may be added to step 2 medication. Cromoglycate or nedocromil may also be tried.

Step 4:

High dose inhaled steroids and regular bronchodilators

Inhaled short acting β agonists as required with inhaled beclomethasone or budesonide 800–2000 µg daily or fluticasone 400–1000 µg daily via a large volume spacer
plus
a sequential therapeutic trial of one or more of
- inhaled long acting β agonists
- sustained release theophylline
- inhaled ipratropium or oxitropium
- long acting β agonist tablets
- high dose inhaled bronchodilators
- cromoglycate or nedocromil.

Step 5:

Addition of regular steroid tablets

Inhaled short acting β agonists as required with inhaled beclomethasone or budesonide 800–2000 µg daily or fluticasone 400–1000 µg daily via a large volume spacer and one or more of the long acting bronchodilators
plus
regular prednisolone tablets in a single daily dose

Outcome of steps 1–3: control of asthma

- Minimal (ideally no) chronic symptoms, including nocturnal symptoms
- Minimal (infrequent) exacerbations
- Minimal need for relieving bronchodilators
- No limitations on activities including exercise
- Circadian variation in peak expiratory flow (PEF) < 20%
- PEF ≥ 80% of predicted or best
- Minimal (or no) adverse effects from medicine

Outcome of steps 4–5: best possible results

- Least possible symptoms
- Least possible need for relieving bronchodilators
- Least possible limitation of activity
- Least possible variation in PEF
- Best PEF
- Least adverse effects from medicine

NATIONAL ASTHMA CAMPAIGN
improving asthma

Working for Healthier Lungs

in association with the General Practitioner in Asthma Group, the British Association of Accident and Emergency Medicine, the British Paediatric Respiratory Society and the Royal College of Paediatrics and Child Health

Adapted from poster designed by Business Design Group

Fig. 24.2 Management of chronic asthma in adults and schoolchildren. (From British Thoracic Society 1997.)

Inhaled bronchodilators

Short-acting beta$_2$ agonists

Salbutamol and terbutaline are the most widely used inhaled bronchodilators. They should be used 'as required', and are often referred to as 'relievers'. If a reliever inhaler is required more than once or twice a day most days then an additional 'preventer' (usually a steroid) inhaler is required.

When talking to asthmatics about their reliever inhaler the following points should be remembered:

- The inhaler itself is not dangerous—but asthma is potentially fatal.
- Appropriate, 'as required' use of a reliever inhaler provides a useful marker of the severity of the condition.
- Frequent usage of a reliever inhaler may indicate severe uncontrolled asthma.
- There is no risk that using the reliever inhaler whenever needed will result in a diminishing response, but worsening asthma will not respond to a reliever inhaler alone—additional treatment is required.
- If the reliever inhaler is not relieving symptoms, urgent medical attention is required.
- If reliever inhaler usage has increased, or is being used more than once or twice a day most days, a review of treatment is required.
- The reliever inhaler can be used 15–20 minutes before sport/exercise to prevent exercise-induced asthma in susceptible individuals.
- A reliever inhaler is normally blue.

Unwanted effects of inhaled beta$_2$ agonists are rare but tremor can occur.

Long-acting (regular) beta$_2$ agonists

Salmeterol and formoterol are long-acting bronchodilators. They are normally used twice daily, and are indicated for asthmatics who are symptomatic despite adequate doses of inhaled steroids. Formoterol is also licensed for once-daily use. These inhalers are often referred to as 'protectors'.

When talking to asthmatics about their protector inhaler the following points should be remembered:

- Protector inhalers should be used regularly and not on an 'as required' basis.
- A reliever inhaler (short-acting beta$_2$ agonist) should be used to relieve break-through symptoms.
- Inhaled steroids (preventer inhalers) should be continued.

- Inhalers containing a combination of a long-acting beta$_2$ agonist and an inhaled steroid are available.

Antimuscarinics (anticholinergics)

Ipratropium and oxitropium are used as regular bronchodilators. Ipratropium requires four times daily administration, oxitropium can be used twice daily. These drugs are more commonly used in patients with COPD than in asthmatics.

Inhaled steroids

The powerful anti-inflammatory actions of steroids ideally suit them to control the inflammatory processes in asthma.

The inhaled route allows small doses of steroid to be used, minimizing the risk of systemic effects. The ideal inhaled steroid's properties would include:

- Poor absorption from the gastrointestinal tract to minimize systemic effects due to the swallowed portion
- Almost complete metabolism in the 'first pass' through the liver
- High topical activity
- Metabolism in the lung to inactive metabolites (absorption from the lung circumvents the 'first pass' through the liver).

Using a spacer device with the steroid inhaler, and/or rinsing the mouth with water and spitting immediately after using the inhaled steroid may further reduce systemic effects.

Beclometasone, budesonide and fluticasone are examples of inhaled steroids. They are normally used twice daily. Budesonide is also licensed for once-daily use. Inhaled steroids are often referred to as 'preventers'.

When talking to asthmatics about their inhaled steroid, the following points should be remembered:

- Inhaled steroids should be used regularly not on an 'as required' basis.
- The dose of inhaled steroid may be increased in line with a self-management plan, e.g. when the asthmatic has a 'cold'.
- Inhaled steroids have no immediate effect.
- Improved asthma control will take a minimum of 3 days and possibly as long as 14 days after starting or increasing the dose of inhaled steroid.
- Steroid inhalers are normally brown, orange or maroon.

Concerns about side-effects may be allayed by reference to:

- The small dose due to the inhaled route
- All steroids not being the same, e.g. inhaled steroids are topically active steroids not anabolic steroids
- Nearly 30 years of clinical experience.

Unwanted systemic effects of inhaled steroids are extremely rare provided that the total daily dose is less than the equivalent of 1000 micrograms beclometasone diproplonate.

Unwanted local effects of inhaled steroids are:

- Oral candidiasis (thrush)
- Dysphonia.

The peak flow meter

The peak flow meter is a simple inexpensive device, prescribable on the NHS, which gives a useful objective measure of airways obstruction in asthmatics. A peak flow meter and its correct use is illustrated in Figure 24.3. The peak flow meter (PFM) measures peak expiratory flow rate (PEFR). PEFR is expressed in litres per minute (L/min). Flow rate of gas through a tube is proportional to the diameter of the tube when the pressure exerted on the gas is constant. Thus the maximum rate at which individuals can expel air from their lungs is proportional to the patency of the tubes in their lungs. A reduced PEFR indicates that there is obstruction to air flow in the lungs.

Normal values are available for PEFR in graph or chart form or on 'wheels'. In adults normal values for PEFR vary by age, sex and height; for children PEFR varies just by height. Normal or average values of PEFR are just that and values of 50–100 L/min above or below a predicted value fall within the normal range. An increase of at least 20% in PEFR following the use of an inhaled short-acting beta$_2$ agonist such as salbutamol is diagnostic of asthma. This is known as a reversibility test. However many asthmatics' PEFR will be normal much of the time, so one-off measurement of PEFR can be of limited value. Of much more value is twice-daily domiciliary measurement of PEFR, recorded on a peak flow diary chart for a minimum of 2–4 weeks. Home monitoring of PEFR is useful in:

- Diagnosing asthma
- Assessing control of asthma on current treatment
- Assessing effectiveness of new treatment
- Ensuring that asthma control is maintained when treatment is 'stepped down'.

Regular use of a peak flow meter is also useful in providing early warning of deteriorating asthma as PEFR may fall significantly before the asthmatic perceives an increase in severity or frequency of symptoms.

The PEFR chart of an asthmatic whose asthma is poorly controlled would typically show an average PEFR lower than predicted, with diurnal variation giving evening peaks and morning troughs. A diurnal variation of at least 20% is diagnostic of asthma.

The peak flow meter is a very useful tool in the self-management of asthma. A self-management plan is a method by which the doctor or other health care professional agrees with asthmatics how they should vary their treatment in response to changes in PEFR and/or symptoms, and when the asthmatic should seek medical assistance.

Self-management plans are particularly appropriate for asthmatics on regular preventative therapy but require them to have a reasonable understanding of their condition and their medication. This clearly requires patient education. Pharmacists have a valuable role to play in patient education and will find they will be most successful if they work as part of a team with the other health care professionals responsible for the care of the asthmatic.

Self-management plans should be written and provide a good basis for discussion between the pharmacist and asthmatic. School teachers may also welcome a copy of an asthmatic child's management plan.

Simplicity is the key to a successful self-management plan and a plan based on PEFR may be based on three different values. These values would be specific to each individual but might be:

1 Set marker to zero
2 Stand up, hold PFM horizontally avoiding touching or blocking the movement of the marker
3 Breathe in deeply then blow into the PFM as fast and hard as possible
4 Note reading, reset marker and repeat twice
5 The peak flow is the highest of the three readings

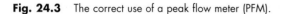

Fig. 24.3   The correct use of a peak flow meter (PFM).

- PEFR 450 or above—NORMAL—use inhalers as prescribed
- PEFR below 450 but above 300—WARNING—double inhaled steroid and continue on higher dose for 2 weeks after PEFR consistently above 450
- PEFR below 300—DANGER—make urgent appointment with doctor.

Self-management plans should be regularly reviewed, ideally at a doctor-, nurse- or pharmacist-run asthma clinic.

Aerosol inhalers

Metered dose inhaler (MDI)

A metered dose inhaler (Fig. 24.4) delivers an aerosol of drug dissolved or suspended in a propellant. Immediately an MDI is actuated some of the propellant rapidly evaporates to produce droplets of appropriate size to be inhaled into the lung. Further evaporation of propellant may occur in the mouth and the so-called 'cold-freon effect' occurs if there is further evaporation of propellant (freon) when the aerosol impacts on the back of the throat. The sensation produced by the 'cold-freon effect' can be sufficient in a minority of individuals to stop the inhalation and means that these individuals cannot use MDIs. The propellants currently used are generally hydrofluoro-alkanes (HFAs). Chlorofluoroalkanes, also known as chlorofluorocarbons (CFCs), were formerly used as propellants, but are now banned by international treaty because of their ozone-depleting properties. Medical aerosols were given exemption from the ban on CFCs, until alternatives were found and tested. Currently the change from CFCs to HFAs is not complete. It should perhaps be noted that whilst HFAs do not have the ozone-depleting effects of CFCs, both CFCs and HFAs are 'greenhouse' gases.

Patients who have previously had CFC-containing MDIs may be concerned when they start using a CFC-free MDI, because the taste and 'feel' of the aerosol is different. These differences are largely due to the fact that most CFC-containing MDIs are suspensions of drug in propellant, whereas most CFC-free MDIs are solutions of drug in propellant. Suspensions of drug in propellant result in nearly all the propellant evaporating after actuation and this can cause the 'cold-freon' effect (see above), but for many people the cooling sensation provides feedback that they are inhaling the drug. Solutions of drug in propellant result in only a fraction of the propellant evaporating after actuation, resulting in a reduced potential for the 'cold-freon' effect but also a different 'feel' for the patient.

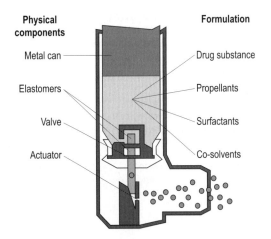

Fig. 24.4   The main elements of a metered dose inhaler.

Patients with concerns about their CFC-free inhalers offer pharmacists the opportunity not only to deal with patients' concern about their inhalers but also to check inhaler technique and asthma control.

Surfactants such as oleic acid and co-solvents such as ethanol may be used to facilitate the production of an appropriate suspension or solution of drug in propellant.

The propellants, which are gases at room temperature, are maintained as liquid by filling under pressure into the metal aerosol canister.

A metered dose is achieved by having an appropriate size reservoir in the valve, which fills by gravity as the valve reseats after each actuation.

The correct method of using an MDI is shown in Figure 24.5.

Common errors in using an MDI include:

- Inability to coordinate actuation of the inhaler with inspiration
- Taking a short, sharp inspiration, instead of a long steady inspiration (this is often at least in part due to not exhaling before using the inhaler)
- Actuating the inhaler twice (or more) on one inspiration.

Breath-actuated MDI

Inhaling through a breath-actuated MDI triggers a mechanism that 'fires' (actuates) the aerosol. These inhalers are particularly useful for those patients who have difficulty coordinating inspiration with actuation of the MDI.

Easi-Breathe is a type of breath-actuated MDI; its correct use is shown in Figure 24.6.

**HOW TO USE A
METERED DOSE INHALER**

1 Remove the cap
2 Shake the inhaler
3 Breathe out gently
4 Put the mouthpiece in the mouth
  and at the start of inspiration, which
  should be slow and deep, press the
  canister down and continue to inhale
  deeply
5 Hold the breath for 10 seconds,
  or as long as possible, then
  breathe out slowly
6 Wait for a few seconds
  before repeating steps 2-5
7 Replace cap

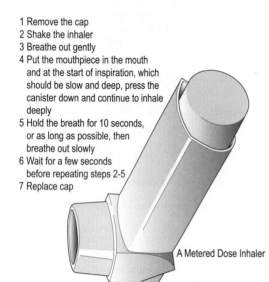

A Metered Dose Inhaler

**ALWAYS DEMONSTRATE TO THE PATIENT HOW TO USE THE
METERED DOSE INHALER**

Fig. 24.5   How to use a metered dose inhaler. (Source:
National Respiratory Training Centre.)

HOW TO USE THE EASI-BREATHE

1 Shake the inhaler
2 Hold the inhaler upright. Open the cap
3 Breathe out gently. Keep the inhaler upright,
  put the mouthpiece in the mouth and close
  lips and teeth around it (the airholes on the
  top must not be blocked by the hand)
4 Breathe in steadily through the
  mouthpiece. DON'T stop breathing when
  the inhaler "puffs" and continue taking a
  really deep breath
5 Hold the breath for 10 seconds
6 After use, hold the inhaler upright and
  immediately close the cap
7 For a second dose, wait a few seconds
  before repeating steps 1-6

Easi-Breathe

**ALWAYS DEMONSTRATE TO THE PATIENT HOW TO USE THE
EASI-BREATHE**

Fig. 24.6   How to use the Easi-Breathe. (Source:
National Respiratory Training Centre.)

Autohaler is another breath-actuated MDI. Using an
Autohaler is essentially the same as using an Easi-Breathe
except that the Autohaler is primed by raising a lever on the
top of the inhaler, whereas the Easi-Breathe is primed by
opening the mouthpiece cover.

Common errors when using a breath-actuated MDI
include:

- Not achieving a sufficiently high inspiratory flow rate to
  actuate the device
- Stopping inhaling immediately the inhaler actuates.

MDI + spacer

A chamber device (spacer) may be attached to an MDI
(Fig. 24.7).

A spacer consists of a plastic chamber with a port at one
end for the MDI and in most cases a one-way valve and
mouthpiece at the other end.

An MDI + spacer is best used by firing a single dose from
the MDI; inhalation should then start as soon as possible.

A spacer may be used with an MDI for the following
reasons:

- To overcome difficulty in coordinating inspiration with
  actuation of the MDI, as the inspirable particles remain
  available for inhalation for some seconds after actuation.
- To decrease deposition of non-respirable particles in the
  oropharynx. The larger particles are deposited in the
  spacer, rather than the oropharynx. This may be particularly important for high-dose inhaled steroids.
- To allow those unable to distinguish between inspiration
  and expiration (e.g. young children) to benefit from
  inhaled therapy by simply inhaling and exhaling across
  the one-way valve.
- To deliver a large dose of bronchodilator in an acute
  attack. The MDI is 'fired' a number of times into the
  spacer and the asthmatic inhales the drug by breathing
  through the one-way valve.

A mask may be attached or be integral to a spacer. The mask
can then be placed over the mouth and nose of babies or

HOW TO USE A SPACER DEVICE
e.g. VOLUMATIC

Single breath technique

1 Remove the cap
2 Shake the inhaler and insert into the device
3 Place the mouthpiece in the mouth
4 Press the canister once to release a dose of the drug
5 Take a deep, slow breath in
6 Hold the breath for about 10 seconds, then breathe out through the mouthpiece
7 Breathe in again but do not press the canister
8 Remove the device from the mouth
9 Wait about 30 seconds before repeating steps 2-8

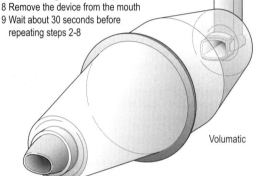

Volumatic

ALWAYS DEMONSTRATE TO THE PATIENT HOW TO USE THE SPACER DEVICE

Fig. 24.7 How to use a spacer device, e.g. Volumatic. Method for patients who can use the device without help. (Source: National Respiratory Training Centre.)

infants to enable them to benefit from inhaled therapy. The correct use of a spacer and face mask is shown in Figure 24.8.

Examples of spacers are Volumatic, Nebuhaler and Aerochamber.

Dry powder inhalers

Medicines for inhalation can be presented as a micronized powder. The powder may be pure drug as in the Turbohaler, or be drug and a carrier powder such as lactose, as in Rotacaps, Diskhaler and Accuhaler.

When a carrier powder is used the drug particles are adhered by weak electrostatic forces to the much larger carrier particles. As the drug/carrier powder is inhaled from the inhaler the small respirable drug particles fly off the larger non-respirable carrier particles. The lactose carrier thus remains in the mouth. Patients using dry powder inhalers that employ a carrier powder should be re-assured

HOW TO USE A LARGE VOLUME
SPACER AND MASK

1 Remove the mouthpiece cover from the inhaler
2 Attach the mask to the spacer mouthpiece. The Laerdal mask attaches to the Volumatic and the new 'McCarthy' mask to the Nebuhaler
3 Shake the inhaler and insert into the spacer device
4 Tip the spacer to an angle of 45° or more to enable the valve to remain open
5 Apply the mask to the child's face covering nose and mouth with as tight a seal as possible
6 Press the inhaler canister once to release a dose of the medication, keep the mask on the child's face to allow 5 or 6 breaths
7 Wait for 30 seconds before repeating steps 3-6
8 When using this method to administer inhaled steroids, remember to wash the child's face after each treatment

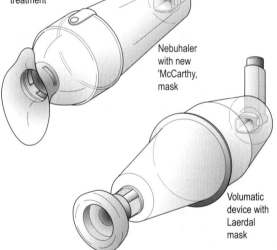

Nebuhaler with new 'McCarthy, mask

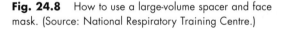

Volumatic device with Laerdal mask

ALWAYS DEMONSTRATE TO THE PATIENT HOW TO USE THE LARGE VOLUME SPACER AND MASK

Fig. 24.8 How to use a large-volume spacer and face mask. (Source: National Respiratory Training Centre.)

that even when using the inhaler correctly they will have carrier powder left in the mouth.

Patients inhaling pure drug from a Turbohaler may experience little or no taste.

The correct method of using the Turbohaler is shown in Figure 24.9 and the Accuhaler in Figure 24.10.

All inhalers are boxed with instruction leaflets. However the best way to learn how to use an inhaler is to have the technique demonstrated, then to attempt to use the inhaler under supervision so that any errors can be corrected. Many patients will benefit from pharmacists providing this

HOW TO USE THE TURBOHALER

1 Unscrew and lift off the white cover
2 Hold Turbohaler upright and twist the grip then twist it back again as far as it will go. You should hear a click
3 Breathe out gently, put the mouthpiece between the lips and teeth and breathe in as deeply as possible. Even when a full dose is taken there may be no taste. (Do not breathe out into Turbohaler)
4 Remove the Turbohaler from the mouth and hold breath about 10 seconds
5 For a second dose repeat steps 2-4
6 Replace white cover
7 A red line appears in the window on the side of the Turbohaler when there are 20 doses left. When the whole window is red the inhaler is empty

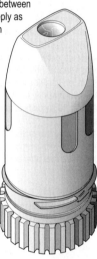

Turbohaler

ALWAYS DEMONSTRATE TO THE PATIENT HOW TO USE THE TURBOHALER

Fig. 24.9   How to use the Turbohaler. (Source: National Respiratory Training Centre.)

service. Similarly for pharmacists to best learn how to provide this service, they too should be shown how to use the inhaler and how to spot common errors. Medical representatives from companies that market inhalers are usually

HOW TO USE THE ACCUHALER

1 Open the Accuhaler by holding outer casing of the Accuhaler in one hand whilst pushing the thumbgrip away until a click is heard
2 Hold the Accuhaler with the mouthpiece towards you, slide the lever away until it clicks. This makes the dose available for inhalation and moves the dose counter on
3 Holding the Accuhaler level, breath out gently away from the device, put mouthpiece in mouth and take a breath in steadily and deeply
4 Remove the Accuhaler from the mouth and hold breath for about 10 seconds
5 To close, slide the thumb grip back towards you as far as it will go until it clicks
6 For a second dose repeat steps 1-5
7 The dose counter counts down from 60 to 0. The last 5 numbers are red

Accuhaler

ALWAYS DEMONSTRATE TO THE PATIENT HOW TO USE THE ACCUHALER

Fig. 24.10   How to use the Accuhaler. (Source: National Respiratory Training Centre.)

more than happy to train pharmacists how to use, demonstrate and check inhaler technique. As part of this service the medical representative will provide placebo inhalers, to allow the pharmacist to demonstrate the correct inhaler technique, instruction leaflets and other patient education material.

The use and care of a dry powder inhaler (DPI) differs from that of an MDI as shown in Table 24.1.

Table 24.1 Differences in the use and care of MDIs and DPIs	
MDI	**DPI**
Coordination of actuation and inhalation required	No coordination required, as the release of powder and inhalation is a two-step process
Long slow inhalation is the ideal to allow vaporization of propellants	Inhalation should be vigorous to disperse drug particles
Should be washed at least once a week to prevent blockage of actuator	Inhalers containing drug, e.g. Turbohaler, must never be washed. Inhalers that do not contain drug, e.g. Rotahaler, may be washed but must be scrupulously dry before use
Exhalation prior to inhalation can be into the inhaler	Exhalation must never be into the inhaler

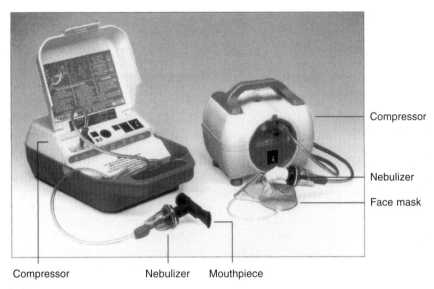

Fig. 24.11 Nebulization equipment.

Nebulizers

Medicines for inhalation can be presented as solutions or suspensions for nebulization. A nebulizing system (Fig. 24.11) usually consists of a compressor supplying compressed air to a nebulizing chamber, which delivers the nebulized drug to the patient via a mouthpiece or face mask. The face mask is most commonly used but when deposition of the nebulized drug on the face is undesirable (e.g. a steroid) then a mouthpiece is preferable, or the face under the mask should be protected with petroleum jelly.

The principle of jet nebulization is shown in Figure 24.12. The gas used to drive the nebulization process may be oxygen or air but in either case a minimum flow rate of 8 L/min at a pressure of at least 69 kPa (10 psi) is required.

Nebulizers are used when high doses of drug are required and/or when the patient is unable to use any form of inhaler. Nebulizers do not require the patient to learn any 'technique' and are effective on normal or shallow breathing.

Nebulizers are used in the treatment of severe acute asthma and this is best done under medical supervision:

- To ensure that an adequate objective (e.g. by measuring PEFR before and after nebulization) and maintained response to treatment is achieved
- To assess if other treatment is indicated, e.g. oral or parenteral steroids
- To plan follow-up and possible review of chronic medication.

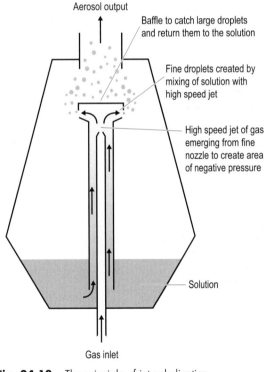

Fig. 24.12 The principle of jet nebulization.

Nebulized treatment may also be used in the latter stages of COPD often in conjunction with domiciliary oxygen therapy. Domiciliary oxygen cylinders do not provide sufficient flow rates to produce adequate nebulization, so a compressor unit should be used.

Drugs for nebulization are normally presented as unit dose vials; examples of these are Nebules and Respules.

Key Points

- A range of inhalation devices is available to deliver drugs directly to the lungs. This has clear advantages for lung conditions such as asthma whilst using much lower doses compared to oral therapy.
- The use of inhalers is technique dependent and patients require training in their use.
- Aerosol metered dose inhalers are the most widely prescribed, but can be difficult to use because they require coordination of inhalation with actuation of the inhaler.
- A range of breath-actuated metered dose inhalers and dry powder inhalers are available which overcome the need to coordinate inhalation with actuation.
- Spacers also overcome the need for coordination and are useful in small children. When spacers are fitted with a face mask, babies can benefit from inhaled therapy.
- Asthma treatment as set out in the BTS Guidelines involves a stepwise approach based on different types of (mainly inhaled) drugs—two of the most important being short-acting bronchodilators (beta$_2$ agonists), also known as 'relievers', and inhaled steroids, also known as 'preventers'.
- Many asthmatics use two or more inhalers, commonly a 'reliever' and a 'preventer' and often a 'protector' in addition. They are most likely to obtain optimal benefit from their treatment if they have some understanding of their condition and the role of their different inhalers.
- Asthmatics who have had appropriate education and training can monitor and self-manage their asthma within agreed limits. The peak flow meter provides an objective measure of lung function to aid this process.
- Asthma is a chronic condition best managed by regular review (as opposed to crisis management).
- Nebulized therapy delivers high doses of drugs to the lung and is often used in severe acute asthma. As severe acute asthma is life threatening, nebulized treatment for this should be under the direct supervision of a doctor or subject to a clear protocol.
- Pharmacists with an understanding of asthma its treatment and the correct use of inhalers can provide advice, education, training and review to patients on inhaled therapy to improve these patients' quality of life.

25

Parenteral products

D. G. Chapman

After studying this chapter you will know about:

The reasons for parenteral administration
The routes available for parenteral administration
The various forms and types of parenteral product
The design of containers and methods of administration of parenteral products
The formulation and uses of parenteral products
Pyrogens
Tonicity adjustment
Large-volume sterile products

Introduction

Parenteral products are dosage forms that are delivered to the patient by a route outwith the alimentary canal. The parenteral route of administration is often used for drugs that cannot be given orally. This may be due to patient intolerance, to the instability of the drug or to poor absorption of the drug if given by the oral route. In practice, parenteral products are often regarded as dosage forms that are implanted, injected or infused directly into vessels, tissues, tissue spaces or body compartments. From the site of administration the drug is then transported to the site of action. With developing technology, parenteral therapy is being used outwith the hospital or clinic environment. Patients are increasingly using it at home and in the workplace, allowing them to administer their own medication.

Parenteral therapy is used to:

- Produce a localized effect
- Administer drugs if the oral route cannot be used
- Deliver drugs to the unconscious patient
- Rapidly correct fluid and electrolyte imbalances
- Ensure delivery of the drug to the target tissues.

Parenteral injections are either administered directly into blood for a fast and controlled effect or into tissues outside the blood vessels for a local or systemic effect. An injection can be administered intravenously to rapidly increase the concentration of drug in the blood plasma, but the concentration soon falls due to the reversible transfer of the drug from blood plasma into body tissues, a process known as distribution. The drug concentration remaining in the blood plasma is affected both by the administered dose and the quantity of drug transferred into body tissues. Thereafter, there is a slower decrease in the drug concentration due to irreversible excretion and metabolism. An intravenous infusion administers a large volume of fluid at a slow rate and ensures that the drug enters the general circulation at a constant rate. In this procedure, the drug concentration in the blood plasma rises soon after the start of the infusion and achieves a steady state when the rate of drug addition equals the rate of drug loss. When infusion is stopped, elimination of the drug from the body by metabolism and/or excretion generally follows first-order kinetics.

Following subcutaneous and intramuscular injection there is a delay in the systemic effects of the drug. The delay is due to the time for the drug to firstly pass through the epithelial cells and basement membrane that forms the walls of the capillaries before entering into the blood. This occurs by passive diffusion that is promoted by the concentration gradient across the capillary wall. Other factors are also important, including the permeability characteristics and number of the capillaries in the area. Most plasma solutes pass freely across the capillary walls, while water-soluble substances such as glucose and amino acids pass through intercellular aqueous spaces of the capillary wall. After passing through the capillary wall the drug concentration in the blood plasma rises to a peak level and then falls due to distribution to the tissues followed by metabolism and excretion.

ADMINISTRATION PROCEDURES

Intravenous injections and infusions

Administration by this route provides strict control of the drug concentration in the circulating blood. The vein that is selected for administering the formulation depends on several factors. These include the size of the delivery needle or catheter, the type and volume of fluid to be administered and the rate of administering the fluid. The fluids are administered into a superficial vein, commonly on the back of the hand or in the internal flexure of the elbow (see Fig. 16.1). The intravenous route is widely used to administer parenteral products, but it must not be used to administer water-in-oil emulsions or suspensions.

Subcutaneous injections

These are injected into the loose connective and adipose tissue immediately beneath the skin (Fig. 25.1). Typically, the volume injected does not exceed 1 mL. Injection sites include the abdomen, the upper back, the upper arms and the lateral upper hips. This route is used if the medicine cannot be administered orally. The drugs are more rapidly and predictably absorbed than when administered by the oral route. Following administration, the site of the injection, the body temperature, age of the patient and the degree of massaging of the injection site affect drug distribution. However, absorption of the drug after subcutaneous injection is slower and less predictable than when administered by the intramuscular route.

Intramuscular injections

Small-volume aqueous solutions, solutions in oil and suspensions are administered directly into the body of a relaxed muscle (Fig. 25.1). Several muscle sites are used for these injections including the gluteal muscle in the buttock, the deltoid muscle in the shoulder and the vastus lateralis of the thigh. In adults the gluteal muscle is often used as larger volumes can be tolerated. In infants and small children the vastus lateralis of the thigh is usually more developed than other muscle groups and is thus used. For rapid absorption of the medicament the deltoid muscle in the shoulder is often used.

Other routes of parenteral administration are described below.

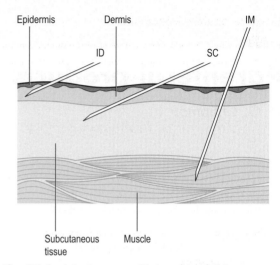

Fig. 25.1 Injection routes. ID, intradermal; SC, subcutaneous; IM, intramuscular.

Intradermal injections

A volume of about 0.1 mL is injected into the skin between the epidermis and the dermis. Absorption from intradermal injections is slow. This route is often used for diagnostic tests for allergy or immunity. It is also used to administer some vaccines.

Intra-arterial injections

The drug is administered directly into an artery. Owing to the fast flow of blood in the artery it is likely that the drug will be rapidly dispersed throughout the blood system. However, manipulative difficulties restrict the use of intra-arterial injections but drugs can be administered by this route to target a specific organ or tissue that is served by the artery.

Intracardiac injections

These are aqueous solutions that are administered in emergency directly into a ventricle or the cardiac muscle for a local effect.

Intraspinal injections

These are aqueous solutions that are injected in volumes less than 20 mL into particular areas of the spinal column. They are categorized as intrathecal, subarachnoid, intracisternal, epidural and peridural injections. The specific gravity of these injections may be adjusted to localize the site of action of the drug.

Intra-articular injections

These are administered as an aqueous solution or suspension into the synovial fluid in a joint cavity. They are often used for the local administration of anti-inflammatory agents.

PRODUCTS FOR PARENTERAL USE

Parenteral products are sterile formulations that are administered into the body by various routes including injection, infusion and implantation.

Injections

These are subdivided into small- and large-volume parenteral fluids. Small-volume parenterals are sterile, pyrogen-free injectable products. They are packaged in volumes up to 100 mL. Small-volume parenteral fluids are packed as:

- Single-dose ampoules
- Multiple-dose vials
- Prefilled syringes.

Single-dose ampoules

Most small-volume parenterals are currently packaged as either ampoules or vials. Glass ampoules are thin-walled containers made of Type I borosilicate glass (see Fig. 9.3). Injections packaged in glass ampoules are manufactured by filling the product into the ampoules that are then heat sealed. To achieve the quality required of these products, the packaged solution must be sterile and practically free of particles. These products are typically prepared in clean room conditions (see Ch. 13). However, the great concern with using glass ampoules relates to the hazards of opening them because the product may become contaminated with glass particles. Opening is easier with glass ampoules with a weakened neck. This is achieved by applying a ceramic paint ring to the ampoule neck. The paint, after a process of heat baking, has the effect of weakening the neck. Even though the subsequent opening of the ampoules is physically easier, a large number of glass particles still contaminate the product. Another ampoule design has a score on the glass at the ampoule neck with a painted dot marker on the opposing side. These are known as one-point cut ampoules. They are easier to open, but glass particles continue to be released when they are opened.

Plastic ampoules are prepared, filled and sealed by a procedure known as blow–fill–seal. This is a four-step continuous procedure in which granules of plastic are heated to a semi-solid state. The plastic is then blow moulded and formed into ampoules. These containers are filled with the product and immediately sealed. This system is only used to package simple solutions. The plastic may take up drug components from the product. When the ampoule is opened by rotating the integral plastic closure, few particles are released into the solution.

Ampoules should have a reliable seal that can be readily leak tested. A good seal will not deteriorate during the lifetime of the product. Medicines packaged in ampoules are intended for single use only. As a result, these products do not contain chemical antimicrobial preservatives. The ampoule must also contain a slight excess volume of product. This is necessary to allow the nominal injection volume to be drawn into a syringe.

Multiple-dose vials

These are composed of a thick-walled glass container that is sealed with a rubber closure. The closure is kept in position by an aluminium seal that is crimped to the neck of the glass vial (see Fig. 9.4). These closures are then covered with a plastic cap. The cap is removed before a needle, attached to a syringe, is inserted through the rubber closure to withdraw a dose of product. The contents of the vial may be removed in several portions.

The glass vial packaging system has the advantage of increased dose flexibility and decreased costs per unit dose. There are also certain disadvantages with the use of glass vials. Fragments of the closure may be released into the product when the needle is inserted through the closure. There is also the risk of interaction between the product and the closure. Repeated withdrawal of injection solution from these containers increases the risk of microbial contamination of the product. These products must, therefore, contain an antimicrobial preservative unless the medicine itself has antimicrobial activity. An example of such a multidose product is insulin. Each dose is withdrawn from the vial when required and administered by the patient.

Prefilled syringes

With these devices, the injection solution is aseptically filled into sterile syringes. The packed solution has a high level of sterility assurance and does not contain an antimicrobial

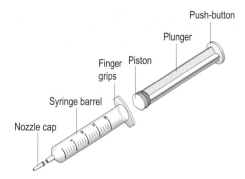

Fig. 25.2 Hypodermic syringe for single use.

preservative. The final product is available for immediate use. Prefilled syringes are expensive and so only limited products are packaged in this way.

Administration of small-volume parenteral products

Hypodermic syringes and needles are extensively used for administering small volumes of parenteral formulations to the patient. These syringes have been sterilized by ethylene oxide gas or, occasionally, by gamma irradiation following packaging. Various sizes of hypodermic syringes are available. They are composed of a barrel, having a graduated scale, together with a plunger and a headpiece, known as a piston (Fig. 25.2). These components are often made of polypropylene, although the piston could be made of medical grade rubber.

FORMULATION OF PARENTERAL PRODUCTS

Vehicles for injections

The drug is generally present in an injection in low concentration. The vehicle provides the highest proportion of the formulation and should not be toxic nor have any therapeutic activity.

Mains water often contains a wide variety of contaminants such as electrolytes, organisms and particulate matter, and dissolved gases, such as carbon dioxide and chlorine. The wide variety of these contaminants causes a problem in the preparation of water for use in injections. This is called water for injections and must be used as the vehicle for parenteral products. It is often used to prepare ophthalmic products but these could be made using purified water.

Water for injections

Water for injections is the most extensively used vehicle in parenteral formulations. Water for injections is well tolerated by the body and ionizable electrolytes readily dissolve in water. Water for injections must be free of pyrogens. It must also have a high level of chemical purity. The *British Pharmacopoeia* (BP 2001) considers that water for injections can only be prepared by distillation in order to produce a consistent supply of the required quality of water.

Preparation of water for injections

The usual method of preparing water for injections in Europe and North America is distillation. Whilst other processes can achieve a similar quality of product, these alternative systems cannot produce a consistent water quality. The source water used in the preparation of water for injections by distillation is usually potable water. This water varies in quality and may be contaminated with dissolved gases, suspended minerals and organic substances, mineral salts, chemicals, endotoxins and microorganisms. The high standards required of water for injections is only achieved if the quality of the source water is improved by suitable pretreatment before it is supplied as feed water for final processing. The pretreatment of the source water usually involves:

- Chemical softening
- Filtration
- Deionization
- pH adjustment.

The water is then treated by reverse osmosis to yield purified water. This water is often used as the feed water for distillation and has a low silica content and a low total organic carbon content. A wide variety of designs of still are used in the production of water for injections. These stills are typically made of stainless steel, although chemically resistant glass could be used.

The single effect still is used to produce volumes less than 90 L/h. This usually fulfils the demands of small-scale production as required by a hospital pharmacy. The single effect still requires de-ionized feed water and has three main structural components:

- An evaporator containing the heater
- A vapour-liquid disengaging section
- A condenser.

When this still is functioning, the feed water in the horizontal evaporator is heated. Steam is produced at atmospheric pressure and at slow velocity. Some steam will condense before it enters a vertical vapour-liquid disengaging unit that is attached to the horizontal evaporator. Baffle plates at the base of the vapour-liquid unit reduces the risk of water droplets being carried in the steam into this unit. The water droplets and the non-volatile impurities are returned to the water in the evaporator. The vapour-liquid disengaging unit often contains a centrifugal device that spins the steam as it rises in this unit. This has the effect of throwing entrapped water droplets in the steam onto the wall of this vertical cylindrical section where it condenses and returns to the evaporator. Only pure steam exits from this unit into the condenser where the heat of vaporization is removed and converts the water vapour to the liquid distillate. Only stills designed to produce high-purity water may be used in the production of water for injections.

In operation the first portion of the distillate must be discarded. The remainder is collected in a suitable storage vessel. Freshly collected distillate is usually free of microbial contaminants and should contain not more than 0.25 international units of endotoxin per mL as determined by the bacterial endotoxin test. However, the distillate is regularly sampled and tested for microbial contamination. It is acceptable if there are less than 10 organisms per 100 mL present at any instance; no *Pseudomonas* bacteria should be present. To ensure that the distillate is of a suitable purity, the electrical conductivity of the distillate is measured. This measurement is used as an indicator of the quality of ionizable materials in the collected water. The electrical conductance should be less than 1.1 µS/cm when measured at 20°C. However, the measurement of electrical conductivity alone as an indicator of water quality can be misleading, as it does not detect silica in the distillate. To conform with the quality standards of the BP (2001) and the *European Pharmacopoeia* (EP 2002) the distillate will also have the following quality limits:

Total organic carbon	Not more than 0.5 mg per litre
Chlorides	Not more than 0.5 parts per million (p.p.m.)
Ammonia	Not more than 0.1 p.p.m.
Nitrates	Not more than 0.2 p.p.m.
Heavy metals	Not more than 0.1 p.p.m.
Oxidizable substances	Not more than 5 p.p.m.
pH	5.0–7.0

Care is required in handling the freshly collected distillate as it is subject to microbial contamination during storage and distribution. Two systems are commonly used for the storage of water for injections: batch storage and dynamic storage.

Batch storage

With this system the water for injections is stored as a batch of discrete unit volumes which may be sterilized. Quality control tests are performed on this batch. Only after the batch is identified as being of suitable quality is it released for use. This system provides maximum product accountability before use. It is, however, an expensive storage system.

Dynamic storage

With this system the storage tank is a surge tank, usually made of quality polished stainless steel. As the level of water for injections in the tank falls then more water for injections is produced and filled into the tank. The fresh water for injections mixes with water remaining in the tank. This system is cheaper and simpler to operate than batch storage. However, it does lack batch accountability and the water may become contaminated through corrosion of the steel tank. Owing to the potential problem with Gram-negative bacterial contamination, it is important that the distillate is stored at 80°C to prevent bacterial growth. Heating the water in the tank is achieved with a steam-heated jacket around the tank.

Surge tanks require sterilization at timed intervals. They are fitted with a filter vent used to equilibrate the tank pressure during filling and emptying the tank. The filter prevents airborne bacterial contamination of the water for injections within the tank.

Distribution

A loop distribution system may be used to deliver the water for injections to the point of use. The water in the distribution system can become contaminated with organisms. As a result, the water in the stainless steel pipes is constantly circulated from the tank to avoid stagnation and to maintain the temperature. This distribution system has one major disadvantage in that the point of use may not require high-temperature water. Thus a cooling system may be fitted close to the point of use. Microbial growth may then occur in the cooled water.

Sterilized water for injections

This is prepared by packing a volume of water for injections in sealed containers. These containers are then moist-heat sterilized which yields a sterile product that remains free of pyrogens. Sterilized water for injections is used to dissolve or dilute parenteral preparations before administration to the patient.

Pyrogens

Water is potentially the greatest source of pyrogens in parenteral products. Untreated pyrogenic water is contaminated with pyrogens and these must be removed before the water can be used in parenteral products. This is achieved in the preparation of water as a vehicle for injections by distillation in the UK. Pyrogens are fever-producing substances. The injection of distilled water may produce a rise in body temperature if it contains pyrogens, while water that is free of this effect is described as apyrogenic.

Microbial pyrogens arise from components of Gram-negative and Gram-positive bacteria, fungi and viruses. Non-microbial pyrogens, such as some steroids and plasma components, also produce a pyrogenic response if injected. The most important pyrogens in pharmacy products are high molecular weight endotoxins that are found in the outer membrane of Gram-negative bacteria. Therefore endotoxins potentially exist in all situations harbouring bacteria.

Freshly prepared parenteral products must not be contaminated with organisms that could produce pyrogens. They must be prepared in conditions that reduce microbial contamination because bacteria contaminating aqueous solutions can release endotoxins. Contaminated solutions will become more pyrogenic with the passage of time. Therefore, these products must be sterilized shortly after preparation.

Endotoxins produce significant physiological changes when injected. Their detection and elimination are very important for manufacturers of parenteral products.

Nature of endotoxins

Endotoxins isolated from the outer membrane of Gram-negative bacteria are composed of three areas. The inner region is composed of lipid A that is linked to a central polysaccharide core. This polysaccharide core is joined to long projections known as the *O*-antigenic side chains. Lipid A is responsible for most of the biological activity of endotoxin. By itself it is not very soluble in water. However, it is

joined to a core polysaccharide by an eight-carbon sugar that acts as a solute carrier for the lipid A in aqueous solutions.

The molecular weight of endotoxin is important in determining its biological activity. In a pure aqueous environment, endotoxin has a relative molecular mass of about 10^6. This is equivalent to the relative molecular mass of a virus particle and is the most common size of endotoxin found in large-volume parenteral formulations. In the presence of magnesium and calcium, the endotoxin forms bilayer sheets or vesicles with a diameter of about 0.1 μm. These small structures can easily pass through a 0.22 μm membrane filter. This size of filter is commonly used in the production of pharmacy products.

Biological activity of pyrogens

The injection of endotoxins and other pyrogens can produce many physiological effects. The most important arising from the use of pharmacy products is the pyrogenic effect, where the lipid A directly affects the thermoregulatory centres in the brain. At high dose levels endotoxin will also:

- Activate the coagulation system
- Alter carbohydrate and lipid metabolism
- Produce platelet aggregation
- Produce shock and ultimately death.

As pyrogens can produce these toxic effects they should never be knowingly injected. Their detection and elimination are very important for the production of parenteral products. The contamination of large-volume parenteral solutions with pyrogens is especially serious, owing to the large volumes that are administered to seriously ill patients.

Although endotoxins are the predominant pyrogen in parenteral formulations, other pyrogenic substances also exist. These agents include peptidoglycan, from Gram-positive bacteria, and bacterial exotoxins, as evidenced by the erythrogenic response produced by *Streptococcus* group A organisms which causes the skin to turn red. Viruses induce a pyrogenic response that often appears like the fever induced by the common cold virus. Moulds and yeasts also produce a pyrogenic effect following intravenous injection.

Tests for pyrogens

The rabbit test included in the BP (2001) and in the EP (2002) is very similar to the original rabbit test included in the 1948 edition of the BP. However, in recent times, alternative tests for bacterial endotoxins have been extensively used. The rabbit test that is used to identify the presence of a wide range of pyrogens does have problems for testing pharmacy products. It is an expensive and slow test that is difficult to perform even in specialized test centres. The bacterial endotoxin test is a specific test for endotoxins of bacterial origin. Bacterial endotoxin is the main pyrogen found in parenteral products and the test is carried out on both the components and the final parenteral products.

Bacterial endotoxin tests

This test as detailed in Appendix XIV of the BP 2001 is commonly referred to as the limulus amoebocyte lysate (LAL) test. It detects or quantifies endotoxins from Gram-negative bacteria. The BP test allows the use of a lysate of amoebocytes from either the American or Japanese horseshoe crab. Not surprisingly, however, in practice the lysate used in tests in Europe and North America is obtained from amoebocytes of the American horseshoe crab *Limulus polyphemus* while the lysate of the Japanese crab (*Tachypleus tridentatus*) is used in tests carried out in Asia. Although six tests are detailed in the BP (2001), these tests can be grouped into one of three types, known as: the gel clot end point, the turbidimetric test and the kinetic chromogenic test. The gel clot end point is based on the formation of a solid gel clot. It is an in vitro test for bacterial endotoxins that does have some advantages, as it is cheap, rapid, simple to perform and sensitive to low endotoxin concentrations. This test is often used by hospital and small-scale manufacturers and is used as a definitive test if doubt exists regarding results obtained by the other test methods.

With the gel clot procedure, a solution containing the endotoxin is added to a solution of the lysate. The reaction requires a proclotting enzyme system and a clottable protein coagulogen that are provided by the lysate. The reaction that takes place is shown in Figure 25.3. The rate of this reaction is affected by several factors, including the concentration of endotoxin, the pH and the temperature. In the test procedure, the lysate is mixed with an equal volume of the test solution in a depyrogenated container, such as a glass tube. The tube is then incubated undisturbed at 37°C for a period of about 60 minutes. The test is a pass or fail test. The end point is identified by gently inverting the glass tube. A positive result is indicated by the formation of a solid clot of coagulin. This clot does not disintegrate when the tube is inverted. A negative result is indicated if no gel clot has been formed. This test needs appropriate positive and negative controls. For a positive control, a known concentration of endotoxin is added to the lysate alone and then repeated with a product sample. As a negative control, water that is

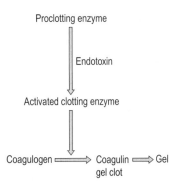

Fig. 25.3 The lysate clotting mechanism.

free of endotoxin is added to the lysate. All the controls must produce appropriate results for the test to be valid. The sensitivity of the assay is limited by the sensitivity of the lysate used in the test. The gel clot test will detect between 0.02 and 1.0 endotoxin units per millilitre. Some recently developed biopharmaceuticals have shown similar activity to endotoxin in this and the other endotoxin tests. Before this test is carried out, it is necessary to determine that:

- The test equipment does not adsorb endotoxins
- The lysate is of suitable sensitivity
- No interfering agents are present.

The turbidimetric test is used in the testing of water systems and for testing simple pharmacy products. The test measures the opacity change in the LAL test due to the formation of insoluble coagulin. An increase in the endotoxin concentration produces a proportional increase in opacity due to the precipitation of the clottable protein coagulin.

The kinetic chromogenic test is an automated test used by commercial parenteral manufacturers to test large numbers of complex products. The test gives an accurate result over a wide range of endotoxin concentrations. The test measures the colour change induced by the release of the chromogenic chemical *para*-nitroanilide. This is released as a byproduct of the clotting reaction during the LAL test. The quantity of *para*-nitroanilide produced is directly proportional to the endotoxin concentration.

Pyrogen testing

The BP pyrogen test involves measuring the rise in body temperature of healthy mature rabbits. This temperature rise is recorded after the rabbits have been intravenously injected with a sterile solution of the test substance. The environment and the equipment used in the test are detailed in the BP (2001). This test can only be carried out where the rabbits can tolerate the test product.

The test itself is preceded by a preliminary test to identify and exclude any animal with an unusual response to the trauma of the injection. With the preliminary test, a warmed pyrogen-free saline solution is injected into the rabbits. The temperature of the rabbits is recorded from 90 minutes before the test to 3 hours after the injection, as specified in the BP (2001). The fever response in the rabbits after the injection with pyrogens follows a biphasic response. After the injection there is a lag time of about 15–18 minutes, which is followed by a rapid temperature rise to a peak within 2 hours. The temperature then falls and is followed by a second rise in temperature. This returns to normal after 6–9 hours. False-positive temperature increases occur with rabbits as a result of:

- Injury
- Badly positioned recording devices
- Distress.

The rabbits may develop a resistance to pyrogens. As a result, they are tested at specified time intervals.

Depyrogenation

Depyrogenation is the elimination of all pyrogens, from the production materials, solutions and equipment. It is achieved by either removal or inactivation of the pyrogens. The main method of preventing pyrogens contaminating parenteral products is strict control of the ingredients used. That is solvents, raw materials, packaging materials and equipment should not be contaminated with pyrogens.

A simple method of removing small amounts of pyrogens from surfaces such as packaging components is by rinsing the surfaces with non-pyrogenic water. As pyrogens are non-volatile, distillation is the principal method of avoiding contamination of water used in parenteral products. This is achieved by positioning a trap, fitted with baffles, in the still. The trap removes the droplets of water by impingement and prevents pyrogens being carried over into the distillate. However, the freshly collected distillate that is initially pyrogen-free water can become contaminated with organisms and pyrogens if stored for more than 4 hours at 22°C. To avoid microbial growth in this water it must be sterilized soon after collection or stored at high temperatures to suppress microbial growth. Pyrogens can be removed from solutions by ultrafiltration that separates pyrogens by a process based on their relative molecular mass. This specialized system has been used to depyrogenate antibiotic

products during their commercial production. These filters are different from the 0.22 μm filters often used in pharmacy production.

Various methods are used to inactivate pyrogens including heat treatment, acid–base hydrolysis and oxidation. High temperature is widely used to incinerate pyrogens especially for glassware, thermostable equipment and formulation components. Dry heat at 250°C for 30 minutes is normally used. The commonly used dry or moist heat sterilization cycles (see Ch. 12) will not greatly reduce the pyrogen burden of parenteral products.

Non-aqueous solvents

Water-miscible co-solvents, such as glycerin and propylene glycol, are used as vehicles in small-volume parenteral fluids. They are used to increase the solubility of drugs and to stabilize drugs degraded by hydrolysis.

Metabolizable oils are used to dissolve drugs that are insoluble in water. For example steroids, hormones and vitamins are dissolved in vegetable oils. These formulations are administered by intramuscular injection.

Additives

Various additives, such as antimicrobial agents, antioxidants, buffers, chelating agents and tonicity-adjusting agents are included in injection formulations. Their purpose is to produce a safe and elegant product. Both the types and amounts of additives to be included in formulations are given in the appropriate monograph in the BP (2001).

Antimicrobial agents

These are added to products that are packaged in multiple-dose vials. They are not used in large-volume injections or if the drug formulation itself has sufficient antimicrobial activity (such as Methohexital Sodium Injection). Antimicrobial agents are added to inhibit the growth of microbial organisms that may accidentally contaminate the product during use. The antimicrobial agents must be stable and effective in the parenteral formulation. Because they are effective in the free form, their activity can be greatly reduced by interaction with components of the injection. Rubber closures have been shown to take up antimicrobial preservatives from the injection solution. Preservative uptake is more significant with natural and neoprene rubber and much less with butyl rubber closures.

Table 25.1 Examples of antimicrobial preservatives used in aqueous multiple dose injections

Antimicrobial preservative	Concentration (% w/v)
Benzyl alcohol	1–2
Chlorocresol	0.1–0.3
Cresol	0.25–0.5
Methyl hydroxybenzoate	0.1
Phenol	0.25–0.6
Thiomersal	0.01

There is concern about the toxic effects of injections containing preservatives. As a result, a low but effective antimicrobial concentration is used in injections. Challenging the product with selected organisms can test the effectiveness of antimicrobial agents. The test procedure will evaluate the antimicrobial activity of the preservative in the packaged product. The test procedure is detailed in BP 2001. Table 25.1 gives details for some commonly used preservatives.

Antioxidants

Many drugs in aqueous solutions are easily degraded by oxidation. Small-volume parenteral products of these drugs often contain an antioxidant. Bisulphites and metabisulphites are commonly used antioxidants in aqueous injections. Antioxidants must be carefully selected for use in injections to avoid interaction with the drug. Antioxidants have a lower oxidation potential than the drug and so are either preferentially oxidized or block oxidative chain reactions. Injection formulations may, in addition to antioxidants, also contain chelating agents. Chelating agents such as EDTA or citric acid remove trace elements which catalyse oxidative degradation.

Buffers

The ideal pH of parenteral products is pH 7.4. If the pH is above pH 9, tissue necrosis may result, whilst below pH 3 pain and phlebitis in tissues can occur.

Buffers are included in injections to maintain the pH of the packaged product. pH changes can arise through interaction between the product and the container. However, the buffer used in the injection must allow body fluids to change the product pH after injection.

Acetate, citrate and phosphate buffers are commonly used in parenteral products.

Tonicity-adjusting agents

Isotonic solutions have the same osmotic pressure as blood plasma and do not damage the membrane of red blood cells. Hypotonic solutions have a lower osmotic pressure than blood plasma and cause blood cells to swell and burst because of fluids passing into the cells by osmosis. Hypertonic solutions have a higher osmotic pressure than plasma; as a result the red blood cells lose fluids and shrink. Following the administration of an injection it is important that tissue damage and irritation are minimized and haemolysis of red blood cells is minimized. Thus, the BP (2001) states that aqueous solutions for large-volume infusion fluids, together with aqueous fluids for subcutaneous, intradermal and intramuscular administration, should be made isotonic. Intrathecal injections must also be isotonic to avoid serious changes in the osmotic pressure of the cerebrospinal fluid. Aqueous hypotonic solutions are made isotonic by adding either sodium chloride, glucose or, occasionally, mannitol. The latter two agents are incompatible with some drugs. If the solution is hypertonic it is made isotonic by dilution.

Some components of injections, such as buffers and antioxidants, affect the tonicity. Other components, such as preservatives, which are present in low concentration, have little effect on the tonicity.

Injection solutions are often made isotonic with 0.9% sodium chloride solution. The amount of solute, or the required dilution necessary to make a solution isotonic, can be determined from the freezing point depression. The freezing point depression of blood plasma and tears is –0.52°C. Thus solutions that freeze at –0.52°C have the same osmotic pressure as body fluids. Hypotonic solutions have a smaller freezing point depression and require the addition of a solute to depress the freezing point to –0.52°C.

The amount of adjusting substance added to these solutions may be calculated from the equation:

$$W = (0.52 - a)/b$$

where W = percentage concentration of adjusting substance in the final solution, a = freezing point depression of the unadjusted hypotonic solution, b = freezing point depression of a 1% w/v concentration of the adjusting substance.

An extensive list of freezing point depression values is detailed in table 6 (pp. 53–64) in the chapter 'Solution properties' in the 12th edition of the *Pharmaceutical Codex* (1994).

EXAMPLE 23.1

A 100 mL volume of a 2% w/v solution of glucose for intravenous injection is to be made isotonic by the addition of sodium chloride.

A 1% w/v solution of glucose depresses the freezing point of water by 0.1°C and a 1% solution of sodium chloride depresses the freezing point of water by 0.576°C.

The depression of freezing point of the unadjusted solution of glucose (a) will therefore be:

$$(a) = 2 \times 0.1 = 0.2$$

A 1% w/v solution of sodium chloride depresses the freezing point of water by 0.576°C (b).

Substituting these values for a and b in the above equation:

$$W = (0.52 - 0.2)/0.576 = 0.32/0.576 = 0.555$$

The intravenous solution thus requires the addition of 0.555 g of sodium chloride per 100 mL volume to make it isotonic with blood plasma.

Other methods that are used to estimate the amount of adjusting substances required to make a solution isotonic include:

- Sodium chloride equivalents
- Molar concentrations
- Serum osmolarity.

Details of these methods are given in the chapter 'Solution Properties' (pp. 64–67) in the 12th edition of the *Pharmaceutical Codex* (1994).

Units of concentration

The concentration of the components in parenteral products may be expressed in various ways (see also Ch. 8):

- *Percentage weight/volume.* Examples include: magnesium sulphate injection 50%, sodium chloride intravenous infusion 0.9%.
- *Weight per unit volume.* Examples include: atropine sulphate 600 micrograms/mL or ephedrine hydrochloride injection 30 mg/mL.
- *Millimoles per unit volume.* Examples include: potassium chloride solution, strong (sterile) contains 2 mmol each of K^+ and Cl^- per mL; Calcium Chloride Injection BP contains 2.5 mmol of Ca^{2+} and 10 mmol of Cl^- in 5 mL.

During the formulation of injections and infusions the units of interest are the ions of electrolytes and the molecules of non-electrolytes. For molecules, 1 millimole (mmol) is the weight in milligrams corresponding to its relative molecular mass. A mole of an ion is its relative atomic mass weighed in grams. The number of moles of each of the ions of a salt in solution depends on the number of each ion in the molecule of the salt.

EXAMPLE 23.2

Sodium chloride has one sodium and one chloride ion. Thus, 1 mole of sodium chloride provides 1 mole of both sodium and chloride ions. The weight of sodium chloride which provides a 1 mmol quantity is 58.5 mg. This weight corresponds to its relative molecular mass and provides 1 mmol of both sodium and chloride ions.

Magnesium chloride has one magnesium and two chloride ions. The weight in milligrams that provides 1 mmol of magnesium and 2 mmol of chloride ions is 203 mg. This weight corresponds to the relative molecular mass of this salt. The quantity of salt in milligrams containing 1 mmol of a particular ion can be determined by dividing the relative molecular mass of the salt by the number of the particular ions that it contains. Weights of common salts that provide 1 mmol are given in table 4 in the chapter 'Solution Properties' (pp. 49–50) in the 12th edition of the *Pharmaceutical Codex* (1994).

Conversion equations

Useful conversion equations include the following:

$$
\begin{aligned}
\text{mg per litre} &= W \times M \\
\text{grams per litre} &= (W \times M)/1000 \\
\text{\% w/v} &= (W \times M)/10\,000
\end{aligned}
$$

where W = the number of milligrams of salt containing 1 mmol of the required ion, M = the number of millimoles per litre.

EXAMPLE 23.3

Calculate the quantities of salts required for the following electrolyte solution:

Sodium	12 mmol
Potassium	4 mmol
Magnesium	6 mmol
Calcium	6 mmol
Chloride	40 mmol
Water for injections	to 1 L

From table 4 in the *Pharmaceutical Codex* (1994; see above), 4 mmol of potassium ion is provided by 4 × 74.5 mg of potassium chloride, which also yields 4 mmol of chloride ions. 6 mmol of magnesium ions is provided by 6 × 203 mg of magnesium chloride, which also yields 2 × 6 = 12 mmol of chloride ions as there are two chloride ions in the molecule. 6 mmol of calcium ions is provided by 6 × 147 mg of calcium chloride, which also yields 12 mmol of chloride ions as there are two chloride ions in the molecule. 12 mmol of sodium ions is provided by 12 × 58.5 mg of sodium chloride that also yields 12 mmol of chloride. The formula can, therefore, be shown as in Table 25.2. It should be noted that the charges on the anions and cations are equally balanced.

EXAMPLE 23.4

Calculate the number of millimoles of dextrose and sodium ions in 1 litre of sodium chloride and dextrose injection containing 5% anhydrous dextrose and 0.9% w/v of sodium chloride.
Use the conversion equation for % w/v calculations.

$$\% \ w/v = (W \times M)/10\ 000$$

From this equation:

$$M = \% \ w/v \times 10\ 000/W$$

For dextrose
As dextrose is a non-electrolyte, $W = 180.2$. Thus:

$$M = 5.0 \times 10\ 000/180.2 = 277 \ \text{mmol}$$

The 1 litre of solution contains 277 mmol.
For sodium chloride

$$M = 0.09 \times 10\ 000/58.5 = 15.4 \ \text{mmol}$$

As 1 mmol of sodium chloride provides 1 mmol of both sodium and chloride ions, 1 litre of the solution will contain 15.4 mmol of both sodium and chloride ions.

EXAMPLE 23.5

Calculate the number of millimoles of magnesium and chloride ions in 1 litre of a 2% solution of magnesium chloride.

$$M = 0.2 \times 10\ 000/203 = 9.85$$

Each mole of magnesium chloride provides 1 mole of magnesium ions and 2 moles of chloride ions. Thus, 1 litre of the solution contains 9.85 mmol of magnesium ions and 19.7 mmol of chloride ions.

SPECIAL INJECTIONS

These are more complex formulations than solutions for injection.

Suspensions

Commonly, suspensions for injection contain less than 5% of drug solids with a mean particle diameter within the range 5–10 µm. Owing to the presence of particles in these formulations, these injections are more difficult to process and sterilize than solutions for injection. During the manufacture of suspensions for injection, the components are prepared and sterilized separately. They are then aseptically combined (see Ch. 13). The final product cannot be filter sterilized owing to the presence of particles in the formulation. Powders for use in sterile suspensions can be sterilized by gas, but gas residues must be avoided (see Ch. 12).

Table 25.2 The formula for Example 25.3						
		Millimoles of				
		Na+	K+	Mg2+	Ca2+	Cl-
Sodium chloride	12 × 58.5 = 0.702 g	12				12
Potassium chloride	4 × 74.5 = 0.298 g		4			4
Magnesium chloride	6 × 203 = 1.218 g			6		12
Calcium chloride	6 × 147 = 0.882 g				6	12
Water for injections to 1 L						
Total (mmol/L)		12	4	6	6	40

Dried injections

With these products the dry sterile powder is aseptically added to a sterile vial. Alternatively, a sterile filtered solution can be freeze-dried in a vial. The dry drug powder is reconstituted with a sterile vehicle before use.

Non-aqueous injections

Drugs that are insoluble in an aqueous vehicle can be formulated in solution using an oil as the vehicle. These formulations are less common than aqueous suspensions. Several oils are used in these formulations, including arachis oil and sesame oil, which are easily metabolized. These viscous injections give a depot effect with slow release of the drug and are administered by intramuscular injection.

LARGE-VOLUME PARENTERAL PRODUCTS

These are parenteral products that are packed and administered in large volumes. They are formulated as single-dose injections that are administered by intravenous infusion. They are sterile aqueous solutions or emulsions with water for injections as the main component. It is important that they are free of particles. During the administration of these fluids additional drugs are often added to the fluids (see Ch. 27). This may be carried out by the injection of small-volume parenteral products to the administration set of the fluid, or by the 'piggyback' method. In this procedure a second, but smaller volume infusion of an additional drug is added to the intravenous delivery system.

Large-volume parenteral products include:

- Infusion fluids
- Total parenteral nutrition solutions
- Intravenous antibiotics
- Patient-controlled analgesia
- Dialysis fluids
- Irrigation solutions.

All of these products have direct contact with blood or are introduced into a body cavity. Large-volume parenterals are variously formulated and packaged and have been used to:

- Restore fluid and electrolyte imbalance in patients suffering from dehydration, shock or injury
- Provide nutrition in circumstances where patients are malnourished, e.g. total parenteral nutrition

- Act as a vehicle for administration of medicines
- Perform dialysis
- Allow irrigation of body parts.

Large-volume parenterals must be terminally heat sterilized. While water for injections is the main component of these products they also incorporate other ingredients including:

- Carbohydrates, e.g. dextrose, sucrose and dextran
- Amino acids
- Lipid emulsions which contain vegetable or semi-synthetic oil
- Electrolytes such as sodium chloride
- Polyols, including glycerol, sorbitol and mannitol.

Most large-volume parenteral fluids are clear aqueous solutions, except for the oil-in-water emulsions. The production of emulsions for infusion is highly specialized as they are destabilized by heat. This results in production difficulties, particularly because the size of the oil droplets must be carefully controlled during the heat sterilization.

Production of large-volume parenteral products

The fluids are produced and filled into containers in a high-standard clean room environment (see Ch. 13). The high standards are required to limit the contamination of these products with organisms, pyrogens and particulate matter. Use of stringent quality assurance procedures is essential to ensure the quality of the products.

In commercial manufacturing facilities large volumes of fluids are used in the production of a batch of product. The fluids are packaged from a bulk container into the product container in highly mechanized operations using high-speed filling machines. Just before the fluid enters the container, particulate matter is removed from the fluid by passing it through an in-line membrane filter. Immediately after filling, the neck of each glass bottle is sealed with a tight-fitting rubber closure that is kept in place with a crimped aluminium cap. The outer cap is also aluminium and an outer tamper-evident closure is used.

When using plastic bags, the preformed plastic bag is aseptically filled and immediately heat sealed. As an alternative, a blow–fill–seal system can be used. This integrated system involves melting the plastic, forming the bag, filling and sealing in a high-quality clean room environment. Blow–fill–seal production decreases the problems with product handling, cleaning and particulate contamination.

Following filling of the product into containers, the fluids are examined for particulate matter and the integrity of container closures established.

Moist heat should be used to sterilize parenteral products, irrigation solutions and dialysis fluids wherever possible. This should be carried out as soon as possible after the containers have been filled. Plastic containers must be sterilized with an over-pressure during the sterilization cycle to avoid the containers bursting.

Containers and closures

Large-volume parenteral fluids are packaged into:

- Glass bottles
- PVC collapsible bags
- Semi-rigid polythene containers.

The containers and closures that are used for packaging parenteral products must:

- Maintain the sterility of the packed fluids
- Withstand sterilization
- Be compatible with the packed fluid
- Allow withdrawal of the contents.

Glass bottles are normally made of Type II glass (Fig. 25.4), but Type I glass is used for products that have a high pH, despite the increased costs. Glass bottles have advantages for packaging these fluids as they are transparent and chemically inert. They may be used for products that are incompatible with plastic containers. Glass bottles also have some disadvantages. They are much heavier than plastic and therefore less transportable. Although they are strong, they are also brittle, and subject to damage during transport and storage. During use they require the use of an air inlet filter device for pressure equilibration within the container. Particles of glass can be released into the injection fluids. Damage to the neck of the bottles may result in contamination of the container contents from the external environment. A further problem with glass containers may occur during moist heat sterilization. This results in contamination of the fluid due to a pressure imbalance between the internal and external environment. Owing to these difficulties with glass containers, plastic containers have become widely used.

PVC collapsible bags are used to package most infusion fluids. They are designed with a port for the attachment of the administration set and an additive port for the addition of small-volume parenteral fluids.

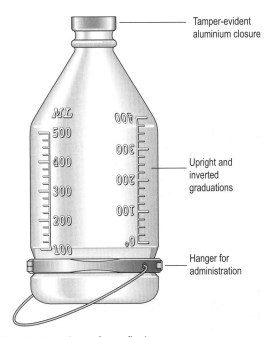

Fig. 25.4 Glass infusion fluid container.

Tamper-evident aluminium closure

Upright and inverted graduations

Hanger for administration

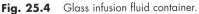

PVC collapsible bags are:

- Resistant to impact
- Flexible and collapse during fluid administration and so do not require an air inlet system.

The disadvantages of plastic bags are:

- They permit a high moisture penetration
- They adsorb some drugs
- They require an extended sterilization time due to the heat resistance of the PVC
- Moist heat sterilization requires air ballasting to avoid pouch explosion.

Semi-rigid plastic containers are used for volumes of 100 mL for electrolyte solutions, 3 L for total parenteral nutrition solutions and up to 5 L for dialysis solutions.

Semi-rigid containers:

- Are more drug compatible than PVC containers
- Are difficult to break
- Do not fully collapse
- Need extended heat sterilization times
- Need air equilibration.

Semi-rigid bags are designed with two ports. One port allows the attachment of the administration set. The other port permits the addition of small-volume parenteral

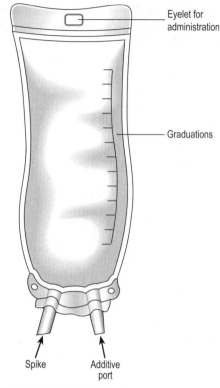

Fig. 25.5 Semi-rigid infusion bag.

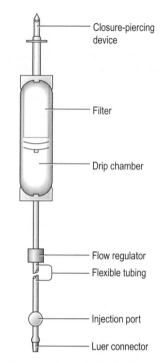

Fig. 25.6 Diagram of a typical administration set. (From BS 2463: Part 2 1989, reproduced with permission.)

products or small-volume infusion fluids. These containers are intended for single use. They have a graduated scale that can be read either in an inverted or upright position (Fig. 25.5). To enable containers of large-volume parenterals to be suspended from a drip stand for administration, bags are made with an eyelet opening that can be pierced to suspend the bag. Glass bottles are supplied with a plastic band that fits around the container to allow the bottle to be suspended during fluid administration.

Administration of large-volume parenteral fluids

All large-volume parenterals are administered to the patient by a parenteral route using a wide variety of administration sets. Most infusion fluids are administered using the standard infusion set specified in British Standard 2463 (Part 2, 1989). These sets are packaged as sterile units intended for single use (Fig. 25.6). Fluid moves through them by gravity, at a rate that is affected by the physical characteristics of the fluid and the fluid pressure, determined by the height of the infusion above the patient. The administration set is made up of a rigid plastic spike that is inserted into the rubber

septum of an infusion container. A filter that removes any particles from the fluid is positioned above a clear drip-control chamber, which aids monitoring the fluid flow rate. These components are connected by at least a 150 cm length of clear flexible tubing. The tubing has a flow regulator and a rubber injection port. The tubing is fitted with a Luer connector for attachment to a needle or catheter that is inserted into the vein of a patient.

Labelling

Batch-produced products have identical labels attached to both the product and the outer packaging carton that is used for transport. With flexible plastic containers, the labelling requirements are commonly printed directly onto the container prior to filling. With bags containing total parenteral nutrition fluids, a label is placed on the bag itself and an identical label is attached to the outer plastic cover on the bag. Labels are attached to infusion fluid containers. The labels on parenteral fluids should include the following details:

- Product identity and details of the contained volume
- Solution strength in terms of the amount of active ingredient in a suitable dose-volume

- Batch number and product expiry date
- Storage requirements
- For total parenteral nutrition (TPN) solutions, the name of the patient, the unit number, ward and infusion rate.

Containers often carry a warning label to discard the remaining product when treatment is completed.

ASEPTIC DISPENSING

Most parenteral fluids are terminally moist heat sterilized. However, some products are aseptically compounded from sterile ingredients in the hospital pharmacy. These products are prepared and dispensed for individual patients. Examples of aseptically prepared products are TPN fluids and the aseptic reconstitution of freeze-dried formulations. These freeze-dried products are often reconstituted using either water for injections or 0.9% sodium chloride injection. Aseptic dispensing is performed in a Grade A clean room environment or a Grade A isolator chamber (see Ch. 13). The dispensing of these products relies on good aseptic procedures to ensure the sterility of the product. Owing to the absence of terminal sterilization it is important that manufacture is performed using rigorous quality assurance procedures. Aseptically dispensed products are given a very limited expiry time.

Infusion fluids used for nutrition

Nutrients can be delivered to patients by intravenous administration. This is known as total parenteral nutrition and should allow for both tissue synthesis and anabolism. Some patients require TPN for prolonged periods. Initially patients are provided with their TPN in hospital. They may then undergo training to allow self-administration at home. This is known as home parenteral nutrition. Information on total and home parenteral nutrition is given in Chapter 28.

Admixtures

These are prepared by adding at least one sterile injection to an intravenous infusion fluid for administration. The injections to be added are packed in an ampoule or vial, or may be reconstituted from a solid. These additions should be carried out using aseptic procedures in a Grade A environment within an isolator cabinet or clean room facility. This environment is required to maintain the sterility of the product and avoid contamination of the product with par-

ticulate matter, microorganisms and pyrogens. Following the additions, a sealing cap may be placed over the additive port of the infusion bag to prevent further, potentially incompatible, additions at ward level. Hospital pharmacies often have a centralized intravenous additive service (CIVAS) as detailed in Chapter 27. These facilities ensure that additions to infusion fluids are carried out in a suitable environment.

Novel delivery systems

Special delivery systems are used to facilitate self-medication by patients in a home environment. Some of these delivery systems are described below.

Infusion devices

There are situations that require strict control of the volume of fluids that are infused into a patient. Accurate flow control with infusion devices is vital for patient safety and for optimum efficacy of the infusion. A range of delivery systems are available that regulate the volume of fluid administered to the patient.

These systems are used both in the hospital and for the self-administration of fluids by patients at home. The selection of an infusion device for the self-administration of medicines by patients requires careful consideration of several factors including:

- Delivery volume and control of flow rate
- Complexity of the administration procedure
- Type of therapy being administered
- Frequency of dosing
- Reservoir volume available in the infusion device.

Infusion devices available include:

- Infusion pumps and controllers
- Elastomeric infusers
- Electromechanical syringe pumps.

All these devices should be:

- Mechanically reliable with accurate flow rates
- Able to provide an output pressure which will not damage the injection site
- Supported with a back-up power supply if electrically operated
- Compact and portable
- Simple to operate for hospital staff and home care patients.

Infusion pumps

These devices use pressure as the driving force to allow administration of fluids into the patient. Infusion pumps, which can be divided into those that move fluid by a piston and valve mechanism and those that move the fluid by peristalsis, are widely used. Infusion pumps are expensive to purchase and operate but allow fluids to be accurately infused into the patient at a slow rate. These devices are becoming more sophisticated with greater electronic controls.

Infusion controller

This is a simple device that can accurately deliver the required fluid volume, although difficulties occur with the administration of viscous solutions. The device relies on gravity moving the infusion fluid down the intravenous administration set. The drop rate in the administration set drop chamber is monitored by a photoelectric mechanism. The device then applies a constriction on the tube of the administration set to give a preselected flow rate.

Elastomeric infusers

These devices are made of a rigid or flexible outer shell with an inner flexible reservoir (Fig. 25.7). The reservoir inside the device is aseptically filled with the fluid. The elasticity of the filled reservoir exerts a constant pressure. This forces the fluid through an integrated flow restriction device that controls the rate of fluid outflow. The tube from the infuser can be connected to an indwelling cannula in a central vein of the patient. These devices are expensive but they are simple to operate and allow easy home care use.

Syringe infusers

These devices are used for controlling the delivery of small volumes of intravenous infusions over a predetermined period of time. The syringe driver is widely used as an infusion controller for the administration of intravenous antibiotics and patient-controlled analgesia. They are often powered by mains electricity, or may be battery operated, although clockwork syringe infusers have limited low-risk applications. Syringe infusers move the syringe plunger by a motor-driven screw forcing the fluid into tubing for delivery to the patient. These small lightweight devices allow the administration of precise volumes of fluids. Syringe devices

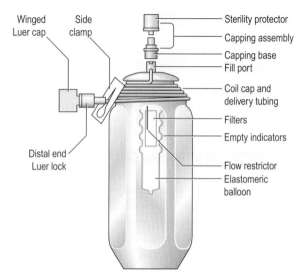

Fig. 25.7 Elastomeric infuser. (Courtesy of Baxter Healthcare Ltd.)

provide good patient home care for patient-controlled analgesia where the drug is often infused over long periods. Patient-controlled analgesia is used by patients to self-regulate the intravenous administration of pain-relieving drugs at controlled intervals. Parenteral administration gives a rapid onset of drug action.

Irrigation solutions

These solutions are applied topically to bathe open wounds and body cavities. They are sterile solutions for single use only. Examples of irrigation fluids are 0.9% sodium chloride solution or sterile water for irrigation. Most irrigation fluids are now available in rigid plastic bottles. Urological irrigation solutions are used for surgical procedures; they are usually sterile water or sterile glycine solutions and are used to remove blood and maintain tissue integrity during an operation.

Water for irrigation is sterilized distilled water that is free of pyrogens. The water is packed in containers and is intended for use on one occasion only. The containers are sealed and sterilized by moist heat.

Peritoneal dialysis fluids

Peritoneal dialysis involves the administration of dialysis solutions directly into the peritoneum by way of an indwelling catheter. The fluid is then drained after a 'dwell-time' to remove toxic waste products from the body. Peritoneal dialysis solutions are sterile solutions manufactured to the same standards as parenteral fluids. The composition of peritoneal dialysis fluid simulates potassium-free extracellular fluid. These fluids are packaged in volumes of 3–5 L in plastic containers that are similar to the bags used for total parenteral nutrition (see Ch. 28).

Haemodialysis

In this dialysis procedure, blood is removed and returned to the patient by way of a catheter, or a double needle arrangement, using a fistula where an artery and vein are joined together. The dialysis procedure involves the use of an artificial disposable membrane within a 'dialyser' machine that acts as an artificial kidney. An electrolyte fluid, simulating body fluid, bathes one side of the membrane with blood from the patient on the other side. There is no direct contact between the blood and the dialyser fluid. Thus fluids for haemodialysis do not require to be sterile or free of pyrogens or particulate matter.

Fluid volumes of 30–50 L are used daily in haemodialysis procedures (see Ch. 28).

Blood products

These products are not usually identified as sterile products although they are commonly packaged as sterile large-volume parenteral fluids. These biological products include albumin, human plasma and blood protein fractions. All these products must be treated to inactivate virus contamination prior to packaging. This is usually achieved by specialized heat treatment or filtration. These products are unstable to heat sterilization. Therefore, they are filter sterilized and then aseptically filled into containers in large-scale production facilities. Most of these products are packed as liquids, although a few blood protein fractions such as factor VIII and factor IX are freeze dried. The collection, management and distribution of these products is carried out by the blood transfusion service.

Key Points

- Convention uses the term 'parenteral' for dosage forms which are placed directly into the body.
- The three main routes are subcutaneous, intramuscular and intravenous, but many others are used in particular situations.
- Parenteral products are sterile forms used for injection, infusion or implantation.
- Glass ampoules are convenient for small volumes, but glass particles can fall into the injection during opening.
- Multiple-dose injections must have an antimicrobial preservative.
- Water for injections must be used as the aqueous ingredient in all injections.
- Water for irrigations is used in large volumes to irrigate body cavities and other areas.
- Pyrogens cause fever and must be eliminated from water for injections and water for irrigations.
- Endotoxins, from Gram-negative bacteria, are a major type of pyrogen.
- Bacterial endotoxin is detected using the LAL tests, whilst pyrogens in general are detected by the rabbit pyrogen test.
- Additives to injections include antimicrobial preservatives, antioxidants, buffers, tonicity adjusters and co-solvents.
- Injection solutions for subcutaneous, intradermal, intramuscular, intrathecal and large-volume intravenous use should be made isotonic.
- Tonicity calculations are normally based on freezing point depression, but sodium chloride equivalents, molar concentrations and serum osmolarity can be used.
- There is a wide range of large-volume parenteral products, including infusion fluids, total parenteral nutrition, dialysis fluids and irrigation solutions.
- All large-volume parenteral products must be sterilized after filling into their final containers.
- Large-volume parenteral products may be packaged in glass bottles, semi-rigid or collapsible plastic containers.
- When aseptic dispensing is required, rigorous quality assurance is essential and a 1-week expiry date is given to the product.
- A range of infusion devices is available for hospital use and to assist patients' self-administration of infusions at home.
- Sterile solutions have other uses, such as in peritoneal dialysis.

Ophthalmic products

R. M. E. Richards

After studying this chapter you should be able to:

Discuss the formulation, preparation and uses of single- and multiple-dose ophthalmic solutions

Discuss the formulation, preparation and uses of ophthalmic ointments

Explain the packaging and labelling requirements for ophthalmic preparations

Advise patients on the use of eye medication and on any adverse effects they experience

Describe the anatomy and physiology of the eye in relation to the administration of medication and the wearing of contact lenses

Explain the properties of contact lenses in relation to their physicochemical composition

Discuss the wearing of and caring for contact lenses and the various products available to facilitate comfort, effectiveness, convenience and safety

Highlight the role of antimicrobial preservatives in ophthalmic products with particular reference to the high-risk microbial contaminants *Pseudomonas aeruginosa* and *Acanthamoeba keratitis*

Advise patients on the possible adverse effects of concurrent medication and the sensible use of cosmetics when wearing contact lenses

Introduction

The human eye is a remarkable organ and the ability to see is one of our most treasured possessions. Thus the highest standards are necessary in the compounding of ophthalmic preparations and the greatest care is required in their use. It is necessary that all ophthalmic preparations are sterile and essentially free from foreign particles.

These preparations may be categorized as follows:

- Eye drops including solutions and suspensions of active medicaments for instillation into the conjunctival sac
- Eye lotions for irrigating and cleansing the eye surface, or for impregnating eye dressings
- Eye ointments, creams and gels containing active ingredient(s) for application to the lid margins and/or conjunctival sac
- Contact lens solutions to facilitate the wearing and care of contact lenses
- Parenteral products for intracorneal, intravitreous or retrobulbar injection
- Ophthalmic inserts placed in the conjunctival sac and designed to release active ingredient over a prolonged period
- Powders for the preparation of eye drops and powders for the preparation of eye lotions.

Medicaments contained in ophthalmic products include:

- Anaesthetics used topically in surgical procedures
- Anti-infectives such as antibacterials, antifungals and antivirals
- Anti-inflammatories such as corticosteroids and antihistamines
- Antiglaucoma agents to reduce intraocular pressure, such as beta-blockers
- Astringents such as zinc sulphate
- Diagnostic agents such as fluorescein which highlight damage to the epithelial tissue
- Miotics such as pilocarpine which constrict the pupil and contract the ciliary muscle, increasing drainage from the anterior chamber
- Mydriatics and cycloplegics such as atropine which dilate the pupil and paralyse the ciliary muscle and thus facilitate the examination of the interior of the eye.

Anatomy and physiology of the eye

Figure 26.1 gives an indication of the relevance of the external structures of the eye and the structure of the eyelids to the application of medication and the wearing of contact lenses.

FORMULATION OF EYE DROPS

The components of an eye drop formulation are given below:

- Active ingredient(s) to produce desired therapeutic effect
- Vehicle, usually aqueous but occasionally may be oil, e.g. tetracycline hydrochloride
- Antimicrobial preservative to eliminate any microbial contamination during use and thus maintain sterility
- Adjuvants to adjust tonicity, viscosity or pH in order to increase the 'comfort' in use and to increase the stability of the active ingredient(s)

- Suitable container for administration of eye drops which maintains the preparation in a stable form and protects from contamination during preparation, storage and use.

The single most important requirement of eye drops is that they are sterile. During the 1940s and 1950s there were several instances reported where microbially contaminated eye drops were used and consequently introduced infection into the eyes being treated. The results were particularly damaging when the contaminating organism was *Pseudomonas aeruginosa* which is difficult to treat successfully and can cause loss of the eye.

Antimicrobial preservatives

It is essential that multiple-dose eye drops contain an effective antimicrobial preservative system which is capable of withstanding the test for efficacy of antimicrobial preservatives of the *British Pharmacopoeia* (BP 2001). This is to ensure that the eye drops are maintained sterile during use

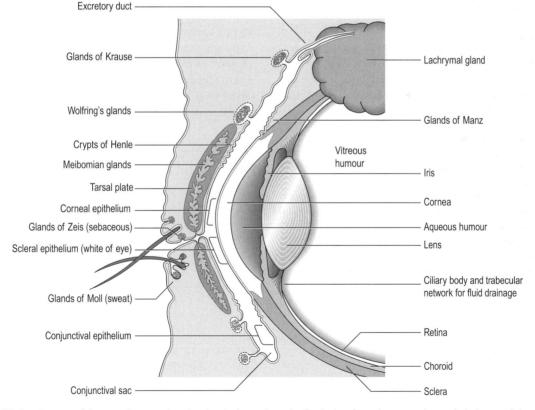

Fig. 26.1 Section of the eye showing the glands which produce the fluids that form the tears, the epithelial sites of drug absorption and the internal sites of pharmacological action.

and will not introduce contamination into the eyes being treated. Normal healthy eyes are quite efficient at preventing penetration by microorganisms. Eyes that have damaged epithelia have their defences compromised and may be colonized by microorganisms. This has to be guarded against. The lack of vascularity of the cornea and certain internal structures of the eye make it very susceptible and difficult to treat once infection has been established.

No single substance is entirely satisfactory for use as a preservative for ophthalmic solutions. The systems that have been used, based on work of the author and others in the 1960s, have formed the basis of effective preservation over the subsequent years.

It should be noted that eye drops supplied for use during intraocular surgery should not contain a preservative because of the risk of damage to the internal surfaces of the eye.

Preservatives which are suitable for a selection of eye drops are given in Box 26.1.

Benzalkonium chloride

This quaternary ammonium compound is the preservative of choice if not otherwise contraindicated for reasons of compatibility or patient sensitivity. It is present in over 70% of commercially produced eye drops and over a third of these also contain disodium edetate, usually at 0.1% w/v.

Rather surprisingly benzalkonium chloride is not a pure material, but is a mixture of alkylbenzyldimethyl ammonium compounds. This permits a mixture of alkyl chain lengths containing even numbers of carbon atoms between 8 and 18 and results in products of different activities. The higher the chain length the greater the antibacterial activity but the less the solubility. Therefore the manufacturer should seek to maximize the activity within the constraints of solubility. This means maximizing the proportions of C_{12}, C_{14} and C_{16}. It should be noted that Benzalkonium Chloride BP contains 50% w/v benzalkonium chloride.

Benzalkonium chloride is well tolerated on the eye up to concentrations of 0.02% w/v but is usually used at 0.01% w/v. It is stable to sterilization by autoclaving. The compound has a rapid bactericidal action in clean conditions against a wide range of Gram-positive and Gram-negative organisms. It destroys the external structures of the cell (cell envelope). It is active in the controlled aqueous environment and pH values of ophthalmic solutions. Activity is reduced in the presence of multivalent cations (Mg^{2+}, Ca^{2+}). These compete with the antibacterial for negatively charged sites on the bacterial cell surface. It also has its activity reduced if heated with methylcellulose or formulated with anionic and certain concentrations of non-ionic surfactants. Benzalkonium chloride is incompatible with fluorescein (large anion) and nitrates and is sorbed from solutions through contact with rubber.

The antibacterial activity of benzalkonium is enhanced by aromatic alcohols (benzyl alcohol, 2-phenylethanol and 3-phenylpropanol) and its activity against Gram-negative organisms is greatly enhanced by chelating agents such as disodium edetate. These agents chelate the divalent cations,

Box 26.1 Preservatives suitable for specific eye drops		
Benzalkonium chloride (BZK) 0.01% w/v	**Chlorhexidine acetate (CHX) 0.01% w/v**	**Phenylmercuric nitrate* (PMN) 0.002% w/v**
Atropine sulphate	Cocaine	Tetracaine (amethocaine)
Carbachol	Cocaine and homatropine	Chloramphenicol
Cyclopentolate		Fluorescein[†]
Homatropine		Hydrocortisone and neomycin
Hyoscine		Lachesine
Hypromellose		Neomycin
Phenylephrine		Sulfacetamide
Physostigmine		Zinc sulphate
Pilocarpine		Zinc sulphate and adrenaline
Prednisolone		(epinephrine)

* The acetate may also be used.
[†] This is preferably used as single dose preparations.

principally Mg^{2+} of Gram-negative cells. These ions form bridges and bind the polysaccharide chains which protrude from the outer membrane of these cells. Thus the integrity of the membrane is compromised and the benzalkonium chloride activity enhanced. This is particularly valuable in preserving against contamination with the most feared bacterial contaminant, *Ps. aeruginosa*.

The surface activity of benzalkonium chloride may be used to enhance the transcorneal passage of non-lipid-soluble drugs such as carbachol. Care must be taken since the preservative can solubilize the outer oily protective layer of the precorneal film. This film has an internal mucin layer in contact with the corneal and scleral epithelia, a middle aqueous layer and an outer oily layer. The oil prevents excessive aqueous evaporation and protects the inner surface of the lids from constant contact with water. The blink reflex helps maintain the integrity of the precorneal film. It is important not to use benzalkonium chloride with local anaesthetics. The combination of the anaesthetic abolishing the blink reflex and the preservative solubilizing the oily layer results in drying of the eye and irritation of the cornea.

Chlorhexidine acetate or gluconate

Chlorhexidine is a cationic biguanide bactericide with antibacterial properties in aqueous solution similar to benzalkonium chloride. Its activity is often reduced in the presence of other formulation ingredients. It is used at 0.01% w/v. Its antibacterial activity against Gram-negative bacteria is enhanced by aromatic alcohols and by disodium edetate. Activity is antagonized by multivalent cations. Stability is greatest at pH 5–6 but it is less stable to autoclaving than benzalkonium chloride. Chlorhexidine salts are generally well tolerated by the eye although allergic reactions may occur.

Chlorbutanol

This chlorinated alcohol is used at 0.5% w/v and is effective against bacteria and fungi. Chlorbutanol is compatible with most ophthalmic products. The main disadvantages are its volatility, absorption by plastic containers and lack of stability at high temperatures. For example, at autoclaving temperatures it breaks down to produce hydrochloric acid which produces solutions of pH 3–4. Although chlorobutanol is more stable at low pH such solutions are not desirable for eye drops.

Phenylmercuric salts

Phenylmercuric acetate and nitrate are organic mercurials and are used in the concentration range 0.001–0.04% w/v. They are slowly active over a wide pH range against bacteria and fungi. Activity is increased by phenylethanol and decreased by disodium edetate. Incompatibilities include halides. Absorption by rubber is marked.

Opinion is against using heavy metals as preservatives if there are suitable alternatives. The organic mercurials should not be used in eye drops which require prolonged usage because such use can lead to intraocular deposition of mercury (mercurialentis).

Thiomersal

This is another organic mercurial and is used at a concentration of 0.005–0.01% w/v. Its action is bacteriostatic and fungistatic. Allergy to this preservative is possible.

Tonicity

Where possible eye drops are made isotonic with lachrymal fluid (approximately equivalent to 0.9% w/v sodium chloride solution). In practice the eye will tolerate small volumes of eye drops having tonicities in the range equivalent to 0.7–1.5% w/v sodium chloride. Nevertheless it is good practice to adjust the tonicity of hypotonic eye drops by the addition of sodium chloride to bring the solution to the tonicity of the lachrymal fluid. Methods for calculating the amount of sodium chloride required are given in Chapter 25. Likewise non-essential increases in the tonicity of hypertonic solutions should be avoided. Some preparations are themselves hypertonic and this cannot be avoided.

If the physiology of the eye is adversely affected, such as when tear film is deficient, or even where hard contact lenses are worn, then the eye surface is more sensitive to variations in tonicity and eye drops should be as near as possible isotonic.

Viscosity enhancers

There is a general assumption that increasing the viscosity of an eye drop increases the residence time of the drop in the eye and results in increased penetration and therapeutic action of the drug. Most commercial preparations have their viscosities adjusted to be within the range 15–25 millipascal seconds (mPas). It should be noted that gently pressing downwards on the inside corner of the closed eye restricts the drainage channel into the nasal cavity and prolongs contact time. This has been recommended to increase the therapeutic index of antiglaucoma medications. Under normal conditions a large proportion of a typical 50 µL drop will have drained from the conjunctival sac (capacity 25 µL) within 30 seconds. There will be no trace of the drop after 20 minutes.

Viscolizing agents include methylcellulose derivatives and polyvinyl alcohol.

Hypromellose

The hydroxypropyl derivative of methylcellulose is the most popular cellulose derivative employed. It has good solubility characteristics (soluble in cold but insoluble in hot water) and good optical clarity. Typical concentrations in eye drop formulations are 0.5–2.0% w/v. Higher concentrations tend to form crusts on the eyelids.

Polyvinyl alcohol

This is used at 1.4% w/v. It has a good contact time on the eye surface and good optical qualities. As well as withstanding autoclaving, it can be filtered through a 0.22 µm filter.

Polyvinylpyrrolidone, polyethylene glycol and dextrin have also been used as viscolizing agents.

pH adjustment

The best compromise is required after considering the following factors:

- The pH offering the best stability during preparation and storage
- The pH offering the best therapeutic activity
- The comfort of the patient.

Most active ingredients are salts of weak bases and are most stable at an acid pH but most active at a slightly alkaline pH.

The lachrymal fluid has a pH of 7.2–7.4 and also possesses considerable buffering capacity. Thus a 50 µL eye drop which is weakly buffered will be rapidly neutralized by lachrymal fluid. Where possible very acidic solutions, such as adrenaline (epinephrine) acid tartrate or pilocarpine hydrochloride, are buffered to reduce stinging on instillation. Suitable buffers are shown in Box 26.2.

Antioxidants

Reducing agents are preferentially oxidized and are added to eye drops in order to protect the active ingredient from

---

> **Box 26.2 Buffers suitable for some specific eye drops**
>
> **Borate buffer (boric acid/borax): pH range 6.8–9.1**
> Chloramphenicol eye drops: BP 1993—pH 7.5
> Hypromellose eye drops: BPC1973—pH 8.4
>
> **Phosphate buffer (sodium acid phosphate/sodium phosphate): pH range 4.5–8.5**
> Neomycin eye drops BPC: 1973—pH 6.5
> Prednisolone sodium phosphate eye drops: BPC 1973—pH 6.6
>
> **Citrate buffer (citric acid/sodium citrate): pH range 2.5–6.5**
> Benzylpenicillin eye drops—pH 6.0
> Idoxuridine eye drops—pH 6.0

---

oxidation. Active ingredients requiring protection include adrenaline (epinephrine), proxymetacaine, sulfacetamide, tetracaine (amethocaine), phenylephrine and physostigmine. With physostigmine, the antioxidant is purely cosmetic as the initial breakdown product is formed by hydrolysis. The antioxidant only prevents the subsequent discoloration of this product produced by oxidation.

Sodium metabisulphite and sodium sulphite

Both may be used as antioxidants at 0.1% w/v. The former is preferred at acid pH and the latter at alkaline pH. Both are stable in solution when protected from light. Sodium metabisulphite possesses marked antimicrobial properties at acid pH and enhances the activity of phenylmercuric nitrate at acid pH. It is incompatible with predinisolone phosphate, adrenaline (epinephrine), chloramphenicol and phenylephrine.

Chelating agents

Traces of heavy metals can catalyse breakdown of the active ingredient by oxidation and other mechanisms. Therefore chelating agents such as disodium edetate may be included to chelate the metal ions and thus enhance stability. It is seen that disodium edetate is a very useful adjuvant to ophthalmic preparations at concentrations of up to 0.1% w/v to enhance antibacterial activity and chemical stability. It has also been used at higher concentrations as an eye drop for the treatment of lime burns in cattle.

Bioavailability

The effect of pH on the therapeutic activity of weak bases such as atropine sulphate has already been indicated under the section on pH adjustment. At acid pH these bases exist in the ionized hydrophilic form. In order to penetrate the cornea, the bases need to be at alkaline pH so that they are in the unionized lipophilic form. Thus at tear pH (7.4) they are able to penetrate the outer lipid layer of the lipid–water–lipid sandwich which constitutes the physico-chemical structure of the cornea. Once inside the epithelium the undissociated free base will partially dissociate. The water-soluble dissociated moiety will then traverse the middle aqueous stromal layer of the cornea. When the dissociated drug reaches the junction of the stroma and the endothelium it will again partially associate forming the lipid-soluble moiety and thus cross the endothelium. Finally the drug will dissociate into its water-soluble form and enter the aqueous humour. From here it can diffuse to the iris and the ciliary body which are the sites of its pharmacological action (Fig. 26.1). Thus it is seen that the most effective penetration of the lipophilic–hydrophilic–lipophilic corneal membrane is by active ingredients having both hydrophilic and lipophilic forms. For example, highly water-soluble steroid phosphate esters have poor corneal penetration but the less water-soluble, more lipophilic steroid acetate has much better corneal penetration. This also explains why the more lipophilic dipivalyladrenaline 0.1% w/v is as active as 2% w/v of the more hydrophilic adrenaline (epinephrine).

Storage conditions

To minimize degradation of eye drop ingredients storage temperature and conditions must be considered at the time of formulation. The stability of several drugs used in eye drops is improved by refrigerated storage (2–8°C) and the following eye drops are recommended for such storage: Chloramphenicol, Eppy, Minims, Mydrilate, Neosporin, Otosporin, Sno-Phenicol and Sno-Pilo.

Containers for eye drops

Containers should be regarded as part of the total formulation. They should protect the eye drops from microbial contamination, moisture and air. Container materials should not be shed or leached into solution neither should any of the eye drop formulation be sorbed (adsorbed and absorbed) by the container. If the product is to be sterilized in the final container all parts of the container must withstand the sterilization process used.

Containers may be made of glass or plastic and may be single or multiple dose. The latter should not contain more than 10 mL. Both single-dose and multiple-dose packs must have tamper-evident closures and packaging.

Single-dose containers

The 'Minims' range manufactured by Smith & Nephew Pharmaceuticals Ltd is the most widely used type of single-dose eye drop container in the UK. It consists of an injection-moulded polypropylene container which is sealed at its base and has a nozzle sealed with a screw cap. This container is sterilized by autoclaving in an outer heat-sealed pouch with peel-off paper backing.

Plastic bottles

Most commercially prepared eye drops are supplied in plastic dropper bottles similar to the illustration in Figure 26.2. The bottles are made of polyethylene or polypropylene and are sterilized by ionizing radiation prior to filling under aseptic conditions with the previously sterilized preparation.

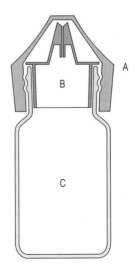

Fig. 26.2 Plastic eye drop bottle. (A) Rigid plastic cap; (B) polythene friction plug containing baffle that produces uniform drops; (C) polythene bottle.

Glass bottles

Most extemporaneously prepared eye drops are supplied in 10 mL amber partially ribbed glass bottles.

The components of the eye dropper bottle are illustrated in Figure 26.3.

The important information to know about the bottle is the glass composition. The bottle is made of either neutral glass or soda glass which has had the internal surfaces treated during manufacture to reduce the release of alkali when in contact with aqueous solutions. The former bottles can be autoclaved more than once but the latter can only be autoclaved once.

Likewise it is necessary to know whether the teat is made of good quality natural or synthetic rubber. The former will withstand autoclaving at 115°C for 30 minutes but will not

withstand the high temperatures of dry heat sterilization. The latter teats, made from silicone rubber, will withstand dry heat sterilization and are suitable for use with oily eye drops. Surprisingly silicone rubber is permeable to water vapour which was not realized initially. As a result aqueous suspensions sometimes became solid cakes! For this reason aqueous eye drops having silicone rubber teats are given a limited shelf life of 3 months. This can be lengthened by supplying the sterile eye drops in an eye drop bottle sealed with an ordinary screw cap together with a separately wrapped and sterilized silicone rubber dropper unit. The dropper is carefully substituted for the cap when the eye drops are about to be used.

Teats and caps are used once only. All components are thoroughly washed with filtered distilled or deionized water, dried and stored in a clean area until required.

Rubber teats sorb preservatives and antioxidants during autoclaving and storage. Generalized quantitative relationships for this process do not exist and it is necessary that individual studies are undertaken during formulation to help counteract preservative and antioxidant loss.

PREPARATION OF EYE DROPS

Extemporaneous preparation of eye drops involves the following:

- Preparation of the solution
- Clarification
- Filling and sterilization.

Preparation of the solution

The aqueous eye drop vehicle containing any necessary preservative, antioxidant, stabilizer, tonicity modifier, viscolizer or buffer should be prepared first. Then the active ingredient is added and the vehicle made up to volume.

Clarification

The BP has stringent requirements for the absence of particulate matter in eye drop solutions. Sintered glass filters or membrane filters of 0.45–1.2 μm pore sizes are suitable. The clarified solution is either filled directly into the final containers which are sealed prior to heat sterilization or filled into a suitable container prior to filtration sterilization. Clarified vehicle is used to prepare eye drop suspensions which are filled into final containers and sealed prior to sterilization.

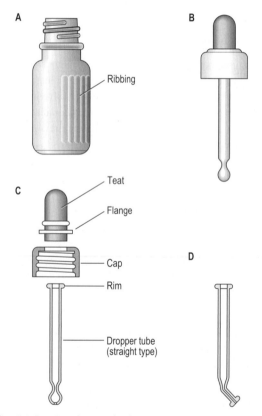

Fig. 26.3 Eye dropper bottle to BS 1679; Part 5 (1974): (**A**) bottle; (**B**) assembled closure; (**C**) components of closure; (**D**) dropper tube (angled type). (Reproduced by permission of the British Standards Institution (complete copies can be obtained from BSI at Linford Wood, Milton Keynes, MK14 6LE).)

Sterilization

This can take the form of:

- Autoclaving at 115°C for 30 minutes or 121°C for 15 minutes.
- Filtration through a membrane filter having a 0.22 μm pore size into sterile containers using strict aseptic technique. Filling should take place under Grade A laminar airflow conditions (see Ch. 13).
- Dry heat sterilization at 160°C for 2 hours is employed for non-aqueous preparations such as liquid paraffin eye drops. Silicone rubber teats must be used.

Immediately following sterilization the eye drop containers must be covered with a readily breakable seal, such as a viskring, to distinguish between opened and unopened containers.

LABELLING OF CONTAINER

Labelling requirements are summarized in Table 26.1 and Box 26.3.

INSTILLATION OF EYE DROPS

- Wash hands.
- Tilt head back and with one hand gently pull down lower eyelid to form a pouch between the eye and the eyelid.

- Hold dropper bottle, or separate eye dropper containing eye drops, above the eye and drop a single drop into the preformed pouch. Do not touch the dropper on the eye or eyelid.
- Release lower lid. Try not to blink more than usual as this removes the medicine from the eye.
- Replace the dropper in the bottle or the cap on the bottle.

Box 26.3   Additional labelling requirements for use in specific locations

All locations
Name and concentration of any antimicrobial present

Hospital: wards
Patient's name. The eye to be treated. Date of opening bottle and/or date to discard (14 days later)

Hospital: operating theatres
Single dose for once-only use. Marked with indication of active ingredient and concentration. No preservative. Outer package fully labelled

Hospital: clinics
Single-dose or multidose used once only

Domiciliary
'Avoid contamination of contents during use'. 'Discard 28 days after opening'. 'Keep out of the reach of children'. Note: If both eyes are to be treated and the patient has an open infection and/or medical opinion dictates, a separate bottle is supplied for each eye and labelled accordingly.

Table 26.1   Labelling requirements for eye drop and eye ointment containers at the time of dispensing. (Based on Department of Health guidance HSC(IS)122 1975 revised by the RPSGB 2001)

Requirement	Include on label
State route of administration	'For use in the eye only'
Fully identify the product	The name and concentration of the active ingredient(s)
Statement on preservation	Confirm presence or absence of preservative
Directions for use	e.g. 'Add one drop to each eye morning and evening'
State an 'in use' expiry date	Day, month, year
Storage requirements	'Store in a cool place' or 'Protect from light'
Identify patient	Patient's name
Date of dispensing	Day, month, year

Note: When the stability of the final preparation requires it, eye drops may be provided in two containers as a dry powder and an aqueous vehicle. The labels should state 'Powder for eye drops' on one container and the directions for the preparation of the eye drops on the other package or container.

Patients who have not used eye drops before need an explanation of how to instil the drops satisfactorily.

FORMULATION OF EYE LOTIONS

As stated in the introduction to this chapter the purpose of eye lotions is to assist in the cleaning of the external surfaces of the eye. This might be to help remove a non-impacted foreign body or to clean away conjunctival discharge. Eye lotions intended for use in surgical or first-aid procedures should not contain antimicrobial preservatives and should be supplied in single-use containers. There is no intention to use an eye lotion to deliver any active ingredient to the eye but rather to remove unwanted gross contaminants from the eye. Thus these preparations should be very simple and the most common eye lotion consists of sterile normal saline. This preparation typifies the requirements of an eye lotion which are:

- Sterile and usually containing no preservative
- Isotonic with lachrymal fluid
- Neutral pH
- Large volume but not greater than 200 mL
- Non-irritant to ocular tissue.

Labels

These should include:

- Title identifying the product and concentration of contents
- 'Sterile until opened'
- 'Not to be taken'
- 'Use once and discard the remaining solution'
- Expiry date.

Preserved eye lotion would need the additional labelling:

- 'Avoid contamination of contents during use'
- 'Discard remaining solutions not more than 4 weeks after first opening'.

The lotions should be supplied in coloured fluted bottles and sealed to exclude microorganisms.

Powders for the preparation of eye drops and powders for the preparation of eye lotions

These powders are supplied in a dry, sterile form for dissolving or suspending in an appropriate vehicle at the time of use

to provide a solution or suspension which complies with the requirements for eye drops or eye lotions as appropriate. The powders may contain suitable excipients to aid dissolution or dispersion, to adjust the tonicity and to improve stability.

FORMULATION OF EYE OINTMENTS

Eye ointments are popular and duplicate many of the therapeutic options offered by eye drops. Ointments have the disadvantage of temporarily interfering with vision, but have the advantage over liquids of providing greater total drug bioavailability. However, ointments take a longer time to reach peak absorption.

Eye ointments must be sterile and may contain suitable antimicrobial preservatives, antioxidants and stabilizers. The *United States Pharmacopoeia* (USP 25) requires these ointments to contain one of the following antimicrobials: chlorobutanol, the parabens or the organic mercurials. It is necessary also that such ointments are free from particulate matter that could be harmful to the tissues of the eye. The *European Pharmacopoeia* (EP 2001) and BP (2001) have limits for the particle size of incorporated solids. For each 10 micrograms of active solid there should be no particles >90 μm, not more than 2 particles >50 μm and not more than 20 >25 μm.

The basic components of an eye ointment are given below:

Liquid paraffin	1 part
Wool fat	1 part (to facilitate incorporation of water)
Yellow soft paraffin	8 parts

Hard paraffin as required to produce required consistency in hot climates.

Containers for eye ointments

Eye ointments should be supplied in small sterilized collapsible tubes made of metal or a suitable plastic. The tube should not contain more than 5 g of preparation and must be fitted or provided with a nozzle of a suitable shape to facilitate application to the eye and surrounds without allowing contamination of the contents. The tubes must be suitably sealed to prevent microbial contamination.

Preparation of eye ointments

Eye ointments are normally prepared using aseptic techniques to incorporate the finely powdered active ingredient or a sterilized concentrated solution of the medicament into the sterile eye ointment basis. Immediately after preparation the eye ointment is filled into the sterile containers which are then sealed so as to exclude microorganisms. The screw cap should be covered with a readily breakable seal.

All apparatus used in the preparation of eye ointments must be scrupulously clean and sterile. Certain commercial eye ointments may be sterilized in their final containers using ionizing radiation.

Preparation of eye ointment basis

The paraffins and the wool fat are heated together and filtered, while molten, through a coarse filter paper in a heated funnel into a container which can withstand dry heat sterilization temperatures. The container is closed to exclude microorganisms and together with contents is maintained at 160°C for 2 hours.

OPHTHALMIC INSERTS

These are sterile solid or semi-solid preparations for insertion in the conjunctival sac. They contain a reservoir of active material which is slowly released from a matrix or through a rate-controlling membrane over a known time period. Ophthalmic inserts each have their own sterile container which is labelled to state the total quantity of active substance per insert and, where applicable, its rate of release.

Monitoring of eye preparations for adverse effects

Pharmacists should be available to counsel patients on the use of their eye medication and advise them about any adverse effects they may experience while using their medicines. Failing to use eye medication appropriately may also have serious consequences. It is important that the pharmacist is able to support the patient in using their medicine correctly and is alert to notice any signs/symptoms of adverse effects, resulting from medication, that the patient may be experiencing in order to give appropriate and timely advice. Table 26.2 indicates the signs/symptoms of adverse effects which may occur with eye preparations used in the treatment of primary open angle glaucoma. In addition to adverse effects associated with the eye, it should be noted that undesirable systemic effects can also occur with eye

medication. Such systemic effects have been reported for certain potent ophthalmic medicines. This is due to excess solution draining from the eye surface through two small channels, the lachrymal canaliculi, into the lachrymal sac and on via the nasolachrymal duct into the gastrointestinal tract. Consequently it is necessary to advise patients to avoid instilling excess eye drops.

Patients who are using an eye drop preparation for a chronic condition may become sensitive to the preservative in the formulation. This may happen with contact lens products also. Changing to a formulation having the same active ingredient but having a different preservative should solve the problem.

CONTACT LENSES AND THEIR SOLUTIONS

The ready accessibility of the eye and its external structures not only facilitates the use of topical medicines in the conjunctival sac and on the anterior surface of the eye but also facilitates the fitting and wearing of lenses on the precorneal film and on the surface of the eye. Optometrists prescribe and fit contact lenses and monitor their use. Pharmacists should refer patients having persistent problems with wearing their lenses to their optometrist.

Popularity, problems, risks

The popularity of contact lenses results from their cosmetic appeal, optical advantages and their usefulness in sporting activities. Many prefer extended-wear soft lenses to daily-wear soft and hard lenses because of their relative convenience.

The problems that occur with the wearing of contact lenses result from inadequate education of the wearer about lens care. Extended-wear lenses in particular have been marketed in a manner which maximizes the volume of sales at the expense of adequate consumer education. That is, the marketing of lenses has overemphasized the convenient and carefree aspects of overnight lenses to the extent of trivializing the wearing of contact lenses. This has often resulted in poor patient compliance with suggested regimens of lens wear and care. It is estimated that more than 50% of those who wear contact lenses care for them unhygienically.

The risks associated with the wearing of contact lenses include recurrent corneal abrasions, corneal scarring and corneal vascularization. However, the most dreaded

Table 26.2   Signs/symptoms of adverse effects which may occur with treatment for primary open angle glaucoma

Drugs used Dose frequency as solutions/suspensions	General signs/symptoms of adverse effects	
	Objective signs	Subjective signs
Beta-blockers	BP—hypotension	Difficulties in breathing
Timolol 2 × daily	Heart rate—slowed	dry eyes
Timolol gel 1 × daily		itchy & watery eyes
Betaxolol 2 × daily		pain after instillation
Carteolol 2 × daily		blurring of vision
Levobunolol 1 or 2 × daily		palpitations
Metipranolol 2 × daily		headaches, dizziness, anxiety
Parasympathomimetics	Heart rate—rarely	Variable blurring of vision
(Miotics)	affected	reduction in night vision
Pilocarpine 4 × daily		transient headache
Ocusert-Pilo * weekly		ocular & periorbital pain
A slow release		twitching eyelids
gel formulation * 24 hourly		sweating, GI upsets—rare
Sympathomimetics	Heart rate—quickened	Smarting & redness of eye
	BP—hypertension	itchy watery eyes
Adrenaline (epinephrine) 2 × daily	conjuntival deposits of oxidized adrenaline[†]	nasal obstruction
Guanethidine 2 × daily	conjunctival fibrosis on prolonged	dilated pupil, could
	guanethidinene use[†]	precipitate acute
		glaucoma—dangerous
		headache, blurring vision
Dipivefrine * 2 × daily		

* these formulations can reduce adverse effects
† these are specific effects

complication is microbial ulcerative keratitis or corneal ulcer, caused by bacterial invasion of the cornea. Left untreated this can lead to loss of vision. Fortunately the natural defences of the cornea are very effective and the normal cornea resists bacterial infection as long as the surface epithelium is intact.

It has been shown that the risk of corneal ulcers is 9–15 times greater for extended-wear lenses worn overnight than for daily-wear soft lenses worn only during the day. The risk increases with the number of consecutive days that lenses are worn without removal.

A serious, but fairly rare, complication that can arise from using non-sterile water in the care of lenses is infection with *Acanthamoeba keratitis*, which is hard to diagnose and to treat and can lead to serious loss of vision.

The aim of formulators and providers of contact lens systems must be to supply the safest possible system with known and acceptable risks; that is, convenience and safety must be the aim.

Relevant properties of the eye

Anatomy and physiology

Figure 26.1 indicates the structures of the eye which are particularly relevant to the use of topical medications, contact lenses and contact lens products. Firstly, it is important to note that the cornea, the lens and the humour compartments are avascular and that this property facilitates the transmission of light and vision. Secondly, exchange of nutrients and waste products in these situations takes place almost entirely by diffusion processes through the aqueous humour, through the lens and cornea and though the lachrymal fluid. Contact lenses reduce the diffusion of oxygen to the cornea and thus can affect corneal metabolism.

Secretions

The secretions of the eye have an important role and influence on the wearing of contact lenses. Tears perform the important functions of lubricating, hydrating, cleaning and disinfecting the anterior surface of the eye. The latter function is performed by the enzyme lysozyme (1,4-N-acetyl-glycosaminidase) which catalyses the hydrolysis of 1,4-glycosidic linkages between N-acetyl muramic acid and N-acetyl-glucosamine in the peptidoglycan layer of the bacterial cell wall. The peptidoglycan layer of Gram-positive cells is accessible to the action of lysozyme.

Lachrymal fluid

The fluid forming the precorneal film is produced by differing groups of glands. It contains mucus (Henle and Manz), water (Krause and Wolfring) and oil (Meibomian, Moll and Zeis). These fluids are stratified in three distinct layers. The surface-active mucoid layer spreads on the corneal surface and associates with the intermediate aqueous layer externally. The aqueous layer is surfaced with an oily layer which lubricates and protects the mucous membranes of the internal lid surfaces.

Tear electrolyte content

This is broadly similar to that of serum except that the potassium ion is approximately four to six times greater (24 mEq/L compared with 4–6 mEq/L in serum). The protein content of tears is mainly albumin and globulin and is approximately a tenth of that in serum (0.7% compared with 7%).

Tear production

Tears are produced in response to four distinct types of stimuli: emotional via psychological factors, sensory via external irritants, continuous via automatic nervous control and systemic via chemicals in the bloodstream affecting the nerves innovating the lachrymal glands.

Tear pH

This is slightly alkaline at 7.2. Tears have sufficient buffering capacity to adjust rapidly the pH of small volumes of weakly buffered solutions to pH 7.2.

Eyelids

These perform a protecting and a cleaning function. The outer margins of the eyelids close slightly before the inner margins and sweep the fluids across the eye towards the lachrymal duct at the inner angle of the eye and from where it can pass via the lachrymal sac into the gastrointestinal tract. Systemic absorption of excess eye medicament may take place through this mechanism. Conversely, by gentle pressure with the tip of a finger, the lachrymal duct may be closed temporarily and eye medicament maintained in contact with the eye surface for a longer period.

Bacterial flora

There is a common misconception that lachrymal fluid is sterile. It has been known since 1908 that staphylococci and diphtheroids can be found regularly in normal conjunctiva. Gram-negative enteric bacilli have also been isolated from the conjunctivas and lids of about 5% of people. This shows that care is necessary when wearing contact lenses to avoid abrading the corneal epithelium.

CONTACT LENSES

Sir John Herschel used a refractive glass shell in 1823 to protect the cornea from a diseased lid. Dr Eugen Fick, a Swiss physician, first used the term 'contact lens' in 1887. Fick's blown-glass lenses were intended to correct defective vision. In 1948 Tuohy introduced the hydrophobic hard plastic corneal lens and in 1962 soft pliable lenses were introduced as the result of work in Prague University. These lenses have been very popular. Gas-permeable hard lenses have also been introduced which allow oxygen perfusion to the cornea. These lenses are more comfortable than the original hard lenses.

The aim in making contact lenses is to produce lenses which will:

- Correct the patient's vision
- Maintain their position on the eye
- Allow respiration of the cornea
- Permit free flow of tears round or through the lens
- Not release toxic substances
- Not introduce microbial contamination
- Be wearable throughout the day
- Be easy to handle and economical to use.

Hard lenses

Methacrylic acid is esterified to produce the basic monomer methyl methacrylate which is polymerized using benzoyl peroxide as catalyst to produce polymethylmethacrylate (PMMA). This is popularly called 'Perspex' and has optical properties similar to spectacle crown glass. PMMA has hydrophobic properties conferred by the large proportion of methyl groups compared to hydrophilic carboxy ester groups. This means that lachrymal fluid does not readily wet lenses made of this material. Therefore the lenses need to be wetted before mounting on the precorneal film to reduce or eliminate patient discomfort. Hence the need for a wetting solution to facilitate wear and the need for a storage, hydrating, decontaminating solution to facilitate care of the lenses when not being worn. The original hard lens composition had some major disadvantages for the wearer. Free passage of oxygen and carbon dioxide to and from the corneal epithelium could not take place. Corneal oedema and distortion were a common result. Thus modern lenses have been designed to be gas permeable. These lenses are physiologically more user-friendly and have greater wearer acceptance.

The original gas-permeable lenses consisted of cellulose acetate butyrate (CAB) which was readily wettable and proved quite acceptable. More recently lenses based on silicone and fluorine have been produced which have greater gas permeability. Silicone methacrylate copolymers are very popular. The silicone composition controls the permeability properties and the PMMA composition controls the degree of rigidity. Similarly fluorosilicone methacrylate copolymers which have very high oxygen permeability properties and good wetting properties are proving to be popular. These gas-permeable lenses are cared for using hard lens solutions. These lenses are less subject than soft lenses to deposits of lipids, protein and other substances from the lachrymal fluid. They also have better optical qualities and are generally easier to care for.

Soft lenses

The hydroxyethyl ester of polymethacrylic acid (poly-HEMA) is prepared. The large number of polar hydroxyl groups confer hydrophilic properties to the polymer. Poly-HEMA is flexible and can absorb about 47% of its own weight of water. Thus lenses of this material are comfortable and easy to wear but more difficult to care for than hard lenses. A particular problem is uptake of antibacterial preservatives and subsequent release and irritancy during wear. Although a wetting solution is not needed, cleaning, storing, hydrating and decontaminating functions are required of solutions.

Copolymers of poly-HEMA with vinylpyrrolidine (VP) are also produced which can absorb up to 80% by weight of water depending on the HEMA/VP ratio. The higher water content lenses have the advantage of greater gas permeability and comfort than the poly-HEMA lenses which may occasionally cause corneal oedema. However, they are more fragile and difficult to care for than poly-HEMA, have a greater tendency to attract deposits, more solution problems and less precise optical properties.

Disposable lenses

It is argued that lens design, life span and manufacturing problems can be overcome by the introduction of disposable lenses. Disposable lenses may be discarded after 1 month, 1 week or even 1 day. The latter would obviate the need for the use of solutions and theoretically increase the safety and acceptability of lens wear. However, the original intention of these lenses was for extended wear without removal. It has already been pointed out that the additional risks that are associated with extended wear make this an unattractive and even dangerous practice. These lenses would seem to offer the greatest advantage to those people who wear lenses on an irregular basis for social and sporting activities and for those children who may need soft lenses.

HARD LENS SOLUTIONS

A 'wetting solution' and a 'soaking/storing/decontaminating solution' are required for the wear and routine care of hard lenses. The first is suitable for placing in the eye but the second must not have contact with the eye.

Wetting solution

Purpose

- Achieves rapid wetting by the lachrymal fluid and thus promotes comfort
- Facilitates insertion of lens
- Provides cushioning and lubrication
- Enables cleaning after removal
- Must be non-irritant during daily use.

Formulation

- Wetting and viscolizing agents—polyvinyl alcohol and hypromellose
- Viscosity 15–20 mPas for comfort
- pH 6.8
- Tonicity 0.9–1.1% sodium chloride
- Antimicrobials—benzalkonium chloride 0.004% plus disodium edetate 0.1%.

Storing solutions

Purpose

- Achieves cleaning and microbial inactivation
- Hydrating.

Formulation

- Surface-active agent not inactivating antimicrobials
- pH 7.4
- Antimicrobials—benzalkonium chloride 0.01% plus disodium edetate 0.1%.

SOFT LENS SOLUTIONS

Cleaning solutions

Purpose

- To remove deposits such as lipoprotein adhering to the lens after wear.

Formulation

- Viscolizing surface-active agent such as hypromellose to enable suitable gentle friction with fingertips.
- Antibacterial—fast-acting benzalkonium chloride 0.004% may be used if contact time is only 20–30 seconds.

Storing solutions

Purpose

- Hydrating
- Cleaning
- Inactivation of microbial contamination.

Formulation

- Isotonic ≡ 0.9% sodium chloride.
- Antibacterial—3% hydrogen peroxide for 30 minutes followed by suitable inactivation with sodium pyruvate, or platinum catalyst, or other suitable method to facilitate subsequent safe wearing of the lenses. Hydrogen peroxide has been reported to have the additional advantage of good activity against *A. keratitis* contamination. However, recent work indicated that the catalytic tablet in a one-step system possibly neutralized the 3% hydrogen peroxide too quickly and thus did not allow sufficient reaction time to kill all the *A. keratitis* cysts in the test system. This reported flaw in the system needs further investigation and correction if necessary to ensure effectiveness against *A. keratitis* which has recently been confirmed as a real if comparatively rare cause of severe corneal infection in wearers of contact lenses in the UK.

Polyquad—a polyquaternium compound has recently been introduced in soft lens solutions because it is not sorbed (neither adsorbed nor absorbed) by lenses and it has low toxicity to corneal and ocular tissues.

(Thermal disinfection is an alternative disinfection process and the American FDA stipulates heating the lenses in a suitable solution in a lens case at a minimum of 80°C for 10 minutes.)

Enzyme protein digest

Purpose

- Occasional cleaning procedure followed by suitable washing and cleansing before wear. Frequency will vary with the individual and their state of health. Influenza or hay fever for example will increase the need.

Formulation

- Proteolytic enzyme, such as papain, as a solution tablet to produce a suitable solution when dissolved in a stated volume of aqueous vehicle.

Lipid digest or combined protein and lipid digest systems are also available.

All-purpose solutions

The all-purpose solutions initially represented a compromise for hard lens wearers finding it difficult to comply with a two-solution regimen. Single-solution lens care systems are now available for soft lenses and incorporate an enzyme cleaner combined with a disinfection solution. Certain all-purpose lens solutions incorporate polyhexamide (polyhexamethylene biguanide) 0.00006–0.0004% as the antimicrobial agent. It is reported to be active against a wide range of bacteria and against *Acanthamoeba*. Such solutions would appear to be gaining in popularity.

Containers

Contact lens solutions are usually packed in plastic containers. It is imperative that the low concentrations of antimicrobials present in these products are not reduced to ineffective levels due to sorption effects with the plastic.

Contact lens storage cases are also of importance to the contact lens wearer. It is important that these containers are kept in a hygienic condition by keeping them scrupulously clean and using the disinfecting/storage solutions strictly in accordance with the manufacturers' instructions.

Advice to patients

General considerations

Contact lens wearers presenting at the pharmacy with a persistent red eye indicating an infection should not be recommended Brolene eye drops. They should be referred to an ophthalmologist. This is to guard against the possibility that the person might have an infection with *A. keratitis*. Such an infection would be more difficult to diagnose after treatment with preparations containing propamidine isethionate.

Disease states leading to a dry eye syndrome such as Sjögren's syndrome, which is mostly confined to menopausal women having osteoarthritis, will also adversely affect the ability of a person to wear contact lenses.

Hard lenses and to a less extent soft lenses interrupt the oxygen supply to the cornea and with prolonged wear produce increasing hypoxia. After approximately 16 hours of wear this corneal hypoxia results in a dip in the corneal glycogen level with resultant oedema. Irritation, itchiness, photophobia and blurred vision can result. The patient should be advised not to overwear the lenses and they may also be recommended to instil sterile sodium chloride 2% w/v every 3–4 hours, after the lenses have been removed, until the oedema has resolved. They should be warned that the hypertonic drops may cause temporary stinging on instillation.

Adverse effects of medicines

Pharmacists should understand medicine-induced problems experienced by patients wearing contact lenses so that they can offer appropriate counselling.

Certain medicines can affect the eye surface and lachrymal fluid production and thereby influence the comfort of contact lens wear. Medication having anticholinergic properties such as sedative antihistamines, chlorphenamine (chlorpheniramine), antispasmodics (hyoscine), tricyclic antidepressants and neuroleptics can all reduce lachrymal fluid production. Diuretics will also reduce tear volume and topical timolol can cause transitory dry eyes. The consequent lack of lubrication may cause lens discomfort and increased lens deposits.

Oral contraceptives may cause corneal oedema, decreased aqueous and increased mucus and protein production and thus lead to lens intolerance. Pregnancy may also be associated with increased lens awareness and discomfort possibly associated with reduced tear flow and changes in corneal thickness and the curvature of the eye. Clomifene and primidone have also been reported to cause lid and corneal oedema.

Cholinergic drugs and reserpine will increase tear volume.

Discoloration, via the lachrymal fluid, particularly with soft lenses, may occur with the administration of certain medicines such as labetalol, nitrofurantoin, phenothiazines, phenolphthalein, rifampicin, sulfasalazine and tetracyclines. Rifampicin for example will stain the lenses and tears orange.

Lenses must be removed before diagnostic dyes such as fluorescein are instilled. In fact it is a general rule that patients should be counselled not to place any ophthalmic preparation onto the eyelids or surface of the eye while contact lenses are in place.

Concurrent use of cosmetics

Lenses should always be inserted before applying eye makeup, nail polish, hand creams, perfumes or using nail polish remover. Aerosol products should be used with caution so that spray does not get between the lens and the eye. All eye makeup should be water based and powders should be avoided. Mascara (not waterproof) should only be applied to the tips of the eyelashes.

The pharmacist should be aware of the various situations mentioned above when offering advice and discussing customers/patients' questions.

Key Points

- Ophthalmic preparations must be sterile.
- Eye drops contain:
  active ingredient
  liquid vehicle free from particulate matter
  antimicrobial preservative
  adjuvants: tonicity, viscosity, pH, antioxidants,
  chelating agents.
- Eye drops are contained in a glass or plastic bottle.
- Eye lotions are:
  isotonic
  neutral pH
  large volume but not greater than 200 ml
  non-irritant
  contained in a fluted, coloured bottle.
- Eye ointments contain:
  semi-solid base
  active ingredient
  antimicrobial preservative
  adjuvants: antioxidants, stabilizers.
- Eye ointments are:
  free from harmful particulate matter
  contained in a metal or plastic tube.
- Ophthalmic inserts:
  contain a reservoir of active material
  incorporate a slow-release mechanism.
- Properties of the eye affecting formulation of products
  include:
  anatomy and physiology
  secretions
  lids
  bacterial flora.
- Contact lenses may be:
  hard lenses including gas permeable
  soft lenses including disposable.
- Contact lens solutions may be:
  hard lenses—(i) wetting and cleaning; (ii) storing and
     disinfecting; or all purpose
  soft lenses:—(i) cleaning; (ii) storing and disinfecting;
     or (iii) all purpose.
- Enzyme cleaning agents are required for all lenses.
- Pharmacists should be able to counsel patients on:
  possible adverse effects of eye medication
  common problems encountered by lens wearers
  adverse effects of concurrent medications
  concurrent use of cosmetics.

Specialized services

K. Sabra (original authors S. L. Hutchinson and D. Graham)

After studying this chapter you will know about:

The nature and formulation of cytotoxic agents

Centralized cytotoxic reconstitution services and the procedures and practices used

Precautions to be taken when preparing and administering cytotoxic agents

Domiciliary chemotherapy programmes

Scope, operation and benefits of a centralized intravenous additive service

The principles of radiopharmacy

Types of radionuclide and their use

Production of radiopharmaceuticals

The production of ^{99m}Tc

Radiation protection

Introduction

Hospital pharmacists now provide a range of specialized services in the field of parenteral medications. These will include cytotoxic medications, intravenous (IV) additives and radiopharmaceuticals. Dosage forms requested by medical staff for individual patient requirements are prepared under aseptic conditions in the hospital pharmacy. This chapter outlines the range of services provided in each of these areas and describes the role of the hospital pharmacist in this work.

PROVISION OF CYTOTOXIC CHEMOTHERAPY

Medicines used in the treatment of malignant disease are cytotoxic in nature. Cytotoxic literally means any substance that is toxic to cells. This cytotoxic effect is not limited to abnormal cells, and can cause harm to healthy cells also.

Cytotoxic medicines act by interfering with normal cell division preventing DNA and RNA replication. The mechanisms of action involved and the relative toxicities of cytotoxic medications differ from one agent to another. Health care workers involved in handling and administration of cytotoxics must have an understanding of cytotoxic agents and the rationale behind their use in the treatment of cancer.

Cytotoxic agents used routinely in the treatment of cancer can be divided into five main groups. Classification is based on mechanisms of action. The groups are described below.

Aklylating agents. These agents act by forming covalent bonds with molecules such as proteins, amino acids and nucleic acids. They can damage cell membranes, deplete amino acid, stress and inactivate enzymes. They stop cell division by forming cross-linkages between DNA chains, thus preventing DNA replication. Examples of alkylating agents are: chlormethine (mustine) hydrochloride, cyclophosphamide, ifosfamide, melphalan, chlorambucil, thiotepa, hexamethylmelamine and busulfan.

Antimetabolites. To allow normal cell division, large reserves of protein and nucleic acids must be built up. For this process to take place, certain essential metabolites must be present. These metabolites form the building blocks for the production of larger molecules. The antimetabolite drugs used in chemotherapy have a similar structure to some of these essential metabolites and can take their place in the nuclear material of the cells inhibiting biological activity. This breakdown in synthesis of essential metabolites and cell components means that cell division will not take place. Drugs in this group include methotrexate, 5-fluorouracil, cytosine arabinoside, 6-mercaptopurine and 6-thioguanine.

Vinca alkaloids. Their main mode of action is to bind to an intracellular protein, tubulin, which is involved in the process of cell mitosis. These agents stop cell division at the second phase of mitosis (metaphase), thus preventing cell reproduction. Cytotoxic agents in this group include vincristine, vinblastine and vindesine.

Antimitotic antibiotics. This is a group of agents used in the treatment of infections, which were in the past found to have an inhibitory effect on dividing tumour cells. Examples of these agents include daunorubicin, doxorubicin and epirubicin.

Miscellaneous agents. This group of agents does not fit into the other above-mentioned categories very easily. However, they have similar modes of action to some agents, e.g. cisplatin and carboplatin have similar actions to alkylating agents but vary in cross-linking mechanism of the DNA strands. Other examples in this group include procarbazine, dacarbazine and etoposide.

Cytotoxic agents can be used individually or in combination. Many oncology centres use a combination of medicines, usually denoted by the initial letters of each medicine used in the regimen, e.g. MOPP which stands for chlomethine (mustine), oncovin (approved name vincristine), procarbazine and prednisone. This combined therapy is used for treatment of Hodgkin's disease. Using more than one cytotoxic agent can be more toxic but may produce an enhanced response and an increased chance of survival for the patient. Further information about these materials and their uses is available in Walker and Edwards (2003).

DOSAGE FORMS USED FOR CYTOTOXIC MEDICINES

Cytotoxic medicines are available in a range of oral dosage forms including tablets, capsules and suspensions. Parenteral cytotoxics are available as freeze-dried powders or sterile solutions, both available in sealed vials. The freeze-dried powders are supplied ready for reconstitution with an appropriate diluent. Examples of cytotoxic products include:

- Cyclophosphamide, available as a sterile white powder in a vial. It is available in a range of strengths and contains sodium chloride to ensure isotonicity after reconstitution with water for injection.
- Methotrexate is available as a clear yellow aqueous isotonic solution for injection or in vials of yellow lyophilized powder of methotrexate sodium ready for reconstitution with water for injection.
- Cisplatin is a yellowish white freeze-dried powder which is reconstituted with water for injection and saline solution.

Parenteral cytotoxics can be administered via the following routes:

- By a syringe
- By slow bolus injection into a cannula or the side arm of an infusion
- By addition of a cytotoxic agent directly into an infusion fluid which is then administered over a predetermined infusion period.

Syringe drivers containing cytotoxic medicines and home care devices are available for use in the community for patients receiving home chemotherapy. This chapter will deal with provision of parenteral cytotoxic medications for hospital and home patients.

DOSE AND SCHEDULE OF ADMINISTERING CHEMOTHERAPEUTIC AGENTS

An explanation is given in Chapter 8 of how to calculate doses on the basis of the patient's body surface area (BSA). Clinical pharmacists specialized in oncology and haematology are now routinely expected to write the chemotherapy prescriptions as well as calculating the doses required. The signature of the treating physician might be required as well.

RISKS INVOLVED FOR HEALTH CARE WORKERS

Over the years there has been concern regarding the handling of cytotoxic agents by health care workers who are involved in the preparation and administration of these medicines. Studies carried out in the past have shown two main areas where health care workers are at greatest risk:

- Local effects caused by contact of cytotoxic agents with skin, eyes and mucous membranes
- Systemic effects caused by inhalation or injection of cytotoxic agents during preparation.

Health care workers handling cytotoxics have in the past experienced symptoms such as dizziness, headaches, lightheadedness and nausea. These effects appear to have been caused by inhalation or ingestion of cytotoxic agents during their preparation. However, on these occasions it was noted that procedures were often carried out under unsuitable conditions such as in small poorly ventilated rooms. As yet the long-term effects of cytotoxic inhalation are not fully understood. Systemic effects appear to pose the greatest risk as cytotoxic agents are said to be mutagenic, teratogenic or carcinogenic.

Today, cytotoxic agents are prepared under strict aseptic conditions, in designated areas within a hospital pharmacy, following guidelines published by the Royal Pharmaceutical Society of Great Britain (RPSGB) in 1983. There precautions ensure that the health and safety of all personnel handling cytotoxics are carefully considered. Pharmacy staff preparing cytotoxic agents must be fully trained in the necessary aseptic techniques and must be fully aware of the precautions that are required when handling cytotoxics. Nursing and medical staff must also be taught strict handling and administration techniques to ensure that they do not expose themselves or their patients to any unnecessary risks. All personnel involved in preparing and handling cytotoxic agents should be given an annual health check by the occupational health department in the hospital to ensure their health is not being compromised by working with these agents.

Published guidelines cover the following areas:

- Personnel handling cytotoxics and preparation areas used
- Techniques and precautions
- Dealing with spillage
- Disposal of cytotoxics
- Labelling, packaging and distribution
- Administration of cytotoxics.

Each of these areas will be discussed in more detail.

PROVISION OF A CYTOTOXIC RECONSTITUTION SERVICE

The guidelines, published in 1983, were intended to give advice to all health care workers handling cytotoxic agents as reconstitution was at that time being carried out by medical staff at a ward level and not in the pharmacy department. The guidelines also advised that the safest option would be to have a centralized cytotoxic reconstitution service.

In 1987 the Cytotoxic Services Working Group was formed. They have produced a manual on how to set up and run a pharmacy-based cytotoxic service. The manual gives information regarding the following areas:

- Facilities and equipment required for cytotoxic reconstitution

- Training required for staff handling cytotoxics
- Documentation required for procedures
- Health and safety requirements.

By 1990, this original manual became *The Cytotoxics Handbook* and has since been updated and republished (Allwood et al 1997) to act as a practical guide for pharmacy staff involved in the reconstitution of cytotoxic agents. *The Cytotoxic Handbook*, together with the RPSGB guidelines, provide the necessary reference material and practical advice to enable hospital pharmacists to set up a cytotoxic reconstitution service.

Why is the pharmacy department chosen to provide cytotoxic agents?

Pharmacy departments in most of the larger hospitals have existing aseptic dispensing facilities (see Ch. 13). These facilities may be utilized to provide adequate compounding facilities for reconstitution of cytotoxics provided strict guidelines on preparation are adhered to. Pharmacy staff are already well trained in aseptic dispensing techniques, recording and checking procedures and ensuring that patients receive the appropriate dose regimens. Pharmacists also have the advantage of having a wide clinical knowledge of cytotoxic agents and a unique knowledge of the stability and formulation requirements of such agents.

A number of these units have a manufacturing licence which allows them to supply other hospitals and home care patients.

Prior to setting up a centralized cytotoxic reconstitution service, several factors must be considered. The existing situation must be carefully examined to determine who currently prepares cytotoxic medicines, where they are prepared and how the procedures are carried out. The information gained can be reviewed and compared with the option of providing a centralized service. The rationale behind this service would be to ensure the health and safety of all health care workers involved in handling cytotoxics and to produce a cost-effective service.

Training required for staff preparing cytotoxics

All personnel involved in preparing and handling of cytotoxics require training in the appropriate techniques. This should include training for pharmacists, pre-registration graduates and all technical staff working in this field. On a practical level, all staff must be aware of the following:

- Procedures required on receipt of a request for a cytotoxic agent
- How to fill out a worksheet and assemble the required materials for cytotoxic reconstitution
- Changing procedures required prior to working in a clean room environment
- General working of laminar airflow cabinets and isolators
- Cleaning and disposal procedures prior to and following aseptic procedures
- Storage and transportation of cytotoxics
- Background information on commonly used cytotoxics
- Local policies and procedures adopted by the hospital trust or health authority. These should be available for consultation and should be adhered to at all times. They should include: health and safety regulations; safe handling procedures for individual manipulative techniques; procedures for dealing with spillage and disposal; advice on storage and administration.

Validation of operator techniques

Prior to commencing work on reconstitution of cytotoxics, an operator's competence in this field must be assessed. This is achieved by validating operator techniques. The operator is asked to carry out broth transfer trials where solutions of sterile broth are transferred from one vial or container to another. The aim of the trial is to carry out aseptic transfer techniques which would routinely be used when preparing sterile cytotoxic products. All work is carried out under strictly controlled aseptic conditions. The vials can then be incubated for an appropriate time (5–7 days) and examined for bacterial growth. This procedure can be used in conjunction with observing the operator at work to deter-

mine operator competence in aseptic transfer techniques (See also Ch. 13).

Each operator undergoing training is required to undertake a predetermined number of broth transfer trials. Operators must achieve negative results (no growth after incubation) on each occasion before they are deemed capable of preparing cytotoxic agents. The number of broth trails undertaken can vary from one hospital to another. It can also be dependent on the level of involvement an operator has in this field. Training procedures should be reviewed on a regular basis and retraining and refresher courses made available to all staff.

Certain handling problems can be encountered when dealing with cytotoxic agents. The formation of an aerosol on removing a needle from a vial containing a cytotoxic agent can be a problem. This is known as 'aerosolization'. Using an inert dye solution such as methylene blue or amaranth in vials instead of the cytotoxic agent can assess operator technique. The presence of the dye will clearly indicate any aerosol formation during the procedure. Using this technique, operator handling techniques can be observed and assessed.

Documentation required for cytotoxics

On receipt of a prescription for a cytotoxic agent a number of procedures must be undertaken. Figure 27.1 shows the areas of work in which a pharmacist may have involvement.

When the prescription is received, it is checked by the pharmacist to ensure that all patient details are in order, dosage calculations are accurate and the dose and presentation are suitable. Drug monographs and data sheets can be consulted to check all details including, for example, shelf life of the reconstituted product and the diluent required.

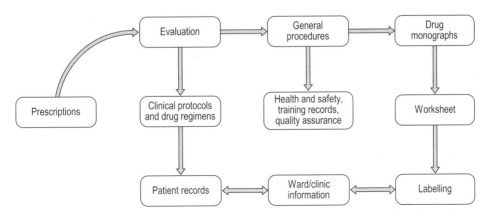

Fig. 27.1 Documentation required for cytotoxic services. (From Allwood et al 1997, reproduced with permission.)

A range of dosage forms is available including syringes, minibags and infusions. The pharmacist in conjunction with medical staff will decide on the most suitable presentation for the patient. The route of administration, the type of cytotoxic agent required and the stability of the final preparation will influence choice of dosage form.

Information from the prescription can be transferred to a dispensing worksheet and details of medicine(s) required, diluent, volume for reconstitution and number of vials required are recorded. Details of batch numbers and expiry date for each product used, time and date of preparation, and expiry of the final product are also required. Finally, a sample label can be attached to the worksheet and the pharmacist will check all details and sign the worksheets. Some cytotoxic agents require protection from light and are sealed in dark-coloured plastic bags to allow protection of the product. In these circumstances labels are required for the outer bag and for the medicine. When the worksheet is complete, the materials required for the reconstitution procedure are collected together and placed in a suitable plastic tray ready for transfer to the designated reconstitution area.

Personnel handling cytotoxics and preparation areas used

In any hospital setting where large quantities of cytotoxic agents are required, preparation of cytotoxics takes place in the hospital pharmacy. A designated area is set aside for the preparation of cytotoxics and is used for this purpose only. A vertical laminar downflow safety cabinet sited in a clean room facility can be used for this purpose (see Ch. 13).

The use of isolators for cytotoxic procedures is on the increase as capital and running costs for isolators are less costly than setting up clean room facilities. Some hospitals place isolators in clean rooms in order to reduce the risk of microbial contamination.

Techniques and precautions

When handling cytotoxics, it is vital that the appropriate protective clothing is worn. Operators using clean room facilities must wear appropriate clean room clothing, with the addition of armlets for extra protection as commercially available suits are known to be permeable to certain cytotoxic agents. When using an isolator cabinet, a full clean room suit is not essential, but appropriate clean room clothing is required. Selection of clothing will be dependent on

the background environment in which the isolator is sited. If reconstitution takes place outside this environment, e.g. by medical staff at a ward level, goggles, mask, apron, armlets and latex gloves should be worn to protect the operator. It is hoped that this latter procedure would be discouraged as the pharmacy department is able to provide a comprehensive service to the wards.

Reconstitution procedures

When carrying out reconstitution procedures, certain precautions must be taken:

- Ampoule necks should be covered with a sterile swab before breaking them open and should be broken facing away from the operator.
- Rubber stoppers on vials should be swabbed with a sterile swab prior to removal of liquid.
- Needles should be covered with the needle cover, or a sterile gauze swab when piercing or withdrawing from a vial or when air is being expelled.
- Luer lock syringes with wide-bore needles should be used for all procedures to allow more efficient removal of liquid and to prevent the build up of pressure in the vial.
- Quills can be used to remove liquid from ampoules as they allow faster flow rates than a needle.
- To ensure that no further additions are made to cytotoxic agents outside the pharmacy preparation area, all completed products in syringe form should be sealed with a blind hub or deadender before removal from the cytotoxic cabinet (Fig. 27.2). An additive plug must be placed on each minibag once additions are complete.

The vials used to contain cytotoxic agents are effectively a closed system. They are sealed vials which contain either a powder which requires reconstitution with a solvent or a liquid which requires withdrawal from the vial into a syringe. In each case, equalization of pressure within the vial is required to allow withdrawal from it. Reconstitution devices are available to help with the reconstitution process. Some devices consist of a small plastic spike attached to a filter. These devices are useful when repeated volumes of diluent must be measured. However, they are capable of making large holes in the rubber bung of cytotoxic medicine vials, thus increasing the risk of leakage of solution from the vial. Another example of a reconstitution device is a 0.2 μm hydrophobic filter venting needle. The CytoSafe needle is a commonly used example of this type of product. This device consists of a needle which is vented to allow equilibrium of pressure between the vial and the syringe. It is useful for

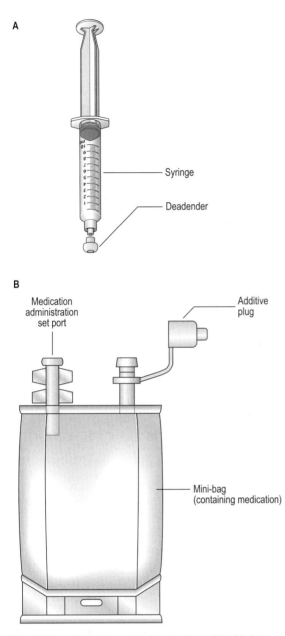

Fig. 27.2 (**A**) Syringe with deadender or blind hub in position. (**B**) Minibag with additive plug.

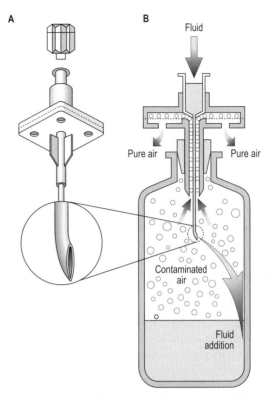

Fig. 27.3 (**A**) CytoSafe needle and (**B**) reconstitution set-up. (Courtesy of Baxa Corporation.)

reconstitution of large vials or when more than one vial is required for a dose (Fig. 27.3). However, care must be taken when withdrawing or adding liquid to a vial as the filter may become blocked.

In the past venting needles (with no filter attached) were used but are no longer recommended due to the risk of leakage of the cytotoxic drug from the vial during reconstitution procedures.

An alternative to using a reconstitution device is to use a 'negative pressure' procedure. This method uses no reconstitution devices and relies solely on the expertise of the operator to ensure proper equalization of pressure within the vial to avoid aerosol formation on withdrawal of the needle. In this procedure the required volume of air for a liquid preparation or solvent for a powder is drawn into the syringe. A small amount of air/solvent is added to the vial and an equal volume of liquid/air is drawn into the syringe. This process is repeated slowly until all the liquid is withdrawn or solvent added. The use of this method avoids build up of pressure in the vial which may result in leakage through the rubber bung. This process is useful for small vials where there is very little room for large filter needles.

Dealing with spillage

During reconstitution procedures, operators must take great care when handling cytotoxic agents and also be aware of the procedures required when dealing with spillage or waste disposal of cytotoxic agents.

In the event of a spillage, the problem should be dealt with immediately. A written policy on dealing with spillages should be known to the operator and must be implemented should one occur. A spill kit should be readily available which contains the required materials to deal with a spill. If the spillage involves a liquid, an absorbent cloth should be used to wipe up the spill and the waste materials placed in a cytotoxic hazardous waste bag. Spillage involving a powder should be wiped up using a damp cloth to ensure that inhalation of powder particles does not occur. All surface areas contaminated by the spillage should be washed with copious amounts of water (sterile water is available in the spill kit). In some instances, manufacturers recommend the use of certain chemicals to deal with cytotoxic spillage as a secondary measure. Manufacturer's literature should be available within the pharmacy and used to obtain appropriate advice in the event of a spillage.

If the spillage has come in contact with the skin, the contaminated area should be washed thoroughly with soap and water. Contact with eyes should be dealt with by irrigation with a sodium chloride eyewash, the incident reported and medical help sought. In the event of a needlestick injury involving direct contact with a cytotoxic agent, the area should again be thoroughly washed and the operator should receive medical attention. All accidents involving spillage should be reported.

Disposal of cytotoxics

All cytotoxic waste materials should be placed in a brightly coloured plastic bag, sealed and labelled with a cytotoxic warning label ready for disposal by incineration or degradation by chemical methods.

Sharp objects including needles, syringes, ampoules and vials should be placed in a sharps bin which is made of rigid plastic and does not allow leakage of cytotoxic waste. When the sharps bin is full, it should be sealed with hazardous waste tape and disposed of safely with other cytotoxic waste.

Nursing staff have the problem of handling excreta of patients who have received cytotoxic medicines. The potential risks involved will vary depending on the medicine used, dosage given, route of administration and the type of elimination profile. Reports suggest that excreta should be assumed to be potentially hazardous for at least 48 hours after cytotoxic administration is complete. Ward staff should be made fully aware of the patients who pose this risk and

should always take the necessary handling precautions. For patients on home chemotherapy, family members should be warned about the potential hazards and advised to exercise extreme caution when handling excreta from the patient.

Labelling, packaging and distribution

Following reconstitution of a cytotoxic agent, the medicine can then be labelled ready for distribution to the ward. Labels must be appropriately designed to show immediately that the container holds a cytotoxic agent.

Labels should include the following details:

- Patient's name and ward number
- Drug name, quantity and final volume
- Vehicle in which the drug is contained (e.g. water for injection)
- Batch number, expiry date and storage conditions required
- Hospital pharmacy name and address
- Infusion rate.

Within each hospital, there should be recommended policies for safe transportation of cytotoxics and local procedures implemented for issue and receipt of medicines.

ADMINISTRATION OF CYTOTOXIC MEDICINES

Medical and nursing staff at a ward level are responsible for administering cytotoxic medicines to patients. The pharmacy department can supply the ward with the medicines in a form suitable for convenient administration to the patient. Medical staff will have access to local hospital policies regarding the safe handling and administration of cytotoxics and are required to adhere to these policies at all times. They are held responsible for ensuring the safety of the patient as well as themselves while administering cytotoxic medicines. As a result of this responsibility, staff chosen to carry out these procedures are usually highly trained personnel who have a wide range of experience in this field and have a good working knowledge of cytotoxic agents. They are able to discuss in detail with patients the procedures being carried out, thereby reassuring them about the medical treatment that they are receiving.

On a practical level, medical and nursing staff must be capable of setting up infusion sets and syringes to avoid leakage of contents and be proficient in injection techniques to ensure that the patient does not suffer from leakage of cytotoxic medicines outside the vein. This latter is known as 'extravasation'. In the event of extravasation occurring, medical staff are trained to stop administration immediately, aspirate and carry out locally agreed policies and procedures which involve, for example, the administration of steroids intravenously or subcutaneously and then topically if required. This procedure is used to prevent irreversible tissue damage. Extravasation kits should be available on hand in the ward to deal with this problem.

PROVISION OF CHEMOTHERAPY AT HOME

Many patients express a desire to have their chemotherapy provided at home. This is now possible with the setting up of domiciliary chemotherapy programmes. Patients have more involvement in the administration of their medicines, are able to spend more time with their families and do not require to attend hospital for regular treatment. If their treatment can be managed at home, hospital beds are available to treat other patients, but this can create an increased workload for the pharmacy department.

The implications for a pharmacy department setting up a home chemotherapy service are wide ranging. Many home chemotherapy doses are supplied for a week at a time. There may be a need to employ more staff and to train new and existing staff in the techniques required for filling the ambulatory infusion devices required for home chemotherapy.

In addition, the stability of the formulations must be considered. Stability data on cytotoxic medicines used routinely in chemotherapy are documented in the ABPI data sheet compendium, *The Cytotoxics Handbook* (Allwood et al 1997), and the *Trisale Handbook of Injectables*. However, fully documented stability data must be obtained for cytotoxic agents administered in home infusion devices before the pharmacy department can take on the responsibility of providing a service to home patients. The pharmacist responsible for the centralized cytotoxics service must have a good working knowledge of appropriate chemotherapy regimens and infusion devices available for home chemotherapy. In certain oncology centres, the pharmacist may also be asked to become involved in training patients in appropriate handling and administration techniques to ensure the health and safety of patients and their carers in the home care environment.

CENTRALIZED INTRAVENOUS ADDITIVE SERVICE (CIVAS)

Breckenridge made recommendations as early as 1976 that hospital pharmacies should be involved in the provision of IV products. However despite the fact that the preparation of IV cytotoxic medicines was taken up, provision of an IV additive service did not take place until the 1980s and then only in a limited number of hospitals.

The setting up of the UK national CIVAS group in 1991 gave more hospital pharmacists the initiative and support for the provision of a CIVA service. By 1993 a CIVAS manual was produced to provide guidelines for hospital pharmacists setting up a CIVA service. Today a large proportion of hospital pharmacists in the UK and many European countries provide a CIVA service.

Scope of a CIVA service

A CIVA service is set up to provide a range of parenteral dosage forms suitable for administration to patients. Medical, nursing and pharmacy staff involved in patient care in this field will decide the range of dosage forms supplied. A CIVA service can provide the following:

- IV antibiotics
- Patient-controlled analgesia
- Ambulatory infusion devices for IV antibiotic therapy at home.

Often a CIVA service is run in conjunction with services which already exist in the pharmacy (e.g. cytotoxic reconstitution and compounding of parenteral nutrition solutions).

Setting up a CIVA service

The same principles adopted when setting up a centralized cytotoxic reconstitution service apply when setting up a CIVA service. A working party can be established consisting of representatives from pharmacy, medical and nursing staff and hospital administrators. The current situation can be assessed to determine the amount of IV doses currently being used, who prepares them and the conditions under which they are prepared. Information can be provided regarding the benefits of a centralized service and any potential problems identified. Often the pharmacy department will initially carry out a pilot study where a limited number of CIVA doses will be supplied to a particular ward or discipline (e.g. two strengths of an antibiotic supplied when required to surgical wards only). After a predetermined time period, the situation could be evaluated and a decision then made either to implement a CIVA service or to continue with ward staff preparing IV doses. If the decision is made to set up a CIVA service, then the pharmacist in charge of this service has a number of factors to consider.

Role of the pharmacist in the provision of a CIVA service

A study carried out by Needle (1995) suggested that pharmacy managers were the main decision makers in terms of initiating a CIVA service. The pharmacist responsible for setting up the service must assess the current situation, including workload, methods for prescribing, preparation and administration. This pharmacist must look realistically at the potential benefits and problems of providing a CIVA service and the implications this will have for the pharmacy, particularly in relation to cost and staff workload. The ultimate aim of any service provided from a hospital pharmacy should be to improve the quality of health care given to the patient. Potential benefits of providing a CIVA service:

- Improved use of hospital resources
- Improved services to the patients
- Improved pharmacy control.
- Quality assurance

Improved use of hospital resources

Pharmacy staff are trained in aseptic procedures and can use their skills to provide a comprehensive range of IV products suitable for administration to the patients by medical and nursing staff. This utilizes pharmacy skills to the maximum and at the same time saves on medical and nursing staff time. Often IV doses have to be made up on the ward by nursing staff or junior doctors who have very little experience in this field and have a limited knowledge of calculating appropriate doses, using the required diluent or preparing IV medicines. Ward facilities for preparing IV medicines are not ideal and increase the risk of the product being contaminated as it is not prepared under aseptic conditions. Using existing aseptic dispensing facilities in the hospital pharmacy ensures that IV products are prepared under the highest possible standards. Better control of ward stocks of IV medicines can be achieved if the pharmacy provides a CIVA service. Each ward can order IV medicines on a daily basis from the pharmacy depending on patient

requirements. This reduces the possibility of medicines being kept on the ward and not used before their expiry date.

Improved services to the patients

When the wards utilize a CIVA service, the pharmacy department prepares the doses, sends them to the ward and patients then receive their medicine on time. All CIVA doses are clearly labelled with appropriate dosage instructions, ensuring that patients receive the correct medication and that it is administered appropriately. This facility allows medical and nursing staff to spend more time with the patients.

Improved pharmacy control

If a CIVA service is set up within a hospital, the pharmacy department can be involved from the very beginning. This allows the pharmacist to have a much greater clinical input to the provision of patient care. The pharmacist can be involved in prescription monitoring and checking, recommending appropriate dosage forms and giving advice on stability of preparations. Under pharmacy control a CIVA service can allow standardization of drug concentrations and improved formulary compliance.

Quality assurance

All procedures used during preparation of CIVA doses will be fully validated and documented. Procedures will also be audited and be subject to in-process monitoring. Staff preparing IV products will adhere to standard operating procedures (SOPs) and published guidelines. Records will be kept for all IV medicines prepared and batch numbers of products used during reconstitution procedures. This ensures that in the event of a product recall or any problems with an IV medicine, pharmacy will hold records of all the necessary documentation.

Potential problems of a CIVA service

- Increased expenditure in the pharmacy including capital expenditure for setting up the service and in provision of staff to prepare the required doses.
- Pharmacy must ensure that they have adequate storage space for CIVA doses that require refrigeration before being transported to wards. Transportation will require to be organized in such a way as to ensure that CIVA doses are not kept out of the refrigerator for prolonged periods of time.

• If pharmacy provides a CIVA service, will they be able to provide an out-of-hours service? If they are unable to do so, will IV medicines have to be made up in advance for weekends? Can these medicines be given a sufficiently long shelf life? Would pharmacists working at weekends know how to make up IV medicines if this is not their normal area for working?

• Certain wards may be difficult to service, e.g. accident and emergency and intensive care, as they may require unusual doses which are not normally provided under the CIVA service. These doses may be required urgently, particularly in an emergency situation. This will put extra pressure on the pharmacy staff and on the facilities, depending on the workload at the time of the request.

• A further complication is the requirement for individualized doses, e.g. in paediatrics. A clinical pharmacist who has specialized knowledge of paediatrics may be able to give advice to staff providing the CIVA service to ensure appropriate dosage regimens are prepared.

• Retrieval and reuse of doses not required by an individual ward can be a problem. Occasionally wards order IV drugs and then dosage regimens are changed at a later stage. There has to be a procedure set in place for retrieval of such doses from the ward to prevent drug wastage.

• Communication requirements must be considered. Good liaison between the clinical pharmacist responsible for the wards supplied and medical staff working in the wards is essential to ensure that orders for CIVA doses are requested on time. Orders for home IV doses may require liaison between health care workers in the community and the hospital sector to ensure that home patients receive adequate supplies of medicines.

Practical considerations when setting up a CIVA service

Preparation areas

Intravenous products can be prepared under aseptic dispensing conditions either in a designated area using an isolator cabinet or using clean room facilities (See Ch. 13).

CIVA dosage forms

Most hospital pharmacies supply IV additives in the form of a preloaded syringe or a minibag. The minibags are small volume infusion bags available in volumes of 50 mL and 100 mL. Medical staff often prefer CIVA doses supplied in minibags as they are easier to administer than syringes.

Reconstitution procedures are usually required as IV doses can be supplied as sterile freeze-dried powders in sealed vials. These vials are then reconstituted with the appropriate diluent and drawn into a syringe or minibag ready for administration to the patient. If minibags are used, a reconstitution device can be used to transfer the diluent into the vial, then, after vigorous shaking, back into the bag again. Throughout this procedure the vial and minibag remain attached via the reconstitution device which has a double-ended needle. One end of the needle is placed through the rubber bung of the vial and the other end is connected into the rubber septum of the minibag (Fig. 27.4).

Prior to removal from the laminar airflow cabinet or the isolator cabinet, all prepared syringes are sealed with a blind hub or deadender and minibags are sealed with an additive plug. This ensures that no further additions are made to the syringe or minibag outside the pharmacy. All products are labelled and sealed into an outer bag before being transported into the ward.

Stability of CIVA doses

Pharmacy departments which have a manufacturer's licence can prepare IV doses for stock and can, in some cases, give products a long shelf life (depending on validated stability data). For non-licensed units the situation is different. Under the Section 10 exemption in the Medicines Act 1968,

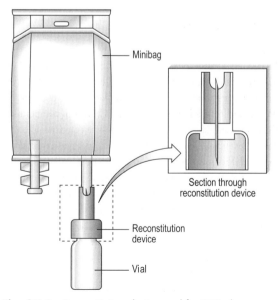

Fig. 27.4 Reconstitution device used for CIVA doses. (Courtesy of Baxter Healthcare Ltd.)

parenteral products can be prepared for stock in advance of a prescription being obtained, provided preparation takes place under the supervision of a pharmacist. Under these circumstances, IV doses can be prepared using aseptic dispensing facilities in the pharmacy, and can be given a shelf life of up to 90 days, providing that microbiological validation data is carried out. In practice, the shelf life given to individual IV medicines will vary. Reference to stability data and manufacturers' guidelines will give detailed information for each IV dose being prepared. Chemical stability data supporting the shelf life must be available for each product being prepared in the pharmacy.

Stability studies have been carried out over the last few years to determine if the shelf life of IV products can be extended. Published evidence suggests that chemical stability of IV products can be prolonged if storage temperature is reduced. Studies show that the shelf life of some products can be extended to 6 months or longer if the IV product is frozen at –20°C. However, not all products are stable in this condition and stability data specific to each product, including dosage form, diluent and presentation, must all be considered. Intravenous medicines stored in minibags and when frozen can be very fragile, hence great care must be observed when handling medicines in this form and in packing them in freezers. Natural thawing time for these IV products will vary and this can be a problem if time is a limiting factor. The use of microwaves to speed up the thawing time has been suggested, but further work in this area is required to validate procedures used.

Storage requirements for IV doses must be carefully considered. If medicines require refrigeration, a designated refrigerator should be set aside in the pharmacy. CIVA doses should be stored there until they are transported to the wards, where they should be refrigerated until required. Refrigerators used in hospital pharmacies are pharmaceutical grade refrigerators. They should have a temperature recorder and should be fitted with an alarm to alert pharmacy staff to any changes in storage conditions. Refrigerators used at a ward level should also be carefully monitored to ensure that adequate storage conditions are achieved. All refrigerated CIVA doses should be allowed to reach room temperature prior to administration to the patient.

Validation of procedures

As with any procedures carried out under aseptic conditions, routine environmental monitoring must be undertaken. This will include the use of settle plates (at least weekly) and contact plates (at least monthly). Air sampling will also take place routinely (monthly) and filter checks should be done at least on an annual basis or in the event of any problems arising. Validation of operator technique will include the use of broth transfer trials and observation of operator techniques. The level of activity and number of staff working in the unit should be taken into account as staff movements are usually the main cause for contamination (see Ch. 13).

Provision of IV doses for home patients

Provision of a CIVA service from a hospital pharmacy will involve a large commitment in terms of staff to ensure that daily requirements are met and that sufficient doses are prepared in advance for an out-of-hours service. However, if provision of IV doses for home patients is considered, more staff may be required to provide this service. Many hospital pharmacies initially set up a CIVA service and are then asked to expand the service to provide services for patients in the community. Some have the facilities and resources to provide IV doses for home patients, others do not. However, with the advances in home infusion devices and greater emphasis being put on health care at home, hospital pharmacies are under more pressure to provide this extended service.

Provision of IV medicines at home using ambulatory devices has meant that pharmacy staff require further training in the filling of these ambulatory devices. A number of different options are available for patients on home IV therapy (see also Ch. 25):

Single-dose infusions. These are administered in the form of a preloaded syringe or minibag attached to an infusion system which is set at a predetermined flow rate to administer the medicine to the patient. These devices can be used for self-administration by patients three to four times daily.

Electronic syringe infusers. These are electric or battery-operated infusion devices used in conjunction with a syringe and tubing to deliver the medicine. The infusers are usually small and lightweight allowing the patients to remain mobile during the infusion period.

Elastomeric infusers. These are disposable plastic units which consist of an inner 'balloon' reservoir surrounded by the outer protective shell. They have a medication entry port and permanently attached tubing. The reservoir can be filled using a one-way Luer lock valve. Filling can take place in the pharmacy and, if required, the line can be primed ready for patient use. An integrated flow-restricting device controls flow rates. Elastomeric devices can be carried by patients in a carrying case or in a pocket.

Slow intravenous push. A needle and syringe are used to deliver the drug by slow intravenous injection over approximately 7 minutes. This is suitable for self-administration by the patient and does not require costly infusion devices.

For all of the above-mentioned methods, the hospital pharmacy can provide the syringes, minibags and elastomeric devices as prefilled products ready for transportation to patients. If large quantities of syringes are required regularly, the hospital pharmacy may use a compounding pump to prepare the quantities required. If hospital pharmacies cannot provide IV doses for home patients, commercial pharmaceutical companies can fulfil this role (see Ch. 28).

RADIOPHARMACY

Radioactivity may be defined as the spontaneous transformation of an unstable nucleus to a more stable nucleus. This transformation involves the release of ionizing radiation which may be in particulate form (e.g. α particles or β particles) or may be in the form of electromagnetic radiation (e.g. γ rays).

Elements that emit radiation are known as radionuclides and have a number of applications in medicine. Radiopharmacy is concerned with the manufacture of radioactive medicines known as radiopharmaceuticals. These have two main applications in medicine:

- As an aid to the diagnosis of disease (diagnostic radiopharmaceuticals)
- In the treatment of disease (therapeutic radiopharmaceuticals).

Diagnostic radiopharmaceuticals may be classified into two types:

- Radiopharmaceuticals used in tracer techniques for measuring physiological parameters (e.g. ^{51}Cr-EDTA for measuring glomerular filtration rate)
- Radiopharmaceuticals for diagnostic imaging (e.g. ^{99m}Tc-methylene diphosphonate (MDP) used in bone scanning).

In diagnostic imaging, γ-emitting radionuclides are used since their interaction with tissue is much less than that of particulate emitters and will cause significantly less damage to tissue. Radiopharmaceuticals are administered to the patient, usually by the IV route, and distribute into a particular organ. The radiation is then detected externally using a special scintillation detector, known as a γ-camera. These are used by nuclear medicine departments to image the distribution of the radiopharmaceutical within the patient's body. Using the γ-camera in conjunction with a computer system it is not only possible to produce static images of an organ, but also to examine how the radiopharmaceutical moves through an organ. These dynamic images describe how the organ is functioning. It is also possible to create images in all three planes, a process known as single photon emission computerized tomography (SPECT).

It is important to note that for the safe production of radiopharmaceuticals, the radiopharmacy must be designed to comply with, and procedures must follow, good manufacturing practice and good radiation protection practice. Radiopharmacists working in this field are part of a multidisciplinary team which includes doctors, physicists and nuclear medicine technicians. As part of this team they not only ensure that the radiopharmaceuticals will give high-quality clinical information, but also that they are safe for both patient and user alike.

RADIONUCLIDES USED IN NUCLEAR MEDICINE

Alpha-emitters

Alpha-decay is the process whereby a nucleus emits a helium nucleus, or α-particle. This commonly occurs with heavy nuclei (e.g. radium-226 $^{226}_{88}Ra \rightarrow \, ^{226}_{86}Ra + \alpha$).

Because they are heavy and positively charged, α-particles travel only short distances in air (~5 mm) and only micrometer distances in tissues. Their ionizing nature would result in a highly localized radiation dose if taken internally and hence they tend not to be used in radiopharmaceuticals.

Some α-emitters (e.g. ^{226}Ra) when encapsulated are used as sealed sources, emitting X-rays or γ-rays for radiotherapy applications. Here the body is exposed to radiation externally in an attempt to treat malignant tumours.

Beta-emitters

Beta-decay occurs in two ways, one that involves the emission of a negatively charged β^--particle, or electron, and the other that involves the emission of a positively charged β^+-particle, or positron.

Table 27.1   Examples of radionuclides used in nuclear medicine

Radionuclide	Radiopharmaceutical	Half-life	Clinical use
β⁻-emitters			
^{131}I	Sodium iodide capsules	8 days	Thyrotoxicosis, thyroid carcinomas
^{32}P	Sodium phosphate injection	14 days	Polycythaemia rubra vera
^{90}Sr	Strontium chloride injection	50 days	Palliation of pain from bone metastases
β⁺-emitters			
^{15}O	^{15}O$_2$ gas	2 min	Brain blood flow imaging
^{18}F	Fluorodeoxy-glucose injection	110 min	Brain glucose metabolism
Electron capture			
^{111}In	Indium chloride solution	67 h	Antibody labelling
^{123}I	Sodium iodide injection	13 h	Thyroid imaging
^{201}Tl	Thallous chloride injection	73 h	Cardiac perfusion imaging
Isomeric transition			
^{99m}Tc	Sodium pertechnetate injection	6 h	See Table 27.2
^{81m}Kr	Krypton gas	13 s	Lung ventilation imaging

β⁻-emitters

Radionuclides which decay by β⁻-decay tend to have nuclei that are neutron rich. They attempt to reach a more stable state by the transformation of a neutron into a proton with the emission of a β⁻-particle.

Despite β⁻-particles having a range in air of up to several metres, their range in tissues is only a few millimetres. Because of this and their highly ionizing nature, β⁻-emitters tend to be used in therapeutic radiopharmaceuticals (Table 27.1).

The principle of therapeutic treatment with radionuclides is to target the radionuclide to a specific tissue within the body in an attempt to selectively damage or destroy that tissue. Ideally therapeutic β⁻-emitting radionuclides should have energies of 0.5–1.5 MeV and a half-life of several days to provide a prolonged radiobiological effect.

The most widely used example of this is ^{131}I-sodium iodide which is used in the treatment of hyperactive thyroid disease and in certain thyroid tumours. Here the physiological property of thyroid tissue is exploited to target the radionuclide to the site of action. Since thyroid tissue avidly takes up iodine in the normal synthesis of the hormone levothyroxine (thyroxine), radioactive iodine is also taken up and held in the thyroid tissue. Hence the radiation damage is targeted to the thyroid tissue specifically and the normal excretion of any excess iodine results in no significant damage to other organs and tissues.

β⁺-emitters

Radionuclides that emit positrons are becoming more widely used in nuclear medicine. In this transformation, a proton-rich nuclide attempts to achieve stability by converting a proton to a neutron with the emission of a positron. The positron is very short-lived, since it interacts with an electron resulting in an annihilation reaction and the conversion of both particles into electromagnetic (EM) radiation. This EM radiation is in the form of two γ-rays, each having an energy of 0.511 MeV, which are emitted at an angle of 180° to each other.

When used in conjunction with a specialized γ-camera with detectors placed 180° apart, it is possible to create images in all three planes with the position of the radiopharmaceutical being very precisely known. This type of imaging technique is known as positron emission tomography (PET). Radionuclides used in PET (Table 27.1) are radioisotopes of naturally occurring elements and hence the radiopharmaceuticals in which they are synthesized have a biological biodistribution identical to the naturally occurring compound. The high cost of producing these radiopharmaceuticals, their very short half-life and the expense of the PET camera, results in this technique being mainly used in medical research.

Electron capture

Nuclei that are proton rich may, as an alternative to positron emission, capture electrons from the atom's electron orbitals. This process results in the transformation of a proton to a neutron within the nucleus. The subsequent re-arrangement of the electrons orbiting the nucleus results in a characteristic emission of X-rays or γ-rays.

Radionuclides which decay by electron capture are useful in diagnostic imaging since they emit γ-rays; examples are given in Table 27.1.

Isomeric transition

Some radionuclides exist for measurable periods in excited, or isomeric, states prior to reaching ground state. This form of decay involves the emission of a γ-ray and is known as isomeric transition. When radionuclides exist in this transitional state they are known as metastable which is denoted by the letter 'm' and written thus: ^{99m}Tc.

A simplified decay scheme for ^{99m}Tc-technetium is shown in Figure 27.5 where ^{99m}Tc's parent radionuclide, molybdenum (^{99}Mo), decays by β$^-$ emission to the ground state ^{99}Tc either directly or indirectly. The indirect route, which is the most common, involves the isomer ^{99m}Tc, which in turn decays from this its metastable state to ^{99}Tc by isomeric transition.

Radionuclides which decay by this process are used in diagnostic imaging since they emit γ-rays (Table 27.1). It should be noted that ^{99m}Tc is the most widely used radionuclide in hospital radiopharmacy today, making up the radionuclide component of around 90% of the radiophar-

maceuticals produced. For these reasons the production processes for ^{99m}Tc-radiopharmaceuticals will be especially emphasized.

Facilities required for the production of radiopharmaceuticals

The majority of radiopharmaceuticals are intended for intravenous (IV) administration, therefore it is of paramount importance that these preparations are sterile. They also contain radionuclides with short half-lives that require their preparation and administration on the same day. Because of the constraints of time, it is not possible to use terminal sterilization by autoclaving and hence these injections must be prepared using aseptic techniques. Here highly skilled operators work with sterile ingredients within clean room facilities containing either laminar flow safety cabinets or isolators. Guidance on the facilities required is given in *Guidance Notes for Hospitals on the Premises and Environment Required for the Preparation of Radiopharmaceuticals* (Department of Health and Social Security 1982).

Principles of radiopharmaceutical production

The physical and chemical properties of ^{99m}Tc make it nearly ideal for imaging purposes as outlined below:

- It has a 6-hour half-life ($T_{1/2}$); long enough to allow imaging to take place in the working day, whilst also short enough that patients are not radioactive for long periods (in 24 hours, or 4 half-lives, the radioactivity will have decayed by 94%).
- ^{99m}Tc emits γ-rays of 140 keV energy—ideal for use with the modern γ-camera.
- There are no particulate emissions that, if present, would add to the patient's radiation dose.
- By purchasing a device known as a ^{99m}Mo/^{99m}Tc-generator, ^{99m}Tc can be made readily available to the hospital site in a sterile and pyrogen-free form.
- ^{99m}Tc has a versatile coordination chemistry and will allow a large number of ligands to complex with it. By using different ligands in the radiopharmaceutical's formulation, the radiopharmacist can prepare a wide range of radiopharmaceuticals, providing for the many different investigations carried out in nuclear medicine departments (Table 27.2).

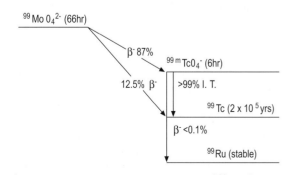

^{99}Mo O$_4$$^{2-}$ (66hr)

β$^-$ 87%

^{99m}TcO$_4$$^-$ (6hr)

12.5% β$^-$

>99% I. T.

^{99}Tc (2 x 10^5 yrs)

β$^-$ <0.1%

^{99}Ru (stable)

Fig. 27.5 Diagrammatic representation of ^{99}Mo decay.

Table 27.2   Examples of ^{99m}Tc-radiopharmaceuticals

Radiopharmaceutical	Organ or tissue of distribution	Main clinical application
^{99m}Tc-sodium pertechnetate	Thyroid	Imaging the thyroid gland and ectopic tissue
	Salivary gland	Dynamic images of accumulation and drainage to show gland function
	Gastric mucosa	Presence of Meckel's diverticulum containing gastric mucosa
^{99m}Tc-methylene diphosphonate (MDP)	Skeleton	Bone metastases from carcinoma of lung, breast and prostrate
^{99m}Tc-macro-aggregates of albumin (MAA)	Lung	Lung perfusion studies most commonly for the diagnosis of pulmonary embolism
^{99m}Tc-exametazime (HM. PAO)	Brain	Regional cerebral imaging in stroke and tumours Diagnosis of Alzheimer's dementia
^{99m}Tc-exametazime (HM. PAO) labelled leucocytes	Infection or inflammation	Identification of abscesses associated with pyrexia of unknown origin Extent of inflammatory bowel disease
^{99m}Tc-tetrofosmin	Heart	Cardiac perfusion imaging
^{99m}Tc-sestamibi (MIBI)	Heart	Cardiac perfusion imaging
^{99m}Tc-tin colloid	Liver	Location of hepatic tumours, abscesses and cysts. Detection of cirrhosis
^{99m}Tc-diethylamine triamine pentaacetic acid (DTPA)	Kidney	Dynamic studies to study kidney function
^{99m}Tc-dimercapto-succinic acid (DMSA)	Kidney	Static imaging showing the kidney structure

The production of ^{99m}Tc—the molybdenum/technetium generator

Radionuclides with long half-lives (e.g. ^{201}Tl, $T_{1/2}$ = 73 hours) can be easily transported from production site to the user hospital. With shorter half-life radionuclides, e.g. ^{99m}Tc, this supply system would be impossible. As a result a device known as the radionuclide generator is used to provide ^{99m}Tc to the hospital site.

Radionuclide generators work on the principle that they contain a relatively long-lived 'parent' radionuclide that decays to produce a 'daughter' radionuclide. The chemical nature of parent and daughter are different, allowing separation of the daughter from the parent.

The molybdenum/technetium generator consists of ^{99m}Mo absorbed onto an alumina-filled column, the ^{99m}Mo being present in the form of molybdate (^{99m}MoO$_4$$^{2-}$). ^{99m}Mo decays to its daughter radionuclide ^{99m}Tc, as pertechnetate, ^{99m}TcO$_4$$^-$ (Fig. 27.5). The amount of ^{99m}TcO$_4$$^-$ grows as a result of the decay of ^{99m}Mo, until a transient equilibrium is reached. At this point the amount of ^{99m}Tc in the column appears to decay with the half-life of ^{99m}Mo (Fig. 27.6).

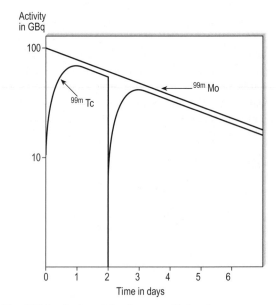

Fig. 27.6   Radioactivity changes with time in a molybdenum/technetium generator column.

By drawing a solution of sodium chloride 0.9% w/v through the column, ^{99m}Tc is removed from the column in the form of sodium pertechnetate, Na^{99m}TcO$_4$. This process is known as eluting the generator and the resulting solution as the eluate. The result of this process is a sterile solution of sodium pertechnetate that may now be used to make ^{99m}Tc-radiopharmaceuticals.

^{99m}Mo remains on the column where it decays to produce further ^{99m}Tc, the equilibrium being re-established about 23 hours after elution. Elution of the generator is repeated daily to provide the radiopharmacy with a supply of ^{99m}Tc for 7–14 days, beyond which the yield of ^{99m}Tc becomes too small to be useful. Hospital radiopharmacies tend to buy generators on a weekly basis to provide a continuous supply of ^{99m}Tc.

Design of a ^{99m}Tc-generator

The design of a typical generator will be described by reference to the Amersham International generator, Amertec II (Fig. 27.7). The main components of this generator are:

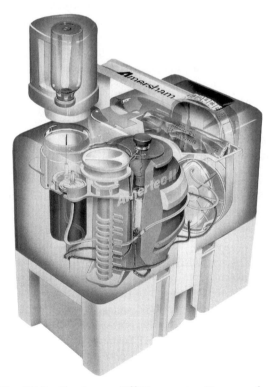

Fig. 27.7 The Amertec II ^{99m}Tc-generator. (Courtesy of Amersham International plc.)

- A 250 mL PVC bag of Sodium Chloride Intravenous Infusion BP 0.9% w/v
- A sterile alumina column to which is bound ^{99m}Mo
- An elution needle
- One 0.22 μm filter and one 0.45 μm filter.

These components are housed within a compact plastic casing. The alumina column is encased in lead to give protection from the radiation.

Operating the generator is fairly straightforward. A sterile evacuated vial, supplied with the generator, is placed in a lead pot designed for the elution process. By placing this on the elution needle, the vacuum draws sterile Sodium Chloride Intravenous Infusion BP 0.9% w/v through the column and into the same vial. When eluate has been collected, air enters the elution vial after first passing through the column. This dries the column as well as removing excess vacuum in the elution vial. The elution process is now complete and the vial may be removed from the generator.

The sterility of the eluates is maintained throughout the useful life of the generator by the following means:

- The eluting solution is terminally sterilized Sodium Chloride Intravenous Infusion BP 0.9% w/v.
- Air entering the system passes through a 0.22 μm hydrophobic filter.
- A terminal eluate filter is placed between the column and the elution needle.
- Between elutions the needle is protected by a single-use, disposable, sterile needle guard.
- The elution of the generator should be carried out in a Grade A environment (see Ch.13).

Preparation of ^{99m}Tc-radiopharmaceuticals

The daily supply of ^{99m}Tc is provided by the elution of the generator, resulting in a sterile solution of sodium pertechnetate that is subdivided to provide the activity component of the radiopharmaceutical. Some nuclear medicine investigations use sodium pertechnetate alone as the radiopharmaceutical (Table 27.2). In this case preparation of Sodium Pertechnetate Injection requires only the subdivision from the generator eluate with perhaps some dilution with Sodium Chloride Intravenous Infusion BP 0.9% w/v. Other investigations, and these are in the majority, use radiopharmaceuticals that involve the chemical transformation of the sodium pertechnetate into another radiochemical form.

In order to make the preparation of ^{99m}Tc-radiopharmaceuticals as simple as possible, commercially available 'kits' are used to manufacture these radiopharmaceuticals. These kits allow the radiopharmacist, in the hospital environment, to transform the pertechnetate, via complex chemical reactions performed within the vial, into the desired radiopharmaceutical. This is achieved by the simple addition of pertechnetate into the vial followed by shaking to dissolve the contents.

A kit consists of a prepacked set of sterile ingredients designed for the preparation of a specific radiopharmaceutical. Most commonly the ingredients are freeze-dried, enclosed within a rubber-capped nitrogen-filled vial. Normally the kit contains sufficient materials to prepare a number of patient doses. In a typical formulation the following may be found:

- The compound to be complexed to the ^{99m}Tc. These are known as ligands (e.g. methylene diphosphonate).
- Stannous ions (e.g. stannous chloride or fluoride) which are present as a reducing agent. The reduction of ^{99m}TcO$_4^-$ to a lower valance state is required to allow the ligands to form a complex with the ^{99m}Tc.
- Other compounds that act as stabilizers, buffers, or antioxidants.

Given below is an example of how ^{99m}Tc-radiopharmaceutical production may be performed. The compounding procedures must be carried out within the facilities described in Chapter 13 using aseptic technique and carried out as 'closed' procedures (GMP).

The production method (Fig. 27.8) involves two simple steps.

Step 1. The freeze-dried kit is reconstituted by aseptically transferring the necessary activity of sodium pertechnetate using a sterile syringe and needle. This step may also include a further dilution of the eluate with a suitable diluent. The amount of activity withdrawn for the reconstitution of the kit vial depends on two factors:

- The number of patient doses to be manufactured.
- The amount of activity required at injection time for each of the patient doses. The calculation would take into account the decay of ^{99m}Tc. Manufacturers normally specify a maximum activity that may be added to the vial.

Step 2. The reconstituted kit is aseptically subdivided to provide each patient dose with sufficient activity to allow proper imaging after administration. As in Step 1, a diluent may be added to the final dose to give the desired radioactive concentration.

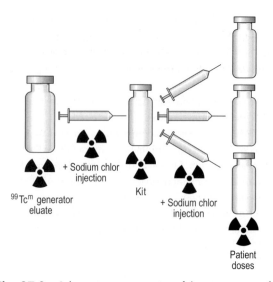

+ Sodium chlor injection

^{99}Tc^m generator eluate

Kit

+ Sodium chlor injection

Patient doses

Fig. 27.8   Schematic representation of the preparation of patient doses of radiopharmaceuticals.

^{99m}Tc-radiopharmaceuticals must be administered on the day of production, for the following reasons:

Sterility.   Aseptically prepared pharmaceuticals should ideally be administered within a few hours of production, in accordance with GMP Section 13.

Radioactivity. ^{99m}Tc has a half-life of only 6 hours.

Radiochemical stability. ^{99m}Tc-complexes are generally stable for a period between 4 and 8 hours after production.

Radiation protection in the radiopharmacy

There are three basic principles to radiation protection:

Shielding.   By placing shielding around the radioactive source the radiation dose rate may be reduced. Materials used as shielding must be appropriate to the type of radiation being emitted by the radionuclide. Plastic, Perspex and metals of low molecular weight like aluminium are appropriate materials for shielding β-emitters. For γ-emitters high molecular weight metals like lead and tungsten should be used. The thickness of shielding material necessary for γ-emitters is dependent on the γ-ray energy—the greater the energy, the thicker the shield required.

Distance.   The radiation dose from a radioactive course is inversely proportional to the square of the distance (i.e. by doubling the distance the radiation dose is quartered).

Time. Minimizing the time spent handling a radioactive source will reduce the radiation dose. It is important for new operators to practise the handling operation prior to working with radioactive materials.

In working practice all three of these principles may be used in isolation or together to reduce the radiation dose to the operator. For example in the dispensing operation outlined in Figure 27.8, all vials containing radioactive material would be contained in a 3 mm lead pot. This will attenuate ^{99m}Tc's γ-rays by a factor of approximately 1000. The syringes used to carry out the transfers would be only half full (i.e. 1 mL of radioactive solution would be transferred with a 2 mL syringe) in order to maximize the distance between the operator's fingers and the source, without compromising the accuracy of the dispensing operation.

The syringes, during the operation, should also be contained within a syringe shield. These are made of materials such as lead, tungsten, lead glass or lead acrylic, the latter two being transparent. Lead and tungsten syringe shields have lead glass/acrylic windows incorporated to allow the operator to see the graduations on the syringe. Alternatively the whole syringe shield may be made of lead glass/acrylic which would have the advantage of giving greater visibility.

Handling the vials outside their lead pots should be carried out using long forceps and not with the fingers. The dispensing process should be carried out over a 'drip tray' that allows easy containment of any accidental spillage. It also should be carried out within a laminar flow safety cabinet or isolator that provides operator protection as well as product protection (see Ch. 13).

The staff working in the radiopharmacy will be constantly monitored to assess their radiation exposure and to ensure compliance with safety legislation. Whole-body dose may be monitored with film badges and the radiation dose to the finger pulp with thermoluminescent dosimeters.

Key Points

- Cytotoxic agents may be alkylating agents, antimetabolites, vinca alkaloids or antimitotics.
- Cytotoxic agents may be given orally (tablets, capsules or suspensions) or parenterally (syringe, slow bolus or IV additive).
- There are risks to health care workers who handle cytotoxics.
- Use of strict aseptic conditions minimizes the risks during preparation.
- Following the RPSGB guidelines and *The Cytotoxics Handbook*, ensure the health and safety of all personnel, including patients.
- Detailed procedures for preparation and use of cytotoxic agents must be drawn up and followed.
- All personnel involved in provision of a centralized cytotoxic reconstitutions service must have full training in procedures, clean rooms, storage and transportation of cytotoxics and all local policies.
- Opening ampoules or the venting or removal of needles from vials carries the risk of escape of cytotoxic material
- Home chemotherapy services place extra demands on the pharmacy department and could also present drug stability problems.

- A centralized intravenous additive service can provide IV antibiotics, patient-controlled analgesia and domiciliary IV antibiotics.
- Pharmacy managers are the main decision-makers in setting up a CIVAS.
- Potential benefits of CIVAS are improved use of resources, services to patients and pharmacy control.
- A number of problems can arise with CIVAS, such as staffing, storage, distribution, out-of-hours and emergency provision and communications.
- Most doses are provided from CIVAS as preloaded syringes or as a minibag.
- Home IV therapy is likely to use single-dose infusers, electronic or elastomeric infusers or a slow IV push.
- Radiopharmaceuticals may be used in therapy or diagnosis, the latter either as tracers or in imaging.
- ^{99m}Tc is the most widely used radionuclide.
- Radiopharmaceuticals are normally administered intravenously and must be produced on the day of use by aseptic techniques.
- A molybdenum/technetium generator will provide a daily supply of ^{99m}Tc for 7–14 days, as sodium pertechnetate.
- Reacting with a suitable ligand can chemically modify sodium pertechnetate.
- Radiation protection should be provided for operators using a combination of shielding, distance and time.

28

Parenteral nutrition and dialysis

K. Sabra (original author S. L. Hutchinson)

After studying this chapter you will know about:

Provision of nutritional support
Indications for total parenteral nutrition (TPN)
Components and compounding of a TPN/home parenteral nutrition (HPN) formulation
Addition of medicines to a TPN or HPN bag
HPN training and potential problems
Administration of a TPN/HPN formulation
The National Total Parenteral Nutrition Group
Introduction to home care for patients on dialysis
Haemodialysis (HD), peritoneal dialysis (PD), including continuous ambulatory peritoneal dialysis (CAPD), intermittent peritoneal dialysis (IPD) and automated peritoneal dialysis (APD)
Dialysis solutions
Provision of services from a hospital renal unit, including home dialysis

Introduction

Today an increasing number of patients are provided with health care services at home. Such services include provision of home parenteral nutrition and home dialysis. This chapter will explore the provision of parenteral nutrition and dialysis for patients in hospital and will explain how these services can be transferred to the home care setting.

PROVISION OF NUTRITIONAL SUPPORT

Studies have shown that up to 50% of medical and surgical patients can suffer from nutritional deficiencies. If nutritional support is indicated, enteral feeding is considered as the first option. Patients can receive nutrients orally or via a tube feed, e.g. by nasogastric feeding. This is only possible if the gastrointestinal tract is functional. If this is not the case, parenteral nutrition may be considered. Short-term (e.g. postoperative) intravenous (IV) administration of fluids such as 5% dextrose saline may be sufficient. This could provide the patient with around 500 calories per day but does not provide any protein, vitamins, minerals or trace elements.

For patients requiring longer-term nutrition, total parenteral nutrition (TPN) may be required. TPN is a method of administering adequate nutrients via the parenteral route. The components of a TPN formulation are added to a sterile infusion bag and administered to the patient via a catheter. Administration can be via a peripheral vein or a central vein. However, TPN fluids are normally highly concentrated mixtures which on a long-term basis could cause damage to peripheral veins. For this reason, peripheral veins are only used for TPN administration lasting up to 2 weeks.

If parenteral nutrition is supplied to patients at home, it is known as home parenteral nutrition (HPN). Patients on HPN administer their nutrition via a central vein. A compounding service providing TPN and HPN formulations is now readily available from a large number of hospital pharmacies in the UK. Commercial pharmaceutical companies also provide home care services for HPN patients.

Parenteral nutrition formulations are prepared under strict aseptic conditions (see Ch. 13) following guidelines published by the Medicines Control Agency (MCA) in *Rules and Guidance for Pharmaceutical Manufacturers* (2002) and by the Department of Health in *Aseptic Dispensing for NHS Patients* (Farwell 1995).

HPN is becoming more popular, particularly for patients who require long-term parenteral nutrition. Guidelines have been published by the British Association of Parenteral and Enteral Nutrition (BAPEN) to ensure that adequate provision is made for patients receiving HPN (Wood 1995).

Patients who are suitable candidates for HPN will be provided initially with TPN bags in the hospital. Therapy will continue until their medical condition is stabilized. They can then undergo appropriate training to enable them to administer their TPN bags at home. However HPN patients may still require to return to the hospital for regular check-ups. This means that pharmacists involved in the care of HPN patients will require a working knowledge of the procedures adopted to provide care for patients in hospital and at home. They may also have to liaise with the patient's GP, the community nurse and other health care workers in this field.

This chapter concentrates on the provision of adult TPN in hospital and at home, although neonatal TPN is available.

INDICATIONS FOR TPN

TPN can be required for finite periods of time or can be required for life. Some of the main indications for TPN are:

- Gastrointestinal disease including: Crohn's disease, ulcerative colitis, pancreatitis and malabsorption syndrome
- Major trauma including: severe burns, severe septicaemia, intensive care patients and acute renal failure
- Major abdominal surgery: severely malnourished patients may benefit from early postoperative parenteral nutrition if surgery has resulted in a non-functioning gastrointestinal tract
- Malignancy of the small bowel
- Radiation enteritis: TPN is considered if enteritis is severe after treatment of a primary malignancy
- High-dose chemotherapy, radiotherapy and bone marrow transplantation. Patients are often ill for a limited time (3–6 weeks) and are unable to eat. TPN can be administered during this period to ensure that the patient's nutritional requirements are adequately met.

Several other conditions may require the nutritional support of TPN, e.g. moderately malnourished patients prior to surgical treatment, patients in a prolonged coma or AIDS patients.

ASSESSMENT OF THE PATIENT IN HOSPITAL

TPN aims to provide patients with all their nutritional requirements in one formulation which can then be infused directly into the body via a central line catheter into the veins. In order to determine exactly what the patient's nutritional requirements are, clinical and biochemical assessment must take place. A patient history is recorded followed by a physical examination to give a clearer picture of the patient's current medical status. Patients' body weight and height can be recorded and comparison made with their ideal body weight which would be available from standard charts. Some hospitals use nomograms which give an estimation of patients' energy and nitrogen requirements taking into consideration their medical condition and body characteristics.

Biochemical assessment will be undertaken initially by performing a number of routine tests which can then be repeated as necessary during TPN therapy. Factors investigated will include blood counts, 24-hour urine analysis, electrolyte and fluid balance.

Each hospital has its own particular way of designing a TPN regimen. Some hospitals tailor regimens to individual patients and carry out a number of calculations to determine baseline requirements for each component. In this way they can build up a formulation by matching up the patient's requirements to commercially available solutions which contain the required components in the correct proportions. During this process careful consideration is given to the patient's medical condition and the necessary adjustments made.

Other hospitals use a range of standard formulations which are routinely used to treat TPN patients. Standard bags can be altered if the need arises: e.g. intensive care patients may require extra nitrogen in the formulation; renal patients may need an electrolyte-free formulation. In general, additions to the finished TPN bags are not recommended in order to minimize microbial contamination.

More recently pharmaceutical companies have introduced a three in one ready-to-use bag. This bag has three chambers, which contain amino acid, dextrose and lipid. When a bag of TPN is required, the seal separating the chambers can easily be broken and the three solutions are mixed together in one chamber. This type of bag can be used when initiating patients on TPN, and also additions of vitamins or electrolytes can be added to the bags prior to usage.

THE NUTRITION TEAM

In most hospitals where TPN is supplied there will be a nutrition team. This team can include the following:

- Consultant
- Senior registrar/registrar
- Pharmacist

- Nutrition nurse(s)
- Dietician(s)
- Biochemist(s).

The role of these individuals in provision of patient care can vary from one hospital to another. In general, the consultant is responsible for prescribing the TPN formulation and liaising with the patient's GP to provide care for HPN patients.

The pharmacist can provide information on aseptic techniques for handling and setting up TPN bags, formulation requirements, potential complications or stability problems, and storage conditions required. In some hospitals, the pharmacist's role can be extended to include the following:

- Training nursing staff in the techniques required for IV administration of TPN fluids
- Helping with patient training for HPN
- Monitoring of patients in HPN clinics.

The nutrition nurse and dietician will together give advice on a day-to-day basis regarding the nutritional status of the patients and advise on necessary dietary requirements. The nutrition nurse can also be responsible for training patients for HPN.

The biochemist can supply results of daily or weekly analysis of patients' urine and electrolyte levels and alterations can then be made to the TPN formulation if required. The nutrition team can meet on a weekly basis to discuss the requirements of patients currently receiving TPN both in hospital and at home.

If HPN is supplied by the hospital pharmacy, patients can be provided with the support of a small group of people, some of whom may be part of the nutrition team. This group usually includes the nutrition nurse, the hospital pharmacist and the patient's GP.

Commercial companies supplying home care services have a nutrition nurse who provides medical care, support and advice (on a 24-hour basis if required), a patient coordinator who deals with the ordering of HPN bags and ancillaries, and a designated delivery person who will supply the necessary equipment and HPN bags to the patient's home.

COMPONENTS OF A TPN FORMULATION

TPN formulations can contain the following components:

- Water
- Protein source

- Energy source—carbohydrate and possibly fat
- Electrolytes
- Trace elements
- Vitamins and minerals.

Baseline water requirements

Water accounts for over 50% of the body weight. To prevent patients becoming dehydrated, daily water losses and gains must be carefully considered. Water can be lost through urine and faeces and through 'insensible losses' through skin and lungs.

Several methods are available for estimating daily fluid requirements, but most take into consideration body weight and measured urine output, and an allowance is made for insensible losses. The average adult requires between 1500 and 3000 mL of fluid per day. A TPN regimen will require to provide this volume of fluid on a daily basis.

Protein source

Protein requirements vary from one patient to another and are highly dependent on the metabolic status of the patient. Undernourished patients requiring parenteral nutrition are generally said to have a negative nitrogen balance. This means that the amount of nitrogen excreted in urine and faeces is greater than the nitrogen administered.

Lack of nitrogen in the body can result in poor wound healing and interference with body defence mechanisms. To overcome this problem, a utilizable source of nitrogen must be administered to the patient. This is achieved by administering amino acid solutions in a TPN formulation. These solutions act as a source of nitrogen and are said to be the building blocks for the formation of proteins in the body. Nitrogen requirements can be estimated from a 24-hour urine collection. This is done by analysing the total amount of urea excreted and by considering the individual patient's body weight and clinical 'type'.

EXAMPLE 28.1

A postoperative surgical patient requires 0.2 g/kg/24 h of nitrogen. The patient weighs 47 kg.

$$\text{Nitrogen requirements per day} = 0.2 \times 47 \text{ kg}$$
$$= 9.4 \text{ g nitrogen}$$

This requirement can then be matched up to commercially available solutions. Each gram of amino

---

acid nitrogen is equivalent to 6.25 g of protein, e.g. Vamin 9 contains 9.4 g of nitrogen. This is equivalent to 60 g of protein and will provide the patient with the required daily nitrogen intake. However, care must also be taken when selecting an amino acid solution for inclusion in a TPN formulation, as most commercially available solutions are hypertonic in nature and have a pH between 5 and 7.4. The pH of the amino acid solution may have an effect on the overall stability of the formulation and must be considered carefully.

Energy sources

Carbohydrates and fats are chosen to provide optimal energy sources for TPN patients. The relative proportions of each will be dependent on the clinical requirements of the patient and formulation considerations. The carbohydrate of choice is normally dextrose and is available in solution with concentrations ranging from 5 to 70% w/v. Like amino acid solutions, dextrose solutions are hypertonic and have a low pH (3–5). If dextrose is required in large quantities (greater than 300–400 g per day), insulin can be administered in the TPN formulation to increase the uptake of dextrose into the body tissues from the bloodstream and to reduce the risk of hypoglycaemia at the end of the infusion period.

The fat component in a TPN formulation is administered in the form of an oil-in-water emulsion. Fat emulsions are isotonic with plasma, have neutral pH and provide a high calorie source in a low volume. As a result, they are often used in combination with dextrose to provide the necessary calorie content, thereby avoiding the potential problems encountered with excessive dextrose administration.

Fat emulsions provide the patient with essential fatty acids and also act as a vehicle for fat-soluble vitamins which may be required in the TPN formulation. Fat is not required in every TPN formulation, but fat deficiency can occur in patients who do not receive fat components for periods greater than 1 month. Depending on individual requirements, patients on long-term TPN may require fat added to their TPN bag daily, on alternative days or two or three times weekly.

Commercially available preparations are based on soya bean oils and are composed of varying combinations of long and medium chain triglycerides. The energy content of commercially available solutions for both carbohydrates and fats is expressed in kcal/litre, e.g. Intralipid 10% provides 550 kcal/500 mL; Dextrose 5% provides 210 kcal/500 mL.

Electrolytes

The main electrolytes of clinical significance in a TPN formulation include sodium, potassium, magnesium, calcium, phosphate and chloride. The requirement for electrolytes can be met in the form of injectable solutions of varying percentage content. Electrolyte content of each is expressed in terms of mmol/L. The individual role of each electrolyte in a TPN formulation is given in Table 28.1.

Trace elements

Trace elements act as metabolic cofactors and are said to be essential for the proper functioning of several enzyme systems in the body. Despite being termed essential, they are only required in very small quantities, expressed in micromoles. The main trace elements required in a TPN formulation are zinc, copper, manganese and chromium. More details on trace element requirements are given in Walker and Edwards (2003).

Vitamins and minerals

Vitamin requirements fall into two categories, fat soluble and water soluble. Four fat-soluble vitamins (vitamins A, D, E and K) and nine water-soluble vitamins (vitamins B_1, B_2, B_3, B_5, B_6, B_{12}, C, folic acid and biotin) are said to be essential.

Vitamins and minerals are normally included in foods taken in orally and must therefore be included in TPN formulations for patients on long-term parenteral nutrition. They are required for several body processes and act as essential coenzymes in carbohydrate metabolism and amino acid and DNA synthesis. Commercially available solutions include Multibionta, Parentovite, Solivito N and Vitlipid N Adult.

COMPOUNDING OF TPN AND HPN FORMULATIONS

Compounding can take place within a hospital pharmacy using aseptic dispensing facilities within a clean room or within a designated compounding unit in a commercial pharmaceutical company.

Preparation and training

For patients in hospital, the consultant will prescribe a suitable TPN regimen. On receipt of the prescription, the

Table 28.1   Role of electrolytes used in TPN formulations. (From Walker & Edwards 2003, reproduced by permission)

Electrolyte	Principal function	Daily intravenous requirement	Symptoms of deficiency	Symptoms of excess	Common sources
Sodium	Main extracellular cation Regulation of water balance Neuromuscular contractility	1–2 mmol/kg	Weakness, lethargy, confusion, convulsions, appetite, nausea and vomiting	Lethargy, coma, convulsions, muscle rigidity, thirst	Sodium chloride Sodium acetate Sodium phosphate
Potassium	Main intracellular cation Regulation of acid–base balance Neuromuscular contractility	1–2 mmol/kg	Muscle weakness, ileus, arrhythmias, alkalosis	Muscle weakness, paraesthesia, bradycardia, nausea and vomiting	Potassium chloride Potassium phosphate
Magnesium	Cofactor for enzyme systems Neuromuscular contractility	0.1–0.2 mmol/kg	Lethargy, cramps, tetany, paraesthesia, arrhythmias, neuromuscular excitability, hypokalaemia, hypocalcaemia	Decreased muscular activity, lethargy, respiratory depression	Magnesium sulphate Magnesium chloride
Calcium	Mineralization: bones + teeth Neuromuscular contractility	0.1–0.15 mmol/kg	Paraesthesia, tetany, fitting, confusion, arrhythmias	Nausea, anorexia, lethargy, muscle weakness, confusion	Calcium gluconate Calcium chloride
Phosphate	Main intracellular anion Acid–base balance Energy	0.5–0.7 mmol/kg	Weakness, tingling	Non-specific effects on calcium balance	Phosphate salts of sodium and potassium, hydrogen
Chloride	Main extracellular anion Acid–base balance	1–2 mmol/kg	Alkalosis	Acidosis	Chloride salts of above cations

pharmacist checks the suitability and compatibility of the formulation, the required volume of each component is calculated and details are transferred to a worksheet. Patient details can be entered into a computer and labels generated for the worksheet and the final product. In the preparation area items required for the compounding process can be collected together in an appropriate tray ready for transfer to the clean room facility. Batch numbers and expiry dates for

each product used are recorded on the worksheet. The pharmacist checks all details, including calculations, before the compounding procedure begins.

Compounding of a TPN formulation is carried out under strict aseptic conditions (in a Grade A environment) using a laminar airflow (LAF) cabinet within a clean room facility. Chapter 13 gives details regarding clean room facilities, gowning-up procedures for entry to clean rooms and working procedures for using LAF cabinets. Standard operating procedures (SOPs) should be available for all staff carrying out aseptic dispensing procedures. Operators will undergo appropriate training including validation of operator techniques by broth fill tests (see Ch. 13) prior to commencing work in the field.

TPN/HPN bags

The components of a TPN formulation are sterile and are prepared under sterile conditions as the formulation is eventually infused directly into the bloodstream of the patient. It is therefore essential that the bags used to hold the TPN formulation are also sterile. In the past, only polyvinyl chloride (PVC) bags were used for TPN formulations. However, because of the problems of leaching of plasticizers from PVC bags containing a fat component, ethylvinyl acetate (EVA) bags (which contain no plasticizers) are now more commonly used. However, EVA bags have been shown to be permeable to oxygen; hence multilayer EVA bags are now available for formulations requiring prolonged storage. These bags are made of layers of plastic with an inert inner layer made of EVA. This arrangement reduces oxygen permeation to a minimum.

Bags are usually supplied with a premounted sterile filling set attached. The filling set consists of a number of hollow plastic tubes (up to six) with a plastic spike attached to the end of each. The spikes are used to pierce the rubber septum of the bottles and bags of amino acids, glucose and fat emulsion to enable filling of the components into the TPN bag. Clamps fitted with air vents are attached to each filling tube to clamp off the source bottles and bags when they are empty. Filling sets are used for compounding purposes only and are disconnected and replaced with a sterile hub before being sent out to the patient. Every HPN bag is supplied with a sterile giving set which allows the bag to be infused into the patient.

TPN bags vary in size, ranging from small 250 mL bags used for neonatal TPN up to 3 L bags for adult TPN. Bags used for HPN patients are identical to those used for TPN in hospitals. Figure 28.1 shows a TPN bag with filling set attached.

Addition of components to a TPN bag

Components are added into the TPN bag in a strictly defined procedure. Small-volume additives can be added directly into large-volume fluids (but not directly into the fat com-

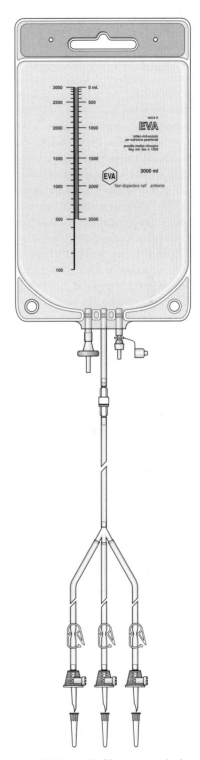

Fig. 28.1   A TPN bag with filling set attached.

ponent) or directly into the additive port on the bag (depending on manufacturers' recommendations). Amino acid solutions and glucose are added into the bag first, followed by any fat emulsion if required. To prevent precipitation of vitamins, they are generally only added immediately before administration.

Filling of the TPN bags can be achieved under gravity. The bag is placed on the floor of the LAF cabinet and the solution components suspended from a retort stand, enabling the solution to flow freely into the bag. If several bags require to be compounded in a limited time period, the bag can be placed in a vacuum chamber to speed up the filling process. Electronic devices, known as compounders, are also available. They are usually under microprocessor control and can be pre-programmed to fill TPN bags with set volumes of individual components. They can be used to achieve rapid filling of a number of TPN bags and are useful devices for compounding neonatal TPN bags where strict control of fluid volumes is required.

When all the components are added, the bag can be clamped off and the filling set removed. A sterile hub replaces the filling set to prevent any further additions being made to the bag outside the sterile production area. The bag is gently shaken to ensure adequate mixing of all components. The TPN bag and compounding materials are transferred back to the preparation area. A visual inspection of the bag is made, including checking of the additive port, for integrity. All necessary documentation is completed and the TPN bag is labelled.

Details to be included on the label are:

- Patient name (ward and unit number if hospital patient)
- Components of the bag (expressed in mmol)
- Total volume (mL)
- Energy content (kcal)
- Nitrogen content (g)
- Infusion rate (mL/h)
- Expiry date and storage conditions.

The TPN bag is then sealed into a dark-coloured outer plastic bag (to protect the formulation from light) and an outer label that is identical to the label on the bag itself is attached.

To maintain stability of the formulated product, it is refrigerated until required. All TPN and HPN formulation must be stored in a designated pharmaceutical grade refrigerator. Cool-boxes packed with ice packs can be used for transportation of formulations to the ward or the patient's home.

COMPOUNDING OF HPN FORMULATIONS BY COMMERCIAL COMPANIES

A designated compounding unit is used for preparing HPN formulations. Conditions used will be the same as those used in the hospital sector (aseptic dispensing facilities in a clean room). If the commercial company does not have its own compounding facilities it may utilize the services of a hospital pharmacy or another industrial pharmaceutical company to compound the HPN bags. The compounding unit must hold a manufacturing licence prior to supplying TPN bags.

Regardless of the compounding arrangements, the commercial company providing the home care service must be in receipt of a prescription for the HPN formulation prior to compounding. The prescription will be the same formulation which the patient initially had during his stay in hospital.

However, when the health care is transferred to the home care setting in Scotland, the patient's GP will take on the responsibility for supplying the HPN prescription. In England and Wales the health authority is responsible for providing the HPN prescription. Subsequent prescriptions will then be forwarded to the commercial company in advance of the patient's requirements. Orders for sundries and ancillaries such as pumps, dressings, needles, etc. will be dealt with by the patient coordinator.

POTENTIAL COMPLICATIONS ARISING DURING COMPOUNDING AND ADMINISTRATION OF TPN FORMULATIONS

The components of a TPN formulation will individually and collectively contribute to the overall stability of the resulting formulation. However, with several hospitals now using standard TPN formulations, many of these problems can be overcome. For hospital pharmacies which have a manufacturing licence, standard bags can be made up in advance of requirements and stored in a refrigerator for periods of 30 days or more. The shelf life given to individual formulations must be based on validated stability studies previously carried out on the formulation.

Individual components of the formulation such as vitamins, electrolytes and fat can cause formulation complications.

Vitamin stability is very poor, particularly in the presence of light and with extended storage time. Stability is also affected by solution pH, hence the need for careful consideration of the overall formulation.

The requirement for administration of calcium and phosphate in a formulation can lead to precipitation of calcium phosphate. This reaction is said to be affected by factors such as the relative amounts of each component present, solution pH, concentration of amino acid solutions present and the mixing process used. To overcome this type of problem, manufacturers of parenteral nutrition fluids can supply tables which give details of the amount of each component that can be safely combined to ensure stability of the formulation is maintained. These tables are specific to an individual formulation and details cannot be interchanged between formulations.

The presence of fat in a TPN formulation can cause stability problems. As storage time increases, the fat component of the formulation becomes less stable, resulting in a process of 'cracking' where the oil and water phases of the emulsion separate out. If the formulation is administered to the patient in this unstable condition, this can lead to potentially dangerous fat deposits arising in the lungs and other body tissues.

The factors a pharmacist must consider when formulating a TPN bag with a fat component are:

- The order in which components are added to the bag
- The types of electrolytes present and their relative proportions—divalent and trivalent cations reduce stability
- The pH of the resultant mixture—higher pH improves stability
- Conditions arising during storage and administration
- The type of plastic bag used—EVA bags preferred.

ADDITION OF MEDICINES TO A TPN OR HPN BAG

Stability studies have been carried out on a number of medicines to determine their compatibility and stability in a TPN bag. So far, studies have confirmed the suitability of only a limited range of medicines which includes: heparin, insulin, aminophylline, cimetidine, famotidine, ranitidine and certain antibiotics. Reference to manufacturers' literature and compatibility studies will provide current recommendations.

ADMINISTRATION OF TPN/HPN FORMULATIONS

For patients requiring TPN for longer than 2 weeks, central venous access is required. During their stay in hospital, patients have a catheter inserted into the subclavian vein under anaesthesia. It has an exit site on the lower chest wall, allowing patients easy access for care of the catheter site.

Catheters can be made of materials such as polyvinyl chloride or silicone. For long-term feeding a permanent catheter (a Hickman catheter or a portacath) is used. It is held in place by a Dacron cuff (an internal woven plastic used to connect arteries and veins under the skin). Good aseptic techniques are essential to ensure that the catheter site does not become contaminated. Infection around the catheter site can be difficult to treat successfully and may eventually result in removal of the catheter and replacement at another site.

Catheter sites should only be used for administration of TPN fluids and not for blood sampling or administration of other medicines. However, in exceptional circumstances (where venous access is limited) the TPN line may have to be used for these purposes. In some instances, a triple lumen catheter can be used with one line being kept for administration of the TPN bag only. To infuse the TPN formulation into the patient, the catheter is connected via an extension set to a volumetric infusion pump. These devices use positive pressure as the driving force to allow accurate infusion at pre-set rates (see Ch. 25).

Adult TPN formulations can have a volume ranging from about 1500 mL to 3000 mL. The infusion period varies from 24 hours in hospital to around 8–12 hours for home patients (as HPN can often be administered overnight). Infusion rate can be calculated by dividing the total volume of the infusion (mL) by the infusion period (hours) giving a rate of mL/hour. Most pumps now have the ability to be programmed to give an infusion rate which 'steps up' at the beginning and 'steps down' at the end of the infusion period, avoiding potential problems with high concentrations of dextrose in the formulation. They are also fitted with an alarm which will alert the patient if a technical fault arises.

POTENTIAL PROBLEMS FOR HPN PATENTS

Mechanical problems

Problems of pneumothorax, or air embolism, are more likely to occur in the hospital environment in the early stages of catheter placement and are dealt with before the patient commences on HPN. However, daily connection and disconnection of the catheter hub may result in cracking and possible leakage of the HPN fluid. Repair kits are available and if used promptly when the problem first arises, catheter replacement may not be necessary.

Internal blockage of the catheter can arise. Patients are taught to flush out the catheter port with heparinized saline to prevent thrombus formation. Blockage of the line arising during administration of the HPN fluid can cause changes in flow rate which are recognized by the pump, and the alarm is activated.

Metabolic problems

Metabolic complications include:

- Problems with electrolyte levels leading to conditions such as hypernatraemia or hyponatraemia.
- Problems with glucose levels leading to hyperglycaemia or hypoglycaemia.
- Balancing of fluid intake (to ensure adequate hydration is achieved).

The majority of the metabolic complications which can affect HPN patients can be overcome by careful monitoring of the patient initially in hospital and with regular check-ups and home visits by the nutrition nurse.

Catheter-related complications

Catheter-related infections can arise as a result of poor management of the catheter exit site. Infection is distinguished by pain, redness and tenderness around the site. To minimize such infections, staff in the hospital are trained to use strict aseptic procedures when changing TPN bags and use of the catheter port is restricted to administration of the TPN bag only. HPN patients are taught the same aseptic techniques and are required to carry out these procedures at all times when changing bags at home. Home care patients are also taught to be aware of their own physical condition and to be alert to any deterioration in their medical condition at the earliest possible time. Patients are asked to contact their nutrition nurse if they experience any signs or symptoms of infection around the catheter site.

Psychological and social problems

Patients receiving TPN in hospital or at home must learn to adapt to the changes occurring in their lifestyle. Some patients have, over a prolonged period of time, suffered from a general deterioration in their health and as a result adapt well to the initiation of parenteral nutrition as it improves their quality of life. Other patients require TPN as a result of major trauma and these patients find the dramatic changes in their lifestyle very difficult to cope with.

While in the hospital receiving treatment, patients have the constant support of medical and nursing staff who can help them to cope with any practical difficulties encountered. When patients return to the home care setting they need continued support to enable them to cope with their HPN therapy on their own. The ability of patients to adapt to HPN is highly dependent on a number of factors:

- Patient's underlying medical condition
- Physical ability and capability of the patient
- Training and counselling prior to leaving hospital
- Home circumstances, particularly support from family members and the patient's GP
- Ability to deal with physical and emotional changes in lifestyle, e.g. dependence on others, potential for mood swings and clinical depression. Disruption to normal sleeping pattern during administration of the HPN bag overnight and loss of 'social' eating can be difficult for many patients, particularly in the initial stages of HPN.

To enable a smooth transition from hospital to home to be achieved, patients require the services of the nutrition nurse and other health care workers to teach them the necessary skills required for handling, setting up their HPN bags and disconnecting them once the procedure is complete.

TRAINING FOR HPN PATIENTS

Health care which can be provided at home has a number of advantages. Patients have a better quality of life and can become more independent as their confidence in providing self-care increases. However, motivation and confidence to carry out the required manipulations at home are essential. Thus training in the hospital environment is required to build up the necessary skills and techniques.

When a patient has been selected for home care a nutrition nurse will begin a training programme with the patient to teach the practical skills required for safe and effective administration of the TPN bag at home. A discharge plan is required for each patient working towards home care. The British Association of Parenteral and Enteral Nutrition (BAPEN), a registered charity formed in 1992, has laid down guidelines for the provision of nutritional care at home. Individual hospitals will develop their own guidelines based on the advice given by BAPEN. The scope of BAPEN includes guidelines on the following matters:

- Details which should be included in a patient discharge plan
- Knowledge and practical skills which must be achieved by patients prior to discharge
- Guidelines for GPs on the provision of HPN
- Advice on how to liaise with patients' GPs to ensure that everyone is aware of their responsibilities
- Information regarding the supplier of the HPN bags and equipment and how this service will be provided.
- Details of appropriate people who patients can contact for advice and help with any problems they have.

The length of time required for training can vary depending on the patient's underlying medical condition and personal approach to training. Patients must be taught aseptic techniques and the importance of ensuring that they are carried out correctly. They must demonstrate their skills and competence on several occasions prior to leaving the hospital. Training will take place during the day initially, then, as the patient becomes more confident with the techniques, overnight feeding will be started. This allows the patient to lead as normal a life as possible and allows some patients to return to a working environment. Areas covered during the training period include:

- Aseptic techniques for setting up and disconnecting the HPN bag
- Care of the catheter site
- How to deal with problems of the catheter blocking
- Setting the pump for infusion of the HPN bag
- Dealing with simple mechanical problems with the pump.

Information booklets on HPN and educational videos can be used with patients to reinforce the training received in hospital.

SERVICES PROVIDED BY HOME CARE COMPANIES

Patients receiving home care will require certain practical arrangements to be put in place before HPN can be initiated. Home care companies who provide services to HPN patients normally provide the following items for patient use: a refrigerator for storing HPN bags; a trolley for patients to set up their HPN bags aseptically; a drip stand and an infusion pump. Patients are required to have adequate storage space

to keep any extra components which may be required for HPN administration and easy access to hand washing facilities for use prior to setting up their HPN bag

SUPPORT SERVICES PROVIDED FOR HPN PATIENTS

Patients will be metabolically stable prior to transfer to the home care setting, hence frequency of monitoring will be reduced to a minimum. Patients can have monthly checkups at the hospital initially, reducing to 3-monthly as they adapt to life on HPN. During visits, patients may be seen by the consultant and the nutrition nurse, possibly at a lipid clinic. Routine monitoring can be carried out during these visits including the following:

- Checking the patient's underlying medical condition
- Reviewing the patient's nutritional status, particularly in relation to their weight
- Routine haematological and biochemical tests
- Checking for any cardiovascular complications
- Reviewing the patient's psychological state.

The nutrition nurse will make home visits if required to check on aseptic techniques and any practical difficulties being encountered by patients and/or their partner or carer.

Patients on HPN can benefit from the support of others undergoing nutrition therapy at home. This is made possible by an organization called 'PINNT' (Patients on Intravenous and Nasogastric Nutrition Therapy). This is a charitable organization which aims to support and bring together people who have similar medical conditions and could benefit from the moral support of others who understand the problems they face. PINNT provides practical help in areas such as provision of portable equipment for people on HPN who wish to go on holiday; help with holiday arrangements including appropriate travel insurance; and general advice on benefits available to HPN patients. A newsletter is produced on a regular basis and close links are kept between PINNT and BAPEN to ensure that patient needs are adequately met.

THE NATIONAL TOTAL PARENTERAL NUTRITION GROUP

Pharmacists in the UK can keep up to date with the working of organizations like PINNT and BAPEN by joining the National Total Parenteral Nutrition Group (NTPNG).

Currently NTPNG has a large membership, most of whom are hospital pharmacists working in the NHS. However, membership also includes dieticians, nutrition nurses, research workers and members of commercial companies who work in the field of TPN and HPN. The NTPNG exists to further the practice of TPN through a number of activities including research, contributing to the work of BAPEN and arranging symposia on practical and scientific developments in the field. This group is also one of five constituent groups which make up BAPEN. Hence good communication is achieved between the different sectors of health care who provide care for home and hospital patients receiving nutrition support.

INTRODUCTION TO HOME CARE FOR PATIENTS ON DIALYSIS

Like HPN, dialysis at home is now a regular occurrence. Patients requiring dialysis at home are those who require treatment for end-stage renal disease (ESRD) or renal failure. For such patients, their options are dialysis in a hospital renal unit, home dialysis or a transplant. However, because there are insufficient kidney donors, patients can require dialysis for prolonged periods.

WHAT IS DIALYSIS?

In a healthy individual the kidney acts as a crude filter removing toxic waste products such as creatinine and urea from the body, whilst retaining the essential components required to maintain the body's natural homeostatic balance. This process is often referred to as an 'ultrafiltration' process. If renal function is impaired, water and electrolyte balance is disturbed, toxic waste products build up in the blood and the patient suffers from fluid overload. An artificial method of allowing this ultrafiltration to take place must be adopted. This is where dialysis can be used.

Dialysis can never completely replace renal function but can be used as a way of removing toxic metabolites, correcting acid–base balance and avoiding fluid overload. The process of dialysis is dependent on the use of a semipermeable membrane which can allow the separation of a mixture of blood and dialysis fluid as it passes over the membrane. Such a membrane is only permeable to water and small ions but is not permeable to blood cells, plasma proteins or lipids (fats). As the dialysis fluid moves over the membrane it

removes water and waste products from the blood restoring the homeostatic balance. Two main types of dialysis exist:

- Haemodialysis (HD)
- Peritoneal dialysis (PD).

Both HD and PD can be carried out in a hospital renal unit or in the patient's home. Patients are constantly monitored and readings of blood pressure and body weight recorded before, during and after dialysis periods.

Haemodialysis

In HD blood is removed from the patient's body and filtered by passing it over an artificial semipermeable membrane known as a 'dialyser' before being returned to the patient's body again. To allow HD to take place an access point into the patient's body is required. This is achieved using a surgical procedure whereby a fistula is created. This involves joining an artery and a vein together to allow blood at arterial pressure to enter the veins near the skin surface. This allows access to the body circulation. Over a period of weeks the walls of the fused artery and vein dilate creating an access point to enable dialysis to take place. The fistula is usually created in the forearm of the non-dominant arm. Usually two needles with a length of tubing attached are inserted into the fistula; one for transportation of blood to the dialyser and the other to carry purified blood back to the patient. Heparin is normally added to the dialysis fluid to prevent the blood clotting.

To achieve HD the patient's blood must pass over a membrane with a large surface area. This allows solutes to be exchanged between the blood and dialysis fluid. Dialysis membranes are sterile disposable membranes made of cellulose or polycarbonate materials. Pressure is applied to the blood to induce the ultrafiltration process and allow removal of excess water. Dialysis machines have preprogrammed cycles to allow dialysis to be achieved as quickly and efficiently as possible.

HD will initially take the form of short dialysis periods which will be repeated on a regular basis to resolve the fluid overload problem. Once the situation is under control, HD sessions can take place at least three times weekly and will last approximately 4 hours.

HD is a much more efficient way of treating renal failure than peritoneal dialysis (PD) and can correct the fluid overload and electrolyte imbalance more rapidly. However a number of factors make it a more complicated procedure for home patients:

• Training for patients can be time consuming and complicated. Specially trained staff are required to teach aseptic techniques for handling the fistula site and administering intravenous medicines.

• Patients must have a restricted diet and fluid intake as urine output between dialysis sessions is minimal.

• Blood loss can arise during dialysis resulting in a 'washed-out' feeling and possibly anaemia.

• A fine balance is required to achieve the correct dialysis concentration to allow sufficient removal of excess fluids. Hypotension can be a problem if short intensive dialysis periods occur too often.

Peritoneal dialysis

In PD the dialysis fluid is passed directly into the patient's body and no blood removal occurs. Dialysis is achieved by passing the dialysis fluid directly into the peritoneum-lined abdominal cavity, leaving it in situ for a predetermined period and draining it back out again. This is known as the 'dwell time'. During this time, the peritoneal membrane acts as a semipermeable membrane allowing exchange between the blood and the dialysis solution. This enables removal of excess water and waste products from the blood, restoring the body's homeostatic balance. This cycle of filling and draining can be repeated up to five times daily.

Fluids are introduced into the body via an indwelling sterile silicone catheter, known as a Teckhoff catheter. The catheter is inserted under anaesthesia using surgical procedures. The catheter is held firmly in position by two Dacron cuffs. The distal end of the catheter has tiny holes in it to allow the dialysis fluid to flow freely into the peritoneal cavity. Patients and medical staff are taught strict aseptic techniques to ensure that the catheter site remains sterile and free from infection.

With PD, the ultrafiltration process is achieved by an osmotic effect created by the presence of high concentrations of glucose in the dialysis fluid. Glucose concentration can be adjusted to achieve the required removal of the excess fluid from the patient.

Three main types of PD exist:

• Continuous ambulatory peritoneal dialysis (CAPD)
• Intermittent peritoneal dialysis (IPD)
• Automated peritoneal dialysis (APD).

CAPD is the procedure which is most widely used by home dialysis patients. When CAPD is initiated, no dialysis machines are required. Dialysis fluids are warmed to body temperature using a bag warmer and allowed to flow into the peritoneal cavity under the influence of gravity. The fluid bag is attached to a drip stand and is suspended approximately 1 metre above the patient's body. Once the fluid is completely drained from the bag into the peritoneum, it remains there for approximately 4–8 hours. The bag can be disconnected and a sterile Luer lock cap placed over the outer catheter site to avoid the risk of contamination (special 'Y' connectors can be used, one for filling and the other for draining). During this time, patients can carry on with their normal daily routine. When the dwell time is over, an empty sterile dialysis bag is reconnected to the catheter site, the bag placed on the floor and the dialysis fluid drained off. Once the process is complete, a new bag is set up. Each cycle of filling and draining is known as an 'exchange'. Patients on CAPD are recommended to carry out between three and five exchanges per day. The longest dwell time can be 8–10 hours overnight.

IPD involves the use of a 'cycling' machine which automatically repeats the fill and drain sequence, avoiding the need for patients to manually change the dialysis bags. The machine can be loaded with a number of dialysis bags, providing a reservoir of dialysis fluid which can be warmed and delivered into the patient in preset volumes. Dwell times can vary (20 minutes or more) but in general, the patient is connected to the machine for approximately 12 hours. Patients can carry out IPD overnight at home or within a hospital dialysis unit. The process is generally repeated two to four times weekly. For home IPD patients a special room must be set aside to accommodate machinery and dialysis fluids. IPD can be costly to set up at home and is not used as a home dialysis method in preference to CAPD. Patient mobility is also restricted owing to the machinery involved; hence IPD is not as popular with patients.

APD or continuous cycle PD (CCPD) involves the use of a machine to perform the dialysis overnight. The machine utilizes a pump delivery system which warms the dialysis fluid prior to administration and delivers a carefully selected volume of dialysis fluid which exchanges throughout the infusion period overnight. The home patient is required to set up the machine every night by connecting it to the catheter site. The main advantage of this type of dialysis is that the patient is free to continue with a normal daily routine and carry out the dialysis overnight. APD is becoming more popular with patients as procedures used do not require constant bag exchanges. However, it still remains a more costly procedure than CAPD for home patients.

Using CAPD as a technique for home dialysis has a number of advantages:

- CAPD is used continuously (dialysis fluid kept in contact with blood for longer periods) hence there is less disruption to the body's electrolyte balance and fluid and dietary restrictions are limited.
- Blood loss is avoided, hence this is a safer technique for anaemic patients.
- CAPD is a relatively simple process to teach patients as no complicated equipment is required.
- It is a useful technique for children as they have a large peritoneal cavity relative to their body mass.
- Blood sugar levels in diabetic patients can be well controlled by the addition of insulin added to dialysis fluids, if required.

However, CAPD also has a number of disadvantages:

- CAPD is not as efficient a process as clinicians would desire. Patients can suffer from nutritional problems due to the peritoneum allowing the loss of large protein and amino acid molecules through the membrane. As a result, CAPD patients can require high dietary input to make up for daily protein losses.
- Obesity can be a problem with some patients due to large quantities of glucose being absorbed from the dialysis fluids. This gives an added complication of potential cardiovascular problems.
- CAPD is contraindicated in patients who have recently undergone abdominal surgery or in those with severe pulmonary disease as dialysis can compromise lung function.
- Peritonitis can develop in CAPD patients.

Home dialysis patients are taught to recognize the signs and symptoms of peritonitis developing, e.g. cloudiness in the dialysis fluid being drained out, abdominal pain, redness or swelling around the catheter site. They are requested to contact the CAPD nurse of the renal unit immediately. If the infection is caught in the early stage, antibiotic treatment can be initiated and may prevent the complications of catheter replacement. If peritonitis becomes a recurring problem, the patient may have to revert to HD.

DIALYSIS SOLUTIONS

Dialysis solutions used for both HD and PD have similar constituents. They are required to contain electrolytes in concentrations similar to those found in normal extracellular body fluid.

Composition of solutions can vary, but in general they contain sodium, calcium, magnesium, chloride ions and a source of bicarbonate ions (usually from lactate or acetate). Glucose is included as a component of dialysis fluids to achieve the necessary osmotic effect during dialysis. Potassium is normally only incorporated into HD solutions, but can be added to PD solutions if required. Owing to the large volumes of fluid required for HD, solutions are normally prepared in the form of a concentrate which can then be diluted with water prior to use.

HD solutions are not required to be sterile as the membrane within the dialysis machine does not permit the passage of bacteria. All PD solutions require to be sterile and are prepared using aseptic techniques and terminally sterilized by autoclaving. Dialysis fluids are compounded by commercial pharmaceutical companies who supply them directly to hospital renal units or to home dialysis patients. Solutions are supplied in sterile plastic bags (similar to EVA bags used for TPN formulations). Bags are available in a range of sizes from 2 to 7 L. Drainage bags used in CAPD must be of larger capacity to accommodate excess fluid removed during dialysis.

PROVISION OF SERVICES FROM THE HOSPITAL RENAL UNIT

Within the unit there will be a multidisciplinary team of people who are responsible for making decisions regarding the treatment required by patients, for providing medical care and support and training patients for home dialysis. This group can meet at least once or twice weekly to discuss the needs of patients in hospital and at home. The following people can be included in this team: consultant, registrar, pharmacist, renal nurses, dietician, social worker and renal technician. The renal team members will all have individual responsibilities similar to those in the nutrition team:

- The consultant/registrar is responsible for prescribing during dialysis and monitoring the patient's clinical condition.
- The pharmacist can have involvement in a number of areas including: advice on aseptic handling techniques and catheter care, clinical assessment of patients, provision of drug information (particularly bioavailability of renally excreted drugs) and ordering and supplying dialysis fluids and ancillaries to home dialysis patients.

- Renal nurses can be responsible for providing nursing care, monitoring the patient's condition and training patients for home dialysis.
- The dietician can provide patients with detailed information on necessary dietary requirements, food and fluid restrictions.
- A social worker is included in the renal team to provide the necessary advice and practical help for patients at home, e.g. housing requirements, care of other family members particularly children, benefits available for patients unable to work while on dialysis.
- The renal technician is responsible for day-to-day functioning of dialysis machines and advising on dialysis fluid concentrations.

- Aseptic techniques for handling the fistula, checking to ensure that it is in working order and keeping it free from contamination
- How to connect up the fistula lines to the dialysis machine and set it up for dialysis (including adding dialysis fluid and setting up the dialysis cycle)
- Injection techniques for administration of medicines and anaesthetics required during dialysis procedures
- Use of heparin to maintain patency of the line and to prevent blood clotting during dialysis.

Many patients find these procedures too complicated to learn and to carry out on a long-term basis. They also require the constant support of another family member to help with the day-to-day practical issues of carrying out the dialysis.

TRAINING FOR HOME DIALYSIS PATIENTS

Training is carried out by a member of the renal team, usually a CAPD nurse as the majority of patients on home dialysis are CAPD patients. The CAPD nurse will provide the training in hospital and can also act as a point of contact for patients once they are home. Patients will have regular home visits from the CAPD nurse to ensure that they are coping with their dialysis at home. Prior to discharge a training room will be used where patients can set up CAPD or HD and practise their techniques and build up the necessary confidence to carry out their dialysis at home. Educational videos and literature can be used with patients to reinforce practical skills learned within the hospital. The length of time required for training will vary depending on the capabilities of individual patients and the techniques being taught.

HD training can take longer than for CAPD as patients have to be taught a wide range of procedures including:

SUPPORT AND SERVICES FOR HOME DIALYSIS PATIENTS

Like HPN patients, home dialysis patients can be provided with their dialysis fluids, equipment and ancillaries by the hospital pharmacy or a commercial home care company. If the pharmacy provides the service, the pharmacist may be responsible for ensuring that all dialysis fluids and ancillaries are ordered and delivered to the patient on time. If a home care company provides the service, each patient will be allocated a patient coordinator whom the patient will telephone to order dialysis supplies. A designated delivery person will deliver dialysis fluids to the patient's home and rotate stock to ensure that it is used in appropriate date order. Companies can also provide a nutrition nurse to give 'on call' advice to patients, but patients are still free to contact their dialysis unit at any time.

Each individual hospital will be affiliated to the Kidney Patients' Association and will encourage patients and their carers to attend regular meetings to provide practical support for home dialysis patients.

Key Points

- Up to half of medical and surgical patients can have nutritional deficiencies.
- TPN/HPN formulations are prepared under strict aseptic conditions.
- Before starting TPN a full assessment of the patient's nutritional needs must be made.
- The nutrition team contribute their expertise to provide good patient care by meeting regularly to monitor patient needs.
- A TPN formulation may contain water, protein, carbohydrate, fat, electrolytes, trace elements, vitamins and minerals.
- Most TPN patients have a negative nitrogen balance and so require amino acids.
- Care must be taken when administering dextrose in a TPN/HPN formulation to prevent problems of hyper- or hypoglycaemia.
- Strictly defined procedures are followed when adding ingredients to TPN bags during preparation.
- Stability of TPN formulations is one of the major issues which must be carefully considered.
- Controlling quantities can minimize incompatibilities such as that between calcium and phosphate.
- TPN bags containing a fat component become less stable on prolonged storage and could result in fat deposits arising in lungs and capillaries if administered in this unstable condition.

- For TPN lasting longer than 2 weeks a central vein should be used.
- A number of problems can arise during TPN/ HPN administration. For HPN patients, adequate training to deal with problems arising at home is essential.
- HPN patients require to make psychological and social adjustments, but can also have an improvement in quality of life.
- BAPEN has laid down standards for home nutritional care which are used as the basis for patient training prior to discharge.
- Dialysis is used to remove toxic metabolites, correct acid–base balance and avoid fluid overload.
- In haemodialysis, the patient's blood is passed over a semipermeable membrane to allow exchange of small solutes with dialysis fluid.
- Peritoneal dialysis uses the peritoneal membrane as the semipermeable membrane, the dialysis fluid staying in the peritoneal cavity during the exchange.
- CAPD has a number of advantages and disadvantages for patients.
- HD solutions do not require to be sterile, but PD solutions must be sterile and aseptic technique used in handling.
- Home dialysis patients will require training and support. Patients are encouraged to join the Kidney Patients' Association.

Wound management, stoma and incontinence products

J. H. Winfield and A. J. Winfield

After studying this chapter you will know about:

Types of wounds
The form and use of dressings
Graduated compression hosiery
Selection of wound management products
The types of stoma and problems associated with them
Different types of stoma appliances
Incidence and causes of incontinence
The management of incontinence and the use of incontinence appliances
Pharmaceutical advice for patients with stoma and continence problems

WOUNDS

A wound may be defined as any damage to the skin. Wounds are caused by mechanical injuries, burns and underlying medical conditions giving rise to ulcers.

After a wound has been cleansed and debris removed, the complex process of wound healing can begin. This involves the growth of fibrous and vascular tissue within the wound and the migration of epithelial cells from the edges of the wound. Normally a hard scab forms at the wound surface and underlying dehydrated tissue slows down the movement of cells. If the wound is kept moist, epithelial cells can move unimpeded and the epidermis is regenerated within half the time.

Types of wounds

However a wound has been generated, treatment will depend largely upon the present condition of the wound. The same wound may go through several stages in the healing process, and the most appropriate choice of wound management product will change accordingly.

Necrotic wounds

Necrotic wounds are covered with a hard, dry, black layer of dead tissue known as eschar (pronounced eskar). It often occurs in pressure sores. The eschar needs to be removed before healing can begin. A dressing which rehydrates the necrotic tissue by retaining moisture would be appropriate here.

Sloughy wounds

Slough (pronounced sluff) is white, yellow or brown soft material formed from dead cells on the surface of the wound. Again, it needs to be removed for healing to occur. The function of a dressing here would be to rehydrate a dry wound or remove excess fluid from a moist wound.

Granulating wounds

Granulating wounds are red, granular and moist. This is due to granulation tissue, consisting of blood vessels, collagen and other connective tissue, being laid down in the base of the wound. The ideal dressing here would promote moist wound healing and provide thermal insulation; wounds heal more quickly at body temperature.

Epithelializing wounds

Epithelializing wounds are pink in colour as a new epidermis is being formed. This occurs within 24 hours with shallow superficial wounds. In others it follows the granulation stage. A suitable dressing is one which provides a moist environment and does not adhere to the wound.

Exuding wounds

Granulating and epithelializing wounds produce varying amounts of liquid exudate, which usually decrease as healing proceeds. A dressing should be sufficiently absorbent to contain excess exudate while still maintaining a moist wound surface.

Infected and malodorous wounds

Infected wounds are often surrounded by red, hot, inflamed tissue, and pus may be present. As infection delays healing, it should be treated. Minor infections can be treated with dressings containing antimicrobial substances. For more serious infection, a course of appropriate antibiotics given systemically is safer than topical application. Infected burns often respond successfully to Flamazine, a hydrophilic cream containing silver sulfadiazine. Infection with anaerobic bacteria also causes an unpleasant odour. Odour-absorbing dressings will help to remove the offensive smell.

TRADITIONAL DRESSINGS

Dressings have been used for centuries and some of these are still in use today. Most are passive in that they cover and hide the wound, but have little impact on the healing process.

Absorbents

Absorbent dressings are used to:

- Clean and swab wounds
- Absorb excess wound exudate
- Apply medicaments to the skin
- Protect the wound from future knocks.

The dressings can be used in the original fibrous form, e.g. absorbent cotton and cellulose wadding. Alternatively, the fibres are spun into a yarn and woven into a fabric, to be used as fabric absorbents. These include gauzes made from loosely woven cotton or combined cotton and viscose. They are used extensively in surgery. A combination of fibrous and fabric absorbents is found in Gamgee Tissue, where absorbent cotton is enclosed in gauze.

Absorbent dressings should not be left directly on a moist wound for several reasons:

- Dehydration of the wound surface
- Adhesion—as the wound exudate dries out it forms a powerful glue between the dressing and the dermis; removal of the dressing destroys new epidermis and causes fresh bleeding
- Formation of capillary loops as new blood vessels grow around the threads of the fabric
- Shedding of fibres into the wound
- Absorption of antibacterial exudate, so removing part of the body's natural defence mechanism
- Strike-through of exudate to the outer surface of the dressing, providing a pathway for bacteria.

Bandages

Bandages are used for retention of other dressings, support and compression, and for treating skin conditions.

Retention bandages

Retention bandages may be extensible (stretch) or non-extensible. Examples of non-stretch products are Open-wove Bandage and Domette Bandage. The latter contains wool which imparts warmth. These have been largely replaced by more conformable bandages. One example is Cotton Conforming Bandage, which is made of cotton crimped mechanically to impart elasticity in both directions. This helps it to retain dressings in difficult positions such as over joints. Tubular bandages in a variety of sizes are a convenient way of retaining dressings on limbs, abdomen and trunk. They are knitted fabrics, some of which include rubber to increase their elasticity.

Support and compression bandages

Support and compression bandages are one-way stretch products. The support and compression they give increase with the weight of the dressing and its elasticity. Non-adhesive products include crepe bandage, where elasticity is imparted by the inclusion of wool and double twisted cotton threads. This gives light support for strains and sprains. Greater support is given by high and extra-high performance compression bandages. The latter incorporate rubber threads in their structure and a coloured thread running down the centre which acts as a guide in their application, to provide even compression. High compression bandages are used in the management of gross varices, post-thrombotic venous insufficiency, venous leg ulcers and gross oedema.

Adhesive support and compression bandages have the advantage of remaining secure once applied. They are useful in the treatment of injured joints and varicose veins, especially in patients who are mobile. Unfortunately, their application and particularly their removal may be painful and may damage fragile skin. Another disadvantage is a possible sensitivity to ingredients of the adhesive, e.g. rubber. Bandages may be:

- Self-adhesive, e.g. elastic adhesive bandage
- Diachylon, e.g. Lestreflex—the bandage is warmed prior to application in order to produce adhesion
- Cohesive, e.g. Coban—the bandage adheres to itself but not to the patient's skin.

Multilayered compression bandaging is more effective than single-layered systems. It involves applying four layers of bandages:

- First layer: a subcompression wadding bandage to absorb exudate
- Second layer: a light support crepe bandage
- Third layer: a light compression bandage
- Fourth layer: an elastic cohesive bandage to keep the other layers in place.

Medicated bandages

Medicated bandages consist of a cotton bandage impregnated with a medicament formulated in a moist paste. They are used in the treatment of skin conditions, such as eczema and inflammation associated with leg ulcers. They may be left in position for up to a week. They are usually covered by a support and compression bandage. Most are zinc paste bandages containing zinc oxide. Additional ingredients include calamine, coal tar (a fungicide), clioquinol and ichthammol (antibacterials). Some also contain *para*-hydroxybenzoates (parabens) as preservatives, to which some patients are sensitive. A preservative-free product is Steripaste. Stockings impregnated with zinc oxide ointment (e.g. Zipzoc) are also available.

Graduated compression hosiery

Graduated compression hosiery performs a similar function to support and compression bandages, but in a more controlled manner. It is designed so that compression is greatest at the ankle and decreases up the leg. It is classified according to the pressure exerted at the ankle, as shown in Table 29.1.

Table 29.1 Classification of graduated compression hosiery

Class	Pressure at ankle (mmHg)	Degree of support
I	14–17	Light
II	18–24	Medium
III	25–35	Strong

Compression hosiery is indicated for the treatment of varicose veins, varicose ulcers and venous insufficiency. Class I hosiery also helps to prevent deep vein thrombosis (DVT) and varicose veins, so is recommended for pregnant women and for long-haul fliers who are at risk of developing DVT.

Garments available on the Drug Tariff are below-knee and thigh-length stockings. Anklets and kneecaps are also available in classes II and III. These are used for the support of soft tissue injuries. Each item is subject to a prescription charge, so a pair of stockings would be liable for two charges.

Measurements required for elastic hosiery are:

- Circumference of the mid thigh
- Circumference of the widest part of the calf
- Circumference of the ankle
- Length of the foot.

Measurements should be made for each leg early in the day, starting at the top.

Adhesive tapes and dressings

Adhesive tapes consist of a backing material coated on one side with an adhesive mass. The backing material may be fabric or a plastic film. Different combinations of backing material and adhesive give products with different permeabilities:

- Permeable—to air, water and bacteria.
- Vapour-permeable:
  Permeable to air and water vapour
  Impermeable to liquid water and bacteria.
- Occlusive—impermeable.

They are used:

- For securing dressings and appliances
- As skin closures for small incisions
- For covering infected wounds to prevent contamination.

Adhesive dressings have an absorbent pad in addition to the adhesive tape. The pad may be impregnated with a suitable antiseptic, such as aminoacridine hydrochloride or chlorhexidine gluconate.

Low-adherent dressings

Low-adherent dressings are either a single layer over which another dressing is placed, or multilayered with the low-adherent layer in direct contact with the wound.

Paraffin gauze dressings

Paraffin gauze or tulle gras dressings are made of cotton and/or viscose gauze impregnated with white or yellow soft paraffin. The soft paraffin reduces dehydration of the wound surface. Antimicrobial medicaments such as chlorhexidine may also be included. Dressings containing antibiotics such as framycetin sulphate should be used with caution because of the potential problems of bacterial resistance and skin sensitivity.

Tulle dressings with a reduced content of soft paraffin are used to treat superficial wounds such as abrasions and partial thickness burns. Those containing the traditional amount are useful in the transfer of skin grafts, when the tackiness of the products is exploited.

Knitted viscose dressings

Knitted viscose dressings (e.g. N-A Dressing, Tricotex) have an open structure, which allows liquid exudate from the wound to pass through to a superimposed absorbent pad. N-A Ultra has a silicone-coated surface, which reduces adherence further. A medicated version of these products is povidone-iodine fabric dressing (e.g. Inadine), where the dressing is impregnated with povidone-iodine ointment as an antiseptic. It may be used on infected superficial burns and other injuries. The orange-brown dressing loses its colour as the iodine is used up, and the decolorized fabric is a visible indication that the dressing needs renewing.

Absorbent perforated dressings

The number of absorbent perforated dressings has escalated in recent years. They are multilayered with the layer in contact with the wound being a perforated plastic film. The film minimizes adherence to the wound while the perforations allow excess exudate to pass through to an absorbent fibrous layer. Some dressings have an adhesive border,

while others need to be secured with separate adhesive tape. Care is required with some (e.g. Melolin) in applying the correct film-side to the wound. They are all used for lightly exuding wounds.

Other low-adherent dressings

Some low-adherent dressings (e.g. Mepilex and Mepitel) incorporate soft silicone in the wound contact layer. Others have thicker absorbent pads, with gauze (e.g. Mesorb) or non-woven viscose fabric (e.g. Surgipad) to reduce adherence to the wound. These can be used on heavily exuding wounds. Another product, Atrauman, is a polyester tulle dressing, impregnated with triglycerides.

Odour-absorbing dressings

Most odour-absorbing dressings contain activated charcoal. This adsorbs noxious materials and so eliminates offensive odour from infected malodorous wounds. A simple example is CliniSorb. This is an activated charcoal cloth sandwiched between viscose rayon and applied on top of another dressing. In Actisorb Silver 220, the microporous activated charcoal cloth contains silver residues. The silver imparts antibacterial properties to the cloth. The dressing may be applied directly to the wound or over a low-adherent dressing. In Carbonet and Carbopad VC, the low-adherent layer is an integral part of the dressing. A charcoal layer is also included in some of the more modern products, such as Lyofoam C and CarboFlex.

A resurrected remedy for infected malodorous wounds is sugar in the form of sugar pastes. These are made from caster sugar, icing sugar, polyethylene glycol and hydrogen peroxide. Sugar exerts an antibacterial effect by competing for the water present in the bacterial cells. Another management strategy is the use of metronidazole gel on fungating malodorous tumours.

MODERN WOUND MANAGEMENT PRODUCTS

Many of the wound management products which have been introduced in the last 25 years affect the wound healing process. Most are vapour-permeable, so enabling gaseous exchange, but not allowing passage of liquid water or bacteria. This prevents dehydration of the wound surface and so provides a moist environment for the formation of granulation tissue and accelerated epidermal regeneration. The

Vapour-permeable dressings

Dry absorbent dressings

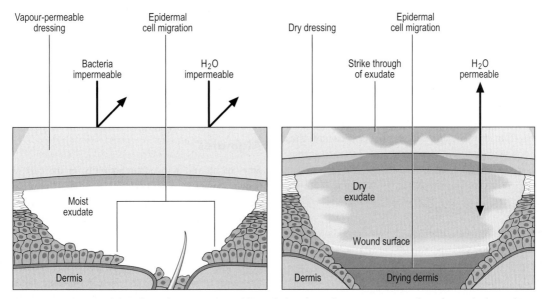

Fig. 29.1 Comparison of the effect of vapour-permeable and absorbent dressings on wounds. (After Coloplast Ltd.)

advantages of these products compared to dry permeable absorbent dressings are illustrated in Figure 29.1.

Vapour-permeable films

Most vapour-permeable films (e.g. Bioclusive, Cutifilm, Opsite Flexigrid, Tegaderm) consist of a thin transparent polyurethane film coated with an adhesive. Some films (e.g. Mepore Ultra, Opsite Plus) have an additional absorbent pad. Others (e.g. Opsite Flexigrid) incorporate a grid for monitoring wound size. Arglaes contains 10% silver ions, which are released in a controlled manner to exert an antibacterial effect.

The vapour-permeable properties of these films enable water vapour, but not liquid water, to pass through from the wound. This occurs at different rates for different products. This may result in the accumulation of excessive exudate under the film. If this occurs, the film should be replaced with a new one, after irrigating the wound with normal saline. Products also differ in their degree of transparency, enabling some wounds to be inspected without removal of the dressing.

Vapour-permeable films are indicated for:

- Use as secondary dressings over alginates or hydrogels
- Lightly exuding shallow wounds, such as minor burns
- Prevention and treatment of superficial pressure sores

- Securing cannulae and catheters
- Use as sterile drapes during surgery.

Foams

Foam dressings are made of polyurethane (e.g. Lyofoam) or silicone (e.g. Cavi-Care). Lyofoam consists of a hydrophobic polyurethane foam sheet, one side of which has been heated under pressure to produce a smooth low-adherent hydrophilic surface. When this smooth surface is placed onto an exuding wound, liquid is absorbed into the 0.5 mm thick hydrophilic layer. As the exudate cannot progress further through the dressing, it maintains a moist wound surface. Eventual lateral strike-through indicates the need for a change of dressing. The 8 mm thick hydrophobic layer is vapour permeable and offers good thermal insulation. It needs to be secured by adhesive tape. This is not necessary with Lyofoam A and Lyofoam K, which incorporate a self-adhesive surround. Lyofoam K also contains a keyhole cut to fit around a catheter or tubing. Lyofoam T performs a similar function as a tracheostomy and cannula dressing. Another product, Lyofoam C, contains a layer of activated carbon within the hydrophobic part, and so is useful for malodorous wounds. The above dressings are used for lightly to moderately exuding wounds. For heavily exuding wounds, the highly absorbent Lyofoam Extra products are more appropriate. Technically, these are foam films—see the next section.

Silicone foam cavity wound dressing (Cavi-Care) is made in situ by stirring the silicone base with a catalyst for 15 seconds, then pouring into the wound cavity. The foam or 'stent' sets in 3–5 minutes, expanding to about four times its original volume. It forms a hydrophobic membrane over the surface exposed to the atmosphere. However, the foam in contact with the wound remains hydrophilic and is able to absorb exudate from the wound surface. The stent may be removed from the wound twice a day for cleaning, then replaced. A new stent is made after about a week, to accommodate wound contraction.

Foam film dressings

Foam film dressings are multilayered products, combining the properties of foams and vapour-permeable films. Most consist of:

- An outer vapour-permeable polyurethane film
- A central absorbent hydrophilic polyurethane foam or membrane
- A low-adherent wound contact layer.

In addition, a hydrogel layer is included in Biatain and the foam in Avance products is impregnated with silver. Most products are available with or without an adhesive border. The latter is preferable on fragile skin.

Most foam films are indicated for lightly to moderately exuding wounds and can be left in place for up to 1 week. Some can be used under compression bandaging and are useful for leg ulcers. Some products are available in a variety of shapes to fit different parts of the anatomy, e.g. the sacrum and the heel, so are useful for pressure sores.

A foam film dressing designed for deeper wounds is Allevyn Cavity Wound Dressing, made of highly absorbent foam 'chips' enclosed in a low-adherent perforated film. Its circular and tubular shapes conform to the shape of the wound.

Polysaccharides

Polysaccharide dressings (e.g. Debrisan, Iodosorb) are tiny spherical beads of glucose polymers. Debrisan is made of dextranomer, manufactured from a derivative of dextran. Iodosorb is cadexomer iodine, which is a hydrophilic modified starch polymer containing 0.9% iodine. When introduced into an exuding wound the beads exert a capillary action on the exudate. Water is absorbed by the beads, while

bacteria and cellular debris become trapped in the spaces between them. The debris is washed away during removal of the dressing.

Beads should not be used on dry or lightly exuding wounds, as they may dry out and be difficult to remove. These products are indicated for infected, sloughy, medium to heavily exuding wounds, especially leg ulcers. As the slippery beads are difficult to use on some wounds, they are also formulated as pastes and an ointment.

Alginates

Salts of alginic acid occur naturally in the cell walls of brown seaweeds, whose healing properties have been recognized by sailors for centuries. Only recently has this been exploited in the extraction of alginates and their subsequent use in wound management.

Alginic acid is a polymer of mannuronic and guluronic acid units. Alginates with a higher proportion of mannuronic acid units form soft flexible gels (e.g. Sorbsan, Algisite M), while those rich in guluronic acid units form firmer gels (e.g. Kaltostat). Alginate dressings are made of non-woven fibres of either 100% calcium alginate (e.g. Sorbsan, Tegagen) or a mixture of calcium alginate and up to 20% sodium alginate (e.g. Kaltostat).

When alginates are placed on moist wounds, there is an exchange of sodium ions at the wound surface with the calcium ions of the dressing. The extra calcium ions help to stop any bleeding. The sodium ions convert part of the insoluble calcium alginate dressing into the more water-soluble sodium alginate. In the presence of exudate the sodium alginate forms a hydrophilic gel over the surface of the wound, providing a moist environment for healing. Dressings may be removed by irrigating with sterile saline. Manufacturers claim any fibres trapped in the wound are biodegraded. Alginate dressings, therefore, should not be used on dry wounds, but are suitable for moderately to heavily exuding wounds.

Alginate dressings are available as:

- Flat non-woven pads—for exuding shallow wounds
- Rope, ribbon, strips or packing—for exuding cavity wounds.

A secondary dressing, such as an absorbent pad or vapour-permeable adhesive film, is needed to cover the alginate fibres. The appropriate choice will be governed by the amount of exudate. With some alginate dressings the secondary dressing is incorporated into the one product. Examples are:

- Sorbsan Plus—includes an absorbent viscose pad
- Sorbsan SA—alginate fibres covered by an adhesive polyurethane foam.

Hydrogels

Hydrogels are three-dimensional networks of hydrophilic polymers, made from materials such as gelatin, polysaccharides and cross-linked synthetic polymers, containing a large proportion of water. They are able to donate water to necrotic and dry sloughy wounds. They also interact with aqueous solutions by absorbing and retaining more water within their structures, without dissolving. Some hydrogels (e.g. Nu-Gel, Purilon) are combined with sodium or calcium alginate, while Granugel contains hydrocolloid powders. There are two types of hydrogels used in wound management:

- Thin flexible sheets (e.g. Geliperm, Hydrosorb, Novogel)—swell as they absorb fluid
- Amorphous gels (e.g. Intrasite Gel, Aquaform, Sterigel)— decrease in viscosity as they absorb fluid until the polymer is dispersed.

The high moisture content of hydrogels maintains a moist wound surface. The amorphous gels are particularly useful in rehydrating necrotic tissue and assisting its separation from underlying healthy tissue, and in treating sloughy wounds. Hydrogels are also indicated for lightly exuding granulating wounds. They cool the wound surface and so reduce pain and inflammation. They are transparent but most need a secondary dressing. One exception is self-adhesive Hydrosorb, covered with a semipermeable polyurethane film; it is available with and without an adhesive border.

Amorphous hydrogels are available in tubes, concertina packs (e.g. Nu-Gel) or applipak (e.g. Intrasite Gel) to facilitate application to awkward places.

Hydrocolloids

Most hydrocolloid dressings (e.g. Granuflex, Comfeel, Tegasorb) are complex formulations containing colloids, elastomers and adhesives. The colloid is the gelling element and absorbent. In most products, it consists of sodium carboxymethylcellulose with some also containing pectin and gelatin. In the sheet form of the dressing, these are present as hydrophilic particles dispersed in a hydrophobic adhesive. The adhesive is bonded to a vapour-permeable polyurethane film, which extends beyond the hydrocolloid

part in some products. An outer polyurethane foam is also present in Granuflex. Aquacel differs in that it is simply a non-woven pad of hydrocolloid fibres only, so requires a secondary dressing when used.

Some hydrocolloids are combined with other materials, e.g. calcium alginate in Comfeel Plus products. Combiderm only has hydrocolloid in its adhesive border, which surrounds an absorbent pad containing polyacrylate granules.

When a hydrocolloid is placed on an exuding wound, the hydrophilic particles absorb fluid and swell into the wound cavity, forming a moist gel at the surface, as shown in Figure 29.2. When the dressing is removed, part of the gel is left in contact with the wound. By covering the nerve endings, the gel reduces pain. The gel often produces an unpleasant odour, about which patients should be warned and reassured.

Most hydrocolloids are available as self-adhesive sheets, which may be square, rectangular, oval, triangular or anatomically shaped for use on the sacrum, heel or elbow. Some products (e.g. Comfeel Plus, Hydrocoll) have

1. Absorption of moisture from wound

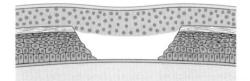

2. Swelling and formation of gel

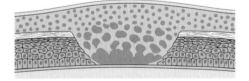

3. Removal of dressing

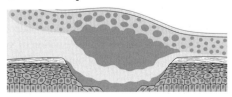

Fig. 29.2 Effect of a hydrocolloid on an exuding wound. (After Coloplast Ltd.)

bevelled edges to prevent the dressing peeling off and to improve the fit in difficult places. For cavity wounds, hydrocolloid powder, paste or ribbon is used in conjunction with the sheet form. Comfeel Plus Pressure Relieving Dressing combines a hydrocolloid sheet with a flexible foam disc, from which central portions can be removed to alleviate pressure on the wound.

Hydrocolloids are used extensively in the treatment of leg ulcers and pressure sores at most stages in the healing process. They rehydrate hard necrotic tissue, which softens and eventually separates. They also remove dead tissue from sloughy wounds. They encourage granulation, but sometimes produce too much granulation tissue. If this occurs they should be replaced by another type of dressing. Most hydrocolloid products are indicated for lightly to moderately exuding wounds. Moderately to heavily exuding wounds can be covered with Aquacel, Combiderm, Cutinova Hydro or Tegasorb. Some dressings are available in a thinner form (e.g. Duoderm Extra Thin, Tegasorb Thin) for use on lightly exuding wounds.

Miscellaneous products

Keloid dressings (e.g. Cica-Care, Mepiform, Silgel) are silicone gel sheets. They are used to manage and prevent hypertrophic and keloid scarring. Application times are increased gradually to acclimatize the skin to the gel sheet.

Dressings based on hyaluronic acid have been developed (e.g. Hyalofill, Seprafilm). Hyaluronic acid is a carbohydrate component of the intercellular matrix of most organs and tissues, including skin. It plays an important role in wound repair. Hyalofill is an ester of hyaluronic acid. It is available as fibrous sheets and rope, which form a thick gel on contact with wound exudate.

Growth factors (GFs) are proteins that bind to receptors on the cell surface. This results in activating cell proliferation and/or differentiation. They include epidermal GFs, platelet-derived GFs, fibroblast GFs and transforming GFs. Attempts to use these in the management of wounds have been fraught with problems, such as their destruction by protein-degrading enzymes in the wound. One product that has reached the market is Regranex, which is a gel containing 0.01% becaplermin. This is a recombinant human platelet-derived GF. It enhances the formation of granulation tissue and is indicated for full-thickness, neuropathic, chronic, diabetic ulcers.

Maggots, particularly sterile larvae of the common greenbottle (e.g. LarvE), are an effective treatment of sloughy, infected or necrotic wounds. The maggots secrete proteolytic enzymes, which break down and liquefy sloughy and necrotic tissue, which they then ingest. They also ingest bacteria, including methicillin-resistant *Staphylococcus aureus* (MRSA). The maggots are left on the wound for a maximum of 3 days.

SELECTION OF AN APPROPRIATE WOUND MANAGEMENT PRODUCT

From the vast array of products, it is increasingly difficult to select the most appropriate wound management product. The number of such products on the *Drug Tariff* has escalated from 29 in 1995 to over 200 in 2002. Many of these products are also in the *Nurse Prescribers' Formulary*. There are limited studies on the comparative effectiveness of products. This is recognized by the National Institute for Clinical Excellence (NICE) guidance on debriding agents for difficult-to-heal wounds. It states that there is insufficient evidence to support one debriding agent over another and choice should be based on patient acceptability, type and location of the wound, and total cost. Many hospitals and primary care trusts have developed wound management formularies in an attempt to rationalize the treatment of wounds.

Table 29.2 gives examples of products that may be used to treat various types of wounds. The examples given do not indicate preferences for those particular products. As new products are continually being developed and names of existing ones changed, it is essential to check with current literature for up-to-date information.

STOMA

There are three types of surgically created stoma, namely ileostomy, colostomy and uroscopy. The reasons for their creation vary, as does the type of effluent produced and the most appropriate appliances to use in their management. These are summarized in Table 29.3.

One-piece or two-piece appliances are used, both being available with closed or drainable pouches. Closed bags are normally used for more solid stools, whilst drainable ones are better with semisolids or liquids. Urostomy bags have a non-return valve to prevent reflux. One-piece products have the skin seal and bag in one item. The hole can be precut or cut by the patient to fit the stoma. Two-piece products have a flange attached to the skin onto which the bag is clipped. These require good skin condition and reasonable dexterity.

Table 29.2   Wound management products for different types of wounds

Wound type	Product type	Examples
Necrotic	Amorphous hydrogel	Aquaform, Granugel, Intrasite Gel, Nu-Gel, Purilon Gel, Sterigel
	Hydrocolloid sheet	Comfeel, Granuflex, Hydrocoll, Tegasorb
	Maggots	LarvE
Sloughy	Sugar paste	
	Polysaccharide	Debrisan, Iodosorb, Iodoflex
	Amorphous hydrogel	Aquaform, Granugel, Intrasite Gel, Nu-Gel, Purilon Gel, Sterigel
	Hydrocolloid—sheet, powder, paste	Comfeel, Granuflex, Hydrocoll, Tegasorb
	Maggots	LarvE
Granulating cavity	Foam	Cavi-Care
	Foam film	Allevyn Cavity
	Alginate—rope, ribbon, strips, etc.	Algisite M, Algosteril, Kaltostat, Melgisorb, Sorbsan, Tegagen
	Hydrogel	Aquaform, Granugel, Intrasite Gel, Nu-Gel
	Hydrocolloid—powder, paste, ribbon	Aquacel, Comfeel, Granuflex
	Hyaluronic acid ester	Hyalofill-R
Granulating and epithelializing		
Moderately to heavily exuding	Low-adherent dressing	Mesorb, Surgipad
	Vapour-permeable film	Arglaes
	Foam film	Lyofoam Extra, Allevyn, Tielle Plus
	Alginate	Algisite M, Algosteril, Kaltostat, Melgisorb, SeaSorb, Sorbalgon, Sorbsan, Tegagen
	Hydrocolloid	Aquacel, Combiderm, Hydrocoll, Tegasorb
Lightly to moderately exuding	Low-adherent dressing	Atrauman, Mepilex
	Foam	Lyofoam
	Foam film	Biatain, Spyrosorb, Tielle, Transorbent, Trufoam
	Alginate	Sorbsan SA
	Hydrogel—sheet	Geliperm, Hydrosorb, Novogel
	Hydrogel—amorphous	Aquaform, Granugel, Intrasite Gel, Nu-Gel, Purilon Gel, Sterigel
	Hydrocolloid	Askina Biofilm Transparent, Comfeel, Granuflex, Replicare Ultra
Epithelializing		
Lightly exuding	Paraffin gauze	Paranet, Paratulle, Unitulle
	Absorbent perforated dressing	Cutilin, Interpose, Melolin, Release, Skintact, Solvaline N, Cosmopor E, Mepore, Primapore, Sterifix
	Other low-adherent dressing	Melolite, Mepitel
	Vapour-permeable film	Bioclusive, Cutifilm, C-View, Hydrofilm, Mefilm, Opsite Flexigrid, Opsite Plus, Tegaderm
	Foam film	Flexipore
	Hydrocolloid	Duoderm Extra Thin, Tegasorb Thin

Table 29.2 *(cont'd)*

Wound type	Product type	Examples
Infected	Antibacterial paste bandage Chlorhexidine paraffin gauze Povidone-iodine fabric Silver-containing product Polysaccharide	Quinaband Bactigras Inadine Flamazine, Actisorb Silver 220, Arglaes, Avance Debrisan, Iodosorb, Iodoflex
Malodorous	Odour-absorbing dressing Sugar paste Metronidazole gel	Actisorb Silver 220, CarboFlex, Carbonet, Carbopad VC, Clinisorb, Lyofoam C Anabact, Metrotop

The main types of product are outlined in Figure 29.3. There are many products available to assist with stoma care and require the largest section of the *Drug Tariff* to detail. Choice of the best appliance for an individual patient is complex and specialized stoma care nurses often provide guidance. Ostomy patients can obtain a prescription charge Exemption Certificate and patients may obtain their stoma care needs from pharmacists, direct from manufacturers or from dispensing appliance contractors.

Problems with stoma

Hypoallergenic adhesives are used, but careful skin care is required. Detergents and disinfectants may cause irritation so washing with water is preferred. This should be followed by patting dry (not rubbing). Leaks may occur if the appliance has not been fitted properly, the skin is uneven or the bag has not been attached properly. Leakage, especially from an ileostomy or urostomy, can damage or irritate skin.

Diet and drugs can affect stoma effluent. A normal, varied diet should be eaten avoiding too much fibre and foods which produce flatus (wind) and odour, such as beans and onions. Yoghurt and buttermilk may reduce odour and flatus; however, most bags have filters to reduce odour. Food can alter the colour (beetroot) and smell (asparagus) of stools and urine.

Drug therapy needs to be considered. Ileostomy patients in particular have a reduced area for absorption. As a general

Table 29.3   Types of osteomy, effluent and normal type of pouch used for each

Ostomy	Reason for ostomy	Type of effluent	Type of pouch
Colostomy descending/sigmoid,	Cancer, diverticular disease, trauma, Crohn's disease	Soft to nearly solid	Closed pouch
Colostomy, transverse	Cancer, diverticular disease, trauma, Crohn's disease	Semiliquid to soft	Drainable pouch with open end and clip
Colostomy, ascending	Cancer, diverticular disease, trauma, Crohn's disease	Liquid to paste-like	Drainable pouch with open end and clip
Ileostomy	Ulcerative colitis, Crohn's disease, trauma, cancer	Liquid, continuous, includes digestive enzymes	Drainable pouch with open end and clip
Urostomy	Cancer, urinary incontinence, fistulae, spinal column disorders	Urine	Drainable pouch with tap

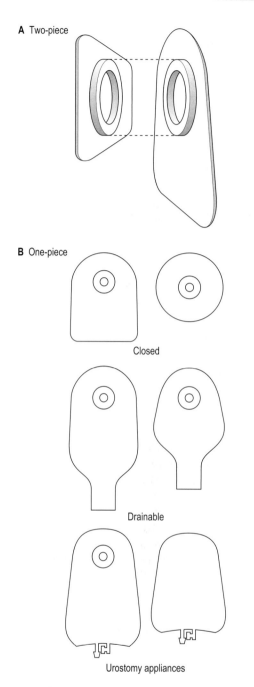

A Two-piece

B One-piece

Closed

Drainable

Urostomy appliances

Fig. 29.3 The main types of one-piece (**A**) and two-piece (**B**) stoma appliances.

rule, modified-release products should not be used. Absorption of oral contraceptives from the terminal ileum is reduced, so other methods of contraception should be used. Constipation may be produced by opioids, anticholin-ergic drugs (tricyclic antidepressants, antihistamines) and calcium and magnesium-containing antacids. Antibiotics, iron and cytotoxics may produce diarrhoea. The same effect can result from excessive drinking if there is a drug-induced dry mouth. Diuretics and antacids should be used very carefully with ileostomists who are already at risk of dehydration. Drugs can also alter the colour of urine and stools. Pharmacists can offer general advice to stoma patients remembering that these patients may be embarrassed or shy. Reassurance of the patient is very important. Patients may be directed to a stoma care nurse or one of the support organizations (Box 29.1).

Box 29.1   Some of the organizations which offer support to ostomy and incontinent patients

British Colostomy Association, 15 Station Square, Reading RG1 1LG. http://www.bcass.org.uk
Ileostomy and Internal Pouch Support Group (ia), PO Box 132, Scunthorpe DN15 9YM. http://www.ileostomypouch.demon.co.uk
Urostomy Association, 'Buckland', Beaumont Park, Danbury Essex CM3 4DE. http://www.uagbi.org
National Advisory Service for Parents of Children with a Stoma, 51 Anderson Drive, Darvel, Ayrshire KA17 0DE
The Continence Foundation, 307 Hatton Square, 16 Baldwin Gardens, London WC1N 7RJ. http://www.continence-foundation.org.uk
Incontact (National Association on Incontinence), United House, North Road, London N7 9DP. http://www.interact.demon.co.uk
ERIC (Enuresis, Resource and Information Centre for children/young adults), 34 Old School House, Britannia Road, Kingswood, Bristol BS15 2DB. http://www.enuresis.org.uk

---

INCONTINENCE

Incontinence is the 'involuntary loss of urine or faeces which is objectively demonstrable and is a social or hygienic problem'. It is very common, but difficult to measure accurately because of social stigma. The prevalence varies with age and gender. Under age 30 years, the incidence is about 30% in women and 8% in men, 30–60 years 25% in women and 6% in men, over 60 years the incidence can be 30–50%. Because of the social stigma, any help offered must be discreet. Sufferers may find it difficult

Table 29.4	Different types and causes of urinary incontinence	
Type	**Features**	**Cause**
Stress	Slight leakage on exertion. Normal voiding	Inadequate sphincter. Oestrogen deficiency
Overflow	Small, frequent escapes. Slow, difficult, incomplete normal urination	Sphincter pressure too large. Enlarged prostate. Diabetes. Nerve damage
Urge	Inability to control passing urine. Nocturnal enuresis	Drugs—diuretics, sedatives. Hypersensitivity. Vaginal atrophy
Reflex	No sensation, sudden voiding	Nerve disease (such as multiple sclerosis, cord injury)
Continuous	Slow leakage all the time	Fistula. Bladder neck or sphincter open
Functional	Inability to reach toilet in time	Disability. Arthritis

to talk about their problem. It is best to use the same words as they use to describe the problem.

The different types and causes of urinary incontinence are shown in Table 29.4. Diuretic use can lead to incontinence due to rapid production of urine. Drugs which increase bladder contraction, such as beta-blockers, or relax the sphincter, such as antiepileptic and psychotropic drugs and muscle relaxants, increase incontinence.

A variety of management techniques are used. Pelvic floor exercises are useful and can be taught by continence advisers, nurses, doctors or physiotherapists. Electrical stimulators are available to strengthen and tone pelvic floor muscles. Bladder retraining, perhaps combined with a drug treatment (such as oxybutynin hydrochloride), can restore an acceptable pattern of micturition. Likewise, scheduled toileting can help, especially for the elderly and bedridden. Constipation can cause urinary and fecal incontinence and should be avoided, preferably by diet and fluid control. Laxatives should be avoided if possible. Inadequate fluid intake can increase urinary incontinence.

Incontinence appliances

A wide range of equipment has been developed to help people where other methods have not prevented their incontinence. Those which can be prescribed in the UK are detailed in the *Drug Tariff*; others have to be purchased. Products can be grouped into four types:

- Absorbents
- External collectors
- Invasive devices
- Intravaginal devices.

Selection of a particular aid will be made on the basis of personal preference, nature of incontinence and other personal characteristics such as sex, age, mobility, dexterity and mental awareness.

Absorbent pads

These can be used by either sex, and may be the only option for many women. Sanitary pads are best avoided. Pads are available for different levels of incontinence. Light pads hold 50–100 mL and can be worn inside a user's own pants. Those for moderate urinary incontinence may be specially shaped, whilst heavy incontinence may require elasticated legs, waterproof backs or plastic garments. Modern fabric design helps the skin stay dry and eliminates odour. Some can hold up to 50 times their weight of water. Chair or bed protection using flat pads may also be required, although several products claim to be adequate for overnight protection.

External collectors

A variety of penile sheaths, dribble pouches and drip collectors are available. Sheaths are either latex-free or made of soft latex and are held on the penis by adhesive, the urine being collected in a drainage bag. Different types of bag are available: leg bags, suspensory bags (carried from the waist for larger volumes) and night drainage bags. Some are equipped with a siphon facility especially for wheelchair users. Users generally need good eyesight and dexterity. Designs for females are generally less satisfactory.

Invasive devices

Women more commonly use urethral catheters, the urine draining into a suitable collecting bag. Catheters, of different designs, are made from latex, plastic or silicone and may be coated with hydrogel or Teflon. Indwelling catheters are held in place by a 'balloon' which is inflated after insertion. Intermittent catheterization may be used by patients who wish to retain control over the process. The catheter is inserted several times a day as required. The risk of bladder infection increases with each insertion or separation of collecting device from the catheter. Patient skill is also required. When an infection occurs, antiseptic bladder washes are normally used. With both external collectors and catheters, care is required to ensure connections to the bag are compatible.

Intravaginal devices

There are a number of moulded plastic devices designed to be worn in the vagina to support the neck of the bladder. They come in different sizes and are claimed to be very effective.

Other relevant information

Some simple physical changes to the living environment may enable the patient to reach the toilet more quickly. Any underlying medical condition requires treatment and some patients may require surgery. Skin care is important. Normal, regular hygiene, using simple soaps, should be adequate for most people. Avoid long periods of contact with wet pads or appliances, which will also help reduce odour. Most regions have continence advisers and there are three national organizations with local branches to give additional support (Box 29.1).

Rectal incontinence

Where a patient first reports fecal incontinence, referral to a GP for investigation is recommended. There are many possible causes including chronic constipation, severe diarrhoea, chronic laxative abuse, stress or emotional disturbance, and physical damage.

Management is equally complex. Loperamide has been used as have other drugs to reduce motility and secretions. Dietary manipulation can also be used. Bowel retraining or biofeedback techniques can be effective for some patients. Where non-operative techniques fail, surgical repair or augmentation may be required.

Key Points

- A warm, moist environment optimizes wound healing.
- Wounds may be classified as necrotic, sloughy, granulating, or epithelializing.
- Wounds may become infected and malodorous.
- Wounds can change type as healing progresses.
- Choice of wound management product is influenced by the type of wound.
- Traditional absorbent dressings should not be left in contact with moist wounds.
- Bandages may be medicated or for support, compression or retention.
- Graduated compression hosiery gives the greatest compression at the ankle.
- Measurements for elastic hosiery are the circumference of the mid thigh, widest part of the calf, ankle and length of the foot.
- Adhesive tapes may be permeable, vapour-permeable or occlusive.
- Low-adherent dressings include paraffin gauze, knitted viscose and absorbent perforated dressings.
- Charcoal is used in dressings and stoma appliances to adsorb offensive odour.
- Modern dressings aim to produce conditions which promote moist wound healing.
- Vapour-permeable films enable water vapour to pass through.
- Foam and foam film dressings have hydrophobic and hydrophilic parts to control moisture at the wound surface.
- Polysaccharide dressings may be used on infected exuding wounds, but not on dry wounds.
- Alginate dressings form a gel over moist wounds and provide calcium ions to help stop bleeding.
- Two types of hydrogel are used in wound management: flexible sheets and amorphous gels. The latter are useful in removing necrotic tissue.
- Hydrocolloid dressings interact with wound exudate to form a moist gel. They are used to treat several types of wounds.
- Stoma appliances may be one or two piece with closed or drainable bags.
- Skin care is important with stoma and incontinence.
- Drug therapy may impact on stoma management.
- Incontinence is twice as common in women as men.
- There are many self-help techniques which can be used by people with a continence problem.
- Incontinence appliances include absorbents, sheaths, catheters and collection systems.
- Newly reported rectal incontinence requires referral to a GP.

30

Medical gases

A. J. Winfield

After studying this chapter you will know about:

Definition, nature and properties of medical gases
Control of medical gases
Equipment used with medical gases
Identification of medical gases
Safety aspects of medical gases
The uses of medical gases
Counselling of patients receiving domiciliary oxygen

Introduction

A medical gas may be defined as any gas which is inhaled by a patient under the direction of a doctor. The use of gases to treat disease was pioneered in the 18th century, notably by Thomas Beddoes. The hope of these early workers that many diseases could be treated in this way was unfounded, but a number of gases are used in modern medical practice.

Oxygen is provided to patients in their own homes by pharmacies which have a contract with the local health authority or board. Details about this will be discussed later. In 2000 the UK government announced a review of domiciliary oxygen services. In hospitals, pharmacists are often involved with the supply of oxygen, nitrous oxide, nitrous oxide/oxygen mixtures, compressed air and vacuum and occasionally more specialized gases. In most hospitals, rather than cylinders being used, a piped system is employed to distribute the gases from a central supply to each bedside. Further details will be given later in the chapter.

Legal aspects

There are many national and international standards, specifications and codes of practice. In the UK, the manufacture of medical gases is controlled by the Medicines Act 1968, to standards laid down in the *British Pharmacopoeia* (BP) and *European Pharmacopoeia* (EP). Ancillary equipment is detailed in British and International Standards (BS and ISO) and various Home Office Specifications. The *Drug Tariff* details domiciliary equipment and services which can be prescribed on FP 10 (GP 10 in Scotland) on the NHS.

THE HARDWARE USED WITH MEDICAL GASES

Unless very large quantities are required, medical gases are stored in cylinders. These are made of steel and are designed to withstand pressures of over 200 bar and in the UK must comply with BS EN 850:1997. Cylinders are filled to a nominal pressure of 137 bar at 14°C. The nominal size of cylinders varies from 36 to 5112 L capacity. The size used for domiciliary oxygen has a capacity of 1360 L, is 930 mm long and 102 mm in diameter, with an empty weight of about 14.5 kg. The British Standard also gives details of the valves used for closing the cylinders. Other equipment can then be added by means of a standard screw thread. This will always include a device for pressure reduction and flow regulation and may also include flow rate measurement and a humidifier before delivery to the patient by mask or nasal catheter.

IDENTIFICATION OF MEDICAL GASES

A colour coding system for identification is given in BS EN 850, which has been accepted by most countries (ISO 32). In devising the system, the cylinder was divided into two parts, the main body and the shoulder at the valve end. The latter part could be all the same colour, or divided into

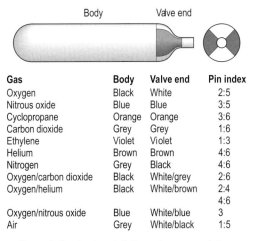

Gas	Body	Valve end	Pin index
Oxygen	Black	White	2:5
Nitrous oxide	Blue	Blue	3:5
Cyclopropane	Orange	Orange	3:6
Carbon dioxide	Grey	Grey	1:6
Ethylene	Violet	Violet	1:3
Helium	Brown	Brown	4:6
Nitrogen	Grey	Black	4:6
Oxygen/carbon dioxide	Black	White/grey	2:6
Oxygen/helium	Black	White/brown	2:4
			4:6
Oxygen/nitrous oxide	Blue	White/blue	3
Air	Grey	White/black	1:5

Oxygen/helium has two pin indices, where oxygen is less
than 20% 4:6, where oxygen is greater than 20% 2:4

Fig. 30.1 Colour code and pin-index methods of
identification of medical gas cylinders.

quarters showing alternate colours. When a mixture of
gases is in the cylinder, they are indicated by these alternating colours. Details for the common gases are given in
Figure 30.1.

The pin-index valve provides an alternative means of
identification. Six possible pin positions, relative to the gas
outlet, are used. A particular gas uses pin positions (usually
two) as detailed in BS EN 850. These are shown in Figure
30.1. In addition, the chemical symbol of the gas is painted
onto the cylinder.

Another difficulty with medical gases can be knowing
how full a cylinder is. For a permanent gas, the pressure is
proportional to the volume, so the use of a pressure gauge
is adequate. Domiciliary equipment is usually calibrated in
'full', 'half', 'quarter'. However, some gases are liquids at
cylinder pressures. In these cases, a pressure gauge would
only show the vapour pressure of the liquid, which will be
constant until the cylinder is virtually empty. This applies to
carbon dioxide, nitrous oxide, ethylene and cyclopropane.
In these cases, weighing the cylinder is necessary.

STORAGE AND DISTRIBUTION

Medical gas cylinders need to be stored in cool dry conditions to avoid rusting and damage to the paint. Care is
required to ensure that there is no confusion between full
and empty cylinders. This may be achieved by the use of
disposable shrink seals and marking empty cylinders clearly.

Pharmacists with contracts to supply domiciliary oxygen
must be prepared to:

- Stock sufficient cylinders to meet demands
- Deliver, set up and explain the use of the equipment and
  cylinders
- Provide a leaflet on the use, care and storage of medical
  gases.

There is also a requirement that a notified PMR (patient
medication records) system is operated and that records of
supply and advice are made to allow for regular audit.

Some patients who require large amounts of oxygen may
use an oxygen concentrator rather than cylinders. Normally
patients considered for an oxygen concentrator would be
using oxygen for 8 hours per day or more (equivalent to
about 20 cylinders per month). Concentrators are not supplied as part of the pharmacy-based domiciliary supply
system, although they are available on prescription. They
operate by using either a molecular sieve or semipermeable
membrane to remove some nitrogen and other gases from
air, thereby producing oxygen-enriched gas for the patient.

Liquid oxygen is used for domiciliary supply in conti-
nental Europe and North America but not in the UK at
present.

Many hospitals have a piped system from a central source
to each bedside being equipped with a self-closing outlet.
Great care is required in the design, installing and testing of
the pipe work to ensure that an adequate flow is available to
all outlets. An engineer and pharmacist normally share this
responsibility. All joints in the pipe work have to be colour
coded to allow identification as shown in Table 30.1. The
gases may be provided either from banks of cylinders when
relatively small volumes are used, or from liquid gas tanks.
With cylinders, there are two banks of cylinders, one of
which is supplying the system. When the pressure falls
below a preset level, automatic switching brings in the
reserve bank of cylinders and allows the empty ones to be

Table 30.1 Colour codes used on joints in hospital piped-gas supplies	
Gas	**Colour code**
Oxygen	White
Nitrous oxide	Blue
Nitrous oxide/oxygen	Blue/white
Carbon dioxide	Grey
Air	White/black
Vacuum	Primrose yellow

replaced without interruption of supply. Hospitals usually use liquid oxygen tanks. These are large insulated tanks, from which the liquid oxygen, at $-183°C$, will slowly evaporate. The process can be speeded up when required by the use of electrical heating coils. Heat exchangers are incorporated to warm the oxygen to room temperature before administration to patients.

SAFE HANDLING OF MEDICAL GAS CYLINDERS

Only suitably trained staff should install oxygen therapy equipment. Before use, cylinders should be in a safe position so that they cannot fall over (either in a stand or clamped vertically). When connecting equipment, care should be taken to ensure that grease does not come into contact with joints as this can lead to spontaneous combustion at high gas pressures. Staff must avoid things like hand cream, oil or grease on fingers when handling equipment. Just prior to connecting the equipment, momentary opening of the cylinder valve blows away any dust or particles. This is known as 'snuffing' or 'cracking'. On tightening the joint, do not use excessive force as this might cause damage to the thread; hand-tightness is adequate. The valve should be turned slowly until fully open, then turned back a quarter turn (so that it is obviously in use). If resistance is excessive, the cylinder should be returned to the manufacturer. Release oils, such as WD40 must never be used. The key should be left in place if it is a spindle key valve in case an emergency closure is needed. All joints should be checked for leaks. This is easiest using a little soapy water which will produce bubbles if there is a leak. Reconnecting the joint may solve any problem, otherwise it must be reported. During use, the pressure should be checked regularly to ensure that there is sufficient gas remaining. After use the valve should be closed immediately. When the cylinder is empty, the valve is closed, the pressure released and the equipment disconnected. The exposed valve should be covered to prevent dust getting into the mechanism.

There are fire and explosion risks associated with all oxygen sources which can be minimized if appropriate precautions are taken. Fire is a potential hazard with oxygen, nitrous oxide and cyclopropane. The latter is flammable and can be explosive at certain concentrations with oxygen or air. Oxygen and nitrous oxide support combustion, so that materials which do not normally burn easily may become flammable in an atmosphere rich in oxygen or nitrous oxide. This will include clothing, bedding and soft furnishings.

Sparks from toys or electrical equipment may be enough to produce violent ignition. Smoking should be banned close to any oxygen equipment.

MEDICAL GASES

Oxygen

Oxygen has many therapeutic uses. The main one is treating hypoxaemia which arises because of underventilation of the lungs (such as in bronchitis, pneumonia, acute severe asthma, chronic obstructive pulmonary disease (COPD), pulmonary oedema and after general anaesthesia) or where the circulation of the blood is inadequate (as in heart failure). Other situations in which it is used include the treatment of carbon monoxide and other poisoning, respiratory depression and respiratory failure. High concentrations of oxygen should be reduced as soon as possible owing to its toxic effects. Oxygen can also be used in special chambers at pressures greater than 1 bar (hyperbaric oxygen) for treatment of carbon monoxide and cyanide poisoning and as part of the treatment of anaerobic infections such as gangrene, in radiation therapy and decompression sickness. The use of hyperbaric oxygen in multiple sclerosis is still controversial.

Oxygen can produce respiratory depression and can be toxic. Symptoms of toxicity include nausea, mood changes, vertigo, twitching, convulsions and loss of consciousness. Patients receiving long-term oxygen should report any of the above symptoms, regular headaches, altered breathing patterns or blue lips or fingernails to their doctor. Changes in the prescribed oxygen flow rate should only be made by the doctor. Retinopathy of prematurity (retrolental fibroplasia) occurs from an excessive use of oxygen with neonates. This produces blindness and was a common hazard in the 1940s and 1950s before the cause was recognized.

Oxygen is produced commercially by fractionation of liquid air. For domiciliary use it is provided in 1360 L cylinders, although smaller ones are available where portability is important. The PD oxygen cylinder (300 L) is compatible with the Drug Tariff equipment and provides enough oxygen for 10–12 hours' supply depending on the method of use but is not currently in the Drug Tariff.

The aim of therapy with oxygen is to increase the amount of oxygen in the lungs without danger to the patient. Most domiciliary apparatus is designed to produce concentrations of up to 28% oxygen in the lungs using a flow rate of 2 L/min ('medium' on standard headset). There are a number of different ways in which the gas can be given to the patient.

Nasal catheters (or prongs) are moulded plastic devices which introduce oxygen into the nostrils whilst leaving the mouth clear and may be more acceptable to long-term patients. Lightweight oxygen masks come in different designs. Those commonly used in domiciliary oxygen therapy may give either a fixed concentration of oxygen, or may be adjusted to provide different concentrations. The so-called constant performance masks produce 28% oxygen to the patient independently of the patient's pattern of breathing and the flow rate used. Examples include the Ventimask MkIV and the Intersurgical 010 Mask. Other masks give variable performances depending on the flow rate used. At 2 L/min it is usually 25–30% oxygen, but at 4 L/min ('high' on the standard headset) up to 40% oxygen can be provided, depending on the pattern of breathing. Examples include the Venticaire Mask and the Intersurgical 005 Mask. Heavy-duty rubber masks are available for more specialized use. Full details of the masks are given in the Drug Tariff.

Instructions for patients

It is important that pharmacists should give adequate instructions to patients to ensure safe and effective use of their oxygen. The amount of information presented will vary and be a matter for judgment when a cylinder is delivered. Patients who may have to connect cylinders themselves will require more information than those for whom the pharmacist carries out the operation. Some of the points which may require to be discussed are listed in Box 30.1. Safety has to be a concern because of the risk of explosion and fire. Cards with 'do not' points are available from BOC Gases Medical for attaching to the cylinders.

Other medical gases

The use of other medical gases is more specialized and so is normally confined to hospital use. A brief summary is given, but further details can be found in Grant (1978) and in pharmacopoeias.

Nitrous oxide

Nitrous oxide is used for analgesia in midwifery, postoperative pain and procedures such as bronchoscopy and as an anaesthetic in dentistry. It has slight addictive properties. Synthesis is by decomposition of ammonium nitrate at high temperature.

For normal analgesia a 50% nitrous oxide/oxygen mixture is usually adequate. This is readily available com-

---

Box 30.1 Precautions when using medical gases about which pharmacists may need to inform patients

Storage
Avoid extreme heat or cold (avoid radiators)
Dry, clean, well ventilated
Away from combustible materials (including vapour rub, skin lotion, aerosol sprays)
Away from sources of ignition

Preparation for use
Never lubricate valve and joints
Ensure seal is intact and remove it
'Snuff' the joint before connecting
Use reasonable force in making connections
Open valve fully at first
Quarter close during use

Leaks
Listen for hissing noise
Do not use sealing compounds on leaks
Report a leak as soon as possible

Use of cylinders
Handle with care, avoid knocks
Ensure cylinder cannot fall over
Observe no smoking or naked lights
Close cylinder valve as soon as therapy is complete
Avoid long lengths of tubing especially on the floor
When empty, close valve and replace cap

---

mercially as a mixture called Entonox. This mixture remains as a gas down to –7°C, below which the nitrous oxide liquefies and collects at the bottom of the cylinder. When it evaporates, the nitrous oxide remains at the base of the cylinder because of its greater density. Thus storage of Entonox at low temperature must be avoided. Where higher concentrations may be required, oxygen and nitrous oxide are mixed from separate cylinders just prior to administration. Some of the equipment allows the patient to control the proportions within externally controlled limits. When inducing anaesthesia, concentrations approaching 100% are sometimes employed. If used for more than a short time this could cause asphyxiation. Nitrous oxide is a non-permanent gas which is present as a liquid in cylinders (critical temperature 36.4°C, critical pressure 72.5 bar). In hospitals nitrous oxide may be distributed by a piped system to bedsides. Nitrous oxide is not combustible, but it does support combustion and will, like oxygen, rekindle a glowing split. There is, therefore, a potential fire hazard as with oxygen and similar precautions should be taken.

Carbon dioxide

This gas is colourless, odourless and tasteless. Commercially it is produced as a byproduct from a number of industrial processes. At concentrations up to 5% carbon dioxide is a powerful respiratory stimulant and vasodilator. It finds limited clinical use in treating respiratory depression by drugs such as depressants, hypnotics and anaesthetics and has been used for treating intractable hiccup. At concentrations above 6%, carbon dioxide produces an increasing central depression and acidosis. A ready prepared mixture of 5% carbon dioxide and 95% oxygen is available. Pure carbon dioxide is a non-permanent gas (critical temperature 31.04°C, critical pressure 73.8 bar) so is present as a liquid in cylinders.

Rapid expansion from the cylinder causes a cooling of the carbon dioxide to below its melting point (−78.5°C) and produces solid carbon dioxide as a 'snow'. This may be collected and shaped for use in cryotherapy of warts, naevi and other skin conditions. Care is required when handling solid carbon dioxide because it 'burns' the skin.

Carbon dioxide dissolves in water to produce carbonated vehicles. These have a sharp taste which has been reported as being useful in masking the unpleasant taste of some liquid medicines.

Helium

Helium is an inert permanent gas prepared from liquefied air or natural gas. It is used for its physical properties, in particular it has a very low density (approximately one-tenth of that of nitrogen) which makes it easier to breathe. A 20% oxygen in helium mixture can be used as a substitute for air in patients with acute upper respiratory tract obstruction.

It has a much lower solubility in plasma than nitrogen and so is used in high-pressure diving. Breathing helium increases vocal pitch and distorts the voice.

Cyclopropane

Cyclopropane is a colourless gas synthesized by reacting zinc with a 1,3-dihalopropane. It is a potent anaesthetic although its use is less widespread than previously. It can form explosive mixtures with air, oxygen or nitrous oxide. It liquefies in the cylinder. Owing to its potency, small quantities only are required and so small cylinder sizes are used.

Key Points

- Medical gases are used in hospital and domiciliary situations.
- The BS EN 850 gives details of cylinders, valves, colour codes, pin-index identification and storage.
- Colour coding and stencilled chemical symbols are used to identify cylinder contents.
- Mixtures of gases are indicated by alternating colours on the valve end of the cylinder, the body having the colour of the main gas.
- The pin-index valve prevents connection of an incorrect cylinder.
- For permanent gases the pressure is proportional to the amount of gas remaining, but for liquefied gases the pressure remains constant until the cylinder is nearly empty.
- Pharmacists with a domiciliary oxygen supply contract must keep agreed stock levels and assist with delivery and installation, provide instructions and keep adequate records.
- Hospital oxygen supplies are designed to avoid any interruption of supply to the patient.
- Medical gases produce fire and explosion hazards which must be minimized.
- Domiciliary patients must be given detailed instructions on the use of oxygen and equipment.
- Oxygen is used to treat hypoxia, carbon monoxide poisoning and respiratory depression and failure.
- Oxygen has the potential to be toxic, so most domiciliary oxygen masks give a maximum 28% concentration.
- Storage of Entonox at low temperature can cause separation of the gases.
- Carbon dioxide is a respiratory stimulant up to 5%, and a central depressant above 6% concentration.
- Helium is used for its low density to aid patients with respiratory tract obstruction.

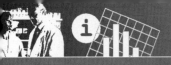

PART 4

USING PHARMACEUTICAL SKILLS IN CARING FOR PATIENTS

31

Clinical pharmacy practice

M. Watson and C. M. Bond (including some material by J. A. Cromarty, J. G. Hamley, J. Krska and A. J. Winfield)

After studying this chapter you will know about:

The development of clinical pharmacy
Aspects of clinical pharmacy practice
Elements of pharmacy services provision
Prioritization and planning of pharmaceutical care
Monitoring patients
Keeping and using patient medication records
Pharmacists and residential care
Assessing quality of pharmaceutical care

Introduction

Pharmacists are society's experts on drugs. Clinical pharmacy aims to help maximize drug efficacy, minimize drug toxicity and promote cost-effectiveness. To achieve this, pharmacists need to work as fully integrated members of the health care team. As team members as well as being members of their own professional body, pharmacists are accountable to patients for the services which they provide. Prior to the development of clinical pharmacy, pharmacists were primarily involved in the supply of medicines. However, as pharmaceutical services have developed, it is possible for pharmacists in all health care settings to develop clinical roles.

Clinical pharmacy can be delivered through activities known as 'pharmaceutical care' or 'medicines management'. In 1990, the term 'pharmaceutical care' was defined as 'the responsible provision of drug therapy for the purpose of achieving definite outcomes that improve a patient's quality of life' (Hepler and Strand, 1990). Although this early definition focused on the use of medicines, it has been developed in recent years and is now regarded as including non-medicine-related care.

More recently, 'medicines management' has been defined as 'a holistic approach to patient care through systematic management of the patient's medicines and a new partnership of structured collaboration with the doctor' (PSNC, 1999). Medicines management does not solely consider drug therapy but provides a wider (holistic) perspective of clinical pharmacy services regardless of setting. In the community pharmacy setting, the purpose of medicines management is to maximize benefit and minimize risk for patients from prescribed medicines by ensuring:

- The safe and appropriate choice of medicines and therapeutic regimens
- Structured discussion with the patient on specified aspects of the medicines and the need for commitment to prescribed treatments
- Systematic collaboration with the prescriber and other members of the primary health care team in addressing patient needs
- Record maintenance and reporting for GPs in agreed format.

Medicines management has been identified as being 'central to the quality of health care'. The Audit Commission's (2001) definition of medicines management in secondary care is that it 'encompasses the entire way that medicines are selected, procured, delivered, prescribed, administered and reviewed to optimize the contribution that medicines make to producing informed and desired outcomes of patient care'.

It is important to note that the terms 'medicines management' and 'pharmaceutical care' are used interchangeably throughout this chapter. These activities form the vehicle for the delivery of clinical pharmacy.

Pharmacists' roles are changing as a result of changes in the NHS, peoples' lifestyles and expectations (Table 31.1). Until recently, the majority of pharmacists within the NHS could have been classified as either community or hospital pharmacists. The former were based in community pharmacies and tended to work in isolation of primary health care teams. Their role was one of supply with little 'clinical' activity. As described above, this situation has changed in

Table 31.1 Types of clinical pharmacy practice in the UK

Type of pharmacist	Setting	Location	Example of activity
Community pharmacist	Primary care	Pharmacy	Medication review
Hospital pharmacist	Secondary care	Hospital	Medication history taking
Practice pharmacist	Primary care	General practice	Development of prescribing policy
Other	Various	Various	See community, hospital and practice pharmacists

recent years. Community pharmacists provide a range of clinical services that may include medication review, health checks (e.g. blood pressure monitoring) and domiciliary services. Hospital pharmacists have a longer history of integration into clinical teams at ward level. Their duties may range from the patient's admission, in the form of medication history taking, to discharge, where discharge counselling is provided and liaison with community services promotes continuity of care.

A third 'type' of pharmacist has emerged in recent years. Practice pharmacists work within, or in association with, general practices. These pharmacists may be employed on a sessional basis or full time, and work closely with practice staff (e.g. GPs, nurses). The clinical services that they provide may include advice to prescribers (which nowadays may include nurses), formulary and protocol development, and medication review. Although the number of practice pharmacists is growing steadily there are concerns regarding their cost-effectiveness.

The origins of clinical pharmacy come from the hospital setting. Nowadays, however, clinical pharmacy services can be delivered in every setting where pharmacists are employed. Many pharmacists now combine different types of employment. For example, some pharmacists may work in community pharmacy but provide sessional work as practice pharmacists in general practices.

This chapter sets the scene for Part 4 of the book. It describes how modern clinical pharmacy practice has developed and the many components and factors associated with clinical pharmacy services, further details of which occur in subsequent chapters.

THE DEVELOPMENT OF CLINICAL PHARMACY

Until the mid 1960s, pharmacists were almost solely involved in the purchase, manufacture and supply of medicines. Then in the USA the development of clinical pharmacy began and a more clinically oriented pharmacy curriculum was developed with the award of a PharmD degree. This affected the practice of pharmacy in the UK. Evidence from studies in the UK began to highlight problems with medication errors at ward level and clinical pharmacy began to develop. Firstly, prescription and drug administration records were introduced, followed by an increasing pharmacy presence on hospital wards. Then masters degrees in clinical pharmacy were introduced, the first in 1976, supported by a textbook. However, it wasn't until the Nuffield Report in 1986 that clinical pharmacy really began to gain momentum. In Table 31.2, the key events in the development of clinical pharmacy in the UK are presented.

The provision of health care in the UK is in a dynamic situation. Many of the current developments and proposed future developments for the NHS are the result of high-profile critical incidents (e.g. Bristol Royal Infirmary Inquiry, Dr Shipman). The Kennedy Report (2001) was published following an inquiry into the high mortality of paediatric cardiac surgery cases at Bristol Royal Infirmary. The conclusions and recommendations of this report have serious and far-reaching implications for the health service at a national level down to the level of the individual health care professional. The report highlights the importance of communication and teamwork, as well as ensuring that methods exist to measure the quality of care.

There are two distinct themes in the report that should be applied to clinical pharmacy services, namely the provision of quality health care, and the maintenance of professional competence through continuing professional development (CPD).

HEALTH CARE QUALITY

The Kennedy Report recommended that there should be agreed and published standards of clinical care for health care professionals to follow and that there should be openness about clinical performance. The report stated that 'patients' safety must be the foundation of quality'.

Table 31.2   Key stages in the development of clinical pharmacy in the UK

Year	Event	Outcome
1976	First UK MSc in clinical pharmacy	Provided trained personnel to develop role
1982	Publication of textbook *Clinical Pharmacy and Hospital Drug Management* (Lawson & Richards 1982)	Provided a resource book in the UK situation
1986	The Nuffield Report (Nuffield Foundation 1986)	'Clinical pharmacy should be practised in all hospitals'
1988	*The Way Forward for Hospital Pharmaceutical Services* (Department of Health 1988)	Action requested from health authorities and health boards re. Nuffield report
1988	'Promoting Better Health' (Secretaries of State for Social Services WNIaS 1987)	Recognition that pharmacists' skills could be used more effectively in community practice
1989	'Working for Patients' (Secretaries of State for WNIaS 1989)	Recognition that pharmacists' skills could be used more effectively in community practice
1992	*Pharmaceutical Care: the future for community pharmacy* (RPSGB 1992)	30 recommendations on the development of NHS community pharmaceutical services
1996	*Primary Care: the future* (Department of Health 1996)	Recommendation that pharmacy staff skills should be used to support self-care of minor illness and provide prescribing advice to other health professionals
1997	Introduction of 4 year MPharm degree with an increased clinical content	All newly qualified pharmacists now had a basic knowledge of clinical pharmacy
2000	*Pharmacy in the Future—implementing the NHS plan* (Department of Health 2002)	Programme for pharmacy in the NHS
2001	*A Spoonful of Sugar* (Audit Commission 2001)	Emphasized the importance of medicines management as part of NHS Trust Boards
2002	The Right Medicine (Scottish Executive 2002)	Made proposals for the integration of pharmacy into the core NHS team, with an emphasis on improving patient care through the involvement of pharmacy

Note: Most of the papers cited above refer to English publications. Other British papers are only cited if they differ substantially from the English documents.

Clinical governance

One of the most important developments for health care in general in the UK was the introduction of clinical governance in the late 1990s. Clinical governance is:

A framework through which NHS organizations are accountable for continually improving the quality of their services and safeguarding high standards of care by creating an environment in which excellence in clinical care will flourish.

There are four main components of clinical governance.

- Clear lines of responsibility and accountability for the overall quality of clinical care
- A comprehensive programme of quality improvement activities
- Clear policies aimed at managing risks
- Procedures for all professional groups to identify and remedy poor performance.

Although clinical governance has been adopted into health service provision within the hospital setting, there has been a much slower recognition of its importance in the community pharmacy setting. However, there is growing awareness of the need for clinical governance in community pharmacy and this is likely to lead to changes and developments in practice in the next few years.

Professional competence

In terms of professional competence, the Kennedy Report recommended that 'as part of all health care professionals' contracts with a trust (or health board) (and part of a GP's terms of service) that they undergo appraisal, continuing professional development and revalidation to ensure that all health care professionals remain competent to do their job'. The report stated 'CPD, periodic appraisal and revalidation must be compulsory for all health care professionals'. Currently, methods exist to assess service and competence, including audit and peer review.

Audit

Professional audit refers to the process of audit carried out within a particular profession, usually by that profession. Clinical audit on the other hand is multidisciplinary in nature and may be undertaken by health care professionals from any discipline. Multidisciplinary audit should also involve the 'customers' of the services being audited, i.e. other health care professionals, clients, patients and their carers. Clinical audit often examines a clinical process which involves a number of different health care professions. Professional and clinical audit is described in more detail in Chapter 43.

Peer review

Assessing the performance of clinical pharmacists involves issues of professional judgment. Peer review methods are appropriate for this purpose. They generate useful subjective measures of performance. This can complement the objective measures of performance achieved through audit. Peer review is often used as part of a professional development programme rather than as part of a formal assessment of clinical pharmacy practice. It involves members of the same profession and should be non-threatening. The aim is to develop the clinical knowledge and skills of pharmacists to improve the quality of their practice.

Future developments in assessing and maintaining professional competence are discussed at the end of this chapter.

Rational medicine use

Drugs should be prescribed to maximize effectiveness, minimize risks and costs, and respect patient's wishes. In other words, prescribing should be rational. Rational prescribing comprises five major components:

- A defensible formulation of the patient's problem
- Clarity of therapeutic intention
- Access to independent data on drugs
- Communication with the patient
- Follow-up.

Many strategies exist to promote rational prescribing, which incorporate some of these major components. There follows a discussion of some of these strategies (Marinker, 1994).

Evidence-based practice

There is an increasing trend and requirement that health professionals should provide evidence-based health care. Evidence-based practice should ideally ensure that available resources are used effectively and efficiently and that variation in clinical practice is minimized. The gold standard of evidence is generally derived from randomized controlled trials (RCTs) which may or may not have been combined as a meta-analysis. The Cochrane Collaboration (http://www.update-software.com/ccweb/default.htm) is an international organization of health professionals and academics who undertake systematic reviews of evidence using established methodology to address some of the many health care questions that arise from daily practice. Pharmacists should refer to the Cochrane Library to identify reviews and trials that may provide evidence that will inform their everyday practice, or that can be used in the development of evidence-based guidelines for pharmaceutical services. Another organization that provides evidence in the form of guidelines and technical appraisals is the National Institute for Clinical Excellence (NICE) (www.nice.org.uk). This is a special health authority that was set up in 1999. Its purpose is to provide patients, health professionals and the public with authoritative, robust and reliable guidance on current 'best practice'.

To provide for the pharmaceutical needs of patient groups and promote rational prescribing, a few key tools are essential:

- Guidelines
- Local policies and protocols
- Prescribing advice
- Evaluated drug information
- Formularies (see Ch. 36).

Guidelines

Guidelines are 'systematically developed statements to assist practitioner and patient decisions about appropriate health care for specific clinical circumstances' (Field and Lohr, 1992). They are a method of influencing clinical behaviour and increasingly these are based on high-quality evidence. The majority of guidelines developed thus far have been intended for medical practitioners. Few guidelines have been produced to promote high-quality pharmaceutical care. A systematic review of guidelines in professions allied to medicine (PAMs) (which included pharmacy studies) concluded that whilst guidelines may change health care provided by PAMs it may not be possible to generalize the findings between different professions and settings.

The adoption of guideline recommendations into professional practice is unlikely to result solely from their publication and dissemination. Active implementation strategies (e.g. educational outreach visits, opinion leaders) are usually required if the guideline recommendations are to be translated into changes in professional behaviour and practice.

Pharmacists can be involved in the development and implementation of guidelines. Multiprofessional guideline development groups should include pharmacy representatives where appropriate. This could be for the development of guidelines for the non-prescription treatment of vaginal candidiasis with over-the-counter (OTC) antifungals, or the treatment of hay fever with OTC antihistamines (see also Ch. 34). Pharmacists can also make substantial contributions to the development of condition-specific guidelines or guidelines for the use of prescription only medicines (POMs).

In terms of guideline implementation, pharmacists may either be the disseminators of the guideline recommendations

or the target of the guidelines. Pharmacists have been used to disseminate prescribing guidelines to GPs, and as an implementation strategy to promote the guideline recommendations to change prescribing behaviour. Pharmacists may also be the recipients of guidelines. For example, with the increasing numbers of medicines that are available for purchase from community pharmacies without a prescription (i.e. OTC medicines), pharmacists need guidance and support to ensure that sales of these products maximize benefit and minimize risk.

Local policies and protocols

Local protocols for the treatment of specific clinical conditions can be derived from national guidelines. A local prescribing policy may also be developed from a local formulary. Adding information about when and how the formulary drugs should be used can achieve this. In some cases, local policies are derived from local data rather than national guideline recommendations. For example, local microbial sensitivity patterns could be used to inform the development of local antibiotic policies. Local policies are also often developed for the quantity of medicines supplied to patients on discharge from hospital to the community. This type of policy would benefit from pharmacist involvement, both from the hospital and community pharmacy settings.

There are many examples of local protocols for the care of particular patient groups. Shared care protocols devised jointly by practitioners working in primary and secondary care are increasing. These help to define the roles and responsibilities of the various health care professionals involved. For example, they may define when patients should be referred to hospital by GPs. They may also state who is responsible for the monitoring of which therapeutic outcomes. Pharmacists should be involved in the development of these protocols since they often apply to patients on long-term medication. Many pharmaceutical services to patient groups would benefit from local policies; examples include the supply of repeat prescriptions and the provision of services to drug misusers.

Patient group directions

The regulatory framework for the way medicines are supplied and administered was recently reviewed. The resulting Crown report laid the foundations for a documented system for the supply and administration of prescription only medicines by professionals other than medical doctors

(Patient Group Directions), and for the prescription of such medicines directly by non-doctors. One of the principles of the recommendations and resultant revised regulations was that patient convenience was increased without compromising patient safety.

A Patient Group Direction (PGD) (sometimes referred to as a group protocol) is a written set of instructions for the supply or administration of medicines, by health care professionals other than doctors, to groups of patients who may not be individually identified before presentation for treatment. It is signed by a doctor (or dentist), a pharmacist and by a representative of the profession to whom the PGD applies, and must be authorized by a health board or NHS trust. It contains information on the medicine(s) and regimens, clinical situation, excluded patients, relevant warnings, follow-up and referrals (see Ch. 15). Examples of PGDs written for pharmacy use might include the NHS supply of nicotine replacement therapies to customers wishing to stop smoking, outside the OTC product license, or for the community pharmacy supply and administration of flu vaccines.

Prescribing advice

Information about individual or practice prescribing is available to most prescribers in the UK. This information needs to be evaluated before it can be used to promote rational prescribing. Pharmacists are frequently called upon to evaluate prescribing data. They can identify ways in which prescribing quality can be improved and/or cost savings can be made. Drug utilization and peer reviews can be used to identify suboptimal prescribing, its causes and solutions. Ultimately, this should result in the development and implementation of local policies (see above) to improve specific prescribing areas.

Evaluated drug information

Evaluation of drug information is covered in Chapter 33.

PHARMACEUTICAL SERVICE PROVISION

It is imperative that the limited resources of the NHS and other health care providers are used efficiently to maximize health care benefits. Drugs prescribed in general practice account for over 10% of NHS expenditure and cost over four times more than hospital-prescribed drugs. Inappropriate or unnecessary medicine use should be avoided not only to minimize unnecessary expenditure but also to minimize iatrogenic effects. Iatrogenic disease has significant implications for the health service. A substantial proportion of admissions to hospital (in particular elderly patients) are attributable to iatrogenic causes. Furthermore, it is estimated that 1 in 20 patients admitted to hospitals in England and Wales each year experience an adverse event, which may have been preventable (Kennedy, 2001). Therefore, everyone who has influence over the use of medicines has a responsibility to ensure that they are used optimally. This is a key area where clinical pharmacy services can be applied. Pharmacists have a major role in determining the use of medicines, both those which are prescribed and those which are used for self-medication.

Clinical pharmacy services are often directed towards individual patients. These may be customers in community pharmacies, inpatients or outpatients in hospitals, housebound patients and clients in residential homes. Clinical pharmacy services can also be provided at a population level. This can include the involvement of pharmacists in the development, implementation and monitoring of methods designed to promote the rational use of medicines (e.g. guidelines, protocols). In the UK, the government has set specific targets for health (DoH, 1999). Pharmacists can contribute to the attainment of these targets by the provision of clinical pharmacy services. The government aims to reduce mortality due to coronary heart disease (CHD) and stroke by 40%, from accidents by 20% and from suicide by at least 20%, all by 2010. These are all areas where pharmacists can make a substantial contribution. A large RCT is underway in community pharmacies in England looking at the effectiveness and cost-effectiveness of medicine management for patients with CHD. If effective and efficient, similar initiatives could be provided for patients at risk from stroke and many other conditions. Medicines are the cause of many accidents, either directly or indirectly. Pharmacists can promote the safe storage of medicines to minimize the risk to children, as well as clients in residential homes. The safe disposal of medicines and related equipment is a service that many pharmacists already provide, e.g. disposal of syringes and needles for drug misusers. The appropriate supply of medicines to individual patients is a core requirement that may simply involve checking a prescription for strength, dose and frequency, or checking that a prescribed drug is not contraindicated as a result of pre-existing disease or concurrent medication. There is growing awareness of the increased risk of road traffic accidents with patients taking specific medicines, e.g. benzodiazepines, antidepressants, opiate analgesics. Pharmacists have a role, and indeed a professional responsibility, to inform patients receiving prescribed medicines and customers purchasing OTC medicines, of the risks associated with their use.

Smoking is the largest preventable cause of poor health in the UK. Community pharmacists in particular are well placed to provide smoking cessation advice and treatment with nicotine replacement therapy (NRT). Of the other health issues being targeted nationally, sexual health, substance misuse (illicit drugs, alcohol) and communicable diseases are examples where clinical pharmacy services can and have been developed.

Needs assessment

There are many diverse groups of patients for whom health care must be planned. This requires that the needs of these groups be assessed. Needs assessment is a multidisciplinary activity, involving social services as well as health care services personnel. The involvement of pharmacists is essential, since needs assessment must include patients' pharmaceutical needs. This refers not only to patients' needs for prescribed medicines, but also their need for other pharmacy services. Access to pharmacies for their self-medication facilities and general advice on health care is important. Counselling and advice on prescribed and purchased medicines should be available, as should compliance aids, where necessary. Particular community pharmacies may be a source of specially manufactured products, e.g. total parenteral nutrition (TPN) bags, or special services, e.g. harm-minimization services for drug misusers. Patients in residential and nursing homes may have unrecognized needs which could only be met through a visit by a pharmacist.

Needs assessments enable pharmaceutical services to be planned. Patients may be unaware of their pharmaceutical needs. Conversely, those who request services are not always those in greatest need. A simple example is housebound patients with chronic diseases for which they are prescribed regular medication. Neighbours may be willing to collect dispensed medicines for these patients, but the patients may need pharmaceutical advice about whether the medicines are appropriate and how to use them optimally. If these patients never visit a pharmacy and a pharmacist never visits the patients, their pharmaceutical needs may not be determined. Thus patients should have a right of access to pharmaceutical assessment, irrespective of their location.

Table 31.3 Identifying patients at whom clinical pharmacy services should be targeted

Characteristics	Examples
Patient	
Age	Very young or elderly
Social circumstances	Living alone, homeless
Pregnancy/lactation	
Mobility/disability	Visual impairment, limited dexterity
Substance misuse	Alcohol, nicotine, illicit drugs
Learning difficulties	Illiterate, innumerate
Communication	Non-native language speaker, deaf
Treatment	
Polypharmacy	
Narrow therapeutic index	Anticonvulsants
Non-prescription medicines	Analgesics, antifungals
Complementary therapies	Homoeopathy
Condition	
Multiple pathology	Rheumatoid arthritis and gastric ulcer
Chronic disease	Asthma, hypertension
Mental health problems	Schizophrenia, depression

The importance of maximizing benefit and minimizing cost has already been discussed. By identifying 'at risk' patient groups, clinical pharmacy services can be targeted and thus used with greater efficiency. In Table 31.3, the characteristics for identifying patients for clinical pharmacy intervention are presented.

Patients with one or more of the above characteristics may have more need for clinical pharmacy input than others. Consequently, the role which the pharmacist plays in their care will differ.

Patient characteristics

Age

The elderly and the very young have special pharmaceutical needs. This is due primarily to different pharmacodynamics and/or pharmacokinetics compared with adults. Elderly patients are more likely to have multiple medical conditions and need multiple drug therapy (polypharmacy), therefore they are at greater risk of adverse drug reactions. Elderly patients are likely to have considerable needs in terms of counselling and advice about their medicines. They may also require additional help in terms of remembering to take their medications, and using them appropriately. The use of compliance devices such as daily or weekly medication boxes can often solve problems of this type. Elderly patients may also have impaired dexterity and should be assessed in terms of their ability to access their medicines. Child-resistant closures should be replaced if necessary. Often the use of larger rather than small medicine bottles is sufficient to enable an elderly patient access to their medicines. Pharmacists should familiarize themselves with the range of devices and aids that are available so that they are well equipped to provide for patients with these difficulties (see Ch. 40).

In the UK, patients aged 75 years and over who live at home should have an annual assessment from a nurse or health visitor. Many such patients have multiple pharmaceutical needs. It is important that the assessor is trained to identify these patients' pharmaceutical needs. A preferable situation would be for the local community pharmacist to become involved in routine assessments of this patient population.

Most medicines are developed and tested in adult populations before they gain their licence. This means there is often little data available regarding the use of medicines in infants and children. The distribution, metabolism and elimination of drugs by infants and children differs from adults for many drugs, and these differences need to be considered prior to the administration of medicines in these populations. The doses that are used in young patients are often a fraction of the adult dose, therefore careful measurement of doses is essential, especially for parenteral and liquid formulations.

Social circumstances

Although the majority of patients live at home, many will at some time experience a hospital stay. Others live in residential or nursing homes, in sheltered housing or in other community-based settings. These patients will experience varying degrees of care. Even within hospital settings there are different groups of patients with different needs. Patients may be grouped according to their major disease state or to their age. For example, patients may be located in renal or in neonatal units. The pharmaceutical needs of these different groups determine how pharmaceutical services are divided

between different units within a hospital. The provision of medicine management services in residential homes is discussed later in this chapter. Homeless patients and the travelling community are likely to have different and perhaps more challenging pharmaceutical needs. Patients who live alone may have difficulty accessing pharmaceutical care, as will housebound patients. All these different social circumstances have implications for the provision of pharmaceutical care.

Pregnancy and breastfeeding

Women who are pregnant, considering pregnancy or who are breastfeeding have differing pharmaceutical needs. Medicines management of these women can maximize benefit and minimize risk to the woman, fetus or child. For example, community pharmacists have a role in promoting the use of folic acid prior to conception to minimize the risk of neural tube defects. The importance of avoiding the unnecessary use of medicines in pregnancy or during lactation is another role where pharmacists can be involved.

Mobility and disability

Many patients will be unable to have direct access to their local community pharmacy due to impaired mobility or disability. As mentioned above, patients may be unable to access their pharmacist in the pharmacy, and may suffer from unmet pharmaceutical needs unless their community pharmacist provides domiciliary visits. Patients with specific disabilities may have greater pharmaceutical needs than others. For example, patients with visual impairment may be unable to distinguish between different medicines, therefore it is the pharmacist's responsibility to address this problem. Patients may have difficulty swallowing, therefore alternative formulations may be needed. Pharmacists can also help to devise methods of assisting illiterate and innumerate patients in taking their medicines safely.

Substance misuse

The medicine management needs arising from substance misuse are discussed in Chapter 42.

Treatment characteristics

Polypharmacy

Polypharmacy refers to the use of multiple medications by an individual patient. As the number of medicines used by an individual increases, the likelihood of drug interactions and adverse drug reactions also rises. The prevalence of many diseases increases with advancing age, therefore elderly patients are more likely to receive polypharmacy than younger patients.

Narrow therapeutic index

Examples of drugs with a narrow therapeutic index that are supplied from community pharmacies include digoxin, lithium and some anticonvulsants, and in the hospital setting also include aminoglycosides. Patients who take drugs with narrow therapeutic indices, e.g. gentamicin, may require a therapeutic drug monitoring (TDM) service. Antibiotic use within hospitals is nearly always controlled by a policy. Similarly, the operation of a TDM service may be subject to a hospital policy.

Condition characteristics

Multiple pathology

Patients (especially the elderly) often have more than one condition or disease that requires pharmacological treatment. A patient may be receiving treatment for hypertension, rheumatoid arthritis (RA) and asthma. Each disease may have implications for other conditions. For example, patients with RA often need an NSAID to relieve their pain and inflammation. However, NSAIDs are associated with hypertension and should be used with caution in asthmatics, therefore careful planning is required to ensure the patient has adequate analgesic cover without exacerbating other pre-existing conditions. The metabolism and elimination of drugs will be altered in patients with impaired renal, hepatic or cardiac function. For example, impaired renal function in patients with RA will influence the range of disease-modifying agents that are appropriate for their treatment.

Chronic disease

Most patients with chronic disease are likely to live at home and will have most of their medicines prescribed by their GP. Patients receiving treatment for chronic disease will often receive repeat prescriptions for their medicines. A repeat prescription is one that is issued to a patient for a particular medicine or medicines, which the patient has received before and which their GP has deemed appropriate for re-issue without requiring further consultation with the patient. Most general practices have repeat prescribing systems which facilitate the issue of repeat prescriptions.

Policies are required to ensure the regular review of long-term medicines and to prevent abuse of the system. Increasingly, pharmacists are becoming involved in improving repeat prescribing systems. It is likely that pharmacists will soon assume more responsibility for repeat prescribing, particularly if the proposed repeat dispensing systems are introduced. This will involve pharmacists in the regular review of patients' medication.

Pharmacists can make considerable contributions to the care of patients with chronic disease. They can provide and collaborate with the provision of chronic disease clinics in general practices. Hospital pharmacists can also provide substantial input to patients with chronic disease. For example, ensuring that RA patients are educated about their treatment and that the medicines are titrated, monitored and appropriate to their needs. Asthma is a chronic disease and all types of pharmacist have a role to play. The practice pharmacist could develop prescribing policies to ensure that patients who should receive inhaled corticosteroids do so. Hospital and community pharmacists can ensure that inhaler technique is satisfactory (see Ch. 24).

With the advancing age of the general population, chronic diseases will become more prevalent. This presents a major opportunity to pharmacists to develop their clinical roles.

Mental health problems and learning difficulties

Patients with mental health problems are a diverse group. Problems may range from the acutely psychotic in a hospital ward to the patient with depression who is living at home. These patients need specialized pharmaceutical input. A considerable degree of collaboration with other health care and social services workers is also required. As an integrated team member, the pharmacist is better able to understand the complex needs of these patients. Other members of the team also require to be fully appraised of the risks and benefits of drug therapy.

Patients with learning difficulties may have special medicine management needs. Various social, clinical and pharmaceutical factors may render this group of patients vulnerable to medicine-related problems. Patients discharged from long-stay care may be at particular risk. Their pharmaceutical needs require to be assessed in the context of their social support. Carers and patients may require advice and counselling on their medication. As with the mental health group, effective liaison between health care sectors and social services is essential.

Hospital admission or discharge can substantially change patients' pharmaceutical needs. The same may be generally true of transfer from one health care setting to another. Patients may require additional medicines, fewer medicines or changes in their drug regimen. Some may also require support on discharge in order to manage their medicines. However, it is likely that some form of long-term medication will need to be continued. Information about these medicines, the patient's progress with therapy and any other special requirements about the medicines should be transferred with the patient. Those responsible for the patient's care in the community should also be informed about any therapy changes made during the patient's time in hospital. Similarly, there needs to be an awareness amongst the community carers and health professionals of any new medical conditions which have developed or new pharmaceutical needs which have been identified since admission. In other words, all relevant information must be transferred with patients when they cross health care boundaries. Clearly, pharmacists have a major role to play in this transfer process. Effective communication between pharmacists across health care boundaries is essential. So too is communication between pharmacists and other members of the health care team.

Prioritization of care

Prioritization of care can be achieved by adopting a systematic approach to practice. The targeting of patient groups and screening of patients within these groups are the first steps in a systematic approach. Targeting was discussed earlier in this chapter.

An assessment of the needs of different groups should form the basis of pharmaceutical resource allocation. In hospitals, this should be agreed with management, clinicians and patient representatives. The type of patient, the nature of care provided and the duration of admission are all factors which feature in the allocation of priorities. As a group, long-stay elderly patients without active care plans often receive lower priority than, for example, patients admitted to a general medical ward with acute renal failure. The high risk of adverse effects associated with cancer chemotherapy is usually reflected by the extent of pharmaceutical input to oncology units.

Many community pharmacists are geographically isolated from the rest of the health care team. Thus, many determine their own priorities for particular patient groups. These priorities should be based upon a combination of professional judgment and current evidence on best practice.

Wherever possible, these priorities should reflect the views of other health care professionals and patients. For example, time might be allocated to counsel all patients newly commenced on metered dose inhalers. Similarly all patients with comprehension difficulties might be targeted to receive compliance aids.

This process of targeting groups of patients for particular attention is a tool to guide the most appropriate use of resources. However, it should always be remembered that pharmacists have a duty of care to every patient and customer.

The screening process involves a quick assessment of the individual patients within a target group. Screening identifies patients or customers who require the pharmacist's immediate attention. For individual patient records, it is important to document the outcomes of the screening process. Such a record may also prove useful for the purpose of management information. Patients screened out at this stage should be subject to periodic review as their need for pharmacist input may change. The processes of targeting and screening are summarized in Figure 31.1.

The skills required to screen patients are gained through experience. Criteria used to screen patients or customers are based upon an assessment of potential risk and benefit to the individual. Some criteria relate to the medicine, others to the patient or customer. Examples include the number of

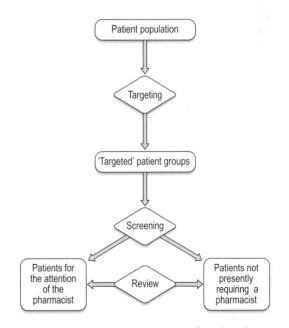

Fig. 31.1 Targeting and screening. (After Clinical Resources and Audit Group 1996.)

medicines prescribed and purchased, the potential for adverse drug reactions, the use of unlicensed or newly marketed medicines, medicines with a narrow therapeutic index, unusual formulations and specialized administration devices. Other criteria are linked with the patient's physical, mental and social condition.

Assessing patients

Targeting particular patient groups and screening patients within these groups identifies patients with potential medicine-related problems. Subject to the availability of relevant clinical information on patients, the pharmacist can make a more detailed assessment. Information from a variety of sources is assimilated and analysed (Table 31.4). The purpose of this assessment is to identify patient and medication risk factors. The patient's pharmaceutical needs are confirmed and actual medicine-related problems are identified.

In most cases pharmacists have access to a minimum of two of the above sources of information—the patient and the prescription. Many community pharmacists have patient medication records (PMRs) for the majority of their patients and hospital pharmacists have access to patients' hospital medical records. Ideally, the pharmacist should try to obtain a medication history directly from the patient. Some carers and representatives may be able to provide a good history. Even where records are available, it is good practice to check with the patient that they are accurate and up to date. Monitoring prescriptions helps to ensure that drug therapy is appropriate. However, it is important to note that, where possible, prescriptions should not be assessed in isolation from other patient data.

A case could be made for taking a medication history from all patients. Usually, however, it is a matter of profes-

sional judgment to identify patients for whom this is important. For example, a review of past and current medicine use is helpful when adverse drug reactions are suspected. Alternatively, the reasons for a patient's failure to respond to therapy may not be clear. Thus medication histories can produce useful information about patients' experience of efficacy and toxicity. Such information, on the one hand, might include the patients' beliefs about medicines from which they feel they derive benefit. On the other hand, the history may reveal important information on allergies and hypersensitivities.

There is a principle here which applies not only to medication history taking, but also to patient counselling and any other form of consultation in which the patient is being assessed. The principle involves considering the patients' perspectives. This may include their beliefs, perceptions, experiences, expectations and wishes. Thus in any consultation, patients may reveal, or may be encouraged, to discuss their perceptions of their disease and/or their therapy. This approach accepts the rights and the autonomy of individual patients. However, it is of fundamental importance, as it enables pharmacists and physicians to form a therapeutic alliance between themselves and their patients. This concept is called concordance and is discussed in Chapter 40. Applying this concept to medication history taking is likely to increase the usefulness of the information obtained. For example, patients may be more inclined to participate and contribute information if they perceive that their views will be listened to, respected and taken into account. This may lead to a more complete and honest picture of which medicines they take and how they take them. A picture of the patient's concerns, for example, may allow the pharmacist to provide reassurance or to dispel unnecessary fears. The pharmacist who is unaware of the patient's concerns is less likely to be in a position of influence.

Table 31.4 Usual sources of information available by health care setting

	Community pharmacist	Hospital pharmacist	Practice pharmacist
Patient	√	√	?
Prescription	√	√	?
Computer records*	–	√	√
Medical case notes*	–	√	√
Patient medication records	√	√	?
Other health professionals	?	√	√

* If community pharmacy becomes part of NHSnet this will change.

Patients should be told the purpose of the medication history and their agreement to it must be obtained. If possible, the pharmacist should prepare for the history taking before interviewing the patient. This may include compiling information on current and past drug therapy, PMRs or medical notes. Carers and relatives may be helpful in the case of young children, or forgetful or confused patients. Equally, access to other health care professionals may help to clarify details.

The interview should be conducted in a setting and in a manner which enables patients to discuss confidential issues. The patient should be asked about their use of all medicines—prescribed, OTC and complementary. The medication history should be documented in the PMR and/or in the patient's medical notes.

In the hospital setting, prescription monitoring is a component of assessing patients for medicine-related risk factors. It is not a substitute for speaking to patients or assessing other sources of patient information. For example, hospital pharmacists usually have easy access to clinical information which would enable them to judge the appropriateness of dose, route and frequency of administration. In the case of gentamicin, however, this would only be possible if the pharmacist also had access to the patient's age, weight and renal function.

In the community setting, the appropriateness of a prescription for ciprofloxacin may be more difficult to discern. The pharmacist would wish to consider whether this was the drug of choice for the indication involved. However, information on the exact indication and results from culture and sensitivity testing may not be available to the pharmacist, but the pharmacist may be aware of the clinical circumstances in which the GP prescribes ciprofloxacin. Indeed the pharmacist may have been involved in helping the general practice surgery to produce its formulary. The community pharmacist would also wish to consider the patient's concomitant drug therapy. This could be established from the PMR or from the patient. If necessary, the pharmacist may have to contact the prescriber to avoid the possibility of an important drug interaction.

Having accessed and evaluated all the available information, the patient's pharmaceutical needs can be identified. The pharmacist then confirms those needs with the patient and health care team. Actual medicine-related problems are identified. A decision is made regarding which problems should be addressed by the pharmacist. Other members of the team may be involved. In hospitals, this might be achieved during a ward round. In community practice, it may necessitate a telephone call or referral to the patient's GP. The hospital pharmacist also requires to consider at this early stage of assessment the patient's discharge plan. Early consideration is designed to accommodate the patient's anticipated pharmaceutical needs and problems on discharge. This is part of a systematic approach to individual patient care. It requires pharmacists to continuously address the changing pharmaceutical needs and medicine-related problems of patients.

Information on patient and medication risk factors and medicine-related problems should be recorded in the form of a patient medication profile. These profiles can be paper-based or electronic record systems. This can be done as a separate pharmacy record or as part of the overall patient record system. Such records are updated as necessary to provide a continuous means of identifying potential medicine-related problems.

PLANNING CARE

Targeting patient groups and screening patients within them are the first two stages of prioritizing care. These processes identify patients potentially in need of pharmaceutical input. The pharmacist then needs to assess them (see above) and plan their care. This should be achieved within the context of the overall clinical management of the patient. Determining priorities for individual patient care is the third stage of prioritizing care. Whether and how this is achieved depends both on the patient's needs and the pharmacist's opportunity.

In an intensive therapy unit (ITU), priorities for patient care are very different from those for long-stay elderly patients. In the former case, patients are treated for life-threatening conditions. Their clinical status may change rapidly. The high priority attached to ITU patients may be reflected in a very much higher pharmacist : patient ratio and a greater frequency of ward visits. Clearly, such a difference in patients' needs has implications for care planning. Pharmacists also have easier access to other members of the health care team in an ITU. Patients in long-stay elderly units may be managed clinically by their GPs to whom the pharmacist may have only occasional direct access.

Problems that occur frequently should be managed with a standard approach, therefore the pharmacist's time might best be used to facilitate the development, implementation and monitoring of local (standard) treatment protocols. A sepsis protocol can guide appropriate antibiotic selection prior to receiving a bacteriology report. Similarly, agreement between community pharmacists and local GPs can be derived regarding the referral of patients with dyspepsia for a medical opinion.

Other staff may manage some commonly occurring medication-related issues. Appropriately trained medicine counter assistants (MCAs) can recommend medicines for the treatment of many common conditions. Nurses may assess patients' inhaler technique and identify individuals who need to be counselled. In these situations, the pharmacist must ensure that staff are appropriately trained and that procedures are followed correctly. This represents appropriate and judicious use of policies, protocols and other trained staff. It creates time for the pharmacist to focus on planning care for those patients most in need of their attention.

Formulating a pharmaceutical care plan

In all interactions with patients, pharmacists require to formulate an action (how they intend to achieve the aim) and a measure that tells them that their aim has been achieved. These are the basic elements of a care plan. They should always be in place, whether or not the care plan is written down. Aims should be agreed with the patient, their carer (where relevant) and/or the other members of the clinical team.

If a patient wishes to buy a 'cough medicine' the aim should be to advise on an appropriate choice. The action would be to identify the type of cough, advise on selection and counsel the patient. The measure of achievement of the care plan would be whether or not the patient took the advice. Whether or not the medicine helped the patient would be the clinical outcome associated with the plan. In the case of this OTC medicine, the pharmacist has a shared responsibility for the outcome of the plan. The pharmacist has to respond to symptoms, make a recommendation and counsel the patient appropriately. The patient then agrees to take the medicine as advised by the pharmacist. This may appear to be a strikingly simple example of care planning. However, even apparently straightforward cases can turn out to be more complex. For example, the cough could have been a persistent dry one in a patient recently commenced on captopril. It is important that the pharmacist establishes concurrent disease states and/or drug therapy. For example, some cough medicines may be contraindicated in diabetic patients or in those taking monoamine oxidase inhibitors.

When providing care in a team situation (e.g. in a hospital ward) the pharmaceutical care plan should be recorded.

This enables the actions of the pharmacist to be coordinated with other members of the team. Preferably, aims should be stated as measurable end-points to be achieved within a definite time scale. An aim may be to ensure that a patient understands how to use a new inhaler. Prior to discharge, the pharmacist would aim to have the patient demonstrate a satisfactory inhaler technique.

The above aims relate to advice on the prescription, supply and administration of medicines. Aims may also be expressed in terms of achieving specified levels of improvement in laboratory or clinical markers of diseases. An aim to prevent drug toxicity may be to ensure that a particular biochemical marker remains within a specified range. For example, the plan might be to measure, at specified intervals, urea and electrolyte levels in a patient prescribed a high dose of furosemide (frusemide).

In considering the most appropriate actions to achieve their aims pharmacists should take account of the following:

- Local formularies or protocols which could assist in the selection of the most cost-effective therapy. For example, formularies may provide advice on the choice of NSAIDs for use in the elderly.
- Underlying disease states, or concomitant drug therapy which could affect the choice or dosage of medicine. For example, the dosage of digoxin in a patient with renal impairment.
- Previous adverse drug reactions, including drug allergies or hypersensitivities. For example, the proposed use of a cefalosporin in a patient with a history of penicillin sensitivity.
- Any requirement of the patient for health promotion (see Ch. 39). For example, a patient who wishes to purchase an antacid for dyspepsia may require advice on posture and eating habits.
- The patients' knowledge and understanding of their medicines and their ability to use them correctly. For example, the geriatric patient on seven medicines being discharged to sheltered housing.
- The patients' level of domestic and/or social independence or support. For example, the blind patient who obtains assistance with her medicines from her partially sighted husband. This will necessitate the use of some form of compliance aid. In such circumstances, effective transfer of information to carers, community-based health care professionals and/or social workers is essential.

The pharmacist's record of an individual patient's medicine-related problems and aims, together with the proposed actions, form a documented pharmaceutical care plan. This allows pharmacists to report their actions and is important for three reasons. Firstly, it provides a medicolegal record. Secondly, it supports continuity of care; this applies whether patients remain in one care environment or transfer from one care environment to another. Finally, it provides a basis for peer review.

Increasingly, there will be attempts to standardize care plans for patients with certain diseases. This is in response to the production of national clinical guidelines.

As standard care pathways emerge, pharmacists will be encouraged to address the needs of individual patients within agreed protocols. However, adherence to guidelines and protocols may not be in the best interests of all patients. For some patients deviations are justified on grounds of contraindications arising from concurrent disease states or concomitant drug therapy. The particular needs of the individual patient should always take priority.

Monitoring patients

Various health care professionals monitor patients to assess their progress with drug therapy. Most commonly this involves doctors, pharmacists and/or nurses. Ideally, a structured process should be used involving care plans with specified targets and review dates. This requires a systematic approach supported by effective communication and collaboration between the health care professions involved.

Where pharmacists are well integrated into the health care team's activities pharmaceutical care planning may be a routine activity. Implementation of the care plan requires agreement between the pharmacist's and health care team's time scales for monitoring or reviewing the patient. The pharmacist then coordinates her actions with those of the patient and the other team members.

Various indicators may be used to monitor a patient's progress against the aims stipulated in the care plan. These include clinical signs and symptoms, biochemical and haematological parameters and, for certain medicines, serum drug levels. Where appropriate, clinical assessment should be used in conjunction with objective measures. In the absence of objective indicators, the pharmacist relies on the clinical assessment of the patient by other members of the health care team. Where there are valid objective measures of the therapeutic or adverse effects of drugs, the pharmacist may assume responsibility for monitoring them and taking appropriate action. This is usually achieved within a jointly agreed treatment protocol or care plan.

Monitoring patients may be carried out for one or more of the following reasons:

- To monitor health promotion measures
- To monitor the progress of disease
- To monitor for drug efficacy and/or drug toxicity
- To monitor the patient's satisfaction with drug therapy.

Monitoring health promotion measures

Health promotion activities may be directed at preventing disease in healthy subjects or minimizing harm in patients with disease. Lifestyle counselling and monitoring of patients with certain chronic conditions is important. For example, patients with CHD should be encouraged to adopt a healthy lifestyle in relation to their diet and exercise. If relevant, they should be monitored and supported through a smoking cessation programme. Some of these patients may also require assistance in reducing their intake of alcohol. Health promotion is dealt with in more detail in Chapter 39.

Monitoring disease progress

The severity and nature of particular disease states may influence treatment choice. For example, some drugs are contraindicated in renal impairment (e.g. metformin) and others require dosage reduction (e.g. atenolol). Patients with deteriorating renal function therefore require close monitoring of their disease.

Monitoring drug efficacy/toxicity

In some cases the efficacy or toxicity of a drug needs to be assessed by a clinician. For example, a psychiatrist may assess the efficacy of an antidepressant. Confirmation of possible visual disturbance due to ethambutol may require the expertise of an ophthalmologist. However, the efficacy or toxicity of many drugs is readily detected through routine laboratory investigations. Careful and frequent monitoring of appropriate biochemical/haematological parameters may confirm efficacy and/or prevent drug toxicity. Blood glucose is monitored in diabetic patients to inform the dosage adjustment of insulin or of oral hypoglycaemic agents. Blood counts are monitored in AIDS patients receiving ganciclovir for the treatment of cytomegalovirus to detect leucopenia and thrombocytopenia.

Patients play an important role in monitoring toxicity. They need to know about and understand the possible side effects of their medicines. Thus the patient on warfarin therapy should be asked to report any signs of unusual or excessive bruising. Patients should be encouraged to be vigilant, even where objective measures of potential toxicity are available to the health care professional. In the case of warfarin, the risks and benefits may be monitored using prothrombin times monitored at anticoagulant clinics. However, the time between clinic visits coupled with many factors that can affect anticoagulant control, could render the patient at risk of serious haemorrhage prior to the next appointment. In such situations the patient's informed vigilance could be potentially life saving.

For a small number of drugs it may be inappropriate or potentially dangerous to monitor patients through clinical signs or symptoms alone. There may be no appropriate biochemical or haematological indicators of efficacy or toxicity. The use of serum drug levels is appropriate for drugs with a narrow therapeutic index and a well-defined target serum concentration range. Interpretation of drug levels should always be made with a knowledge of medication and dosage history, sampling times and relevant clinical details of the patient. Targeting particular drug levels by the application of pharmacokinetic principles can often result in a quicker and safer route to efficacy than that achieved by clinical assessment alone. This activity is known as therapeutic drug monitoring (TDM). For example, in the case of certain anticonvulsants, efficacy could be monitored solely by seizure frequency. To do so, however, could put the patient at risk. A TDM service facilitates the achievement of effective serum levels of anticonvulsants whilst minimizing the risk of toxicity.

A more detailed consideration of the prevention, detection, monitoring and reporting of adverse drug reactions is provided in Chapter 32.

Monitoring patient satisfaction

Patients should be asked about how they are getting on with their medicines. The patient's response to open questioning may express satisfaction and/or concern. A patient's level of satisfaction need not parallel responses to drug therapy indicated by more objective measures, however it is important. If patients are dissatisfied with their drug therapy they may stop taking their medicine. This could arise if they do not perceive a treatment response or if adverse effects are suspected. Their decision to stop taking their medication may well be justified. However, a patient may be responding to his treatment but not feeling any better. A suspected adverse effect may turn out to be an unrelated symptom requiring

further investigation. It is extremely important, therefore, to maintain a dialogue with patients about their drug therapy. If no specific indicator of drug efficacy or toxicity is being investigated such dialogue may be the only form of monitoring to take place. It also helps to sustain any established concordance (see Ch. 40) between patients and their pharmacist and/or doctor.

Review

Outcomes from the pharmaceutical care plan are evaluated against the aims that were specified at the formulation stage. Where the aims are achieved, assurance is provided of the resolution of medicine-related problems. Where specific aims are not achieved, the pharmaceutical care plan is reviewed. Either the outcome achieved is accepted as being the best achievable for the patient, or an alternative plan is proposed. Pharmaceutical care planning requires to respond continuously to changes in the clinical status and requirements of patients.

Transferring care

In the course of a single acute care episode, a patient may interact with several professionals in different settings. Patients suffering from several chronic diseases are likely to be involved with a large number of health care professionals in primary and secondary care. Transfer of the care of patients between professionals and between health care sectors may be planned or occur in an emergency. Whatever the circumstance, every effort should be made to maintain continuity of care. This requires effective communication between professionals within and between health care sectors.

Continued review of the care plan

Whenever a patient is transferred to a different care environment or to the care of another pharmacist, the pharmaceutical care plan should be reviewed. Proposals should be made to deal with any unresolved medication-related issues and with any new ones that are linked to the transfer of care. Consideration should be given to the change in environment, the level of patient support and shared-care protocols. Priority should be given to ensure that supplies of medicines are available. Sufficient information should be given to the patient, carers and other health care professionals to enable care to continue as planned.

Counselling and advising the patient or carer

The pharmacist should ensure that the patient or their carer understands the medication regimen and is able to administer it correctly. Where appropriate, compliance aids such as calendar cards should be considered. Special labelling should be requested for patients with visual impairment. Consideration should be given to any particular needs of ethnic groups. The patient should be advised on the disposal of discontinued medicines.

Self-medication schemes operate in some hospitals. This usually involves the pharmacist counselling selected patients on their knowledge, understanding and use of medicines at an early stage during their admission. These patients are then given responsibility for administering their own medicines prior to discharge. This enables the patients to manage and monitor their drug regimen. Outside these formal schemes, patient counselling seeks to ensure that all patients are able and prepared to take their medicines as prescribed.

The principle of applying objective measures to monitoring progress and outcomes also applies to the assessment of patients' knowledge and understanding of their medicines. It is all too easy to tell patients how to take their medicines. It is also important to check that they actually have the ability to use their medicines properly. There is particular scope for confusion when patients are discharged or transferred. For example, on admission a patient could be taking Largactil. In hospital she is changed to generic chlorpromazine and is issued with a supply on discharge. No explanation is given to the patient, who subsequently takes both forms of the drug and inadvertently overdoses. Similar problems can occur when a medicine is discontinued during a hospital stay. The patient may be unaware that the medicine has been stopped and continues to take it on returning home. There is more on counselling in Chapter 38.

Communication between health care professionals

As patients are transferred from one health care environment to another, continuity of care relies on the identification of, and effective communication with, professionals to whom responsibility is transferred.

Where a pharmacist is providing care to a patient, it is his duty to ensure that the element of care is continued when the patient is transferred. This is equally so whether the patient is transferred from an acute medical admissions ward to a general medical ward, from one hospital to another, or from hospital into the community. On hospital discharge, a pharmacy discharge summary can conveniently be transferred with the patient to the community pharmacist. There are recommended formats for information to be provided on transfer of patients both into and out of hospital. The Royal Pharmaceutical Society of Great Britain (RPSGB) has developed documentation to facilitate this two-way communication between hospital and community pharmacists.

The confidentiality of information relating to a patient and the patient's family should be respected throughout the transfer process. This also applies to the personal wishes of the patient. For example, patients should be asked which community pharmacy they routinely use. It is important to explain to patients the advantages of using one community pharmacy. This is particularly true for patients with complex medication needs. Such patients include those receiving TPN, pain control or dialysis, and those taking multiple medication for one or more chronic diseases (e.g. cystic fibrosis).

The community pharmacist's computerized PMR is a unique record of patient information. While the GP may be aware of what has been prescribed, some prescriptions are never dispensed. In addition, GPs are unlikely to have any record of the OTC medicines taken by patients. Most patients consistently have their prescriptions dispensed at the same pharmacy. The community pharmacist is therefore ideally placed to provide information to enable a complete medication history to be taken on admission of patients to hospital.

CASE STUDY 31.1

A. Poor transfer of care

Mr Brown, a regular customer in the pharmacy, asked to see the pharmacist. He was pale and quite upset. For several years he had taken antacids for indigestion. In the last 3 months he had little relief and during the last week had been feeling sick. On that morning he had been sick and the vomit was brown. Mr Brown's medication record listed only the antacid which he had been buying and bendroflumethiazide (bendrofluazide), which was prescribed for control of blood pressure. The community pharmacist advised the patient to see his doctor immediately. The doctor admitted Mr Brown to hospital for urgent investigation of the problem. On admission, no record was made of Mr Brown's bendroflumethiazide (bendrofluazide), since he had forgotten to bring his

---

supply with him. Although asked about medicines, he was confused and thought that the hospital doctor was only interested in medicines for indigestion. He was diagnosed as having a duodenal ulcer and discharged on ranitidine 300 mg daily. He continued to smoke, had 'several pints with his mates' on Friday nights and drank milk whenever he was bothered with indigestion. Six months later he was still taking the same dose of ranitidine and still complained of indigestion. He routinely took his ranitidine after breakfast. During a routine check his blood pressure was found to be high.

This example illustrates the potential for problems on transfer of care. Although each of the professionals involved dealt with his or her part of the problem, the overall quality of care was less than adequate. Because the GP failed to inform the hospital doctor about bendroflumethiazide (bendrofluazide), this was missed in hospital and thus was not included on the discharge prescription. No mention was made on the discharge prescription of the duration of treatment with ranitidine. The receptionist amended the repeat prescription, deleting bendroflumethiazide (bendrofluazide) and adding ranitidine. No one gave the patient health promotion advice and no one informed the community pharmacist about the continuing care of the patient. The community pharmacist did not query the cessation of bendroflumethiazide (bendrofluazide) therapy.

The scenario depicted in the case study below indicates how Mr Brown might have fared in different circumstances.

B. Effective transfer of care

Having recognized the potential seriousness of Mr Brown's condition, the pharmacist referred him to his family doctor. Mr Brown was given a copy of his PMR which he was advised to keep and show to his doctor. On referring Mr Brown to hospital, the GP included an up-to-date medication history in the referral letter. Consequently an accurate medication history was taken on admission and bendroflumethiazide (bendrofluazide) was continued. Having been diagnosed as having a duodenal ulcer, he was discharged on ranitidine 300 mg at night. The family doctor was informed that treatment should be continued for 8 weeks and then reviewed. Since the patient was infected with *Helicobacter pylori*, a course of eradication therapy was recommended to be commenced once the ulcer had been healed.

Before discharge, the hospital pharmacist gave Mr Brown a detailed explanation of his treatment. Advice was also given regarding sensible eating and drinking and the need to stop smoking. A pharmacy discharge summary was sent to the community

pharmacist. The treatment plan was described and reinforcement of health promotion advice was recommended.

Six months later Mr Brown's ulcer had healed and his blood pressure was well controlled. *H. pylori* had successfully been eradicated and he was symptom free. He had adopted sensible eating and drinking habits. With the assistance of nicotine patches suggested by the community pharmacist, he had also significantly reduced the number of cigarettes he smoked each day.

PATIENT MEDICATION RECORDS

There has been a tradition of pharmacists keeping records on certain types of medication. Often this was keeping notes about types of insulin or the supply of oxygen cylinders. There has also been the legal requirement to record certain types of prescription and classes of drugs. In recent years there has been a marked increase in the use of records to include a wide range of patient groups and medicines. It has been claimed that 95% of pharmacists keep records, many on all patients. They are commonly called patient medication records (PMRs). The value of these records has been recognized by the UK government who currently pay pharmacists who have completed appropriate training a fee for keeping PMRs.

There are three types of PMR in use in the UK—cards, computer-based systems and 'smart cards'. Each has its advantages and disadvantages. Card systems rely on handwriting. The National Pharmaceutical Association (NPA) has produced a card that enables most of the information to be recorded easily. Cards are stored in a box file, usually in alphabetical order. Computer-based systems are commercially available as 'add-ons' to labelling programs, having been refined since their introduction in the early 1980s. They cost more to purchase and update, but give greater flexibility than the card system. This is the main system used in pharmacies today. 'Smart cards' are still experimental. They use a chip to record patient data on a card that the patient carries with her. Technology is developing rapidly in this area so that large amounts of data can be stored on a credit card-sized smart card. However, there is as yet no standardization and they are only being used in local trials. This method has the potential to carry a lot of medical information about the patient and could have all medicines included in the record, irrespective of where they are dispensed.

Computer-based systems

The RPSGB includes guidelines on pharmacy computer systems in *Medicines, Ethics and Practice*. This gives valuable guidance about the hardware and software aspects of installing a system, as well as addressing issues such as supplier support, multi-user systems, data standards, compatibility and the maintenance of databases. The types of data which the programme should be capable of storing are summarized in Table 31.5. Modern systems also allow the addition of a range of other information. This could include pregnancy, breastfeeding, smoking status and other characteristics or risks. They also have a facility to flag the patient the next time the record is accessed.

The programmes are structured as a number of separate files. These are normally a patient file, a prescription file, a drug file, a dosage instruction file (for labelling) and a doctor file. In operation, the computer links two files by a common set of data, called the linking field. Thus, for example, when a new prescription is entered, the computer would access a number of files. It would go to the patient file to check name and address and any special notes. The drug file would be checked for the drug strength and dosage. Both the patient file and drug file would be used to check for drug interactions and the instruction file would be used if the same label is required. On completion of dispensing the information is stored in the appropriate file and can be accessed in a very flexible way. Thus, for example, it would

be possible to produce lists of all patients on a particular drug, all residents in a residential home, or all patients recorded as having a particular medical condition.

It is essential that any entry can be corrected if it is found to be incorrect. It must also be recognized that each entry takes up space on the computer disk. On older machines the hard disk memory may be restricted, and so it is necessary to either store on floppy disks or delete records. Some programmes will carry out deletion automatically against predetermined criteria, such as after 6 months for most patients, but after 2 years for patients aged over 60 years. It is good practice with any computer system to make regular back-up copies of the data. When data are archived, the Consumer Protection Act requires that they are kept for 10 years. The Department of Health specify that data be stored for at least one year and preferably two. It is essential that there is easy access to any archived data.

The ease of use of computer-based PMRs has led to a widespread use. However, some pharmacists may wish to limit the records to certain groups of patients, particularly when setting up a new system. In such a process, it is advisable to have clear priorities. The NHS contract only requires records for patients over the age of 60 years. Apart from this group, other priority groups could include children under 12, patients in receipt of domiciliary services or living in a residential or nursing home, some disease groups (asthmatics, epileptics), patients with special needs (penicillin sensitivity, regular multiple therapy, confusion, needing

Table 31.5   Types of data to record on a PMR system (based on RPSGB guidelines 1996)

Information	Data
Should record	
Patient	Name, address (including postcode) and telephone number
	Age and date of birth, sex
	NHS number
GP data	Name, identification number
	Practice name and telephone
Medicine	Name, strength, form, quantity
	Dosage regimen
	Date dispensed
Useful	
Patient	Exempt prescription charges
	Child-resistant closures unacceptable
	Drug sensitivity/allergy
	Chronic illness
Medicine	Product licence (for generics), batch number

compliance aids), or patients on certain groups of drugs (H_2 antagonists, anticoagulants, oral contraceptives, steroids, antihypertensives). The ideal is to include all patients.

Data Protection Act

In 1998, the Data Protection Act was introduced in the UK. The act made new provision for the regulation of the processing of information relating to individuals, including the obtaining, holding, use or disclosure of such information. The Act makes specific reference to 'sensitive personal data', which in the context of pharmaceutical care includes personal data consisting of information as to a 'person's physical or mental health or condition, or his sexual life'. The following definitions have been summarized from the Data Protection Act. 'Data' means information which is being processed, or recorded with the intention that it should be processed, or recorded as part of a relevant filing system or with the intention that it should form part of a relevant filing system. It is clear that this Act includes data that are used and recorded by pharmacists for the provision of pharmaceutical care. The 'Act' refers to persons who (either alone or jointly or in common with other persons) determine the purposes for which and the manner in which any personal data are, or are to be, processed. A 'data subject' means an individual who is the subject of 'personal data'. Therefore, patients would be data subjects and personal data would relate to any data that the pharmacist uses, accesses or records that make the patient identifiable. In general, the Data Protection Act states that data should be used for the purpose for which it was collected. It also states who should know about the collection, retention and use of these data. Pharmacists should refer to the Act for full details and to interpret how it affects their professional practice. Many hospitals and health authorities (boards in Scotland) have data protection advisors to whom pharmacists should refer their queries.

In the UK, the Data Protection Act must be complied with when using a computer-based PMR system. The user of the computer system must register with the Data Protection Registrar. The data stored can only be used for the purpose(s) for which they are registered, although they can be used for research providing that an individual cannot be identified. The Act is designed to protect an individual's right to confidentiality and the accuracy of the data. Patients must give their permission before a PMR can be created and they have a right to either see the whole record or receive a complete copy. Some ethical and legal problems can arise. An example is whether the parents, the child or both have the right to see the record of a teenage child.

In this example, there are detailed differences in the law across the UK. The Act also requires that the system is secure to prevent unauthorized access to the data. The Access to Health Records Act (1990) is also relevant for pharmacists in terms of PMRs and other patient records that they might maintain.

Access to Health Records Act

In 1990, the British Government introduced the Access to Health Records Act. The Act states who can have access to a patient's health record. Patients can request access to their health records, or their representative can make the request on the patient's behalf. Health professionals who hold records on patients are required to make the record available, within a reasonable period of time, to the patient if requested to do so. The health professional is also required to provide suitable explanation of the record if it is expressed in terms that are 'not intelligible without explanation'.

Uses of PMRs

Patient medication records have many uses some of which are discussed in the following section.

Dispensing

The major use of a PMR is during dispensing a prescription. Computer-based systems have the capability of confirming the prescriber and that the name and address on the prescription and PMR match. The computer can be used to check for the safety and appropriateness of each item against the data on file, including drug interactions and any recorded contraindications and allergies. Doses may be checked, particularly for consistency with previous occasions of dispensing. Any notes on the patient's record, such as a need to avoid child-resistant closures, can be seen to optimize efficiency. When the item to be dispensed is a simple repeat of a previous prescription, most systems allow automatic label preparation. Finally, a single key stroke will update the record. Thus it provides a very efficient way of checking the safety of the prescription for the patient. In doing so, the ideal is that the record should be checked over a period of at least 2 years for any patient over 65 years and for 3 months for other patients.

In addition, the computer record can improve the efficiency of service provided in a number of ways. For example, the frequency of counselling or checking inhaler technique can be noted and a reminder flashed on the screen.

Where generics are being dispensed, the source can be recorded in order to provide the same one where possible and so avoid anxiety in the patient if the appearance is different. These facilities are useful for a regular pharmacist but are invaluable for a locum pharmacist. The record can also help if errors are made or if information is missing from a repeat prescription, because drug name, dose, strength, quantity and instructions will all be recorded. However, the intention of the prescriber must always be confirmed.

Drug interactions

The PMR can also be used to recognize drug interactions and is often cited as one of the most important facilities of these systems. However, there are a number of possible problems with these programmes. In order to operate effectively the programme must be able to recognize drugs that are entered either by proprietary or generic name. The database used by the computer must be compiled from a reliable source and updated regularly. Interactions vary in their severity and potential to cause harm. Not only do the interactions vary, so do individual patients' susceptibility to them. This is recognized by most of the interaction programs, although the extent of discrimination varies between programmes. Studies have demonstrated that different programmes produce different information about the same combination of drugs. In extreme examples this can range from major interaction to no interaction. The RPSGB guideline indicates that any interactions programme should alert to every interaction listed in the current edition of the *British National Formulary* (BNF) and must be able to highlight any potentially hazardous interactions. There is a danger that people will rely on the computer, but the guidelines make it clear that the pharmacist still has personal responsibility for verifying the safety of any combination of drugs prescribed for a patient.

Increasingly, electronic point of sale (EPOS) systems are being used in pharmacies which can be linked into the PMR system. As a result, the records will include OTC medicines as well as dispensed medicines. This is important from a safety point of view, especially as more drugs are deregulated. However, information on OTC interactions is less well developed and the public still have to be convinced about the use of PMRs when they wish to purchase a medicine.

Other uses

The other uses of PMRs derive from either the ease and flexibility of access to the information or from the nature of the information that is stored. There are a number of reasons why a pharmacist may not be able to dispense all the medicines requested on a prescription. This is usually due to the quantity ordered exceeding the amount in stock, especially when there has been a deliberate decision to keep stock low because of the high cost or short expiry date of the medicine. It could also arise because of a supply problem or heavy demand leading to a need to 'ration' the supply. Regardless of the reason for the shortfall, the amount of the medicine which remains outstanding due to shortage can be 'flagged' in the PMR. Most PMR systems have a facility for recording this, producing a note for the patient and the label for the balance when it is available. This has a clear management advantage. It can be used, if thought necessary, to review the optimum stock levels of particular products. Decisions about stock levels can be difficult to make, because many factors influence them, including time to resupply and cost of items (see Ch. 5). The usage patterns of drugs can be analysed using the data in the PMR. Whilst this will not be the only information needed in order to reach a decision, it is important and can readily show the normal level of demand and any seasonal fluctuations.

The importance of producing and recording information on medicines is discussed in the section on 'Residential care', especially the section 'Regular visits by the pharmacist'. The computer is able to combine the records of all the patients in a specific residential home, both for general information and as a prelude to a visit to that home by the pharmacist.

Another facility that may be useful for residents of homes, or for other patients, is that PMR systems can produce medicine administration records. These are used with monitored dosage systems to provide the name, strength, form, quantity and administration times for each medicine. Compliance charts are not dissimilar in that they also record the same information on paper for a patient or carer. They are used to act as a reminder or to record that the administration has taken place.

Invoices may be required for supplies made to surgeries and other similar places. The computer can generate these easily. Patient information leaflets (PILs) can be produced by some programs. As with drug interactions, it is the responsibility of the pharmacist to ensure the accuracy of the information. Whilst the pharmacist could add the text, the RPSGB guidelines advise against this.

Pharmacists are now part of the adverse drug reaction reporting scheme using the Yellow Card Scheme. The use of PMR systems to keep records of adverse drug reactions will enable the pharmacist to recognize a problem and hence report it using the Yellow Card Scheme.

PMR systems are also useful for product recalls. It is important to trace all product recall medicine that has been supplied. Most PMR systems have the facility for recording product source and batch number. In the event of a recall, this information would allow the pharmacist to know exactly to whom the medicine had been dispensed, together with their addresses and the date of dispensing. This makes recovering the product much more efficient.

Pharmacists may find it useful to keep health-related data that they have determined should be part of their service. Thus, for example, a diary-like record could be made for smoking cessation, blood pressure monitoring, peak flow measurement or blood cholesterol measurement.

Most PMR systems also have a facility for stock ordering to ease the business management aspects of community pharmacy.

Advanced uses of PMRs

More advanced uses of PMRs have been suggested which make direct use of the information, or draw upon it together with other related information. As discussed in Chapter 40, patient compliance with prescribed medication can be a problem. The PMR contains information about the quantity of medicines dispensed over a period of time and the frequency of dosage intended. Thus it is possible to see if this pattern corresponds with what would be expected from the prescription. This does not prove or disprove compliance, but may give a pointer to a problem and lead the pharmacist to ask further questions. A related use is when the method of administration requires a special technique, such as with a pressurized aerosol. It is advisable to check on the patient's technique regularly, but not necessarily every time a prescription is dispensed. A 'flag' can be placed in the PMR reminding the pharmacist to speak to the patient after a set number of prescriptions.

Some facets of health promotion require the identification of patients who are 'at risk', but the main difficulty is making contact with them. One way of doing this may be by using the PMR. It can work by using the drugs that are being prescribed, together with the other information that is stored on the PMR. For example, influenza vaccination is recommended for elderly people and other high-risk groups. The PMR can easily identify elderly people. It can also identify people who have respiratory disease, either by using the notes, or from the drugs that they have been prescribed. Whichever way they are recognized, a flag on the PMR

means that the next time these patients have a prescription dispensed, they can be asked whether they have had the vaccination.

Problems with PMRs

A number of problems with PMR systems have been mentioned already, such as variable information about drug interactions. There are a number of other problems, both technical and practical. Most systems are designed for use by one operator at a time. This may be inadequate. For example in a busy pharmacy where there is more than one pharmacist, multiple access would be required. This need also arises where EPOS is being used, or where the pharmacist wants to have the PMR available at the area in the pharmacy where patient counselling is taking place as well as in the dispensary. Systems are being developed to allow these additional facilities.

The greatest problem with PMRs in pharmacies is that they are often incomplete. Patients are not required to use the same pharmacy every time and they may also purchase General Sales List (GSL) medicines from non-pharmacy outlets. As a result, several different pharmacies may have incomplete records for the same person. In the UK, one large multiple company has a system that interlinks all its stores. Apart from this, at present there have been no initiatives towards interlinking records to produce a more complete record. Likewise, there has been no move towards a scheme in which a patient must register with one pharmacy. The smart card form of PMR has the potential to overcome this serious limitation, if the technical aspects can be standardized. However, even that may not be the complete answer, because the card is ultimately dependent on patients carrying it with them at all times.

The ideal situation would be for all of community pharmacy IT systems, including the PMR, to be linked into the NHSnet. This is now scheduled for 2005. The first planned use of this link is to transmit prescription information electronically from the prescriber to the dispensing pharmacist, ultimately removing the need for a paper prescription form. Advantages of this link include the quick and accurate transmission of information, with the electronic information also capable of generating the dispensing label and updating the PMR. Various models of more advanced integrated systems have been proposed whereby each NHS patient would have an electronic health record to which different health care professionals would have different levels of read and write access. Thus a pharmacist would not only be able to access the current prescription electronically but would also be able to see previous dispensings, whether by themselves or another pharmacy, and would have access to at least some of the patient's medical record including drug history and diagnosis as a minimum. The majority of pharmacists would like access to other items such as hospital letters and test results, but it is likely to be some time before the public and the rest of the health care team would support such a radical change. Similarly, in the longer term, pharmacists will be able to write to the record information on non-dispensed items, date of dispensing, problems identified and OTC sales made. This latter component is particularly important given the increasing range of potent OTC drugs now available without a prescription and the use of which should be conveyed to the GP to inform his own management of the patient. At the moment there is clear evidence that the GP does not always remember to ask for this information, nor for the patient to give it. This results in the potential for therapeutic duplication (e.g. of two 'prescriptions' for NSAIDs), or for drug interactions (e.g. purchase of OTC aspirin by a patient on warfarin).

RESIDENTIAL CARE

As a result of the White Paper 'Caring for People' (1989) and the National Health Service and Community Care Act (2002), there has been a progressive reduction in the number of long-term hospital beds combined with a move to care for patients in the community. Private, local authority and voluntary residential care facilities have been developed to accommodate these changes. Residential homes can be categorized into three groups (Table 31.6). Community pharmacists who have undertaken suitable training and who have signed an agreement to provide clinical pharmacy services to residential homes receive payment for their services.

Medicine administration in homes

Where possible residents should have complete control of all their medicines, both prescribed and OTC. In such situations, the pharmacist should be alert to the potential need for assistance with maintaining compliance (see Ch. 40). However, within homes there is often some form of centralized control over prescribed medicines. There are two basic approaches to medicine administration using centralized control—direct administration and redispensing. With direct administration, a suitably qualified member of staff gives residents their medicine directly from the original pack. In redispensing, the dose is placed in a suitable container for the resident to take, often at a meal table. There are advantages and disadvantages of both methods, which are summarized in Table 31.7. Whichever method is used, pharmacists should be prepared to give advice to ensure that, as far as possible, errors or omissions do not arise. Apart from the actual methods of administration to be used, this will require that adequate records are kept. In addition, it will also need to link with wider issues such as delivery, storage and disposal of medicines and the methods of stock control.

Documentation and recording

It is necessary to have some form of formal recording of medicines in a home for a number of reasons. These include the problems created by a large number of staff, often on shift work, use of relief staff and the large quantities of medicines that will be handled at any one time. In addition, the use of records will facilitate the smooth and effective operation of medicine administration. It is generally accepted that at least three types of record should be used. These are:

- A medicines record, which is used as a central record of ordering and receiving medicines. Its main function is in

Table 31.6 Types of residential home accommodation	
Type of accommodation	**Clientele**
'Sheltered'	High level of independence
Residential homes	Elderly residents with greater needs than those in sheltered accommodation but who also have some degree of independence
Nursing homes	People with specific medical requirements
Other	Children, mentally ill, physical and learning difficulties

Table 31.7   Advantages and disadvantages of redispensing and direct administration

Redispensing	Direct administration
Two-stage process	Single-stage process
Higher risk of error	Lower risk of error
Lower staff time	Higher staff time
Can be prepared in advance	Prepared with resident
Resident has to remember to take medicine	Resident told to take medicine
Consumption not seen	Consumption seen
Distribution is rapid	Distribution is slow
Little help available to resident	Help available to resident

effective stock control to ensure that patients do not run out of medicines.

- The medication profile is a record for each patient. The information required will be the same as that on the patient's PMR and may be computer generated. It will, therefore, include information such as allergies, in addition to details of current and past medicines.
- The administration record is used to record the giving of a medicine to a resident. Ideally this should be on the same sheet as the medication profile, so that checking the actual administration with the prescriber's instructions is facilitated. Many computer systems can produce these sheets. The time and nature of each dose administered are recorded and signed by the member of staff. Over time a complete profile is built up. This indicates the giving of the medicine, but can only guarantee its use where the member of staff gives it directly to the resident and sees that it is taken or used.

Storage and control of medicines

Unless residents look after their own medicines, there will be a need to keep large quantities of medicines centrally. This must be in a manner that will avoid confusion, be secure and provide appropriate conditions for the storage of the medicines.

Two main types of storage are used—medicine cupboards and trolleys. Ideally a cupboard should be specially designed and lockable, and the person in charge keeps the key. Medicine trolleys should be stored in a room not normally accessible to residents and fastened to a fixed object when not in use. The storage conditions for medicines must be considered. In particular, there may be the need for refrigerator storage. It is not necessary to have a refrigerator dedicated to medicine storage in residential homes, but it must be lockable and medicines should be kept separate from other items in a mixed-use refrigerator. The temperature inside storage cupboards should be checked and the trolley storage point should not be near a radiator. There is no need for special storage of controlled drugs, except in nursing homes which must comply with the Misuse of Drugs Act.

Procedures for administering medicines

Ideally any procedures should apply to all medicines, both prescribed and OTC. Procedures should minimize the risk of errors. Key stages are summarized in Box 31.1. The giving of medicines at meal-times can cause many problems. These include identification of residents, the person being absent, omitting or forgetting the medicine. More significantly, administration times may not correspond with meal times, for example when it is required half an hour before food. Such

---

Box 31.1   Preparation stages for administration of a medicine

1. Check the identity of the patient
2. Check the resident's medication record, especially ensuring that the dose has not already been given and noting any changes made by the doctor
3. Identify the medicine and check that the label has the resident's name and corresponds with the medication record
4. Administer the medicine, or place it in receptacle for giving to resident
5. Endorse the medication record immediately
6. Record any reason why a dose is not taken

---

practical issues will need to be discussed by the pharmacist and resolved with the home administrators.

Ordering and delivery of medicines

Most medicines used by residents are supplied using repeat prescriptions. A 1-month supply is normally prescribed. Ideally, residential home staff will know when to order a repeat prescription using the medication profile of the patient and the stock level. This can be reinforced by agreement about the minimum stock level to allow adequate time for prescription preparation, collection, dispensing and delivery. Once agreed, a time for reordering can be marked on the administration record. Sometimes situations arise when there is an urgent need for a medicine, or when a repeat medicine is required before the prescription has been received. Procedures should be developed for dealing with these types of situations.

Disposal of unwanted medicines

Medicines that are no longer used because treatment has been discontinued or completed should be destroyed. If a resident dies, medicine disposal should not be undertaken for a minimum of 1 week in case the coroner requires it. The overall responsibility for the disposal of unwanted medicines should lie with the pharmacist and arrangements with the home must ensure that this occurs. Medicines must not be flushed down the toilet or put in the dustbin. Both pharmacist and responsible person in the home can initial the medicines record. In no situation should medicines be kept by the home for use by other residents.

Regular visits by the pharmacist

Clearly, the use of protocols for recording, administration, storage and disposal of medicines requires the pharmacists spending time with the home administrators. The amount of time will vary with the size, nature and needs of each home. There is also a requirement for regular pharmacist visits, with appropriate records, as part of the remuneration package.

The pharmacist should check the medication records on a regular basis. This helps to ensure that residents are receiving the medication profile intended by their doctor, that the stock levels correspond with the entries in the medicines record and that any changes in treatment have been correctly introduced. At the same time, expiry date checks should also be made. These routine matters can be used as a discussion point between the pharmacist and home staff about the

safe and effective use of medicines and how to deal with problems that arise.

In addition, the pharmacist can use regular visits to develop other aspects of the service to the home. The pharmacist could assume a more clinical role by reviewing the medication profiles of patients. This can be particularly useful when a new resident enters a home. The process helps to identify problems arising with combinations of medicines, dosage form or selection of drug. Where problems are identified and corrected, the care of the resident is improved.

Contact with residents

As for all patients receiving dispensed medicines, clients in residential homes are entitled to expect their pharmacist to provide information and advice about their medicines. They should not be denied this because of the surroundings in which they live. Thus direct contact with residents can become part of regular pharmacist visits and could be especially useful when a person first takes up residence. This allows informal discussion, probably with more time available than in the normal community pharmacy situation. During this time it will be possible for the pharmacist to answer questions and ask about any problems which the person is experiencing. Ideally, residents should be counselled by the pharmacist each time a change of medication occurs. As with any similar situation, the pharmacist can also assess whether the patient might benefit from the use of a compliance aid (see Ch. 40). Likewise, the pharmacist can determine whether the patient is having other difficulties with their medicines, e.g. with swallowing tablets, which might lead to a suggested change in dosage form or regimen. In homes where residents are allowed to use their own OTC medicines, the pharmacist can use this time to discuss the needs of the patient, respond to any symptoms and offer general advice.

Staff training

In the preceding discussion, contact with staff in the home has, by implication, been limited to the senior, responsible personnel. These people may have qualifications and experience that enable them to easily appreciate what is being discussed. However, on a daily basis it is usually the less qualified or less experienced carers who have contact with the residents and who may have to operate the procedures for the administration of medicines. Thus it is important that all levels of staff in a home have an adequate level of knowledge and understanding about medicines and how to operate the agreed procedures. There is a need for training that ensures all staff are at a suitable level of proficiency. Training should be provided at the start of employment or a new initiative, and should be reviewed, repeated and maintained as required. Technically, this is the responsibility of the district pharmaceutical officer or chief administrative pharmaceutical officer. In practice, general training may be provided by the health authority or board, or it might become the responsibility of the community pharmacist. As the relationship between the pharmacist and staff develops, ongoing training is likely to become the responsibility of the pharmacist as a result of the expressed needs of the latter. There are a number of potential topics that are summarized in Box 31.2. The level at which training takes place should match the ability and need for comprehension by the staff.

Procedures

All staff involved in medicine supply and administration to residents must understand the record-keeping system: why it is there, how to use it, how to check the medicine and dosage, and how to record that a dose has been given. Failure to appreciate the operation of the system and its importance will result in meaningless records and potential danger to the residents as the risk of confusion and error increases.

Medication formulations and devices

Staff in residential homes should be aware of the different types of formulation used. They should be aware of what should and should not be done with the different formula-

---

> ### Box 31.2 Summary of suitable training topics for residential home staff
>
> Administration procedures for medicines
> Record keeping
> Acquisition of medicines
> Disposal of medicines
> Storage of medicines
> Types of pharmaceutical formulation
> Handling of different types of medicine
> Fate of drugs in the body
> Side-effects of drugs
> Sources of information and explanation of technical terms
> Use of OTC and household medicines
> Differences in legal classification
> Safe use of medicines

---

tions. For example, staff need to be aware that some tablets can be split or crushed and others that should remain intact, e.g. enteric-coated preparations. With liquid formulations, staff need to know how to shake a bottle effectively and how to measure a dose accurately. With more specialized dosage forms, such as eye drops and inhalers, staff will need to know how to administer them. Practical sessions spent handling different types of products will be beneficial.

Information sources

Some form of reference material should be available in each residential home. The *British National Formulary* (BNF) is a useful source, but the language is technical and may not be helpful to untrained staff. Thus, training sessions could include the explanation of technical terms.

Drugs and their effects

It is useful that staff have an awareness of the basic concepts of pharmacokinetics. This should not be advanced, but it should establish the concepts of absorption, metabolism and excretion. This can be developed to give an appreciation of why different dosage regimens are used and why it is important to adhere to them. A further development of these ideas can be used to give an appreciation of side-effects, why they arise and how they can be minimized. Both the kinetics and side-effects of drugs can be taught using drugs which are used regularly in homes as examples.

Other aspects of training

Staff in residential homes need to be aware of the legal restrictions on the supply of medicines. They must understand that medicines prescribed for one resident should not be given to anyone other than for whom they were prescribed. It is useful to establish that POMs, irrespective of their dosage form, must be treated with the same respect. The use of OTC medicines for trivial complaints can be discussed, together with advice on what to use and when to seek further advice. The use of household remedies and other related products could be discussed. Training is best given on a little-and-often basis. Large blocks of information are unlikely to produce the desired effect.

Advice for pharmacists

The ultimate responsibility for the provision of pharmaceutical services to residential homes lies with the district pharmaceutical officer or chief administrative pharmaceutical officer. Depending on the local situation, the community services pharmacist or equivalent may undertake the day-by-day management of residential home services. This includes an inspection role. It may also include pharmacist training, draft protocols for pharmacists to use with homes and the provision of centrally organized training for home staff. In addition, pharmacists can obtain further guidance from various sources such as the RPSGB, NPA and the centres for postgraduate or post-qualification pharmaceutical education (distance learning).

DEFINING THE LEVEL OF THE PHARMACEUTICAL CARE SERVICE

In the hospital setting, clinical pharmacy services may be based on written service specifications. These are produced in conjunction with management and other clinical care staff. Patient representatives should also be consulted to ensure that services are designed to meet patient needs. Specifications describe and define the level of service offered to various groups of patients. Clinical pharmacists' objectives should be based on these service specifications. The extent to which pharmacists meet these objectives can then be determined by various processes. These include performance appraisal, peer review, professional audit and clinical audit.

In the community setting, pharmacists may produce a patient information leaflet describing the professional services offered by the pharmacy. This is part of the requirement for receiving a professional practice allowance. At the present time, the professional services offered by the majority of community pharmacists may be less well defined than those provided by hospital pharmacists. However, community pharmacists are now required to participate in audit in order to qualify for their professional practice allowance and this may assist in the development of services.

The RPSGB's Statement of Principles and Standards of Good Practice for Hospital Pharmacy in the UK complements standards included in an Appendix to the Society's Code of Ethics. Pharmaceutical officers in the NHS have also defined standards of practice for hospital pharmacists. These documents recognize the need to produce more detailed local clinical pharmacy standards.

A structured, systematic and evidence-based approach to individual patient care is recommended throughout this chapter. If properly documented, this approach is capable of generating data required for the assessment of clinical pharmacy practice. At best, the data would comprise fully documented pharmaceutical care plans and outcomes for every patient. Currently, this is unrealistic, however some hospital pharmacy services generate pharmaceutical care plans for selected priority groups of patients.

One of the most common methods of assessing clinical pharmacy practice is the recording of interventions. These are usually actions by a pharmacist to clarify prescription or administration charts, to promote drug efficacy or economy in the use of medicines, or to prevent or minimize the risk of adverse effects. Whilst this may demonstrate what pharmacists are capable of, it does not generate objective data on their practice. In such a system, pharmacists record only what they observe and see fit to act upon. There are no records of patients for whom there was no pharmaceutical intervention. Pharmacists may also select to omit unsuccessful interventions or those where they lacked confidence. Thus, there is no opportunity to subject these aspects of the pharmacist's performance to independent scrutiny. Another major deficiency of the system is that it is often based on a contribution made retrospectively by the pharmacist. It could be argued that, if appropriate contributions are made prospectively, then the need for interventions would decrease. This would be good clinical pharmacy practice. However, practice has often been assessed on the basis of both the number and nature of pharmacists' interventions.

Assessing clinical pharmacy practice

As members of the health care team and their own professional body, pharmacists are ethically and professionally accountable to patients and clients for the services that they provide. Assuring the quality of these services involves consulting the 'customers'. These may be the patients, carers, clients or other health care professionals. There is a need to involve each through continuous quality improvement (CQI) initiatives.

Quality may be described as a level of excellence that gives complete customer satisfaction. It also ensures that a product or service is fit for the purpose intended (CRAG, 1996). Quality assurance (QA) is achieved through a combination of all the activities and functions associated with achieving quality. Pharmacists have been familiar with this concept for some time, particularly in relation to the quality of medicines (see Ch. 6). More recently, QA has been concerned with assessing clinical pharmacy services.

The role of quality and clinical governance was discussed earlier in this chapter. Health care organizations are broadening the scope of their efforts to ensure quality, which involves a move towards CQI. This approach to quality considers systems within the organization as a whole. It focuses on processes and the need to generate objective data on which the quality of services can be judged. The philosophy of CQI demands that all staff have a responsibility to strive for improvement in the services that they provide. Thus within the community pharmacy this might include the manager/pharmacist, the dispenser/technician and the shop assistants. However, what patients might be equally concerned with is how well the community pharmacy service interacts with the other services involved in their care. CQI includes both intra- and inter-professional processes. As illustrated by the case study in the earlier section of this chapter, the latter can make or break the overall quality of patient care. When assessing clinical pharmacy practice, therefore, processes involving the pharmacist require to be examined in the context of total health care. In keeping with this has been the move within the NHS towards multidisciplinary audit (see Ch. 43).

The Kennedy Report recommended that greater priority should be given to:

- The development of skills in communicating with patients and colleagues
- The development of teamwork
- Clinical audit and reflective practice.

The report also recommended that education, training and CPD of all health care professionals should include joint courses between the professions.

Medicine counter assistants and OTC prescribing

In the community pharmacy setting, the pharmacist cannot be available to deal with every OTC transaction. In 1995, the RPSGB issued a statement that a written protocol should be available in each pharmacy that covers procedures for the supply of OTC medicines. The protocol should define the procedure for when advice on treatment for a medical condition is sought. Since 1996, pharmacy staff who regularly sell medicines should have completed or be undertaking an accredited training course (Royal Pharmaceutical Society 1996). These measures help to ensure that pharmacy staff are trained and have procedures to follow. Introduction of formal standard operating procedures is a further step in this process (see Ch. 6). Staff can then deal appropriately with certain customers' needs and know when to refer the patient to the pharmacist. In this way the pharmacist can prioritize their time. The pharmacist's time can be spent dealing with patients in need of direct pharmaceutical care.

Key points

- Clinical pharmacy aims to maximize drug efficacy, minimize drug toxicity and provide cost-effectiveness.
- Pharmaceutical care and medicine management use an holistic approach to patient care using a systematic management of medicines and partnership with other health care professionals.
- Clinical pharmacy may be practised in hospital and community settings and by working with GPs.
- Professional competence can be demonstrated by audit, peer review and interaction with patients, carers and other health professionals.
- Rational use of drugs requires an evidence base and may use guidelines, local policies and protocols, patient group directives, standard operating procedures and prescribing advice.
- Many factors are important when targeting clinical pharmacy, including patient characteristics, nature of therapy and the condition(s) being treated.
- Patient characteristics include age, social circumstances, pregnancy or lactation, mobility or disability, substance misuse and learning and communication difficulties.
- Patients taking drugs with a narrow therapeutic index, several drugs, having chronic and multiple pathologies are in particular need of pharmaceutical care.
- Assessing patients by attempting to identify individuals with potential medicine-related problems, then identifying actual problems using medication history and other information.
- When problems are identified, realistic aims for pharmaceutical care are set and a plan devised to achieve them, together with monitoring markers.
- Particular problems arise when patients move from one care setting to another, requiring high levels of communication between the different professionals involved.
- Most community pharmacies keep computer-based patient medication records (PMRs) as part of the NHS contract.
- The records kept are subject to the Data Protection Act and the Health Records Act.
- The PMR gives prompts during dispensing, especially for drug interactions, and can be used for, stock control and targeting health promotion.
- Patients in residential care have as much right to pharmaceutical care as any other patient.
- Apart from filling prescriptions, residential homes require input from pharmacists on a range of their medicine-related activities.

- As part of a contract with a home, pharmacists should make regular visits, offer advice and training, monitor medicine storage, dispose of unwanted medicines and discuss issues of concern.
- A structured, systematic and evidence-based approach to patient care must be continually reviewed through processes such as continuous quality improvement.

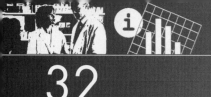

32

Adverse drug reactions

J. Krska

After studying this chapter you will know about:

The classification of ADRs (adverse drug reactions)
Factors affecting the incidence of ADRs
Recognition and assessment of ADRs
Monitoring systems, including the Yellow Card scheme
The role of the pharmacist in preventing, detecting and reporting ADRs

Introduction

Adverse reactions are a recognized hazard of drug therapy. However, since the problem was first addressed in the 1950s, the number of potent prescribed drugs in use has increased dramatically. In addition, the incidence of adverse drug reactions (ADRs) is known to rise with age. This, in combination with the proportionately increasing ageing population, signifies the growing importance of ADRs.

Patients themselves are becoming more aware of potential side-effects of their drug therapy. The pharmacist, along with the prescriber, has a duty to ensure that patients are aware of the risks of side-effects and a suitable course of action should they occur. With their detailed knowledge of medicines, pharmacists have the ability to relate unexpected symptoms experienced by patients to possible adverse effects of their drug therapy.

The reporting of adverse reactions to drugs is certainly not new and has taken place haphazardly throughout history. However, interest in ADRs and their monitoring has increased greatly since the association between thalidomide, a hypnotic, and limb deformities in babies was made in the early 1960s. Until then, thalidomide was thought to be a safe hypnotic and was prescribed during pregnancy with disastrous results. ADR reporting systems were introduced in most developed countries following this tragedy. Although these systems encourage physicians to report suspected

ADRs to all drugs, they suffer from underreporting. Another problem is that reports should ideally include details of non-prescription medicines used by the patient; however, very often these details are unknown by the doctor. Pharmacists in the UK, as in other countries, are permitted to submit reports of suspected ADRs to the Committee on the Safety of Medicines (CSM). Community pharmacists are encouraged in particular to submit details of suspected ADRs involving non-prescription medicines and herbal medicines. The practice of clinical pharmacy also ensures that ADRs are minimized by avoiding drugs with potential side-effects in susceptible patients. Thus pharmacists have a major role to play in relation to prevention, detection and reporting of ADRs.

INCIDENCE OF ADRs

Many studies have assessed the incidence of ADRs in the community, in hospital and as a cause of hospital admission. However, the absence of standardized criteria for identification and assessment of such problems means that estimates of incidence vary widely. It is therefore often difficult to compare such studies.

Hospital inpatients

The risk of ADRs increases when a patient is hospitalized, owing to the high number of drugs prescribed per patient at any one time. Approximately 10–20% of hospitalized patients are thought to have experienced an ADR during their hospital stay.

Primary care

Estimates of the incidence of ADRs in general practice vary widely, from 2% to over 40%, depending on the study methodology. More studies are required to assess the true incidence of the problem in primary care. ADRs are a potential contributory factor to patients not taking medicines appropriately, therefore their perceptions of experiences which could be ADRs are important. Methods of studying patient perceptions are relatively new, but could be of value in obtaining a more realistic picture of the frequency of ADRs when drugs are used in actual practice.

Hospital admissions

Approximately 5% of all hospital admissions are due to ADRs, although estimates of drug-related admissions range from 3 to 27% depending on the patient population studied. This represents a significant cost to the NHS in terms of bed occupancy and treatment of these adverse effects. A small number of studies have investigated drug-related hospital admissions in children, with admission rates for ADRs in the region of 2–3%.

Drug-related deaths

Up to 3% of deaths in hospital inpatients are thought to be due to the adverse effects of drugs. Of those patients admitted to hospital due to ADRs, the death rate is approximately 5%. The CSM receives reports of fatal suspected ADRs and 476 such reports were received in 1995. The top three drugs most commonly associated with fatal suspected reactions in that year were clozapine, diclofenac and ethinylestradiol.

A large proportion of these ADRs are considered to be preventable through good prescribing practice—mainly by individualizing dosage, and avoiding inappropriate and unnecessary drug therapy. In order that pharmacists can make a valuable contribution to the identification, monitoring, reporting and prevention of ADRs to both prescription and non-prescription drugs, they should have a thorough understanding of the aetiology and classification of ADRs.

THE CLASSIFICATION OF ADRs

An ADR is defined by the World Health Organization (WHO) as 'a noxious, unintended effect of a drug that occurs in doses normally used in humans for the diagnosis, prophylaxis or treatment of disease'. This does not incorporate any ADR which occurs as a result of error, although many reported ADRs are in fact due to errors in administration or drug choice. ADRs can be classified into two types.

- Type A (augmented) reactions
- Type B (bizarre) reactions.

Type A reactions

Type A reactions are due to known pharmacological actions of the drug. These may be:

- Excessive effects of the intended pharmacological action of a drug, e.g. haemorrhage with anticoagulants.
- Unwanted pharmacological actions of a drug, e.g. antimuscarinic effects of tricyclic antidepressants which can result in blurred vision, tachycardia, dry mouth and urinary retention.
- Withdrawal reactions, which may occur with abrupt withdrawal of some drugs after prolonged use, e.g. rebound insomnia with hypnotics, acute adrenal insufficiency with glucocorticoids.
- Delayed adverse effects such as vaginal adenocarcinoma in the daughters of women who received diethylstilbestrol during pregnancy for the treatment of threatened abortion. A full table of drugs which may have harmful effects in pregnancy can be found in Appendix 4 of the *British National Formulary* (BNF). The period of greatest risk for producing congenital abnormalities is considered to be from the 3rd to the 11th week of pregnancy. Since many women are unaware of their pregnancy at this stage, care should be taken in prescribing or recommending non-prescription medicines for all women of childbearing age.

Some Type A reactions may be a result of failure to individualize dosage. Although the patient may be prescribed a dose within the normal recommended range, impaired renal or hepatic function affects clearance of the drug and may result in adverse effects. This type of ADR could be considered to be preventable. The ability of other drugs and disease states to increase susceptibility to ADRs is also of importance in their prevention. The predictability of ADRs is an important factor in selection of a drug for an individual patient. Therefore a knowledge of factors influencing the likelihood of any patient experiencing a predictable ADR is important.

Type B reactions

Type B reactions are unexpected effects which are unrelated to the known pharmacological actions of the drug. Many of these reactions have an immunological basis, e.g. anaphylaxis with penicillins. Others are due to genetic abnormalities such as drug-induced haemolysis in patients with glucose-6-phosphate dehydrogenase deficiency, when given oxidative drugs. For some Type B reactions, the cause is

Table 32.1 Characteristics of adverse drug reactions	
Type A	**Type B**
Normal, augmented response	Abnormal, bizarre response
Predictable from pharmacology	Unpredictable from pharmacology
Dose related	Not dose related
Reasonably common	Uncommon
Seldom fatal	Often causes serious illness or death

unknown. These allergic drug reactions are idiosyncratic and normally unrelated to dosage. Management of such ADRs, therefore, usually requires stopping the offending drug. Type B reactions are often associated with serious illness and death, but are relatively rare. At other times, only mild urticaria or pyrexia may be experienced. The differences between the two subgroups of ADRs are highlighted in Table 32.1.

FACTORS AFFECTING THE INCIDENCE OF ADRs

Obviously any individual patient who uses a particular drug is very unlikely to experience all the ADRs that the drug is capable of causing, nor do individual ADRs affect all patients. It is useful to have a working knowledge of the incidence of specific ADRs to assist patients in understanding the risks of particular treatments. Currently there is no requirement for incidence rates to be included in the Summary of Product Characteristics. Pharmacists should also be aware of the main factors which influence the occurrence of ADRs so that they can identify patients most at risk.

Multiple drug therapy

An obvious association exists between the number of drugs being taken and the risk of experiencing an ADR. Some studies have shown a sharp, disproportionate, rise in ADRs with increasing numbers of prescribed drugs, suggesting that there may be more than additive effects occurring. Interactions between the drugs being taken may contribute to this situation. Indeed there are many instances of ADRs occurring as a result of one drug altering the effects of another when taken concurrently. Probably the most common type of issue arises from concurrent administration of two or more drugs with similar adverse effect profiles which can be additive. The likelihood and severity of reactions is increased as a result. Interactions can also involve changes in absorption, distribution and metabolism which result in increased risk of toxicity. Some examples of interactions which can result in ADRs are given in Table 32.2.

Age

The incidence of ADRs is known to rise with age. Changes in pharmacokinetics and pharmacodynamics associated with age may be partly responsible. It is not clear, however, whether age itself is an independent risk factor, although there is evidence of increased sensitivity to some drugs. The increase in some ADRs seen with ageing may be partly due to the elderly taking a greater number of prescribed medicines than younger age groups. Multiple pathology in the elderly may also contribute.

Neonates also have reduced drug clearance, resulting in increased risk of ADRs. A well-known example is the 'grey baby' syndrome with chloramphenicol. Another common adverse reaction in neonates is respiratory depression due to opioids given to the mother during labour. Children also handle drugs differently from adults and can have increased susceptibility to adverse effects from some drugs.

Table 32.2 Examples of ADRs arising from interactions between drugs		
Type of interaction	**Drugs involved**	**Effect**
Pharmacodynamic	Digoxin, beta-blockers	Increased risk of bradycardia
	Alcohol, CNS depressants	Increased sedative and other CNS depressant effects
	Diuretics, alpha-blockers	Increased hypotensive effects
Pharmacokinetic	Cimetidine, warfarin	Increased risk of over-anticoagulation
	Thiazides, lithium	Increased risk of lithium toxicity
	SSRIs, theophylline	Increased theophylline toxicity

Multiple disease states

Some disease states may alter a patient's response to drug therapy and may influence susceptibility to ADRs. Patients with particular disease states may be more likely to experience an ADR with certain drugs. Examples include patients with peptic ulcer disease being at increased risk of bleeding when prescribed non-steroidal anti-inflammatory drugs and those with asthma who may suffer bronchospasm with beta-adrenoceptor blocking drugs. However, in severely ill patients it is also possible that effects related to their disease states may be attributed in error to ADRs.

Type of drugs prescribed

Some drugs are more likely to cause ADRs than others. ADRs may also be more likely to occur when the drug regimen includes medicines with a narrow therapeutic index. Examples of such drugs include digoxin, anticoagulants and insulin. Many commonly taken drugs have been implicated in ADRs serious enough to warrant hospital admission. Those most commonly involved are cardiac drugs, diuretics, non-steroidal anti-inflammatory drugs, corticosteroids, anticoagulants, antimicrobials and psychotropics.

Dosage

Many Type A ADRs seem to be dose-related and can be managed by a reduction in dose of the drug in question. Individualization of drug therapy is essential in avoiding these ADRs. Examples of dose-related adverse effects are drowsiness and ataxia with antiepileptic drugs such as phenytoin, phenobarbital and carbamazepine.

Route of administration

If drugs are given too quickly by the intravenous route, ADRs can arise especially with drugs which act on the heart. The problems can be reduced by giving intravenous injections slowly. For instance, rapid intravenous injection of digoxin may cause nausea and arrhythmias and for this reason should be avoided.

Formulation

ADRs can be due to excipients in pharmaceutical formulations, e.g. colouring agents, sweeteners and preservatives, or to contaminants, such as eosinophilia-myalgia related to

L-tryptophan. Changes in formulation of digoxin resulting in changes in particle size which affected bioavailability led to toxicity in patients previously stabilized. Similarly a change in capsule diluent from calcium sulphate to lactose increased bioavailability of phenytoin, again leading to toxicity. Differences in bioavailability between products for some drugs can result in unexpected ADRs if patients switch from one formulation to another.

Gender

Some ADRs appear to occur more frequently in females, particularly those involving the gastrointestinal tract. The reason for this is unknown.

Race and genetic factors

Differences in susceptibility to ADRs have been demonstrated between races. This is probably due to differences in genetics which can affect drug metabolism and disposition. Such differences are also important within races. For example, those who are deficient in the enzyme glucose-6-phosphate dehydrogenase (G6PD) are more susceptible to toxicity from certain drugs, including quinolones. There are racial differences in the prevalence of G6PD deficiency, with African, Middle Eastern and South East Asians having a higher incidence than other races. Differences between individuals in the cytochrome P450 enzymes which metabolize many drugs account for considerable differences in ability to metabolize commonly used drugs, such as warfarin, many antidepressants, antipsychotics and beta-adrenoceptor blocking drugs. Developments in genetic typing will in future enable an individual's susceptibility to ADRs to be identified prior to initiating therapy.

Patient compliance

Non-compliance with drug therapy, which can be defined as the extent to which the patient follows a prescribed regimen, may also play a part in ADRs. Taking too much of a drug may lead to adverse effects or unexpected drug toxicity.

RECOGNITION AND ASSESSMENT OF ADRs

Pharmacists and other health care professionals responsible for a patient's drug therapy should be constantly vigilant for any new symptoms which may be drug related. Once a suspected ADR has been detected, a causal relationship between the drug and symptom should be established. Causality assessment is used to determine whether the adverse event is definitely, probably or possibly due to the drug. The following factors are important:

- Temporal relationship with drug use
- Type of reaction (A or B)
- Nature of reaction
- Exclusion of other possible causes
- Dechallenge (removing the drug)
- Rechallenge (re-starting the drug)
- Diagnostic tests, e.g. plasma drug concentrations.

In order to establish a causal relationship, patients must be questioned on their use of all other drugs, including non-prescription drugs. Several algorithms have been developed to standardize the assessment of the relationship between the suspected drug and the adverse event. Some are detailed and time-consuming and have a limited application in practice. Ultimately, a degree of clinical judgment is needed to determine whether an adverse event could be due to a drug. Table 32.3 shows the criteria used in assessing the relationship between drug and ADR. The classification of an ADR depends on which criteria are satisfied. For example, for an ADR to be categorized as 'definite', all five criteria must be satisfied.

It should be noted, however, that it is sometimes difficult to apply these criteria in practice. It is seldom ethical to rechallenge a patient who may have had an ADR. In some cases, the adverse effect is not reversible, so is unlikely to disappear on rechallenge. Depending on the adverse event experienced, the time of onset may vary from minutes to years. Difficulties may arise in relating the symptoms to a drug years after it was first prescribed. It is important to recognize that certainty about causality is not essential for reporting of ADRs to authorities.

DETECTION AND MONITORING SYSTEMS

Although all new drugs undergo clinical trials to demonstrate efficacy and detect adverse effects, (see Ch. 34), only the most common ADRs, likely to be Type A reactions, will probably have been detected by the time the drug is marketed. In addition, clinical trials are unlikely to have been carried out on some groups of patients, such as the elderly or pregnant women. Pharmaceutical products must therefore be monitored after marketing to identify any more unusual, serious or delayed adverse effects.

THE UK YELLOW CARD SYSTEM

The Committee on Safety of Medicines (CSM) superseded the Committee on Safety of Drugs after the Medicines Act in 1968. The CSM is responsible for the assessment of new drugs before clinical trials and marketing have taken place. They also manage a spontaneous reporting system which asks doctors and, more recently, pharmacists to report all suspected reactions to new products marked with a black triangle in the BNF, the *ABPI Medicines Compendium* and the *Monthly Index of Medical Specialities* (MIMS). Doctors and pharmacists are also asked to report all serious suspected reactions to established drugs, even if it is considered that the adverse effect is well recognized. A serious suspected ADR is defined as one which is fatal, life-threatening, disabling, incapacitating, results in or prolongs hospitalization, congenital abnormality or is 'medically significant'. As well as drugs, the reporting scheme also applies to contact lens fluids, vaccines, intrauterine contraceptive devices, surgical or dental materials and absorbable sutures.

In addition to reporting serious known reactions and all reactions to 'black triangle' drugs, hospital pharmacists are

---

Table 32.3   Criteria to determine a causal link between drug and symptoms

Criteria	Likelihood of ADR			
	Definite	Probable	Possible	Unlikely
Known ADR	Yes	Yes	Yes	No
Time of administration related to onset of reaction	Yes	Yes	Yes	No
Disappears on dechallenge or dose reduction	Yes	Yes	Yes	No
Symptoms unexplained by clinical condition of patient	Yes	Yes	No	No
Symptoms reappear on rechallenge	Yes	No	No	No

requested to focus their reporting on drugs which are initiated and monitored within specialist hospital units, such as drugs used for the treatment of AIDS, haemophilia and cancer. Community pharmacists are requested to focus their reporting on non-prescription medicines and both licensed and unlicensed herbal medicinal products. The Medicines Control Agency (MCA) is particularly interested to receive reports on ADRs in children, the elderly, pregnancy and delayed effects.

Standard report forms or 'Yellow Cards', shown in Figure 32.1, are located inside the back cover of the BNF, MIMS, *ABPI Medicines Compendium* and on prescription pads. They are also downloadable from the MCA website. These were changed in 2000 to remove the necessity to include the patient's name and date of birth to comply with confidentiality guidelines. A local identification number is sought instead, which may be a Community Health Index (CHI), practice or hospital number. The consent of the patient is not required in order to submit a Yellow Card. The minimum details required for submission are:

- Patient initials and an identification number
- The identity of the reporting doctor or pharmacist
- The suspected drug, dose, route of administration, start and stop dates and indication
- The nature, treatment and outcome of the suspected ADR and its start and stop dates
- The seriousness of the reaction, to be completed using tick boxes.

Yellow Cards also request additional information which may not always be available. These include:

- Patient details—age, sex, weight
- Other drugs taken in the last 3 months, including self-medication and herbal remedies
- Other relevant information including medical history, investigations, allergies and suspected drug interactions.

It is important that pharmacists are not reluctant to report suspected ADRs because they do not have all the details listed above. This problem has resulted in serious underreporting by doctors in the past. Other reasons for doctors underreporting include lack of time, fear of litigation, lack of self-confidence and complacency. Such factors may also apply to pharmacists, however it is an important part of their role in providing a pharmaceutical service.

In addition to the voluntary reporting of ADRs, pharmaceutical companies are responsible for reporting reactions to their licensed products. If a doctor or pharmacist contacts a company for information in relation to a suspected ADR, the company is legally obliged to report serious cases to the CSM within 15 calendar days, regardless of any lack of patient details and causality. There are four basic requirements which constitute a valid report in this situation—the name of the reporter, an adverse event, an identifiable patient and a suspect drug. As well as reporting ADRs to the CSM, pharmacists and prescribers should report ADRs to drug manufacturers. All manufacturers are interested to receive such information about their products. Many are also active in carrying out postmarketing studies on their products. (see Ch. 34) Indeed the CSM expects this for many new products. If serious ADRs are suspected during any company-sponsored postmarketing surveillance, the company's medical department must be informed as well as the CSM.

The CSM receives over 20 000 ADR reports annually. A system capable of capturing, retrieving and processing the Yellow Card data has been developed, known as ADROIT (adverse drug reaction on-line information tracking facility). This database allows rapid processing and analysis of the reports to identify any potential safety issues. The Yellow Card scheme has been successful in identifying both common and rare reactions and can also provide early warnings of possible ADRs. For example, in 1999/2000 over 430 potential safety issues were investigated and led to changes in product information for over 750 medicines.

Some drawbacks to spontaneous reporting systems such as this do exist:

- The incidence of a particular ADR is unknown owing to a lack of information on the number of patients exposed to the drug. A rough estimate can be calculated from the number of prescriptions dispensed.
- There is considerable underreporting.
- Some bias may be introduced if there is a tendency to report ADRs which are well publicized.
- ADRs which are as yet unknown are difficult to spot and so may be prone to underreporting.

Some countries (USA, Germany) allow reporting of ADRs directly from patients, although this has provided little in the way of useful reports. Patients are not allowed to report directly to the CSM in the UK, but should be encouraged to discuss suspected ADRs with their doctor or pharmacist. Recent research has shown that many more patients experience common adverse effects from prescribed medicines than report them to their doctors. (Jarernsiripornkul et al 2002).

Feedback from CSM

Analysis of data collected by the CSM spontaneous reporting scheme takes place routinely. Recently discovered

In Confidence

COMMITTEE ON SAFETY OF MEDICINES

M C A
MEDICINES CONTROL AGENCY

SUSPECTED ADVERSE DRUG REACTIONS

If you are suspicious that an adverse reaction may be related to a drug or combination of drugs please complete this Yellow Card. For reporting advice please see over. Do not be put off reporting because some details are not known.

PATIENT DETAILS   Patient Initials: _____   Sex: M / F   Weight if known (kg): _____
Age (at time of reaction): _____   Identification number (Your Practice / Hospital Ref.)*: _____

SUSPECTED DRUG(S)
Give brand name of drug and batch number if known

	Route	Dosage	Date started	Date stopped	Prescribed for

SUSPECTED REACTION(S)
Please describe the reaction(s) and any treatment given:

Outcome
Recovered ☐
Recovering ☐
Continuing ☐
Other ☐

Date reaction(s) started: _____   Date reaction(s) stopped: _____

Do you consider the reaction to be serious?   Yes / No

If *yes*, please indicate why the reaction is considered to be serious (please tick all that apply):

Patient died due to reaction ☐   Involved or prolonged inpatient hospitalisation ☐

Life threatening ☐   Involved persistent or significant disability or incapacity ☐

Congenital abnormality ☐   Medically significant; please give details: _____

OTHER DRUGS (including self-medication & herbal remedies)
Did the patient take any other drugs in the last 3 months prior to the reaction?   Yes / No

If *yes*, please give the following information if known:

Drug (Brand, if known)	Route	Dosage	Date started	Date stopped	Prescribed for

Additional relevant information   e.g. medical history, test results, known allergies, rechallenge (if performed), suspected drug interactions. For congenital abnormalities please state all other drugs taken during pregnancy and the last menstrual period.

REPORTER DETAILS
Name and Professional Address: _____

Post code: _____   Tel No: _____
Speciality: _____
Signature: _____   Date: _____

CLINICIAN (if not the reporter)
Name and Professional Address: _____

Post code: _____
Tel No: _____   Speciality: _____

If you would like information about other adverse reactions associated with the suspected drug, please tick this box ☐

* This is to enable you to identify the patient in any future correspondence concerning this report

Please attach additional pages if necessary

Fig. 32.1   A Yellow Card.

ADRs and other important points are communicated to doctors, dentists, pharmacists and coroners via the *Current Problems in Pharmacovigilance* bulletin, which is issued four times yearly by the CSM and the MCA. Urgent issues such as drug withdrawals as a result of ADRs or very serious newly identified ADRs may involve direct communication via the Drug Alert system or by post.

OTHER DETECTION AND MONITORING SYSTEMS

Anecdotal reports (case reports)

Case reports from individual clinicians are often published in the medical literature and may be important in detecting new ADRs. These single reports usually require further studies to confirm an ADR, but some serious adverse effects have been brought to light by this mechanism. Notable examples include the oculomucocutaneous syndrome due to practolol and agranulocytosis caused by chloramphenicol. A series of detailed reports about cases which have already been submitted on Yellow Cards were reported regularly in *Pharmacy in Practice*. These can be useful in learning about assessing causality and which cases to report.

Cohort studies (prospective studies)

A 'cohort' of patients taking a specified drug is identified in this type of study. They are then monitored for adverse effects. A control group is identified, which is drawn from the same population but is not taking the drug, in order to compare the incidence of adverse effects detected. It is fundamental that the two groups being compared are at equal risk of developing adverse effects, so must be of similar age, sex, overall morbidity and so on. It is also crucial to include accurate data about drug exposure, i.e. the doses used and duration.

Case control studies (retrospective studies)

These studies involve a group of patients with symptoms which it is suspected may be due to an ADR. The patients are investigated to see if they have taken the drug in question. The prevalence of drug taking is compared to that of a control group who do not have the specified symptoms. Again the two groups must be comparable and, for the association to be made with confidence, accurate information about drug exposure is required. Due to the retrospective nature of these studies, there

is reliance on adequate record keeping to provide this data. If patients themselves are used as the source of information about the amount, timing and duration of drug intake, then it is important to be aware of the difficulty in recalling such information which could lead to bias. Another key difficulty in case control studies is the need to exclude patients who are at increased risk of developing the symptoms being studied.

Despite their difficulties, these studies are useful for determining whether there is an association between a drug and an adverse effect, but only once the relationship has been suspected. They cannot detect new ADRs. They are most often of value for testing hypotheses generated by spontaneous reporting. Case control studies have been important in confirming associations between venous thromboembolism and oral contraceptives, phocomelia and thalidomide and the adverse gastrointestinal effects of aspirin and NSAIDs.

Record linkage studies

Patients' medical records are used to match drugs prescribed with adverse effects experienced in record linkage studies. These studies may be particularly useful for identifying long-term adverse effects of drugs. Prescription event monitoring is an example of this type of study. This involves the identification of patients who have been exposed to a drug through dispensed prescriptions. The general practitioners with whom they are registered are then requested to submit details of all events occurring since drug exposure and details of stopping the drug if applicable. In this way events which occur with greater than usual frequency can be identified as potential ADRs and investigated further using case control or cohort studies.

The General Practice Research Database is a valuable source of information on morbidity and treatment including drugs prescribed, which covers around 4 million patients in the UK and can be accessed by researchers wanting to undertake such case control studies. The UK NHS enables valuable studies such as these to be undertaken, because patients register with a single GP who is the custodian of a single medical record. In many other countries, patients use different health care practitioners on different occasions and the multiplicity of records about drug therapy which results can create difficulties in ascribing particular drug consumption and effects to patients.

Hospital-based population studies

These are useful for determining the incidence of ADRs in hospitalized patients, or on admission to hospital. Some use automatic signals from laboratory data and prescription chart review in a systematic programme. An example of this type of scheme is the Boston Collaborative Drug Surveillance Program, which involves selected hospitals in several countries. Due to the inclusion of all patients, incidence rates for ADRs can be calculated and causality assessment is improved; however the studies are expensive.

International ADR reporting

The World Health Organization Collaborating Centre for International Drug Monitoring was established in 1968. The centre collates spontaneous ADR reports from participating national centres and aims to increase early recognition of new and unexpected ADRs. By combining reports from many countries all over the world, very rare adverse reactions can be detected.

Patient-centred studies

Postmarketing surveillance of medicines can be carried out using information supplied by patients. This is feasible for both prescribed and non-prescription medicines. Questionnaires are supplied to patients or telephone interviews conducted which focus on the occurrence of symptoms which could be ADRs. Various methods can be used to identify cohorts of patients, such as patient medication records (PMRs) in community pharmacies or general practice databases. For non-prescription drugs, patients who purchase these from community pharmacies can be included in studies. These systems have been piloted in Canada, the USA and Scotland and may provide a valuable method of detecting ADRs which complement other systems.

Non-prescription medicines

Since prescription medicines supplied through the NHS are recorded in medical and pharmacy records, their use can be traced and associations made with symptoms which could be ADRs. However non-prescription medicines are obtainable from many outlets, including pharmacies, and there is no requirement for these purchases to be recorded in either medical or pharmacy records. It is good practice to include these records on PMRs when purchases are made from pharmacies and, for patients who take multiple prescription medicines, this provides a valuable source of information which can be used to prevent ADRs arising from duplication or interactions.

In the UK, more prescription medicines are being re-regulated to increase the range of medicines available without prescription. There is evidence that patients do not always use these medicines optimally, (Krska et al 2000; Sinclair et al 2000) possibly because they are often perceived as safe due to their availability without prescription.

Community pharmacists have an important role to play in reporting ADRs to non-prescription medicines, which are currently seriously underreported. By establishing computer records of non-prescription product purchases and therefore defining a population of users of particular products, it would be feasible to involve pharmacists in postmarketing surveillance studies such as event monitoring, case control or cohort studies.

THE ROLE OF THE PHARMACIST

Pharmacists have an important contribution to make in the prevention, identification, documentation and reporting of ADRs.

Identification and documentation

Pharmacists should be looking out for potential ADRs during the course of their work with patients, whether in hospital or community practice. Hospital pharmacists, during their routine reviews of prescriptions, should always be alert for possible factors which could indicate an ADR. Examples are:

- Excessive therapeutic effects of medicines
- Abnormal laboratory values which could be ADRs
- Prescriptions for products which may be used to treat ADRs (Table 32.4)
- Drugs being discontinued, particularly if alternative drugs are prescribed for the same indication.

Pharmacists in primary care can be similarly alert when dispensing prescriptions or reviewing medication. Often in seeking the indication for a newly prescribed or purchased product, the presence of an ADR is uncovered. This is an important reason for the pharmacist to be involved in the sale of non-prescription medicines. The pharmacist is then in a position to prevent recurrence of the reaction.

Pharmacists should also be alert when there are alterations to a patient's drug regimen. A drug may be discontinued owing to adverse effects. If so, this should be recorded. Patients are often more open about their experiences with medicines to pharmacists than to doctors. It is,

Table 32.4 Drugs which may be used to treat ADRs	
Drug products	**Possible reason for use**
Antacids	Gastrointestinal side-effects of NSAIDs or other drugs
Laxatives	Constipation from opioids or tricyclic antidepressants
Antimuscarinics	Parkinsonian side-effects from antipsychotics or antidepressants
Antihistamines	Allergic reactions such as rashes
Hydrocortisone cream	Skin reactions
Topical skin preparations	Skin reactions
Hydrocortisone injection	Bronchospasm or cardiac shock

therefore, important that hospital pharmacists have direct contact with patients and are able to obtain relevant details from them to allow assessment of potential ADRs. In community practice, pharmacists may see patients more frequently than GPs and they are often the health care professionals most able to identify ADRs.

Documentation of confirmed and suspected ADRs is poor, both in hospital and in the community. In hospital, ADRs should be recorded in medical notes, nursing notes and on prescriptions. In the community, they should be recorded in the pharmacist's PMR, but also and equally importantly, in the patient's medical notes and the practice computer. This requires informing the patient's GP of the suspected ADR. The minimum information needed is the suspected medicine and the reaction which occurred. If an ADR is confirmed at a later date, the records should be modified to include this. Consideration should also be given as to whether a report to the CSM is appropriate.

By being vigilant in recording this information themselves and in ensuring that others do so, pharmacists can play a major role in preventing patients from being unnecessarily exposed to the same or similar medicines again. The accuracy of recorded information is equally important in preventing patients from having potentially useful medicines withheld because there is a suspicion of a previous reaction. A common example is the use of the term 'penicillin allergic', often recorded in medical notes of patients who may have experienced type A reactions of minor importance, such as diarrhoea or skin irritation. Penicillins of all types will not be available to this patient, which could have important consequences if a serious infection occurs.

Monitoring and reporting

Pharmacists can actively improve the low reporting rates which the Yellow Card system suffers from. Not only should

they report ADRs themselves, but they should act as facilitators by encouraging physicians to report ADRs and assisting in completing Yellow Cards. Preregistration students are not permitted to report ADRs. Hospital pharmacists with direct involvement in patient care are permitted to report. Discussion with the relevant clinician is recommended, but pharmacists may wish to exercise professional judgment if the clinician advises against submission of a Yellow Card report. The name of the clinician responsible for the patient's care should be included on the form. Some hospital pharmacists are involved in running in-house ADR reporting schemes to support each other in deciding when cases should be reported to the CSM. They may also collate and distribute information to doctors and other pharmacists on the most common ADR problems locally.

ADRs reported by pharmacists in primary care must also provide the name of the patient's GP, as the CSM may require to contact the GP for further information. Cards can be submitted either to the CSM directly or to a regional monitoring centre. These are located in Wales, West Midlands, Mersey and the Northern Region and one has been established in Scotland.

PREVENTION

Since many ADRs are preventable, a major part of the pharmacist's role in ADRs should be to reduce the occurrence of the problem. Pharmacists in all branches of the profession are currently involved in improving the use of medicines in patients through:

- Identifying potential side-effects of drug therapy.
- Avoiding unnecessary polypharmacy by encouraging and carrying out review of therapy already prescribed. Review enables the identification of medicines no longer

required, those that have no clear indication, those prescribed for adverse effects which could be prevented by changes to therapy, and duplication of similar medicines. Medicines that may initially have been indicated but have become unnecessary may be highlighted in this way. For example, a patient taking a NSAID may have been prescribed concurrent therapy with ranitidine for prophylaxis of NSAID-induced duodenal ulcer. On stopping the NSAID, the ranitidine may be inadvertently continued.

- Choosing the least toxic drugs where possible.
- Careful consideration of the dosage requirements for individual patients.
- Ensuring that therapeutic drug monitoring or other appropriate laboratory tests are carried out.
- Checking for a history of allergy or previous reactions to a drug.
- Checking for drug interactions and advising on what action to take—increasing or decreasing the dose of one drug, monitoring the patient, replacing one drug with another. For example, the metabolism of theophylline may be reduced by cimetidine, leading to an increase in the serum level. If prescribed, advice should be given on the avoidance of adverse effects by either reducing the theophylline dose, or by careful monitoring of the serum theophylline concentration. A request for cimetidine in a patient taking theophylline should be met with an offer of an alternative H_2 antagonist. By also explaining the reason for this, future purchases of potentially interacting products may also be prevented.
- Education of patients on their drug regimen, especially when new treatments are initiated. This should include specific details of any medicines available without prescription which should be avoided. In the above example, a patient prescribed theophylline should be educated about not purchasing cimetidine and cough remedies which contain theophylline.
- Encouraging patients to complete courses of medication and dispose of unused drugs to prevent hoarding and sharing of drugs.
- Encouraging patients to report any new symptoms.
- Questioning the patient on any new drug therapy, including non-prescription medicines.

- Advising the patient of expected side-effects of therapy and a safe course of action should they occur.
- Taking drug histories, which may identify previous adverse effects or allergies to particular drugs.
- Drawing up formularies and prescribing protocols to ensure appropriate selection of medicines, and appropriate use in a given situation.
- Advising on simplifying dose and drug regimens to encourage good compliance.

Further developments which may help in the prevention of ADRs may include routine sharing of information between primary and secondary care, both on admission to hospital to prevent ADRs occurring during hospitalization, and on discharge from hospital, which should help minimize ADRs in the community. Information shared on discharge should include reasons for a drug being stopped or changed in hospital, dose changes, new drugs prescribed. Discharge planning schemes in hospitals should ensure that all patients are educated in their drug regimen, especially where new treatments have been initiated. Patients seeking treatment in community pharmacies should be questioned to establish whether any relationship exists between newly prescribed drugs and recently occurring symptoms. The use of one particular pharmacy should be encouraged. Patients having prescriptions dispensed at different pharmacies may be at greater risk of ADRs since the pharmacist will not have a complete picture of the patient's drug regimen.

Although ADRs are unwanted effects of drug therapy, for many drugs, the risk of adverse effects is small compared to the likely benefits of treatment. When adverse effects are experienced, however, patients may be left in a worse condition than before they used the medicine. They can also contribute to reduced medicine taking, leaving the patient with less than optimal treatment. Pharmacists are ideally placed to play an active role in the prevention of ADRs. The benefits to patients in terms of reduced suffering, hospitalization and anxiety are considerable. Significant resource savings to the NHS could also be achieved through reduced hospitalization rates for ADRs, and reduced treatment costs.

Key Points

- Adverse drug reactions (ADRs) may be 'augmented' (Type A) or 'bizarre' (Type B).
- Type A reactions may be due to excessive or unwanted pharmacological effects, withdrawal reactions, delayed effects or failure to individualize dosage.
- Many Type B reactions have an immunological or genetic basis and are normally unrelated to dosage.
- At the time of marketing a new drug, not all ADRs may be known.
- Factors influencing ADRs include multiple drug regimens, multiple disease states, type of drug, route, formulation and dosage, age, gender, race and extent of compliance with medicines.

- Causality of an ADR can be categorized using set criteria.
- The Yellow Card scheme is used by the CSM as one type of postmarketing surveillance.
- Pharmacists can play an important role in identifying, documenting, monitoring and preventing ADRs in their routine practice.
- Pharmacists should report suspected ADRs to the CSM or to regional monitoring centres on Yellow Cards.
- Hospital pharmacists should report particularly ADRs to drugs initiated and monitored within hospital specialist units.
- Community pharmacists should report particularly ADRs to non-prescription medicines and herbal products.

33

Medicines information

A. Lee

After studying this chapter you should know about:

The UK Medicines Information Service
Key drug information resources for practice
Usefulness and limitations of key drug information sources
Primary, secondary and tertiary literature—advantages and disadvantages
The Internet as an information source
Systematic search strategy
Critical appraisal of drug information
Approaches to handling a request for information

Introduction

The first part of this chapter outlines the basic drug information skills required by all pharmacists and the specialty of medicines (formerly drug) information in the UK. The second part reviews the key drug information sources used in pharmacy practice and the approach to take when handling a request for information.

Background

Drug information provision is an essential part of pharmacy practice. This has been the case for many decades but it has become increasingly important in the age of evidence-based medicine and patient empowerment. When pharmacists hear the term 'drug information' they often picture a formalized centre or service that provides, organizes and manages drug information within a given locality. However, drug information activities are inherent in any pharmacy practice. As experts on medicines, all pharmacists have a responsibility to provide information and advice about any medicine supplied by them or under their authority (Royal Pharmaceutical Society of Great Britain's (RPSGB) 'Code of Ethics and Standards'). Health professionals, patients,

carers and the public regularly ask pharmacists for information and advice and it is vital that this should be reliable, accurate and up to date. In today's NHS there is greater emphasis on the contribution that pharmaceutical advice and prescribing support can make to medicines management, and consequently the involvement of pharmacists within primary and secondary care teams is increasing. To carry out these roles effectively pharmacists need to know how and where to find information, how to evaluate it, and how to put it into practice.

Drug information provision may be patient specific, as an integral part of pharmaceutical care, e.g. where the pharmacist uses information and knowledge to support individual patient care through clinical problem solving. Information or advice given in response to questions or enquiries about medicines is referred to as 'reactive' information. 'Proactive' (active) drug information involves the preparation of newsletters, bulletins, websites, etc. in an attempt to educate or raise awareness of key therapeutic issues. It may also be population based, to assist in decision making and evaluating medicines use at a macro level (e.g. formulary development). Activities requiring drug information skills are shown in Box 33.1.

Box 33.1   Activities requiring drug information skills

Solving patient-specific clinical problems
Critical evaluation/appraisal of the literature
Effective provision of verbal and written information to the public
Clinical guideline development
Drug policy management (e.g. formulary management, drug use evaluation or audit)
Preparation of bulletins and newsletters
Managing the entry of new drugs into health care
Adverse drug reaction/event management
Continuing professional development

Information explosion

The amount of medical information available to practitioners is overwhelming and a vast body of this is drug-related. The term 'information explosion' was first used in the context of biomedical literature over 40 years ago and still the overall amount of drug information grows at an alarming rate. There is an expanding range of information sources that can help answer drug-related questions: textbooks, journals, research studies, manufacturers' literature, formularies, full-text databases, treatment guidelines, websites and many more! Finding the piece of information relevant to a clinical problem can be like finding a needle in a haystack; it is difficult for the practitioner to know which source is best for a specific situation.

Clinical governance

The principles of clinical governance mean that all health professionals working in primary and secondary care need to address the quality of the services they provide. Components include quality improvement (e.g. audit, risk management, continuing professional development) and evidence-based practice. The requirement for all health professionals to make an ongoing commitment to continuing professional development (CPD) recognizes the fact that much of the knowledge we acquire as undergraduates will rapidly go out of date after qualifying. There is a continuing drive to ensure that practice, including drug therapy, is evidence based (see Chs 34 and 36). It has been suggested that UK pharmacists are not using enough evidence in their practice; an RPSGB working party on getting research into pharmacy practice concluded that in general pharmacists

were not bringing enough evidence from clinical trials, from systematic reviews of their own activity or from advances in basic science into their daily work.

Doctors' information needs

We have known for many years that the source of drug information used most often by doctors is pharmaceutical industry representatives. There is also evidence that doctors faced with a clinical problem are much more likely to consult their peers for advice than carry out a literature search or ask a pharmacist (Table 33.1). In one key study, the doctors' own perception was that they used reference sources a lot, but in fact they were more likely to consult other doctors. Recent research has shown that many clinicians lack the skills or time to practise evidence-based health care: that is, formulate answerable questions, identify and acquire the best evidence to answer the question, and integrate the findings with clinical expert and patient factors to extract a 'clinical bottom line' or answer. There is also evidence of a large unmet need for drug information, particularly in primary care. In a review article on doctors' information needs, Smith concluded that when doctors see patients they usually generate at least one question (Smith, 1996). Most of these questions are about treatment and around a quarter concern drug therapy. He also concluded that these questions usually go unanswered, even though they could be.

A recent US study analysed questions asked by over 100 family doctors (GPs) regarding patient care and found that 19% of questions related to medicines (Ely et al 1999). The most common resources used to answer questions included textbooks and colleagues; formal literature searches were

Table 33.1 Doctors reported and observed use of information sources. (From Covell et al 1985)		
Information source	**Percentage use**	
	Reported (n=182)	**Observed (n=80)**
Print sources	62	27
General and specialty textbooks	25	3
Pharmaceutical textbooks	14	9
Journals	18	7
Human sources	33	53
Specialist doctors	18	24
Pharmacists	6	3
Other	5	21

rarely performed. A follow-up study categorized the obstacles encountered when doctors attempted to answer these questions with evidence (Ely et al 2002). Six important obstacles were identified: difficulty modifying the original question; the excessive time required to find information; difficulty selecting an appropriate search strategy; failure of identified resource to answer the question; uncertainty as to when a search is complete; and inadequate translation of evidence into a clinically useful statement.

MEDICINES (DRUG) INFORMATION SERVICES

Drug information provision has traditionally been a responsibility of the pharmacy profession, although initially this was confined to pharmaceutical issues such as dosage, formulation and stability. Specialization in drug information resulted from the expansion of pharmacists' involvement with patient care in the clinical pharmacy era. The first drug information centre was established at the University of Kentucky, USA in 1962. This centre aimed to support, assist and promote rational drug therapy, as well as to provide comprehensive information to allow physicians and dentists to evaluate and compare drugs.

In the UK the first specialist drug information centres were established within hospital pharmacy departments in 1969 and within 10 years most hospitals had such a centre. Services were developed as a tiered structure of regional and local centres and individual pharmacists, with each level of the tier acting as a back up to the one below. The fundamental philosophy of the service was that drug information pharmacists should work together in a coordinated way to avoid duplication of effort and this remains a guiding principle today. In 2000 the service changed its name, in response to customer opinion, from Drug Information to Medicines Information, at the same time as a new strategy for the service was launched.

The UK Medicines Information (MI) Service aims to support the safe, effective and efficient use of medicines by the provision of evidence-based information and advice on the therapeutic use of medicines. The service has two broad functions:

- To support medicines management within NHS organizations
- To support the pharmaceutical care of individual patients.

At present the MI service is provided by a network of about 250 local centres based in the pharmacy departments of most hospital trusts. There are also 16 regional/area centres in England and Scotland and national centres in both Northern Ireland and Wales. These centres work together to provide a 'virtual' national service. They are all staffed by pharmacists and technicians with clinical expertise and skills in locating, assessing and interpreting information about medicines.

Pharmacists based in both primary (community) and secondary (hospital) care are the first-line providers of information and advice to patients and health professionals, but also have information requirements for themselves. Local medicines information centres provide an enquiry answering and advisory service as a back up to these pharmacists and direct to other health professionals. They also have a role in providing proactive information and supporting drug and therapeutics committees. At the next level, regional centres support local centres and may help answer enquiries referred to them from around the region. Generally, they provide more proactive information services than local centres, and also coordinate regional activities and provide input to the national network. Many regional centres also provide a local service to the hospital or trust where they are based.

The core function of the MI service is to provide a rapid and efficient enquiry answering service on all aspects of medicines use. In general, enquiries relate to the selection, availability, dose and administration of drugs for a wide spectrum of patient ages and disease states. Many also relate to adverse drug reactions, drug interactions and complementary medicines. The most frequent categories of enquiry received are shown in Box 33.2. Enquiry answering is referred to as 'reactive' drug information provision. In order to facilitate this work, information is gathered from in-house files, databases, libraries and leading biomedical and pharmaceutical journals. Most centres store details of enquiries they have previously answered on electronic databases, to avoid duplication of effort. In the early days many enquiries were straightforward requests for information. Now they are more complex, often requiring specific advice on therapy in individual patients. In addition, as part of the national network, designated specialist centres have developed expertise on the use of medicines in special patient groups that is used to the benefit of the network as a whole.

Pharmacists from the regional centres meet regularly within the UK Medicines Information Pharmacists Group (UKMIPG). This group coordinates the production of shared national information products, formulates strategy, and develops education materials and training programmes. Other products of national collaboration include the Pharmline database, a new medicines information scheme, and standard policies and procedures for use in all centres.

Box 33.2   Categories of drug information enquiry

Choice of therapy (including indications and
   contraindications)
Adverse effects
Administration and dosage
Product information, availability
Drug interactions
Drugs in pregnancy
Drugs in breastfeeding
Complementary medicine
Identification of tablets and other dosage forms
Pharmaceutical (stability, compatibility, formulations)
Pharmacology (including pharmacokinetics)

Over time, medicines information services have become much more advisory, producing proactive information, such as new product assessments, detailed comparisons of medicines within therapeutic classes, and critical appraisals of clinical trials, to a range of customers. In the last few years a national UKMI website (http://www.ukmi.nhs.uk) has been developed, to function both as an information resource and a portal to regional websites. The site is accessible by health professionals in primary and secondary care, although some sections are password protected for access by medicines information pharmacists only. The website allows access to a wide range of materials including frequently asked questions (FAQs), patent expiry database, current awareness bulletins, therapeutic guidelines and information on UKMI policies and practice relating to standards of service, quality assurance and risk management.

SOURCES OF DRUG INFORMATION

All pharmacists need to know how and where to find relevant information when dealing with a clinical problem or answering a medicines-related enquiry from a patient or health professional. There is no single reference source that can be used to answer all questions. Pharmacists need to become familiar with the key reference sources that are useful for common types of questions (e.g. drug interactions, side-effects, drug use in pregnancy). Different types of information sources can be consulted; these are usually classified as primary, secondary or tertiary. Tertiary sources include textbooks, drug compendia, full-text electronic books and databases, and published review articles.

Secondary reference sources include abstracting and indexing systems of the primary literature (e.g. the Medline database). Primary reference sources are those in which new information, usually in the form of research, is published such as articles in scientific journals. The categorization of resources into this classification used to be relatively straightforward. However, technological improvements in the delivery of information have blurred the situation somewhat; many tertiary, secondary and primary sources can be accessed in a range of format, e.g. hard copy, CD-ROM, web-based, microfiche.

Tertiary drug information sources

Textbooks and other tertiary sources provide an overview of a topic in condensed readable form. The information contained in tertiary sources can change based upon new information or knowledge documented in the primary literature. There is a wide range of published textbooks covering all aspects of pharmacy, medicine and therapeutics. Key tertiary drug information sources include *Martindale: the complete drug reference*, *British National Formulary* and the *Medicines Compendium*. There are also textbooks covering specific subject areas such as drug interactions, adverse drug reactions, pharmaceutical compatibility and stability, complementary medicines, and drug use in specific patient populations (e.g. children, the elderly, renal impairment, pregnancy and breastfeeding). Textbooks are important for locating established knowledge or information that is not rapidly changing; they are generally updated and published as a new edition only every 3–4 years. An important exception to this rule of thumb is the BNF, which is published every 6 months. Table 33.2 lists some of the key tertiary drug information resources for practising pharmacists in the UK.

Tertiary references should be the first port of call when trying to find background information on a subject. They present the user with a manageable document that is prepared from a vast amount of published information. With the advent of the electronic age, however, many people seem to have forgotten that it can be quick and easy to find information in a book. Books are easy to handle, readable, contain concise information and indexed. Their biggest disadvantage is the fact that they are out of date as soon as they are published. In general, it can take 5 or more years for new research findings to filter through into medical textbooks. Time constraints in editing and publishing mean that it takes a year or more between the author's submission of a manuscript and publication of the textbook. Because the

Table 33.2 Key tertiary drug information sources for pharmacy practice

Type of resource	Comment	Frequency of hard copy (i.e. textbook)	Formats available
Core resources on medicines			
Martindale: the complete drug reference. (Pharmaceutical Press, London)	Foremost information source on drugs and medicines worldwide. Provides encyclopaedic facts about drugs and medicines including information on nomenclature, physical and pharmaceutical properties, actions and uses and adverse effects. Includes information on herbal medicines and synopses of disease treatments.	Every 3 years (textbook) Electronic versions are updated more frequently than the textbook	Textbook, CD-ROM, online database, part of the Micromedex suite of programs
British National Formulary (BNF). (Produced jointly by the British Medical Association and Royal Pharmaceutical Society of Great Britain)	Authoritative resource on medicines in the UK. Content determined by a joint formulary committee of consultants and pharmacists. Details medicines on the market, with special reference to their uses, cautions, contraindications, side-effects, dosage and relative costs. Reflects current best practice as well as legal and professional guidelines relating to the use of medicines. Information included on the special requirements of children, the elderly, pregnant and breastfeeding women and patients with renal or hepatic impairment. Drug interactions and their clinical importance are also covered.	Every 6 months	Textbook, CD-ROM, Internet, web-enabled. BNF.org (Internet version intended for use by health professionals from home or during private study) eBNF (for standalone PC or small network) WeBNF (intranet version of the BNF designed for networking within large organizations with a facility for linking with local and area formularies).
The Medicines Compendium (Datapharm Communications Ltd, supported by the Association of British Pharmaceutical Industry (ABPI))	Formerly published for over 20 years by the ABPI as the Compendium of Data Sheets and Summaries of Product Characteristics. The new Medicines Compendium contains the Summary of Product Characteristics (SPCs) which describe the properties, effects and warnings about medicines written to guide both healthcare and pharmaceutical industry professionals in the safe and appropriate use of medicines. Information is included on drug presentations,	Current textbook expected to be the last edition	CD-ROM—quarterly updates internet (http://www.emc.vhn.net)—updated daily

Table 33.2 (cont'd)

Type of resource	Comment	Frequency of hard copy (i.e. textbook)	Formats available
	indications, dosage, administration, contraindications, use during pregnancy and pharmaceutical excipients. The source of the information has been approved by the Department of Health's Medicines Control Agency or equivalent European Medicines Evaluation Agency.		
Patient information leaflets	The patient information leaflets included in proprietary medicine packs can also be downloaded from the electronic Medicines Compendium website.	N/A	http://www.emc.vhn.net
Monthly Index of Medical Specialities (MIMS) (Haymarket Medical Publications Ltd, London)	An independently written prescribing guide aimed at GPs. Sent free of charge to GPs and available to other professions on annual subscription. Consists of short monographs on proprietary preparations and a range of useful tables (e.g. skin sensitizers in topical steroids, preservatives in ophthalmic preparations) and summaries of current treatment guidelines.	Monthly	Electronic version available on subscription
OTC Directory (Proprietary Association of Great Britain (PAGB), London)	Detailed guide to over-the-counter medicines aimed at community pharmacists and GPs.	Annual	On-line version available at http://www.medicine-chest.co.uk
Pharmacology			
Goodman and Gilman's Pharmacological Basis of Therapeutics (McGraw Hill, London	US text on the pharmacology behind the therapeutic application of drugs. Does not always reflect practice in the UK.	Every 3–4 years	Also available on CD-ROM
Pharmacotherapy			
Avery's Drug Treatment (Speight T, Holford NHG, eds, Blackwell Science, Oxford)	Disease-orientated textbook on therapeutics. Includes detailed information and evidence-based guidelines on optimum therapy. It also includes information on the relevant economic considerations in pharmacotherapy.	Every 3–4 years	Textbook only

Table 33.2 (cont'd)

Type of resource	Comment	Frequency of hard copy (i.e. textbook)	Formats available
Clinical Pharmacy and Therapeutics (Walker R, Edwards C, eds, 3rd edition, 2003. Churchill Livingstone, Edinburgh)	Aims to help pharmacy students, pharmacists and other health care professionals understand clinical disorders and promote the safe, appropriate and effective use of drugs. Each therapeutic section contains case studies designed to encourage application of therapeutic principles.	Every 3–4 years	Textbook only
Pharmacotherapy: a pathophysiologic approach. (DiPiro JT, Talbert RL, et al eds, 4th edition, 1999. Appleton and Lange, New York)	Another US text focusing on disease states, epidemiology, pathophysiology, clinical presentation and therapeutic management.	Every 4 years	Textbook only
Applied Therapeutics—the clinical use of drugs (Koda-Kimble MA and Young LY, eds, 7th edition, 2001)	US text covering all aspects of the clinical use of drugs. Uses a format of case presentations, questions and fully referenced answers. The presentation can sometimes make it difficult to locate specific information.	Every 4 years	Textbook only
Drug and Therapeutics Bulletin	Monthly bulletin published by Which? Ltd (a subsidiary of Consumers' Association). It gives rigorous and independent evaluations of drugs and other treatments aimed at doctors and pharmacists.	Monthly (by annual subscription)	CD-ROM—complete archive of content since January 1993. Updated twice a year. Also available on CD-ROM with BNF and Medicines Resource Centre (MeReC) Bulletin. Which? Online (http://www.which.net/health/dtb/) gives a summary of articles in the current issue and an index of articles published since 1994.
Drug interactions			
Drug Interactions (Stockley I, ed., 6th edition, 2003. Pharmaceutical Press, London)	Standard UK reference source on drug interactions listing mechanisms of drug interactions, clinical importance and management.	Every 2 to 3 years	Electronic version available late 2002

Table 33.2 (cont'd)

Type of resource	Comment	Frequency of hard copy (i.e. textbook)	Formats available
Adverse drug reactions			
Meyler's Side Effects of Drugs (Dukes MNG, Aronson JK, eds, 14th edition, 2000. Elsevier Science, Amsterdam)	Standard reference source on adverse drug reactions. Information presented as monographs on drug classes.	Every 4 years	CD-ROM—updated twice yearly
Meyler's Side Effects of Drugs Annuals	Companion texts to the above published annually. Each annual provides a critical survey of worldwide publications on adverse drug reactions, with extensive references to the literature.	Annual	CD-ROM—updated twice yearly
Current Problems in Pharmacovigilance	Drug safety bulletin produced by the Medicines Control Agency and the Committee on Safety of Medicines. Mailed to all doctors, dentists, pharmacists and coroners in the UK. Provides alerts to problems with medicines and advice on using medicines safely.	Four times a year	Full content available on Committee on Safety of Medicines website in pdf format (http://www.mca.gov.uk/ourwork/monitorsafequalmed/currentproblems/)
Children's doses*			
Medicines for Children (Royal College of Paediatrics and Child Health and Neonatal and Paediatric Pharmacists Group, 1st edition, 1999)	UK paediatric formulary. Aims to assist those who prescribe, dispense or administer medicines to children. It includes recommendations on which medicines to use and detailed monographs on individual drugs with information on appropriate doses.	Every 3 years. 2nd edition due autumn 2002	Electronic version in development

ª Particular care is required in the calculation of doses suitable for children. Standard reference sources such as the BNF and the Summary of Product Characteristics are often inadequate because many medicines are not licensed for use in children.

knowledge base in many areas of therapeutics is rapidly changing, the information contained in textbooks may be too old to be useful. This problem does not apply, however, to those textbooks available in computerized full-text as these can be more regularly updated, usually every few months. The information contained in textbooks may not be as comprehensive as the reader would like; this may be due to factors such as restriction on chapter length or the degree of emphasis that the author has placed on each topic. Because they cover topics very broadly, textbooks are often poorly referenced, indicating only the most significant papers to support or refute a stated case. The reader must also be aware that the information presented in a textbook is subject to the opinion, evaluation and bias of the author. It is often assumed that what is written in a textbook must be accurate; in fact, the author(s) may not have comprehensively searched, analysed or interpreted the information. A reluctance to use textbooks may be an unwanted spin-off from evidence-based medicine, as a consequence of increased awareness of secondary sources such as Medline. Textbooks are an important reference source that should not be overlooked.

Reviews and systematic reviews

Review articles that summarize a particular topic are considered tertiary reference sources, although they usually contain more current information about a specific topic than textbooks. Some journals feature review articles rather than original research publications (e.g. *Drugs*, *Drug Safety*). In addition, publications such as the *Drug and Therapeutics Bulletin* and the *Adverse Drug Reactions Bulletin* fall into this category.

Review articles have the same inherent limitations as textbooks. For this reason, an approach is needed that limits bias and provides the user with a comprehensive overview of a topic. The systematic review is a technique providing a comprehensive overview of original information that involves precise methods (i.e. methodological quality, precision, validity) of identifying and rejecting studies to be included in the review. As a result of these methods, the information evaluated has limited bias and reliable results. The Cochrane database of systematic reviews is recognized worldwide as a repository of high-quality systematic reviews.

Full text databases

The Micromedex Healthcare Series is a suite of full-text databases covering clinical and drug information produced

---

> **Box 33.3   Tips for evaluating tertiary information sources**
>
> Consider the following:
> - Is the author experienced in the field or topic of discussion?
> - How recently was this edition of the textbook published?
> - Is the reference clear, concise and easy to use?
> - Is it referenced appropriately?
> - Is the information relevant to the topic in question?

by Micromedex in the USA. Drugdex is the best known of these databases. It is a collection of detailed, referenced monographs written by a team of clinicians including pharmacists. These monographs provide comprehensive information gathered from the world's medical literature on most drugs in therapeutic use in the USA. Other databases included relate to drug use in pregnancy (Reprorisk System), complementary medicines (AltMedDex System) and toxicology (Poisindex). These databases are available by annual subscription on CD-ROM and via the Internet. Users need to satisfy themselves that the information contained in US and other overseas systems is appropriate to UK practice. There are other examples of full-text databases including those produced by FirstDatabank in the USA.

Pharmacists should evaluate tertiary information sources critically (Box 33.3); the resources selected should contain the most current and relevant information addressing the topic.

Secondary drug information sources

Secondary drug information sources can be used to systematically locate various types of published literature. In general these are resources that index and/or abstract literature from biomedical journals. Alerting systems provide a means of current awareness by scanning selected journals as soon as they are published, writing brief but informative abstracts and making them directly available to the customer. In this way the user can maintain a superficial knowledge of new developments published in a large number of journals. These resources are generally searchable electronically but may also be available in hard-copy format. The key advantages and disadvantages of secondary sources are shown in Box 33.4.

Inpharma is a useful alerting system aimed at pharmacists. It is a weekly publication providing rapid alerts to

Advantages:

Provide rapid access to the primary literature

Provide a large spectrum of information on specific
topics

Journals covered are generally of a high standard

Ability to link concepts to perform complex searches

Most resources have a facility for provision of routine
updates on selected topics (selective dissemination
of information)

Disadvantages:

The time period between article publication and
inclusion in secondary sources (lag time) varies
between databases (e.g. weeks to months)

User needs to have access to primary sources

The number of journals indexed by each system
depends on the scope of the database

Command language varies between databases

The user needs to be familiar with a particular
database's structure and terminology and to have
proficient search skills in order to search effectively
(training)

Need for user to be proficient in sifting through the
sources listed on a particular subject to find the most
relevant information

Not suitable for browsing

Can be expensive to access relative to tertiary sources

news on drugs and drug therapy distilled from over 1600 international medical journals and the most important medical meetings and conferences. Inpharma is available on annual subscription in a range of formats including hard copy, CD-ROM, via the Internet and on-line via the Dialog corporation (an on-line host provider). Reactions is a similar publication that concentrates on adverse effects and drug interactions.

Indexing systems

There are many different bibliographic biomedical databases. Medline and Embase are the best known of these but there are many others, often with a different scope. For example, there are databases focusing on toxicology, complementary medicine, etc. Bibliographic databases contain citations or documents created by detailed indexing of biomedical journals. Each citation is broken down into sections or fields containing a separate piece of information

about the original article (e.g. title, authors, source, abstract, keywords). The database content can be searched systematically, allowing the user to view a brief description of the information within most citations. Most secondary systems are provided in different formats, such as the Internet, online via host providers and on CD-ROM.

Electronic databases such as Medline are firmly established as an essential tool in research and for ensuring evidence-based clinical practice. With the introduction of new search interfaces, such as Internet-based searching, Medline is easier to use than ever before. Its efficient use, however, is greatly enhanced by a clear understanding of the principles that lie behind the database and its indexing language.

Searching bibliographic sources

Searching is the interaction between the user and the computer system with each communicating in turn. The search or question must first be translated into the 'indexing language' of the database (most use a controlled vocabulary or thesaurus for indexing papers). Free text may be used but the search is not as precise and all possible synonyms have to be included to be sure of retrieving all the relevant information. Before starting the search, it is important to define a clear question or statement that needs to be addressed, e.g. how effective are ACE inhibitors in the treatment of heart failure. The next step is to choose appropriate subject headings or keywords to include in the search. These can then be combined in the search using the Boolean operators (and/or/not) to produce a set of relevant citations that can be limited further if required. The Medline and Embase databases also feature the use of subheadings (i.e. several common concepts such as adverse effects, diagnosis, therapeutic use and surgery are covered by subheadings appended to the subject heading or keyword) which can be used to focus the search to the specific question. Details included in the citations vary according to the database searched but will generally include authors, title of the work, publication source, date and location and often an abstract of the manuscript. Systems that include abstracts must be used with care; although they may be reasonably accurate and offer some detail, they do not normally provide the basis for an answer to a request for information. Abstracts are usually written by the article's authors so there is normally no criticism of methods, results or conclusions.

Biomedical databases such as Medline are essential tools in evidence-based practice. The ability to use these sources is an important skill that can enhance clinical pharmacy practice. To search these databases effectively it is useful to have a clear understanding of the principles that lie behind the database and its indexing language. It is also essential to carefully scan the documents retrieved to obtain the most relevant citations. New users may be able to work through on-line tutorials to learn how to make the best use of these databases.

Abstracting systems

Medline. Produced by the US National Library of Medicine, the Medline database is widely regarded as the premier source for bibliographic and abstract coverage of biomedical literature. MEDLINE encompasses information from *Index Medicus*, *Index to Dental Literature* and *International Nursing*. Coverage dates back to 1966 and more than 11 million records from more than 4300 journals are indexed; abstracts are included for about 51% of the records. Journals covered are published in the USA and 70 other countries. Most records are from English language sources or have English abstracts. Some core pharmacy journals, including *The Pharmaceutical Journal*, are not covered. The database is updated daily, although lag time between publication and entry on the database can be up to several months.

The Medline database can be accessed on CD (either on a standalone computer or on a local network) or over the Internet. There are various CD versions of the database, of which Ovid and SilverPlatter are the most common. Medline systems available via the Internet include PubMed and BioMedNet. These versions of Medline differ in their presentations and search systems, but the database is the same in each case, as are the principles of searching it. The controlled vocabulary or thesaurus of terms used to search Medline is known as MeSH or Medical Subject Headings.

The overlap between Medline and Embase varies with subject, but on average the overlap in journal coverage is about 40–50%.

PreMedline. PreMedline is the National Library of Medicine's in-process database for Medline. It contains very recent records not yet indexed and added to Medline, so is an excellent source of current and recent information. It is updated daily.

Embase. Embase is the Excerpta Medica database, produced by Elsevier Science. It is a major biomedical and pharmaceutical database indexing over 4000 international journals. Coverage dates back to 1974 and it includes over 8 million records. There is particular emphasis on European literature and it is renowned for extensive coverage on drug research, pharmacology and pharmaceutics and for in-depth

indexing. The controlled vocabulary for searching (using Emtree) is distinct from that used by Medline. More than 80% of recent records include full author abstracts. The database is updated daily and the lag time between publication and database entry is generally shorter than with Medline.

The overlap between Medline and Embase varies with subject, but on average the overlap in journal coverage is about 35%.

OVID. OVID Technologies is a provider of information systems including a wide range of electronic journals and textbooks, bibliographic databases and other systems for health professionals. The OVID network or platform is increasingly used by libraries and hospitals, so the Ovid interface is well recognized by many users. Not all databases on Ovid are provided in full, for example Embase coverage dates only from 1980. An online tutorial for Medline searching via the OVID interface can be found at http://www.mclibrary.duke.edu/respub/guides/ovidtut/.

Pharm-line. The Pharm-line database (http://www.pharm-line.com) is an abstracting system covering drugs and professional pharmacy practice. NHS medicines information specialists produce it. Pharm-line is an excellent starting point for pharmacy practice research, particularly if it has been carried out in the UK. The database includes abstracts of articles on pharmacy practice and the clinical use of drugs from over 100 major English language pharmaceutical and medical journals. You can find a list of journals covered at http://www.druginfozone.org/Pharmline/Pharmline/journals/journals.html. All medicines information centres in the UK have access to Pharm-line and to the user guide that gives detailed search instructions.

International Pharmaceutical Abstracts. The International Pharmaceutical Abstracts database (http://www.ashp.org/ipa/), produced by the American Society of Health-System Pharmacists (ASHP), offers comprehensive coverage of world pharmacy literature from 1970, including pharmacy practice and education. It covers 750 pharmaceutical, medical and health-related journals published worldwide. The scope of the database ranges from clinical pharmacy to legislation, sociology, economics, ethics and information processing and literature. Coverage includes abstracts from state pharmacy journals, ASHP meetings (from 1988), with the records updated monthly. International Pharmaceutical Abstracts is searchable through various interfaces, including online (e.g. Dialog), CD and the Internet (e.g. Ovid).

The biggest drawback to the use of this database is its relatively high cost. ASHP has introduced web-based searching of International Pharmaceutical Abstracts (Pharmsearch from IPA at http://www.ashp.org/ipa/pricing.html). The pricing structure recognizes that users may not wish to subscribe in full and includes the option of paying for 'access blocks' (equivalent to 100 search commands) that can be used over an 18-month period. This system covers journals with a greater emphasis on pharmacy-orientated subjects than any other system. It is updated monthly.

Iowa Drug Information Service – indexing/full-text system. This system is produced by the Iowa Drug Information Service. It covers about 200 leading English-language medical and pharmaceutical journals but only those articles relating to drug therapy in humans are indexed. The system allows access to the full text of the articles indexed. The IOWA system is available on CD-ROM and the Internet. Before 1998 the system was available on microfiche and online.

Cochrane Library. In addition to databases like Medline, the Cochrane Library is a useful collection of databases to search. It is published quarterly and is designed to provide evidence for health care decision making. The Cochrane Collaboration is an international network that is committed to preparing, maintaining and disseminating systematic reviews of the effects of health care. The Cochrane Library has four main databases:

- The Cochrane Database of Systematic Reviews (CDSR). This is a database of Cochrane reviews that are highly structured and systematic reviews that concentrate on randomized controlled trials. These systematic reviews are prepared by members of the Cochrane Collaboration.
- The Database of Abstracts of Reviews of Effectiveness (DARE). The DARE database is critically appraised by reviewers at the NHS Centre for Reviews and Dissemination at the University of York, UK. It includes structured abstracts of systematic reviews from around the world.
- The Cochrane Controlled Trials Register (CCTR). This lists controlled trials selected by Cochrane Collaboration contributors and other sources. This is part of an international effort to hand search the world's journals and create an unbiased source of data for systematic reviews.
- The Cochrane Review Methodology Database (CRMD). This is a bibliography of articles and books that discuss the science of research synthesis.

Synthesis journals. In response to evidence-based practice, new journals have been created to focus on evidence-based philosophies. *ACP Journal Club* and *Evidence Based Medicine* are both excellent secondary publications

for searching for evidence. These journals provide abstracts and commentaries of previously published, clinically applicable research. Articles in these journals are selected on strict quality criteria.

Clinical Evidence is a compendium of the best available research findings on common and important clinical questions, updated and expanded every 6 months. It is available on subscription as hard copy, CD-ROM and via the Internet.

Primary drug information sources

Primary literature forms the foundation of the literature hierarchy, i.e. it is the source of information from which secondary and tertiary information sources are developed. It includes original publications and consists of research studies, case reports, editorials and letters to journal editors. The reader is able to critically appraise and analyse the study or article in order to develop a conclusion on its merits. The quality of medical journals is variable: examples of high-quality primary literature resources include the *British Medical Journal*, *Lancet*, *New England Journal of Medicine* and the *Journal of the American Medical Association*. Primary reference sources of particular relevance to pharmacy include the *Pharmaceutical Journal*, *Annals of Pharmacotherapy*, *International Journal of Pharmacy Practice* and *American Journal of Health-Systems Pharmacy*. Most articles submitted to these journals undergo a process of 'peer-review' before they are accepted for publication. During this process journal editors take into account the unbiased views and suggestions of experts to assess and improve the quality of the report. Even the best journals contain some material, such as letters and short reports, that have not been refereed. Some journals do not adopt a peer-review process and occasionally publish studies that are not scientifically robust.

The advantages of the primary literature are that it contains current, original and 'cutting-edge' information. The main disadvantages are that there may be flaws in study methodology or investigator bias (a particular problem for studies sponsored by pharmaceutical manufacturers). The fact that an article appears in print is no guarantee that its findings are valid. Another problem is the length of time it can take before new information presented in the scientific literature gains wide acceptance throughout the medical community. Studies need to be critically appraised before firm conclusions about their implications for practice can be drawn, and this requires some knowledge of scientific methods and statistics.

Critical appraisal of published papers

Pharmacists must have a clear understanding of the principles of critical appraisal or literature evaluation. Readers interested in more detail on this topic may find the following websites useful: http://www.shef.ac.uk/~scharr/ir/units/critapp/index.htm and http://cche.net/userguides/ therapy.asp

There are three stages in appraising a study:

- Understanding the purpose of the study and considering if the way the research was designed appears to be consistent with the purpose
- Studying how the research was actually carried out and deciding if it seems to have been done properly
- Seeing the findings of the research and judging if the conclusions reached are supported by the findings.

The first points to consider when reading a clinical trial paper are the aims and design of the study. The introduction should briefly describe the full background to the study, including work previously published. The aims and objectives should also be detailed in this section. Has a precise aim been described in the title or introduction, and is the design appropriate to the study question?

It is also worth checking for any reference to sponsorship of the research and the authors' affiliations, both of which could potentially alter the emphasis which may be put on the study. The presence of a statistician among the authors may give some reassurance on the statistical aspects of the paper, especially if they were involved in designing the study.

The most important section of any clinical trial paper, and the one many readers skim over, is the methods section. Scrutiny should reveal exactly how the study was performed, in sufficient detail to enable other researchers to repeat the experiment. If inappropriate methods are used, then misleading results and conclusions will be obtained. In particular, the methods section should fully describe the following:

- The types of patients included, how many were excluded from the study and why. Patient age, sex, whether they were selected from hospital or general practice, severity of disease, other disease states and drugs must also be described.
- The treatments given, including each treatment formulation, route of administration and how doses were selected. The method of assessing patient compliance with the treatment should also be described.
- The methods used to measure the effects of treatment. Where possible accepted and standardized methods should be used.

- The control group with which the drug under study was compared. Ideally comparison should be made with the standard treatment and placebo. This standard treatment should be the best available. In certain studies the use of a placebo would not be acceptable. Examples would be when studying the use of drugs in the treatment of cancers or pain control.
- The method of allocating treatments to patients. To prevent bias a random design should be used whereby each patient has an equal chance of receiving any of the available treatments. If this is not done, patients could be given treatments in the anticipation that they will respond in a certain way, thereby introducing bias into the study. Several methods of achieving a random design are available and the particular method used should be described.
- The method selected to ensure blindness. If the patient or investigator knows which treatment is being given, this may affect the response or measurement. To prevent this, a double-blind technique should be used, whereby neither the patient nor investigator knows the treatment being given. The method of achieving double-blindness in the study should be described.
- The number of patients included in the study. In the past the number of patients in a trial was often chosen depending on the amount of money or time available for the study. As a result many of these trials included too few patients to allow differences between treatments to be identified. The number of patients to detect a clinically important difference between treatments can be calculated. These details must be included in this section.

Three factors may influence the outcome of a clinical trial: chance, bias and a true comparison between treatments. Use of appropriate statistical tests to analyse results quantifies the probability that the observed result occurred by chance alone. One of the researcher's most important aims when designing a study is to take steps to eliminate all sources of bias, which may occur at any point during a trial.

The end-points chosen for the trial should be clearly defined, and in the case of 'surrogate' or indirect measures of a drug's action, should be widely recognized as valid markers of response. For example, the reduction of blood pressure by any drug is widely accepted to prevent strokes and other direct complications of hypertension. However, evidence of better sputum penetration by one antibiotic compared to another does not necessarily predict a superior clinical response.

The results section of a paper should be closely scrutinized to ensure that all patients who entered the study are accounted for at the end, whether or not they completed the study. This is important because patients may drop out of the study for reasons related to treatment, such as adverse effects. For this reason, statistical analyses are considered to be more robust if they are done on an 'intention-to-treat' basis, where data are included from all patients, even those who did not complete the study. This more closely approaches the 'real life' situation, where some patients are not compliant with therapy. An analysis which only includes those patients who were perfectly compliant with therapy to the end of the trial is likely to give an overestimate of the effectiveness of the intervention.

It is also important to consider whether the results described actually answer the study question. Occasionally, the result of a secondary end-point becomes the main focus of the analysis and discussion because it has shown a favourable effect of the study drug. However, such results should be viewed with caution, as they may be less valid than those relating to the primary end-point which the study was specifically designed to explore. Similar criticisms may be applied to subgroup analyses which were not originally planned in the study. If a set of data is analysed and re-analysed enough times, a positive result may arise purely by the laws of probability. Such 'data dredging' may point to a need for further investigation in a subset of patients, but cannot be relied upon alone.

Even if a trial is well designed, the way in which the results are presented may be inappropriate, leading to false claims of the effects of the drugs under study. When reviewing the results section, particular attention should be paid to the following:

- Graphs can be distorted to make the differences between drugs appear much greater than they actually are. This approach is sometimes used in promotional material and is described later in this chapter.
- All statistics included should be appropriate. Inexperienced readers can easily be misled by studies which analyse results using inappropriate statistical tests. If in doubt, it is best to consult a statistician for advice.
- Failure to account for all patients. Patients may withdraw from studies for many reasons, including side effects or worsening of the condition. The reasons for all withdrawals must be clearly described.

The discussion section should outline the importance of the findings, indicating any changes in practice which may occur as a result. Limitations of the study, such as problems in recruiting suitable patients, should also be highlighted at this point. The discussion should lead to the main

conclusions of the study which should be justified from the study design and results. The references section is the final section and must reflect the available relevant literature, not simply those studies agreeing with the views of the authors.

The Internet

Internet technology has made a huge impact on both work and leisure over the last 5–10 years and health care is no exception. It provides access to an enormous volume and range of information that previously was inaccessible or too poorly organized to be searched easily. Within pharmacy, it is a rich source of information and resources for students, lecturers, researchers and practising pharmacists. The key advantage is that the Internet allows cheap and easy access to a huge amount of information. Examples of the types of resource available include electronic publications, original documents, information on organizations (professional bodies, universities, government, industry, voluntary organizations), news services and discussion rooms and mailing lists. It is also increasingly used as a medium by which users can access bibliographic and factual databases (e.g. Medline, IOWA Drug Information System, Micromedex). Although a lot of information can be accessed free of charge, some resources require annual subscription or membership of a professional organization.

There are obvious disadvantages to the plethora of unregulated information on the Internet. The information may be written by a leading expert and well documented with a complete bibliography, but anyone can post information regardless of their background. Consequently the information is of variable quality, accuracy and currency. There is a large volume of factually incorrect and out-of-date information that causes considerable information 'noise'. Another drawback is that the information is not well organized. This makes it difficult for practitioners to determine which information is usable and credible. Since it would be impossible to regulate the Internet, health professionals and patients should be aware of how to make the most of it. Before starting a search, the user should consider whether the Internet is the best place to look for the information required; a textbook may be a faster and easier route to relevant information. In some situations the Internet is particularly useful; for example, when you already have a citation or Internet address to a website, for news or current topics not yet in the published literature, and when company-specific information is needed. Searching is relatively easy, but, as with other sources, a planned search is more likely to be productive than simply browsing or surfing.

There are important provisos for Internet searching:

- The sheer amount of information available is daunting
- Access and navigation can be time consuming
- Information may be out of date, incorrect, biased or deliberately misleading
- It may give an inappropriate perspective (especially true in health care where much of the information for the public originates from the USA)
- It is essential to review information found critically
- Many useful sites are subscription only.

The most common way to search the Internet is via a search engine or directory. A search engine, such as Alta Vista (http://www.altavista.com), automatically creates listings from the content of pages on the world-wide web. A directory, such as Yahoo! (http://www.yahoo.com), uses human editors to create listings from the descriptions that the provider of a page submits to it. As well as general search engines and web directories, gateways are an important tool to ensure that a search is focused on high-quality information. A gateway is a site providing links to websites organized by subject area with a short description of the sites. These links have been assessed against specified quality criteria. There are several excellent subject gateways for medicine and pharmacy: OMNI (or Organizing Medical Networked Information) is a UK-based subject gateway to quality medical and health information; Medical Matrix is a free online directory of selected medical sites, primarily aimed at US health professionals; Pharmweb is a comprehensive gateway for topics relevant to pharmacy.

As for effective searching of bibliographic databases, there are search techniques that can be helpful to the Internet user. The information found must be filtered and appraised when evidence-based facts are required. Some tips for using the Internet effectively are given in Box 33.5. A detailed discussion of search techniques is outwith the scope of this chapter but the reader is directed to the following on-line tutorial on Internet information skills for pharmacists, pharmacy academics and pharmacy students (http://www.sosig.ac.uk/vts/pharmacist).

A list of useful website links for pharmacists can be found at http://www.druginfozone.org/links/links.html

Expert opinion

In most instances expert opinion refers to consultation with a respected colleague, a specialist in the field or a supervisor. Expert opinion differs from the other sources of information in that it incorporates clinical experience. This can

---

Box 33.5   Tips for using the Internet

Become familiar with search techniques and the range of information available

Plan your search strategy

Use sites you know are trustworthy (e.g. sites of professional societies) and that give details of who produces them and when they were last updated

Understand the need to critically evaluate resources you find on the Internet

Establish who is responsible for the resource and what expertise or qualifications they have in the field

Don't use information from a site that is not convincingly authoritative (using inaccurate, unverified health information could have disastrous consequences)

Be aware that the Internet can be volatile—information can change or disappear without warning

---

be helpful because it allows for the answer to be focused to the exact clinical question, something that is often not possible with the results of clinical trials. The major disadvantage is the susceptibility of the opinion to bias, as it is not based on systematically collected information.

OTHER INFORMATION SOURCES

Pharmacists should be aware of the information sources described below.

Royal Pharmaceutical Society of Great Britain Information Centre

There is an Information Centre based at the Royal Pharmaceutical Society Headquarters in London comprising the Library and Technical Information Service. The information pharmacists in the Technical Information Service can help answer scientific and technical questions relating to pharmacy practice or continuing education from members from any branch of pharmacy. The subject scope includes advice on the usage and availability of proprietary and other medicinal products, adverse drug reactions and interactions, and the identification of medicines from overseas. Further details can be found at www.rpsgb.org.uk/infocentre/home.htm. The Royal Pharmaceutical Society Library in Edinburgh specializes in pharmaceutics and quality control.

National Pharmaceutical Association (NPA) Information Services

The NPA has an information service for members only. The department is a complete reference centre, skilled at assisting members with a wide range of pharmacy practice-related questions such as drug information, NHS matters and law and ethics. Further details can be found at http://www.npa.co.uk.

The pharmaceutical industry medical information departments

All pharmaceutical companies can provide extensive information on their products. This source of information can be particularly important for new products, when there is often a lack of published information.

Pharmaceutical manufacturers' promotional material

The pharmaceutical industry spends millions of pounds annually on advertising their products in increasingly sophisticated ways. Pharmacists should be able to critically analyse this type of material, looking 'beyond the gloss' to the message behind, in order to evaluate the claims made.

Promotional material makes extensive use of imaginative graphics designed to catch the reader's eye long enough for the message to be assimilated and retained. When the background illustrations and graphics are ignored, it is surprising how often advertisements contain an uninformative or vague statement by way of a headline. Such content suggests that the advertisement's aim is purely to reinforce prescribers' awareness of a particular brand name.

Any claims made about a medicine should always be supported by references, which should be sought out and read to check that they are quoted accurately. Occasionally papers may be misquoted or single statements/phrases from a paper cited out of context such that their original meaning may be distorted.

The source of references is also important; they may be 'data on file', or reports from sponsored symposia. Even published clinical trials should be checked to see whether they are authored or funded by the company whose product is being advertised. Papers that are very old or from obscure journals should arouse suspicion. The quality of references is more important than the quantity.

Graphs and other illustrations are tools which advertisers use to great effect, and therefore should be carefully studied.

Some common 'tricks' which have been used include not starting both axes of a graph or bar chart at zero, using inappropriate scales on axes and extrapolating lines beyond the final plotted point. It is important to be sure that the data displayed in such an eye-catching fashion are actually of clinical relevance, and not obscure laboratory data which have no practical application. This consideration is particularly important when statistical significance is being used to support an advertising claim.

Finally, beware of the use of non sequiturs in the text of advertisements; that is, where two unconnected statements are used in such a way as to imply a connection. For example, a drug may be described as being the most potent of its class, implying that this confers some superiority over other drugs, which of course it does not. Similarly, claims for superior bioavailability over a competitor drug mean nothing unless it is proven to translate into an improved clinical response.

ANSWERING ENQUIRIES ABOUT MEDICINES

As discussed previously, answering enquiries or dealing with requests for information forms an integral part of the daily routine for all pharmacists. This process involves gathering the relevant information, analysing and evaluating it, applying it to the enquiry or clinical problem, and delivering or communicating an answer or response. These steps are the same for a pharmacist practising in primary care, hospital or a medicines information centre. Questions range in complexity from the straightforward to the highly complex but in all cases the advice or information given can improve patient care. Table 33.3 summarizes a systematic approach to dealing with an enquiry.

Dealing with questions remotely, e.g. via the telephone, requires special communication skills. When approached for information or advice about a medicine, unless the pharmacist already knows the enquirer, the first step is to establish who is asking the question. Courtesy and politeness are essential from the beginning to get the caller's confidence and make them feel at ease. It can be very helpful to know something about the enquirer's professional background and position so that the answer can be tailored according to their needs and level of comprehension. For example, with a question about the appropriate dose of a medicine in a patient with renal impairment, the depth of the answer provided will be different depending on whether the question

Table 33.3   Summary of systematic approach to dealing with an enquiry

Stage	Approach
Receive the enquiry	Note contact details (i.e. name, status, department, contact phone number, etc.)
Determine and clarify the question	Elicit background information (i.e. patient details, medication history, disease states, etc.)
Classify the question	E.g. drug interaction, adverse drug reaction, drugs in pregnancy, choice of therapy
Search	Be familiar with available sources Develop search strategy and conduct search
Evaluate	Appraise/evaluate Extract pertinent information
Formulate an answer	Document sources used Abstract statements pertinent to the answer Prepare a concise, relevant and logical summary
Communicate the response	Consider the best way of answering the question, e.g. written answer may be needed for complex enquiries Express the response clearly and confidently Be prepared to clarify as much as necessary Make sure the message is received and understood

is asked by a consultant in renal medicine or a student nurse on the renal ward. Secondly, the background to the question needs to be established, taking into account all relevant information, such as patient details and medication history. Background information helps to clarify the question and is a critical step in the process. The question directly asked may not be a true reflection of the problem that the enquirer is faced with, or the background details can change the approach that should be taken. For example, a pharmacist may be asked 'Can I use ciprofloxacin in a patient who is allergic to penicillin?'. This question could be answered 'yes' at face value, but it may be that the patient has a medical condition that contraindicates the use of ciprofloxacin, or is taking another medicine that has the potential to interact with it. Similarly, the face value answer to the question 'Does sildenafil interact with the antidepressant paroxetine?' may be 'no' but the pharmacist should be expected to ascertain that paroxetine may itself be a cause of erectile dysfunction and that changing the patient to another antidepressant may be a more appropriate course of action.

Enquirers usually volunteer too little information and the pharmacist needs to ask for the relevant details in a tactful and friendly manner. Inadequate background and knowledge may result in the significance of the problem being missed. The type of background information that may be useful is shown in Box 33.6.

Box 33.6   Useful background information

Patient age, sex, weight
Medication (including dose and duration of therapy)
Diagnosis, relevant medical history
Liver and renal function
History of adverse drug reactions
Pregnant, breastfeeding

Before ending the conversation the pharmacist should be clear what the question is and why it is being asked; details can be confirmed by restating the request. It can also be useful to know which sources the enquirer has already checked. It is important to develop a time line for when the response is needed. If you are unable to help immediately you should say so and agree to return to the caller at a mutually convenient time. Before beginning the search, the request should be classified into a category (Box 33.2). This will allow the pharmacist to plan an appropriate search strategy, taking into account the available resources and the specific resources that are appropriate for particular types of question.

Systematic search strategy

The usefulness of a specific information source depends on the relevance and validity of the information and the work it takes to obtain it. In practice, when we attempt to find information relevant to a clinical problem our goal is to find the most useful information in the shortest time. The most useful information will be relevant to the problem, accurate, and it should be located with little work. This concept is often described as the usefulness equation:

$$\text{Usefulness of information} = \frac{\text{Relevance} \times \text{Validity}}{\text{Work to access}}$$

Validity is the likelihood that the information is true or accurate. Conclusions based on results of well-designed clinical trials are more likely to be valid than those drawn for observations in clinical practice. But it is not enough to accept evidence at face value simply because it has been published in a well-known journal or comes recommended from a specialist. Work to access relates to the time and effort that must be spent extracting the information. The ideal information source will be directly relevant, contain valid information and be accessed with a minimum amount of work. Table 33.4 shows an estimate of how existing information sources score against these criteria. Expert-based sources, such as the advice of a colleague, are appealing because the work needed to access the information is low. However, the information may have low validity or relevance and should be used cautiously.

Given the huge range of information sources available, it can be difficult to identify the most appropriate source relevant to a particular enquiry. It is useful to adopt a systematic search strategy (Box 33.7). Tertiary sources relevant to the topic should be consulted first; these may not answer the question but should at least put the subject in context, describe current practice and highlight problems. If one source contains information that provides the basis of an answer to the question then the pharmacist should attempt

---

Box 33.7 Search strategy tips

Classifying the question to help focus the search
Start with the most appropriate tertiary source
Try to verify answer with a second tertiary source
If no information found, proceed to appropriate
    secondary resources to locate pertinent primary
    literature
Use of two secondary sources is preferred
When assessing primary literature, remember the
    evidence hierarchy (see Ch. 34)

---

to verify this using another source if possible. If tertiary sources available do not provide an answer to the question the search should progress via secondary sources to locate primary literature. Because journal coverage varies with different secondary systems, it is important to use more than one secondary source for a thorough search.

The pharmacist needs to assess the information retrieved with respect to its quality and relevance to the enquiry. Data evaluation is critical, particularly when conflicting information is found in the literature. All references used should be documented and a concise, relevant and logical summary written. It is also worth thinking about potential follow-up questions from the enquirer; e.g. if you are going to recommend that a medicine should be stopped as it may be the cause of an adverse drug reaction, then the enquirer is likely to want to know about suitable alternatives. It is essential to communicate the answer effectively. If the enquirer does not clearly understood the answer then all the time you have spent working on the problem has been wasted. Sometimes there is no clear-cut answer to a question within the resources

---

Table 33.4 Usefulness of commonly used drug information source

Information source	Relevance	Validity	Work	Usefulness
Evidence-based, regularly updated textbook (e.g. Martindale, Stockley (2002), *Meyler's Side Effects of Drugs*)	High	High	Low	High
Standard textbook	High	Low	Low	Moderate
Colleagues	High	Moderate	Low	Moderate
Journal articles	Low	High	High	Low
Collections of systematic reviews	Moderate	High	Moderate	Moderate
Evaluated databases (e.g. Micromedex)	High	Moderate–high	Low	Moderate–high
Internet	Moderate	Moderate	Low	Moderate
Medline search	Moderate	High	High	Moderate–high

available; however, you may still feel able to provide informed advice or comment in the light of existing knowledge. The pharmacist has a professional responsibility to clearly inform the enquirer when a particular course of action is more desirable or safer from the patient's perspective.

In medicines information centres it is essential to document fully the enquiry, the relevant references used and the answer given. These details may be called upon should a medicolegal issue arise. Enquiry data is usually entered into an electronic database so that it may be used if the same or similar enquiry arises at a later date. Six examples of enquiries that could occur are given below.

EXAMPLE 33.1

A local GP asks you (as the local community pharmacist) for some information about a new topical preparation of tacrolimus in the treatment of atopic dermatitis. She is interested because some of the patients at the practice eczema clinic have asked her about this product.

Approach to enquiry
In general textbooks are not helpful for finding information about newly marketed products. The printed copy of the *British National Formulary* (BNF) may not include relevant information as it is produced only every 6 months. MIMS or electronic information sources may be helpful. In this situation it would be reasonable to provide the GP with general information such as a copy of new product information from the *Pharmaceutical Journal* or promotional material from the manufacturer. An article providing an overview of new drug treatments for eczema, such as a *Drug and Therapeutics Bulletin* article, if available, would be ideal.

EXAMPLE 33.2

A local GP asks you (as a primary care pharmacist) to give a short presentation to a group of GPs at a practice development meeting on the place of COX-2 selective non-steroidal anti-inflammatory drugs (NSAIDs) in therapy.

Approach to enquiry
In this situation it would be essential to carry out a thorough search looking for relevant articles. The BNF and Martindale would be good starting points, bearing in mind that these are relatively new medicines. Secondary sources should then be searched but, as there is a large volume of published literature, your initial focus should be review articles. There may also be

published guidance on these agents (e.g. NICE guidance or SIGN guidelines). You will need to spend time reading and critically evaluating the information found before preparing your talk. If possible, the views of one or two local experts (such as a rheumatologist or gastroenterologist) might be helpful to give you a better understanding of some of the issues involved.

EXAMPLE 33.3

A patient asks you (as the community pharmacist) how leflunomide works.

Approach to enquiry
There may be hidden reasons for the patient asking such a specific question about leflunomide's mode of action. In practice you would question the patient further to explore any concerns or worries they may have, rather than simply answering the question at face value. Often patients with chronic diseases, such as rheumatoid arthritis, have a very good understanding of drug therapies. In fact, some interested and informed patients may have a better knowledge than the pharmacist or may have already searched the Internet or other sources before asking the question. If a 'knowledge gap' is identified then the pharmacist has a responsibility to find out more about the topic so that the patient can be given up-to-date and accurate advice.

EXAMPLE 33.4

A consultant physician asks you (as a hospital clinical pharmacist) about the dose of cyclophosphamide to use in a patient with Goodpasture's syndrome.

Approach to enquiry
If you are not familiar with this medical condition then the first step should be to find out more about it from a general medical textbook such as the *Oxford Textbook of Medicine*. Standard tertiary sources such as Martindale or pharmacotherapy texts should then be checked for information on the usual treatment and the manufacturer's Summary of Product Characteristics for cyclophosphamide should be reviewed. As a clinical pharmacist you may wish to ask your local medicines information pharmacist whether there is information on file about this treatment. For this enquiry it would also be important to search Medline and Embase in case new information has been published since the textbooks were written.

EXAMPLE 33.5

A consultant dermatologist asks you (as a pharmacist in the medicines information centre) about a patient who has developed lupus erythematosus that may be drug induced. The patient is taking three medicines (lansoprazole, atorvastatin and diltiazem) and she would like to know which of these is the most likely cause of the reaction.

Approach to enquiry

In this case the pharmacist may need to find out a bit more about lupus erythematosus before going any further. Standard reference texts should then be checked (e.g. Martindale, *Meyler's Side Effects of Drugs*, Micromedex) and the Medicines Compendium to check the adverse reactions section for each of the medicines the patient is taking. For a comprehensive answer to this question it will also be necessary to search secondary sources such as Medline and Embase. The search should be planned carefully beforehand, taking into account ways of narrowing the search down if too many citations are found and ways of broadening it out if very little is found. It is important to remember that a comprehensive search for this question should involve searching for the drug classes the patient is taking and not only the specific agents (i.e. although you may find no case reports of atorvastatin as a possible cause of lupus erythematosus there may be several published case reports with simvastatin, which would be relevant to the question asked). The pharmacist should also encourage submission of a Yellow Card report to the Committee on Safety of Medicines, if appropriate.

EXAMPLE 33.6

A customer asks you (as the community pharmacist) for figures on the UK incidence of Lyme disease after tick bites. The customer is from Germany, where the incidence of this disease is high. He enjoys walking in the countryside and would like to know what the relative incidence of Lyme disease is in the UK.

Approach to enquiry

A community pharmacist is unlikely to be able to answer this question from available tertiary or even secondary sources. The Internet is a good first-line resource for this type of question. For example, there may be useful information from government organizations or regional public health departments. Remember that you will need to critically evaluate any information found to assess whether it is reliable.

Key Points

- All pharmacists have a responsibility to provide information and advice about any medicine supplied by them or under their authority. It is vital that this information should be reliable, accurate and up to date.
- Pharmacists need to be familiar with the key reference sources that are useful for common types of questions (e.g. drug interactions, side-effects, drug use in pregnancy) and to be able to critically appraise and evaluate the information found. A systematic search strategy should be adopted when dealing with enquiries or clinical problems.
- Remember, the worst question is the one that is not asked. Continue to question drug therapy issues as this can only enhance your experience, expand your knowledge and, most importantly, benefit your patients. Never settle for poor or inadequate answers.

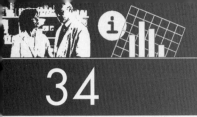

34

The evaluation of medicines

J. Krska

> After studying this chapter you will know about:
>
> **Safety, efficacy and economy**
> **Premarketing studies**
> **Postmarketing studies**
> **Evidence-based medicine**
> **Drug utilization review and evaluation**
> **Evaluation of non-prescription medicines**

SAFETY, EFFICACY AND ECONOMY

The volume, potency and complexity of modern medicines are increasing. The need to compare the therapeutic efficacy (i.e. benefits) of medicines with their potential to cause harm (i.e. risks) remains of paramount importance. With the cost of medicines and related services increasing, economic evaluation is also important. Pharmacists play a major role in the evaluation of the safety, efficacy and economy of medicines use.

At a macro level, the pharmaceutical industry decides which line of drug development would best serve its interests. Clinical trials are necessary to evaluate medicines before they can be marketed. Pharmacists participate extensively in such studies and also contribute to postmarketing surveillance (see Ch. 32). Society and its health care systems are faced with difficult decisions on which specific patient populations to treat, or which expensive new drug therapy to approve for use. Increasingly, such decisions are based on economic evaluations which include evidence of benefits and risks, estimated for potential patient populations (see Ch. 35). Pharmacists are involved extensively in providing independently evaluated information on drugs (see Ch. 33) and selecting drugs for formularies, clinical guidelines and local treatment protocols (see Ch. 36). The ability to evaluate medicines and information about medicines is therefore a key skill for practising pharmacists.

At an individual patient level, each clinician (doctor, pharmacist or nurse) requires to assess the relative risks and benefits of each medicine for individual patients. This involves consideration of factors which can affect drug disposition, efficacy and safety, such as concurrent disease states or drug therapy, risk of untreated disease or affordability. As pharmacists become more involved in selecting treatments, the importance of these skills increases. Furthermore, pharmacists are frequently involved in evaluating the use of medicines selected for individual patients by other prescribers. This involves the skills of drug use review and evaluation.

PREMARKETING STUDIES

In most countries evidence of safety, efficacy and quality must be presented to government-appointed regulatory authorities before a new drug can be marketed. In the UK, the Committee on Safety of Medicines (CSM) requires to be satisfied with such evidence before a product licence can be granted.

Prior to clinical trials in humans, the pharmacokinetics and pharmacodynamics of any new drug are studied. This involves preclinical evaluation in animals to indicate therapeutic and possible toxic effects in humans. However, there are often substantial interspecies differences in drug handling and in drug response. This usually results in the need for screening in more than one animal species. The relationship between the effects of drugs in animals and humans is often poor and necessitates cautious and stepwise trials in humans.

Phase I trials

These first trials are normally carried out in healthy adult volunteers. Their main purpose is to determine the drug's toxicity profile and to assess tolerability. A dosage range is tested initially with a stepwise increase in drug dose being given to successive volunteers. Subjects in Phase I trials are intensively monitored to determine the nature and severity of any predictable dose-related adverse effects. Pharmaco-kinetic data are usually generated from both single- and multiple-dose studies.

The safety data obtained from Phase I studies suffer from a number of limitations. The subjects are healthy adults and unlikely to have compromised drug handling ability. Thus the potential risks of using the drug in patients at extremes of age, or in those with poor hepatic or renal function, are not tested. There are also relatively few of them (e.g. 50–60), so only very common adverse effects are detected.

Phase II trials

Phase II trials commence while Phase I studies are still running. They are carried out in relatively small groups of target patients and tend to be performed within hospital-based departments specializing in particular areas of medicine. Their main aims are to establish efficacy and to confirm an effective dose in closely monitored and con-trolled conditions. Phase II studies give the first indication of the likely value of the drug in patients, i.e. its efficacy. There is less emphasis on safety assessments during this phase, but the results will enable a therapeutic ratio, i.e. the balance between efficacy and safety, to be determined. Double-blind randomized controlled trials use a control group with a matching placebo to assess the effectiveness of new drug therapies. Phase II studies also inform the design of Phase III studies which are more comprehensive. Phases II and III combined may study 1000–2000 patients. The regulatory authorities closely control Phase II and Phase III studies, for which clinical trial certificates or exemptions are required.

Phase III trials

These are the better known trials of safety and efficacy. They are generally large-scale comparative trials with other treat-ments or with placebo. Where appropriate, such trials should have a randomized controlled design which is gen-erally accepted as the best method of conducting clinical research. Assigning each patient randomly to either the new treatment or the control helps to prevent bias in the inter-pretation of each patient's progress. Other aspects of the design of clinical trials are discussed in Chapter 33.

Phase III trials generate data on both efficacy and safety. They are the main source of the information which appears

ultimately in the Summary of Product Characteristics (SPC) for the drug. The conduct of clinical trials is subject to guidelines which cover ethical issues, the trial design, the roles of the various investigators and sponsoring company and the storage and analysis of data.

Safety is assessed by close monitoring of clinical signs and symptoms during scheduled clinical examinations and consultations. This is complemented by relevant laboratory investigations. Baseline pretreatment data are compared with data obtained during periods of treatment with the study drugs. However systematic assessment of symptoms experienced by the patients included in the trials is not always carried out. The use of a systematic checklist for patients to complete has been suggested. With the numbers of patients involved in Phases II and III, these trials are capable of identifying only Type A adverse drug reactions that affect 1 in ≥ 250 patients studied. Type B adverse drug reactions, which are neither pharmacologically predictable nor dose related, tend to be rare (see Ch. 32). The larger number of patients involved in postmarketing surveillance studies are required to detect these types of reactions.

POSTMARKETING STUDIES

Most countries operate a system of postmarketing surveil-lance which involves spontaneous reporting of adverse effects to a central point. An example of this is the Yellow Card system in place in the UK, operated by the Medicines Control Agency (see Ch. 32). Such schemes provide early warning signals of potential problems and can lead to hypotheses about associations between a drug and an effect. These can be tested using retrospective (e.g. case-control studies) or prospective studies (e.g. cohort studies). These are also outlined in Chapter 32.

Safety assessment of marketed medicines (SAMM studies)

Formal studies to evaluate the safety of medicines which are sponsored by the pharmaceutical industry are known as SAMM studies. A SAMM study is defined as a formal investigation conducted for the purpose of assessing the clinical safety of marketed medicines in clinical practice. The conduct of these studies is also subject to guidelines. SAMM studies use the standard methods of case-control and cohort studies, but may also involve further randomized clinical trials (see below).

Patient reporting of adverse drug reactions

In some countries, patients may submit reports of events or symptoms which they believe to be due to using a particular drug. This is not the case in the UK, although there is increasing acceptance of the belief that the patient's experiences should be reported. A systematic checklist of symptoms can be useful for enabling patients to report their experiences (Jarernsiripornkul et al 2002). The majority of patients who report using such a checklist identify known side-effects. Therefore the potential value of this system lies in determining the incidence of adverse events in clinical practice.

Further clinical trials against other drugs/treatments

Most drugs are marketed having been subject to clinical trials in relatively few patients, which may have excluded certain patient groups. Furthermore, trials may have been conducted against placebo to demonstrate efficacy, but there may be no data on the comparative efficacy of a new drug versus an existing treatment for the same condition. In addition, basic research may highlight new theories of how diseases may be treated which require older drugs to be tested for efficacy in conditions where they have not been used previously. Examples of this are the trials required to assess the efficacy of aspirin for prophylaxis against stroke and beta-adrenoceptor blockers in heart failure. As with any other clinical trial, the design is important and the randomized controlled design is considered to be the most appropriate.

EVIDENCE-BASED MEDICINE

As a result of all these clinical trials, many published reports of these and other studies of efficacy and safety appear every year. However many drugs are available for which there is in fact little evidence of efficacy in certain conditions and much drug use is based on historical practice or anecdote. Prescribers are increasingly encouraged not to use such medicines. The practice of evidence-based medicine ensures that therapies are assured of efficacy and safety. Evidence-based medicine (EBM) is an approach to practice which seeks to identify the available evidence to answer specific clinical questions, critically appraise it and apply it to situations, whether in relation to individual patients or to populations. There are five stages as outlined by Sackett et al (2000):

1. Formulate an answerable question
2. Identify the best evidence with which to answer the question
3. Critically appraise the evidence for its validity, impact and applicability
4. Integrate the results of the appraisal with clinical expertise and patient factors
5. Evaluate the previous four steps for effectiveness and efficiency.

Detailing the skills necessary to practice EBM is outwith the scope of this book, however pharmacists should be aware of what is involved. An answerable question is one which includes three aspects: an intervention (often a drug), a disease state or population of patients and an outcome. For example, 'what are the effects on mortality of treatment with lipid-lowering drugs in patients with coronary heart disease?' The second stage involves making a systematic search of the literature to identify publications which may help to answer the question. There are several important databases available which must all be searched to ensure that publications have not been missed. Ideally any search should include Medline, Embase and International Pharmaceutical Abstracts. Skills of critical appraisal are important to ensure that the publications identified are of good quality, but it is also valuable to grade the evidence according to the study design and any important flaws in it. An example of grades of evidence is given in Table 34.1. The highest grading is given to meta-analyses of randomized controlled trials. Meta-analysis involves the pooling of data from studies which are sufficiently similar enough in terms of inclusion and exclusion criteria and outcome measures used. This provides a pooled estimate of effect as well as permitting comparison of results from many similar studies, but is an extremely labour-intensive process.

The next stage is to apply the evidence to the situation, be that an individual patient or a population. For individual patients, there may be many factors present which mean that the evidence cannot be applied directly to them or others, which means that clinical judgment is required in its application. To apply evidence to populations may involve using it to develop a guideline or protocol, which will assist many prescribers in delivering evidence-based therapies. On reviewing how effective and efficient the work to date has been it is important to reflect on the question formulated. If there was not evidence to provide an answer, was this because the question was too broad or narrow or is it really

Table 34.1   A new system for grading recommendations in evidence based guidelines, after Harbour and Miller (BMJ 2001; 334–336)

Level of evidence	Description
1++	High quality meta-analyses, systematic reviews of RCTs or RCTs with a very low risk of bias
1+	Well-conducted meta-analyses, systematic reviews of RCTs or RCTs with a low risk of bias
1–	Meta-analyses, systematic reviews of RCTs or RCTs with a high risk of bias
2++	High-quality systematic reviews of case-control or cohort studies High-quality case-control or cohort studies with a very low risk of confounding, bias, or chance and a high probability that the relationship is causal
2+	Well-conducted case control or cohort studies with a low risk of confounding, bias or chance and a moderate probability that the relationship is causal
2–	Case-control or cohort studies with a high risk of confounding, bias or chance and a significant risk that the relationship is not causal
3	Non-analytic studies, e.g. case reports, case series
4	Expert opinion

that there is little evidence? It is also useful to reflect on the search terms used and the efficiency with which databases are searched. Generally there is a large amount of effort involved in undertaking a critical appraisal of all evidence identified. However often when pharmacists become involved in making decisions about drug choice, they can access critical appraisals already carried out by others who use explicit criteria for their searching and appraisal. A selection of the most frequently used sources is given in Table 34.2.

Table 34.2 Some useful sources of evidence-based reviews

Source	Format
Cochrane library of reviews	Web-based/CD-ROM
Best Evidence	Web-based/CD-ROM
Effectiveness Matters	Paper
Bandolier	Web-based
Evidence based medicine	Journal
Clinical evidence	Book/CD-ROM
Evidence-based medicine reviews	Web-based

National organizations for evaluating medicines

In England, there are several centres which undertake evidence-based reviews of health care interventions, including drugs. They use systematic approaches which are published and produce information which pharmacists can use to ensure best practice is delivered. The Cochrane Collaboration was established in 1993 and is an international organization which produces systematic reviews through groups of volunteers with expertise in particular areas. Many pharmacists contribute to these review groups and reviews are available not just of medicines, but also of other pharmaceutical interventions. The NHS Centre for Reviews and Dissemination based at York University undertakes reviews, while the Health Technology Assessment programme, which includes pharmaceuticals, aims to provide information and identify further research needs. More recently the National Institute for Clinical Excellence (NICE) provides guidance on the use of drugs to the NHS, which is based on published evidence.

In Scotland, The Health Technology Board issues statements on NICE guidance and also undertakes reviews of new technologies including drugs. The Scottish Medicines Consortium also provides evaluated information on all new products. Some other sources of useful information are given in Chapter 33.

Terms used in evidence-based medicine

While all clinical trials provide data in terms of efficacy and safety, there is increasing use of similar methods of expressing results which enables comparisons between studies and therefore between drugs involved in different studies. These terms apply to studies in which two or more interventions are compared. Those most commonly used are summarized in Table 34.3.

The relative risk (RR) of an event (such as an improvement in symptoms or an adverse event) is the ratio of the proportions of events in the two groups in a study. It expresses the risk of an event occurring in the experimental group compared to that in the control group. An alternative is the odds ratio (OR), which is the ratio of the odds of an event occurring in the experimental group compared to that in the control group. The odds of an event occurring are calculated as the number of patients who have an event over the number who do not. Some studies quote a figure for relative risk reduction (RRR). This is simply the amount by which an intervention reduces the risk of an event relative to treatment offered to the control group, which may be placebo. It is expressed as a percentage. The absolute risk reduction (ARR) is the difference in the proportions of events between the two groups in a study, also expressed as a percentage. Number needed to treat (NNT) is more easily related to clinical practice, because it is expressed as the number of patients who must receive the intervention in order to have the desired outcome or benefit. NNT is the reciprocal of ARR. It is possible to express adverse events in a similar way, as relative risk increase (RRI), absolute risk increase (ARI) and number needed to harm (NNH).

DRUG UTILIZATION REVIEW AND EVALUATION

So far this chapter has concentrated on evaluating medicines in terms of efficacy and safety for the purpose of making decisions about whether to use a drug for a given condition. It is equally important to measure whether medicines are being used appropriately. Their proper use increases the quality of patient care and promotes cost-effective health care.

Drug utilization review (DUR) is the assessment of patterns of drug use in a particular clinical context. Drug use evaluation (DUE) incorporates qualitative measures and emphasizes outcomes, including pharmacoeconomic assessment. Drug use evaluation can identify problems in drug use, reduce adverse drug reactions, optimize drug therapy and minimize drug-related expenditure.

It is usually necessary to be selective in the drugs chosen for study, as much of this work is time-consuming. Selection may be on the basis of high cost, wide usage or changes in usage, known or suspected inappropriate use or potential for improvements in patient care. Evaluations of the use of expensive drugs which are also widely prescribed, such as ulcer-healing drugs or antibiotics, are common. These are also examples of drugs for which DUR or DUE would be useful on the grounds of suspected inappropriate use. Studying the use of hypnotics and anxiolytics would be valuable, because these drugs, although many are inexpensive, are widely used and often this use can be inappropriate. Changes in legislation can result in changes in the way medicines are used, e.g. alteration of the legal classification. Patterns of utilization often also change when a new product

Table 34.3 Terms used in evidence-based medicine

Term	Definition
Relative risk	$\dfrac{\text{Proportion of events in experimental group}}{\text{Proportion of events in control group}}$
Odds ratio	$\dfrac{\text{Number experiencing event/Number with no event in experimental group}}{\text{Number experiencing event/Number with no event in control group}}$
Where treatment reduces probability of a bad outcome:	
Relative risk reduction	$\dfrac{\text{Proportion of events in control group} - \text{Proportion of events in experimental group} \times 100}{\text{Proportion of events in control group}}$
Absolute risk reduction	Proportion of events in control group – Proportion of events in experimental group
Number needed to treat	$\dfrac{1}{\text{Proportion of events in control group} - \text{Proportion of events in experimental group}}$

is marketed. Drug use review can provide information on what these changes are and drug use evaluation can determine whether they are beneficial.

Drug utilization review

Drug utilization review developed in the 1960s and focused on the description of which drugs were being used and their costs. A classification system for drugs and a system for quantifying use were developed to enable comparisons between populations. These were the Anatomical Therapeutic Chemical (ATC) system and the Defined Daily Dose (DDD), developed by the Norwegian Medicinal Depot. These systems were subsequently recommended by the World Health Organization (WHO) for international use. In the UK, drugs are more frequently classified by their place in the *British National Formulary*, but DDDs are widely used. There is a DDD for every drug on the market, which is based on the average recommended daily maintenance dose for the drug when used for its most common indication in adults. It is expressed in g, mg, microgram, mmol or units or as the number of tablets for combination products. The Nordic Council on Medicines now sets the DDD for every drug in conjunction with the WHO.

Early hospital DUR programmes developed in the USA in the 1970s focused on antibiotic use and involved the development of standards for the use of each drug or group of drugs. These were then used as criteria against which the actual use of the drugs could be measured. This form of DUR is therefore very similar to clinical audit (see Ch. 43). Most DUR in the UK involves the study of patterns of drug use and the associated costs.

Drug use evaluation

Drug use evaluation programmes relate the use of drugs to patient outcomes and often include interventions to ensure appropriate drug use. Such programmes are potentially of much greater benefit than drug utilization review. They can be retrospective, concurrent or prospective. Retrospective DUE requires, and may be compromised by a lack of, good documentation. It usually has little effect on the treatment of the patients included in the review. Concurrent or prospective DUE can be much more valuable as an aid to improving drug use, since changes in prescribing can be implemented after or even during the evaluation. In carrying out either DUR or DUE, prior agreement of the clinicians is essential, since the findings may be critical of their practice.

There are various levels at which the use of drugs can be studied. These range from very broad measures with little detail, usually obtained from routinely collected data, to expensive methods, in which a great deal of useful information is obtained on individual patients.

Methods

Using drug purchase records

The simplest level of information about which drugs are being used is obtained from drug purchase records. Both hospital and community pharmacies use computerized systems for purchase, which means these data are readily available. This type of information provides no clues as to how the drugs are being used, but can often point to potential areas which may need further investigation.

Various units can be used for the measurement of drug purchases, e.g. cost, number of containers, number of dosage units or number of DDDs. Whatever units are used, drug purchases can be compared between pharmacies or over time.

Using drug issue records

A more detailed record of drug use can be obtained from the drugs issued from pharmacies, either those dispensed from community pharmacies or those issued to wards in hospitals. Again, computerization allows these data to be obtained easily.

In the community, the data are captured when the NHS prescriptions are priced by the Prescription Pricing Authorities in England, Wales and Northern Ireland or the Information and Statistics Division in Scotland. The data are then issued to prescribers as Prescribing Analysis and Cost (PACT) in England, Practice Audit Reports and Catalogues (PARC) in Wales or Scottish Prescribing Analysis (SPA). Data at this level are used to allow individuals to compare their drug use to that of a 'norm', such as the health authority (England) or health board (Wales, Scotland, Northern Ireland) average. Data combined for a group practice is most frequently used by pharmacists in reviewing the drugs prescribed by the practice's GPs and nurses in terms of frequency and cost. An example of the type of data available is shown in Table 34.4. It is important to remember that this data is derived from dispensed prescriptions, so excludes any prescriptions written but not presented by patients for dispensing.

The units used for the measurement of drug issues include those used to measure drug purchase. Additional ways of measuring drug use which are presented to prescribers are the average cost per prescription item and the average cost per patient. Comparisons between prescribers can be made using these methods and also using DDDs, the latter focusing on

Table 34.4   Example of prescribing data available from PACT report for Drug Use Review.
Top 5 BNF sections by cost for a general practice

BNF Section	£	Costs compared with: HA (%)	Costs compared with: Last year (%)	No.	Items compared with: HA (%)	Items compared with: Last year (%)
Lipid-regulating drugs	12 248	−6	33	305	−25	0
Ulcer-healing drugs	11 829	−11	3	588	−7	9
Nitrates, calcium blockers and potassium activators	11 650	12	−1	789	−12	−3
Antidepressant drugs	11 491	9	18	833	8	19
Antihypertensive therapy	9 909	−3	13	661	0	27

quantities rather than cost. The quantity of a drug prescribed is usually expressed as the number of DDDs prescribed per 1000 people over a period of time. For example, the DDD of diazepam is 10 mg. It may be found that, in one area, diazepam is used with a DDD of 2000/1000/year. This means that for every 1000 people, 2000 doses of diazepam were prescribed in a year. This is equivalent to 2 doses per person per year. By using DDDs, not only are quantities prescribed accounted for, but also an allowance is made for the frequency of administration. It is also possible to use the prescribed daily dose (PDD). This represents the average prescribed dose for a drug's main indication. The PDD may be the same as the DDD for some drugs, but the two measures may differ for drugs such as analgesics.

In some hospitals, it may be possible to link data from pharmacy issues to individual clinicians. This will increase with the expansion of on-line computer prescribing in hospitals. Often the data can only be applied at ward level, but this can still be helpful in developing and monitoring ward-based policies on drug use.

Using prescription records

More detailed information from prescriptions, which includes the actual dose prescribed and the concurrent medication, can be obtained in community pharmacies from patient medication records. However, without patient registration and the recording of non-prescription medicines purchased, these are incomplete. In hospitals, this level of data will only be easily obtainable with computer prescribing. Manual data collection from prescriptions is time-consuming, but provides information on the doses of drugs used, the extent of polypharmacy, the frequency of prescribing errors and drug interactions.

None of the above methods of data analysis can be used to determine the use of drugs in relation to indication and outcome. The information which they provide is incomplete and any suggestions of prescribing being inappropriate based solely on this type of data should be made cautiously. Prescribing advisers do advocate the use of prescribing indicators, which are an indicative measure of the quality and cost of prescribing. They use the standard measures already mentioned, but involve specific ways of combining data to enable more useful comparisons to be made. Some examples of prescribing indicators are listed in Box 34.1. The main purpose of prescribing indicators is to raise awareness of what is being prescribed and to highlight areas for more detailed methods of investigation, such as by examination of medical records.

Using medical records and trained investigators

In order to obtain information about the decisions behind the use of particular drugs and their effectiveness, it is necessary

---

Box 34.1   Examples of prescribing indicators

Percentage generic prescribing
Number of prescriptions for drugs of limited clinical value
Inhaled steroids + cromoglicate as % of these + beta-agonists
Inhaled β agonists as % of oral + inhaled β agonists
Bendroflumethiazide (bendrofluazide) 2.5 mg as % of total (2.5 + 5 mg)

Amoxicillin as % of amoxicillin + co-amoxiclav
Single diuretic as % of single + combination
Amount of hypnotic + anxiolytic drugs expressed in DDDs
Four top NSAIDs as % of all NSAIDs
Four top beta-blockers as % of all beta-blockers

to examine medical records. This requires expertise and time and can often be frustrated by the inadequacy of record keeping. Some hospital units and most general practices have computerized patient records, which allow links to be made to the drugs prescribed. In order to link the use of drugs to disease states it is also necessary to have a standardized method of classifying diseases. The most commonly used method in the UK is the Read Code. Increasingly in both hospitals and primary care links are also available to computerized laboratory data, which enable the use of drugs and, for example, monitoring of renal function or serum drug levels to be studied. Many systems, however, are poorly developed or underutilized, with the result that the records are often inaccurate or incomplete. Clearly, it is not possible to compensate for either a lack of data or inaccurate data. However, small retrospective studies undertaken manually can still be of considerable value in determining whether drugs are being used appropriately and effectively. These studies usually involve the use of trained investigators reviewing medical records. With the emphasis on National Service Frameworks and Clinical Standards which specify treatment to be given to patient populations, there is an increasing requirement for complete and accurate computerized data to be available in medical records. As piloting of an electronic health record extends, this data will become available to pharmacists and will facilitate greatly the evaluation of medicines use.

Prospective evaluation of drug use using trained investigators avoids the problem of inadequate records, by allowing data to be recorded and questions to be asked at the time of drug use. While this is likely to change prescribing behaviour, it may also help to improve the use of drugs. It can involve the patient, which thus provides a full picture of drug use, including outcomes and compliance. These latter methods are expensive, but pharmacists, often as part of their normal activities, may carry both out.

EVALUATION OF NON-PRESCRIPTION MEDICINES

Published information on the epidemiology of self-limiting minor illnesses is limited. Similarly, data on the pharmaco-epidemiology of the medicines used in self-treatment of these minor illnesses is limited. The number of such medicines which can be bought from pharmacies or other outlets is increasing. Many former prescription-only medicines have been deregulated to pharmacy medicines. Some former pharmacy medicines are now on the general sales list. These changes make medicines more available to the public. At the same time information on their use becomes less available.

Manufacturers of non-prescription medicines collect data on sales, which provide a global overview of which medicines are being purchased. Community pharmacists are requested to report suspected adverse drug reactions to non-prescription medicines (see Ch. 32). Drug use review requires similar methods to those used for prescription medicines, namely study of drug purchase or supply and data stored in pharmacy medication records. Drug use evaluation of non-prescription medicines is increasing, with the use of patient questionnaire methods. Such studies do show that use is often inappropriate. However currently these studies involve distribution from community pharmacies and therefore do not include the use of medicines purchased from other outlets. As increasing numbers of potent medicines become widely available without prescription, the requirement for a practical yet scientifically robust method of evaluating both the use of and adverse reactions associated with these medicines increases.

Key Points

- Pharmacists are involved extensively in evaluating medicines, their use and information about medicines.
- The Committee on Safety of Medicines (CSM) requires evidence of safety, efficacy and quality before granting a product licence for a new drug.
- Clinical trials take place in three phases: Phase I determines the basic toxicity and tolerability, Phase II establishes efficacy and confirms the dosage, Phase III determines safety and efficacy on a larger sample.
- Postmarketing studies enable comparisons to standard therapies, establishment of new indications and are required to establish many adverse reactions to drugs.
- Evidence-based medicine seeks to identify the available evidence to answer specific clinical questions, critically appraise it and apply it to individual patients or to populations.
- There are several organizations in the UK providing evaluated evidence of the efficacy, safety and economy of medicines.
- Drug utilization review (DUR) assesses the patterns of drug use in particular clinical situations.
- Drug use evaluation (DUE) relates drug use to patient outcome.
- Methods for studying DUR and DUE include the use of drug purchase records, drug issue records, prescription records, medical records and specifically designed recording systems.
- Patient questionnaire methods can provide useful information about the use of non-prescription drugs.

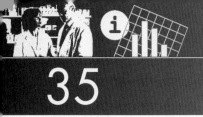

35

Pharmacoeconomics

J. Silcock

After studying this chapter you will be able to:

Define economic evaluation and the concepts of scarcity, choice and opportunity cost

Describe some methods of economic evaluation and their application to practical health care decision making

List common methodological errors made in the conduct of economic evaluations

Understand and critique economic arguments about the use of medicines and pharmacy services

Conduct economic evaluations

Have an awareness of some advanced aspects of evaluation including discounting, sensitivity analysis and models for decision analysis

Introduction

Pharmacoeconomics can be described as the application of economic evaluation to medicines and pharmacy services. Economic evaluation is the comparative analysis of alternative courses of action (interventions) in terms of their costs and consequences. For economic evaluation to be valid:

- Two or more interventions are considered simultaneously, but this may include placebo, best current practice, 'do nothing' or 'watchful waiting'.
- All the active interventions considered must be clinically effective.
- Costs and consequences must each be identified, measured and valued.

Costs in this case are not 'disadvantages' or 'adverse events', they are items of resource that are used or saved. Consequences are health effects, e.g. blood pressure, stroke incidence, mortality or quality of life. Cost data may be collected prospectively alongside a clinical study (primary evaluation) or retrospectively to combine with previously published clinical data (secondary evaluation).

Four general methods of economic evaluation are described in detail and examples relevant to pharmacy are given. However, economic evaluation can be costly, time consuming and hard to understand. A step back is appropriate to consider basic economic principles and the fundamental need for economic evaluation.

BASIC ECONOMIC PRINCIPLES

Scarcity and choice

Resources such as land, labour and equipment are scarce (finite) compared to their possible uses, which are infinite. Therefore, no person or organization is capable of achieving all the good things that they desire and some hard choices must be made. These choices may concern the fundamental direction of a person's career or an organization's responsibilities. They may also be more mundane choices about how best to achieve a particular goal. For a person their salary is one measure of the resources available to them. They might not be able to afford both a new car and an exotic holiday, but must choose which they would get the most pleasure (utility) from. Alternatively, they may get a loan (borrowing from their future income) so that they can enjoy themselves today and pay tomorrow. An organization, like a hospital or primary care trust, has a budget to fund new and existing activities. Periodically, the use of this budget should be reviewed to make sure that patients' health gains from the mix of activities are maximized. Decision-makers should be mainly interested in clinical effectiveness and value for money, but they may have other concerns such as legal restrictions, policy guidance and public relations.

Opportunity cost

When we make choices about personal or workplace activities we usually spend money to engage appropriate resources. Resources are used up in the production of goods and services. Money itself is not a resource, but it is a store of value, a measuring tool and a means of exchange. To consider the amount of money spent the 'cost' of our decision is a little narrow-minded. Economists would argue that the true cost (opportunity cost) of an activity is the utility from other activities that we can no longer afford. Thus, the opportunity cost of a person's car is not £10 000, but might be the pleasure of 2 weeks on an exclusive tropical holiday island which was not taken. Similarly, the opportunity costs of one hip operation might be two coronary artery bypass grafts not performed. Acting to minimize opportunity cost, therefore, ensures that the utility we do obtain from using resources in a particular way is maximized. We call this efficiency, which is of two types: technical and allocative.

- Technical efficiency is about achieving particular goals on a fixed scale in the most appropriate way, e.g. comparing a range of interventions, including medicines and lifestyle changes, within a programme to reduce blood pressure.
- Allocative efficiency is concerned with choosing the right goals in the first place (e.g. coronary heart disease prevention or treating lung cancer) and the most appropriate scale for a health care programme.

Changing the scale of a health care programme might involve treating more people or treating the same people more intensively. The scale of a health care programme is normally limited by the allocated budget. Therefore, if the scale of a health care programme increases, then more resources must be found from elsewhere in the health care system or wider economy. Changes in the scale of a health care programme should be informed by an appropriate method of economic evaluation.

Few diseases are left completely untreated (because it would not be fair or equitable) but normally efficiency demands that most of our scarce resources are used to maximize health gains for the greatest number of people. This philosophy is called utilitarianism. If people whose health status cannot be improved by health care are treated, then there are fewer resources to help those who can benefit.

Supply and demand

Most people wouldn't consciously consider 'minimizing opportunity cost' in their everyday lives. But they would usually try to get the most utility from the smallest amount of expenditure—which is the same thing more simply expressed. The price of goods and their availability are relied on as indicators of quality and desirability. The price mechanism for allocating resources works well if there are many buyers and sellers, each with similar accurate information about the goods and services on offer. After purchase consumers can usually decide if their prior judgments about value for money were correct and if not alter future decisions accordingly. The role of price in controlling supply (from producers) and demand (from consumers) was described by Adam Smith (an 18th-century founder of classic economic theory) as an 'invisible hand' that guides our decisions. However, the market for health care (unlike that for cars and package holidays) doesn't work very well. The reasons for this include:

- Health is demanded but cannot be directly provided.
- The link between health care and improvements in health is uncertain.
- We don't know when we will be ill.
- Providers of health care have more information than consumers.
- Insurance companies or governments often pay for healthcare—not consumers.

Compare the nature of the market for health care with something simple like the market for apples:

- You can buy an apple rather than a machine or service that makes one.
- It is easy to judge the quality of the apple you buy both before and after purchase.
- You might know that you wish to eat an apple every day—to keep the doctor away!
- If you eat a bad apple you can avoid that variety or the seller in future.
- You usually pay for the apple directly—and bear the opportunity cost of purchase, perhaps the orange that you can no longer afford.

When normal markets don't work well economic evaluation can step in as a substitute for price or a 'visible hand' to assist decision-makers. The costs measured and valued in economic evaluation are analogous to the costs of production for a normal good or service. The consequences measured and valued in economic evaluation are analogous to the utility consumers enjoy when using a normal good or service.

METHODS OF ECONOMIC EVALUATION

The basic steps in all economic evaluations are:

- Clarify the economic question, with particular regard to technical or allocative efficiency and list the interventions that will be compared.
- Obtain the best clinical and economic evidence possible.
- Identify and carry out the simplest form of evaluation that is capable of answering the economic question.
- Identify the key variables that influence the results of the evaluation and test the influence of any assumptions or guesswork.
- Present the results clearly and in a form that decision-makers may easily adapt to suit local circumstances.

All the techniques of economic evaluation involve an explicit consideration and calculation of resource use, to ensure that health care expenditure has the maximum possible impact on health status. However, each method of evaluation handles consequences (or health effects) differently.

Because the methods differ in the way that they handle information about clinical effectiveness, some people think the available health effect data determines the method of evaluation. In fact the most suitable method depends crucially on the type of efficiency question being asked (Table 35.1).

Principles of costing

The viewpoint (perspective) of an economic evaluation determines the breadth of cost identification. Typical viewpoints are: a single health care organization, the whole health care system and society. For the same set of interventions, taking a different viewpoint can result in radically different economic conclusions. To give an example, the health system costs of warfarin monitoring do not vary much between large laboratories and local doctors' surgeries. However, patients' travel costs vary considerably. Resources used directly in health care interventions may include:

- Skilled workers, e.g. doctors, nurses and pharmacists
- Equipment, e.g. computers, medical scanners and beds
- Space in which to work including heat, light and rent
- Consumables, e.g. medicines, syringes and dressings.

If available, market prices are used to value these resources, e.g. wage rates and manufacturers' list prices. However, value added tax (VAT) is excluded because it is a 'transfer payment'. That is, it goes directly to the government without buying or using up any resources. Wages rates would be the total employers' costs (adjusted for holidays and hours worked) not the workers' take-home pay. For a typical health care intervention we might expect wages to account for 70% of costs and medicines a further 10%. Medicines might be valued using manufacturers' list prices or hospital contract prices, depending on the perspective taken.

Costs borne outside the health care system (e.g. by patients and carers, or in other sectors of the economy like social care) may be less likely to have accepted and accessible market prices. Voluntary care costs, for example, might be valued using an average societal wage rate. Patients' public transport costs would be clear enough, but for car travel an appropriate mileage rate needs to be agreed or calculated. The productivity of patients going back to work should normally be excluded from costings. This is because any gains or losses in productivity flow from health status changes, which will be separately valued.

When identifying costs for groups of interventions that will be compared, any costs that are identical for all interventions may be safely ignored. This is because economists are more interested in marginal costs (differences or changes in cost) than average costs (total costs of production). It is the costs of change and the differences between alternative interventions that are most relevant for practical and effective decision-making.

Table 35.1	Choosing a method of economic evaluation			
Method	**Efficiency question**	**Budget**	**Scope**	**Outcomes**
CMA	Technical	Fixed	Single service	Identical
CEA	Technical	Fixed	One speciality	Unidimensional
CUA	Technical or allocative	Fixed or open	Health service	QALYs
CBA	Allocative	Open	Whole economy	Money value

Health care interventions often incur costs over a number of years and the duration of two alternative interventions may be different. So timing is an important factor in many costings and is accounted for in a number of ways. Firstly, all costs are counted in a base year, usually the first year of the intervention. Costs are not inflated to account for price rises over the course of the interventions. This ensures that all costs reflect real resource use and not nominal monetary values. Secondly, future costs are 'discounted' back to the base year. In general terms, this reflects a preference to put off costs rather than pay straightway. The rationale and principles are not easy to describe concisely, but to give a practical example £1000 spent in year 1 is considered to be worth about £952 in year 2 and £907 in year 3. Thirdly, capital costs (durable equipment) are apportioned over the lifetime of the equipment. For example, the 'equivalent annual cost' of a piece of equipment purchased for £500 and lasting 5 years is approximately £115. This allows a fair comparison of inventions with different levels of up-front and recurring costs.

Discount rates (5% in the above examples), discount factors and equivalent annual costs are influenced by economic theory and government guidance. They are usually given in special tables but may also be calculated from first principles. Costs from past economic evaluations or other countries cannot be applied today or in the UK without some adjustment. This is most easily achieved if the original evaluator lists all the costs identified and the number of resource units used. The total value of costs can then be easily recalculated to reflect current local circumstances.

Whether consequences that occur in the future should be discounted like costs is open to debate. In practice, consequences are rarely discounted but in theory they probably should be. Without consistent discounting it is particularly hard to fairly compare health promotion interventions (with up-front costs and far-off consequences) with normal clinical treatments.

Cost-minimization analysis

Cost-minimization analysis (CMA) is the simplest, most straightforward and least expensive form of economic evaluation. It is conducted according to the principles of costing outlined above and is appropriate when:

- Two or more interventions have been shown to have exactly the same health effects.
- The budget for producing these health effects has been granted and is fixed

This is a question of technical efficiency and the intervention that costs the least is usually preferred because spare resources can be used to treat more patients or be reallocated to other programmes. Choosing a more expensive option must be justified because using additional resources to achieve the same outcome takes resources away from other programmes where they might achieve something positive.

Lowson, Drummond and Bishop (1981) compared different methods for providing domiciliary oxygen using CMA. The effectiveness of oxygen was considered the same whether provided in cylinders or by concentrator (see Ch. 30). Concentrators were cheaper for most patients despite high purchase and maintenance costs, but this result was sensitive to the number of patients in an area who needed therapy. Malek (1996) used CMA to investigate glyceryl trinitrate spray provided in transparent and opaque canisters. Transparent canisters were found to be cheaper overall because patients knew exactly when to replace them.

CMA might also be used to compare branded and generic medicines, or different formulations of the same medicine, but its practical applications are fairly limited.

Cost-effectiveness analysis

Cost-effectiveness analysis (CEA) is the most commonly used type of economic evaluation for medicines. It is appropriate when:

- The health effects of two or more interventions are not identical but are measured in the same units, e.g. mmHg (blood pressure) or mmol/L (cholesterol).
- The budget for producing these health effects has been granted and is fixed.

This is a question of technical efficiency and is often appropriate within a particular health care programme, e.g. alternative interventions all designed to reduce myocardial infarction and stroke. However, CEA can only deal with one aspect of quantity or quality of life at a time. Each intervention has an average cost–consequence ratio. The differences between interventions listed in increasing order of cost are expressed as incremental cost–consequence ratios or 'incremental cost–effectiveness ratios' (ICERs). The ICER, rather than the average cost–consequence ratio, should be the main guide to decision-making.

A study has compared the cost-effectiveness of intensive pharmaceutical intervention in assisting people to stop smoking (Sinclair et al 1999). In a randomized controlled trial the control was normal practice and the intervention involved intensive support incorporating stage of change assessment and follow up. The main economic results are summarized in Table 35.2. The average cost per quitter was £743 in the control group and £573 in the intervention group. However, the change from current practice to new practice is of most economic interest and the incremental cost per quitter was £300. In this case, the incremental cost–consequence ratio is calculated as follows:

Cost (intensive) – Cost (normal) = Change (cost)
Consequence (intensive) – Consequence (normal)
    = Change (consequence)
Incremental cost–consequence ratio
    = Change (cost)/Change (consequence)

This is important because the ICER always more clearly identifies the implications of a particular decision. In this case, since the normal service is already provided and incurs some costs, the extra costs of providing the new service are reduced compared to its average costs. This makes the change to intensive counselling more desirable.

CEA is the most widely used type of economic evaluation and is often relevant when adding an economic component to a randomized controlled trail (RCT). The consequences used in CEA are always naturally occurring units. Some other examples include: accidents prevented, falls, death, stroke and myocardial infarction. These measures are often clinical indicators or intermediate outcomes, e.g. blood pressure reduction is a predictor of subsequent effects such as stroke and health-related quality of life (HRQoL).

The use of clinical indicators can be problematical, not least because the choice of indicator critically affects the results of an evaluation. It is not unknown for researchers to perform several analyses using different indicators and publish the set of results that is most favourable to a new intervention. The most appropriate indicator or outcome should be chosen before a study commences. This caveat also applies to purely clinical studies.

The most effective intervention can also be the cheapest. This is said to dominate more expensive and less effective interventions, making an ICER meaningless. Without prior knowledge of likely costs and consequences it is often difficult to know which method of economic evaluation (if any) will be most appropriate.

Cost-utility analysis

Cost-utility analysis (CUA) is a useful form of economic evaluation but more difficult to perform than either CMA or CEA. It is appropriate when:

- The health effects of two or more alternatives can be measured in terms of overall impact on quality and quantity of life.
- The budget for producing these health effects has been granted and is flexible.
- A budget has yet to be granted and a sensible allocation must be decided.

CUA is a special form of CEA in which the consequences are quality adjusted life years (QALYs). QALYs are calculated by multiplying years of survival in a health state by a 'health state utility' that indicates its quality. The utility value is 0 for 'dead' and 1 for 'full health'. Surveys have determined intermediate values for typical health states. A patient's particular health state may match one already valued or a patient may self-assess their health state using a simple instrument.

The advantage of the QALY is that it incorporates quality and quantity of life in a way that allows comparison of interventions from different clinical areas; e.g. nurse-led asthma clinics and domiciliary visits by pharmacists to improve compliance in older people. By contrast, the consequences in CEA measure only quality or quantity, they are unidimensional, in a single clinical area. This means that CUA can answers questions of technical efficiency and allocative efficiency within the health sector.

Imagine that Figure 35.1 illustrates the impact of low-dose and high-dose drug treatment for a disease, that no

Table 35.2	Cost-effectiveness of smoking cessation counselling (per 100 service users)					
	Cost*	No. of quitters	Cost per quitter*	Extra cost*	Extra quitters	Incremental cost per quitter
Normal	5495	7.4	743	-	-	–
Intensive	6874	12	573	1378	4.6	300*
* Cost in pounds sterling 1995 prices.						

Table 35.3	Illustration of costs per QALY			
	Cost per QALY	QALYs	Average cost per QALY	Incremental cost per QALY
No treatment	0	0	–	–
Current treatment	1000	1	1000	1000
Low dose	5000	6	833	800
High dose	10 000	7.2	1389	4167

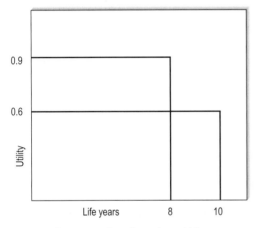

Fig. 35.1   Illustration of quality adjusted life years.

treatment leads to immediate death and that current best practice allows 2 years of life at a health status utility of 0.5. The impact of the treatment options on cost per QALY is shown in Table 35.3. Given this data, there is a good case for implementing low-dose treatment, if it can be done within the current budget. Its incremental cost per QALY is lower than the average cost per QALY of current treatment. Whether high-dose treatment should be implemented or not presents a more difficult issue. The incremental cost per QALY shows significant movement and the overall budget is more likely to increase. So our decision depends on a judgment about whether £4167 is a reasonable cost per QALY. One way to do this is by comparison with published cost per QALY league tables (Table 35.4).

A practical decision might involve the treatment of hyper-cholesterolaemia by diet or drugs. Obviously, people with the highest levels of cholesterol benefit most from treatment. Therefore, as drug use is extended to people with lower cholesterol the marginal consequences decrease. The con-sequences may be valued in life years gained (in CEA) or

QALYs (in CUA). A decrease in marginal consequences leads to an increase in the incremental cost–consequence ratio (i.e. the treatment becomes less cost-effective). Economics doesn't tell us when to stop expanding drug use, but does allow the implications to be assessed.

Cost-benefit analysis

Cost-benefit analysis (CBA) is the least common economic evaluation of health care. It is appropriate when:

- The welfare effects of two or more alternatives can be expressed as a global willingness to pay.
- A budget has yet to be granted and a sensible allocation between different sectors of the economy must be decided.

In CBA consequences are valued using monetary units, which reflect the value of health status improvement and not the cost of health care. The alternative that offers the largest net consequence (value of consequences minus costs) is preferred. This technique can answer questions concerning allocative efficiency across the whole economy. In principle at least, the largest net consequence rule can help us decide whether to build a new hospital or a new road.

Table 35.4 Examples of incremental cost per QALY. (Selected from Briggs & Gray 2000)	
Intervention	**Cost per QALY***
Pacemaker for atrioventricular block	700
Kidney transplantation (cadaver)	3000
Heart transplantation	5000
Haemodialysis at home	11 000
Haemodialysis at hospital	14 000
* Cost in pounds sterling.	

There are three ways to place a monetary value on consequences: implied values, the human capital approach and willingness-to-pay. Implied values are taken from insurance companies, court awards for accidents or risk premiums we pay people to do dangerous jobs. For example, travel insurance companies may state how much they will pay for the loss of an eye or limb, and these values could be applied to the consequences of ophthalmic and vascular surgery respectively. Although implied values are one way to put a publicly acceptable monetary value on health effects, they do not exist for all possible consequences, may not be adjusted regularly and may be unpredictable.

The human capital approach places a value on human life that is equivalent to an individual's future income stream. This has the disadvantage of judging that the life of a managing director is worth more than that of a shop floor worker. This is unpalatable for most health care professionals and not widely applied. However, surveys do suggest that the general public value the lives of the very young and old less highly than the lives of productive workers with families. It has also been suggested that traditional societies tend to sacrifice weaker members first in times of hardship.

Willingness-to-pay (WTP) is the preferred way to place a monetary value on consequences. WTP surveys require good descriptions of interventions and associated health effects, which are presented to disease sufferers or the general public. After reading the description people are asked for a monetary valuation of the scenario, which may incorporate preferences about the method of treatment, information provided by medical tests and actual clinical outcome. The willingness-to-pay question may be open ended with no suggested values or may ask the person to choose from one value in a range.

In practice, people tend to have difficulty distinguishing the concepts of 'cost of production' and 'value in use'. Therefore, they often place a higher value on the things that apparently cost the most (in resource terms), rather than those things that they would prefer to have. In the UK, with its tradition of free health care, people also tend to treat WTP questions with some mistrust. In all societies we might be concerned that WTP is related to income or ability to pay (ATP). The relationship between WTP and ATP will only produce a biased evaluation if the health state preferences of rich and poor people are different.

A few useful CBAs do exist in the medical literature, but the term cost-benefit analysis is sometimes used in a general way to describe any form of economic evaluation. WTP may be a useful technique for valuing pharmacy services, par-ticularly when the health effects on many individuals are small or hard to describe. By contrast, the effects of open heart surgery, which has a major impact on a few people, are easy to describe and evaluate. WTP also allows people to put a value on the process of care not just its outcomes, e.g. the consequences of fetal ultrasound pictures and unsuccessful cycles of IVF.

MODELLING AND SENSITIVITY ANALYSIS

A lack of cost and consequences data for many complicated health care interventions presents the analyst with problems. Sometimes this can be resolved using clinical and economic modelling, the most common types being decision trees and Markov models.

A decision tree maps out the alternatives being compared in as much detail as possible. Figure 35.2 shows the start of one possible tree, outlining options for the treatment of dyspepsia. Cooke (1999) has produced some simple decision trees related to clinical pharmacy. Usually the decision tree starts with a decision node (by convention a square). This is because most health care starts with a decision about whether one alternative or another is the most appropriate course of action. Subsequent probability nodes (by convention circles) show the chances of each possible consequence occurring. At each probability node the sum of probabilities is 1, that is, a 100% chance that something will happen.

A range of interventions and their possible consequences can be mapped out clearly in a decision tree. Once the options are clear, probabilities can be attached to them either using new trial data or information from the existing

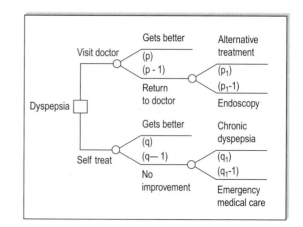

Fig. 35.2 Example of a decision tree.

literature. For each option we may also identify and state costs. At the end of each route through the decision tree there should also be a terminal node (by convention a triangle) associated with a final outcome. Taken together these steps mean that a cost–consequence ratio for each initial decision can be calculated and easily adjusted when new information becomes available. Computer software to help draw and analyse decision trees makes their use particularly attractive for sensitivity analysis and the comparison of three or more interventions.

Sensitivity analysis is the act of changing assumptions about the value or probability of costs and consequences, to determine whether or not the results of an evaluation are sensitive to such changes. Even without the help of a decision tree or computer software, evaluators should highlight any assumptions they make about costs and consequences, and list the key variables that influence their recommendations.

Markov models are helpful, when decision trees are not sufficient, for complex interventions and chronic diseases where the same decisions recur constantly. A disease is divided into health states (e.g. good health, bad health, death) and during a chosen period of time each individual is given a probability of moving from one state to another. Estimates of resource use and health effects are also attached to each state and transition. The model is then cycled to produce long-term estimates of cost-effectiveness in hypothetical patient cohorts.

Many health care professionals are distrustful of modelling and hypothetical data. However, in some cases it is the best information we have. These techniques should not be rejected out of hand, but instead questions asked about the assumptions made to produce the model and the accuracy of typical clinical scenarios. Better information is better than nothing at all and modelling can be a great deal better than a badly designed trial.

APPRAISING ECONOMIC EVALUATIONS

Economic evaluations are produced mainly by: academic health economists, pharmaceutical companies (marketing and R&D staff) and health care professionals. This complicates the appraisal of published studies. Health economists produce the most robust evaluations, but their methods are likely to be the most complex and hard to understand.

Evaluations from pharmaceutical companies need to be appraised carefully to ensure objectivity, particularly when marketing staff are involved. Health care professionals are likely to focus on realistic practical problems, but may be less familiar with good evaluation practice. Additionally, there are national differences in the conduct of evaluations with US researchers more likely to focus on costs than consequences.

Overall the quality of published economic evaluations in the medical and pharmacy literature is disappointing but improving. Just as with clinical literature, methodological details require close examination to ensure the validity of the results for local decision-making. However, as experience of economic evaluation has grown, journal editors have been able to identify better reviewers and apply more stringent methodological criteria that are widely accepted.

An assessment of internal validity (evaluation quality) involves, among other things, answers to the following questions:

- Is the study well designed and executed?
- Do I trust the authors and place of publication?
- Are the conclusions clear?
- Are the conclusions consistent with my interpretation of the results?

There is less agreement about the assessment of external validity, or the practical usefulness of evaluations. Evaluators can help by adopting the decision-maker's perspective, and questions to ask could include:

- Are the interventions considered realistic? (local or best practice)
- Are my patients like those in the study? (age, sex, deprivation)
- If true, are the results important? (clinically and economically)
- Can I implement the recommendations within available budgets?

It is also important to ensure that any current treatment strategies are optimized, since it may be better to ensure best current practice before moving further on. If an evaluation promises savings from the adoption of a new intervention, then local assessment is needed to see if these can actually be achieved. Evaluators don't necessarily have all the answers and local decision-makers or clinicians may be able to devise more efficient ways to improve health outcomes.

CONCLUSION

Economics may be simply described as the science of choice. Economic evaluation usually tries to give decision-makers better information about the implications of choices that they make. Sometimes we talk about priority setting in health care (or 'rationing') as if it's a bad thing, but choices are inevitable and it is better for them to be informed. Pharmacists may need to conduct economic evaluations and certainly need to understand them.

> **Key points**
>
> - Pharmacoeconomics applies the principles of economic evaluation to pharmacy.
> - Some of the basic economic concepts are scarcity, choice and opportunity cost which can be applied to the medical field.
> - There are recognized steps in carrying out any economic evaluation.
> - Application of the principles of costing may be straightforward but can be difficult, especially when applying 'discount'.
> - Cost-minimization analysis (CMA) is applied when outcomes are the same and relative cost is the variation.
> - Cost-effectiveness analysis (CEA) is applied when both outcomes and cost can vary and is frequently applied in pharmacy and medicine.
> - Cost-utility analysis (CUA) involves the concept of quality of life to assist in informing resource allocation.
> - Cost-benefit analysis (CBA) is complex, but should allow informed resource allocation within the whole economy, not just in health.
> - CBA may use implied values, human capital or willingness-to-pay methods.
> - To accommodate decision-taking in health care, modelling and sensitivity analysis methods can be used.
> - Any published pharmacoeconomic analysis requires careful appraisal to ensure the internal and external validity.

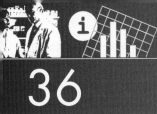

36

Formularies and guidelines

J. Krska

After studying this chapter you will know about:

Definitions of formularies and guidelines
The development and structure of formularies
Benefits of formularies and guidelines
Formulary development
Formulary management systems
The use of prescribing data in formulary development and management
Guideline development and use
Changing practice
Auditing performance

Table 36.1 Examples of formularies

Purpose	Example formulary
General use	British National Formulary
Hospital formulary	Dundee Teaching Hospitals Trust Drug Formulary
General practice	Practice Formulary (Royal College of General Practitioners, Northern Ireland Faculty)
Joint formulary	Grampian Joint Formulary
Nurse prescribers	Nurse Practitioners' Formulary
Dentists	Dental Practitioners' Formulary
Developing countries	WHO essential drugs list

Definitions

The modern definition of a formulary is a list of drugs which are recommended or approved for use by a group of practitioners. It is compiled by members of the group and is regularly revised. Drugs are usually selected for inclusion on the basis of efficacy, safety, patient acceptability and cost. Drugs listed in a formulary should be available for use. Information on dosage, indications, side-effects, contraindications, formulations and costs may also be included. An introduction, giving information on how the drugs were selected, by whom and how to use the formulary is usually provided. Some examples of useful formularies are given in Table 36.1.

A formulary may be thought of as a prescribing policy, because it lists which drugs are recommended. Prescribing policies should, however, be much more detailed than a formulary, giving details of drugs which should be selected for use in specific medical conditions. Examples of prescribing policies in common use are antibiotic policies, head lice eradication policies and malarial prophylaxis policies.

A guideline contains more detailed information derived from research or expert opinions about how a service should be delivered or patients treated. Some examples of practice guidelines which apply to pharmacists are those on counselling and advice on medicines and appliances in community pharmacy practice and those for clinical pharmacy practice in hospital and primary care. A clinical guideline is a series of systematically developed statements to assist practitioner and patient decisions about appropriate health care for specific clinical circumstances. There are many clinical guidelines available. Some are developed nationally, such as by the Scottish Intercollegiate Guidelines Network (SIGN), British Thoracic Society, British Society for Haematology and so on. Others are developed by smaller groups such as Area Drug and Therapeutics Committees.

BENEFITS OF FORMULARIES AND GUIDELINES

Drug costs are a major component of the total cost of the NHS and are constantly rising. As the resources of the NHS are finite, it becomes increasingly necessary to contain the escalation in drug costs. A lot of evidence has accumulated to show that drugs are not always prescribed appropriately. Therefore some of the expenditure on drugs could be reduced if prescribing were improved. Formularies, which recommend specific drugs and exclude others, are one means by which this can be achieved. Prescribing policies assist prescribers in using the drugs in a formulary and specific treatment protocols make them even more useful. Clinical guidelines help to ensure that the treatment of patients is based on evidence of best practice. Used together, formularies, clinical guidelines and treatment protocols can ensure that standards of prescribing are both uniform and high quality. All these are tools used to promote rational and cost-effective prescribing.

Rational prescribing

Prescribing which is based on the four important factors of efficacy, safety, patient acceptability and cost should be rational. While there may be many drugs available to treat any particular condition, the process of selecting the most appropriate one for any individual patient should take account of all these factors, plus patient factors, such as concurrent diseases, drugs, previous exposure and outcomes. The four factors can also be applied to selection of drugs to treat populations of patients and it is for this situation that formularies and guidelines are developed. Providing drug selection is based on good quality evidence of efficacy and toxicity, formularies and guidelines then assist in making decisions regarding individual patients.

Cost-effective prescribing

Formularies often provide information on the cost of products to help users to become cost-conscious. Local formularies usually include only a small proportion of the drugs listed in the *British National Formulary* (BNF), often between 200 and 500. If prescribers only use the range of drugs included in a local formulary, the range stocked by pharmacies can decrease, which reduces unnecessary outlay. Using a restricted range of drugs may allow pharmacists to buy in bulk those which are prescribed, further reducing costs. Formularies also encourage generic prescribing which, for some drugs, may reduce costs even further. If fewer products are stocked, monitoring of expiry dates becomes easier and cash flow may improve. Any money saved on hospital or on GPs' budgets by using a formulary may be used in other ways to benefit patients. For example, there is good evidence that many patients would benefit from receiving

lipid-lowering therapy. In a cash-limited budget, the cost of this prescribing could be offset by reducing prescribing of drugs for which there is little evidence of efficacy, such as peripheral vasodilators. Recommending the use of more cost-effective alternatives to some expensive modified-release formulations is another way in which formularies can give guidance on what to prescribe to reduce expenditure. In addition, as safety is also a key factor in drug selection, formularies may contribute to reducing the incidence of adverse drug reactions, which often carries a high cost.

Educational value

Compilation of a formulary or guideline involves researching the literature to gather evidence of efficacy and toxicity. For those involved this is a highly demanding task, but one which results in a great deal of educational benefit. For users of formularies and guidelines, there are also benefits. Prescribers who use a restricted range of drugs should know more about those drugs and their formulations through frequent use. Those who use guidelines will become familiar with the current evidence of what is best practice. There are also benefits for the patient, as prescribers' increased knowledge should reduce the risk of inappropriate prescribing, which could have led to adverse effects, interactions or lack of efficacy. Many guidelines are available to patients directly and allow them to become involved in managing their conditions in line with best practice.

Continuous care

A local formulary which has been compiled by prescribers and pharmacists in both primary and secondary care results in the same range of drugs being prescribed whether patients are at home or in hospital. This makes continuing drug treatment easier. As patient packs become increasingly available, patients may be more likely to use their own drugs during a hospital stay. A joint formulary helps this, as there is less chance of drug therapy having to change to comply with a different formulary on admission to hospital. Similarly guidelines which apply to both primary and secondary care ensure that the same standard treatments are used, whatever the setting.

FORMULARY DEVELOPMENT

Formularies take a very long time to produce; a period of several years is not uncommon. Obtaining everyone's opinions and discussing the drugs to be included is the main reason for this prolonged time. A formulary then needs to be updated regularly if it is going to be useful, which is a further time commitment. There are two basic ways of producing a new formulary; either start from scratch or modify an existing one. Adapting another formulary to suit local needs is much less time consuming than starting from scratch. Although much can be learned from looking at someone else's formulary, simply deciding to adopt it without any changes is not a good idea. Producing a formulary is an educational process, during which all concerned learn from each other's experience and update their clinical pharmacology and therapeutics along the way. Producing a formulary brings a sense of ownership, which encourages commitment to it and increases the chance of it being used. Local needs should also be addressed by a local formulary, so copying someone else's may not be satisfactory.

Many local formularies are produced by Area Drug and Therapeutic Committees (ADTCs). These include senior professionals and managers from both primary and secondary care, including pharmacists. While small subgroups of local experts may do most of the work, the opinions of potential users should also be sought. This is a very important point in formulary development. The people expected to use a formulary must have the opportunity to give their views on its content. If their opinions are not asked, they may feel that it does not apply to them and will be less likely to use it. Small formularies, such as that for one general medical practice, should involve all the prescribers in that practice with a pharmacist. These may draw on the work of ADTCs.

Content

The formulary should start with an introduction, giving the names of those who have compiled it, stating who is expected to use it and explaining its format. It is important to state whether all the drugs included are recommended for all users and if not, how different recommendations can be distinguished. The BNF, for example, lists drugs the Joint Formulary Committee considers less suitable for prescribing in small type. Local formularies may choose to place restrictions on some drugs, for use by specialists only, for certain indications or in certain locations only. These drugs should be easily distinguishable from the others in the formulary. A list of contents and an index should be included to make the formulary easy to use.

Most formularies follow the BNF, listing their drugs in the same order and by therapeutic indication or pharmacological class. Reference to the relevant BNF section is helpful if a local formulary is designed to be used in conjunction with the BNF. Users can be directed to read the monographs there for information on dosage, indications, side-effects, contraindications and precautions. Some formularies include all this information, but only for the recommended drugs. Other important information which may be given is drug costs and the reasons for selection of the drugs included.

Drug costs are one of the factors taken into account when compiling a formulary (see below). The price of a drug can be expressed in several different ways. The prices given in the BNF are the prices of different pack sizes or for 20 doses of generics at Drug Tariff prices. The cost of a period of treatment may be more useful if comparisons are being encouraged. A suitable period may be 1 day, 1 month (28 days) or a standard course of treatment (e.g. 5 days for antibiotics). Since the price of the drug usually varies with the pack size, this may not be as easy to calculate as it first appears. A further complicating factor is the differing prices in hospital and community. If a formulary is designed to be used in hospital only, the hospital price may seem most relevant. However, the price of the drug may be different in general practice and patients may take the drug while living in the community for much longer than they take it in hospital. Therefore the price in community is also of relevance, especially in joint formularies.

When large numbers of prescribers are to use a formulary, it is possible that not all of them will have been consulted about its content. If that is the case, providing explanations of how drugs have come to be included in a formulary is of particular importance. Many formularies state the general basis of drug selection as being efficacy, safety, patient acceptability and cost. Sometimes additional information is given about specific drugs. The BNF gives this type of information in introductory paragraphs to each section. An example is that most other thiazides have no advantages over bendroflumethiazide (bendrofluazide), but are more expensive. It may be desirable to reference the formulary to give readers the opportunity to see the evidence on which statements such as these are based. It may also be useful to explain local preferences, particularly in the case of antibiotic selection, which should take local microbiological sensitivities into account.

Some or all of the formulary may be presented as prescribing policies. Again this is most likely for antibiotics, but may extend to any group of drugs. If this approach is taken, details of which drugs are to be used in specific medical conditions should be given. It may be necessary to include alternatives and the particular occasions when they should be used. In a prescribing policy, details of the recommended dosage, route and method of administration and duration of therapy should also be included.

A local formulary may have sections relating to prescribing in certain types of patients, such as the elderly, children, those with renal or hepatic impairment or in pregnancy and breastfeeding. As there is little point in reproducing the BNF, the content of these sections, if included, should be local recommendations, like the rest of the formulary.

Presentation

The appearance of a formulary is an indicator of the importance attached to it by those who have produced it. If it is presented on a few tattered sheets of paper, those who are expected to use it are unlikely to have a great deal of respect for its content. This may lead to poor adherence to its recommendations. It is therefore worth creating a document which is attractive and looks professionally produced.

The size of the formulary document should also be considered. Ideally, it should be pocket-sized, perhaps compatible in size with the BNF, to make it easy to use the two together. A large document which cannot be carried around is much less likely to be available when needed. This again may result in its recommendations being ignored. Ensuring that the formulary is up to date is extremely important and its presentation must allow for this. Loose-leaf binding will enable easy updating, but relies on everyone modifying their own copy.

The formulary should be easy to use, to encourage prescribers to refer to it when necessary. This will be helped by a contents list, which means the pages have to be numbered. Arranging the drugs in the same order as the BNF will also help to make the formulary easier to use, as prescribers should be familiar with this order. Using different typefaces and print size can make a formulary easier to use. Highlighting the drug names in some way can be useful, as often the name of the recommended drug may be all that someone is seeking (Fig. 36.1). Colour can add to the appearance of the formulary, but also adds to the cost. The cover of the formulary must be durable enough to withstand regular use, so should be of card rather than paper.

Increasingly local formularies are available in electronic form, as is the BNF. This makes them more attractive to prescribers who use computers and also makes studying adherence easier.

Selection of products for inclusion

It is important to decide at the outset the range of indications which the formulary should cover. Most hospital formularies

do not attempt to include drugs to treat all possible conditions. Some deliberately exclude certain drugs, such as those used in cancer chemotherapy and anaesthetics. These areas are extremely specialized, so drugs in these groups are never likely to be used by most prescribers. A formulary for use in general practice should aim to include enough drugs to treat between 80% and 90% of all common conditions which present to a GP. It is also useful to include emergency drugs, such as those which should be carried by GPs in their emergency bags. Clearly if a formulary includes all the available drugs, as does the BNF, it will not only be bulky, but also will not have many of the advantages that a local formulary can provide. It should be possible to cover most needs, either in hospital or general practice, with about 300–500 drugs. In selecting drugs for inclusion in a formulary, it is important to remember that recommendations are being made to treat the majority of the population. However, individual patients' needs and preferences should, where possible, be taken into account. This means that there may be individuals for whom the recommended formulary drug is not suitable, but the formulary should attempt to make provision for most commonly encountered situations. An example would be the inclusion of a histamine H_2 antagonist which does not inhibit cytochrome P450, to cover the situations when a patient is also taking a drug which is metabolized by this route.

As already stated, most formularies include drugs on the basis of efficacy, safety, patient acceptability and cost, but other factors are also usually considered. A list of factors which influence selection of drugs for inclusion is given in Box 36.1.

The most important factors are efficacy and toxicity. Drugs which are included in a formulary must be effective,

---

Box 36.1   Factors influencing selection of drugs for inclusion in a formulary

Efficacy for the indications to be included in the formulary

Side-effect profiles and contraindications of individual drugs

Interaction profiles of individual drugs

Pharmacokinetic profiles of individual drugs

Acceptability to patients—taste, appearance, ease of administration

Formulations available

General availability, including generic availability

Cost

Usage patterns

1.4 ANTIDIARRHOEAL DRUGS

CODEINE PHOSPHATE
LOPERAMIDE

Codeine phosphate (*tablets, solution*) is the cheapest, effective antidiarrhoeal. It is suitable for short-term use only because of the risk of CNS side-effects and dependence.

Loperamide (*capsules, mixture*) may be used as an adjunct to rehydration in acute diarrhoea and for chronic diarrhoea in adults. It is less likely to cause central side-effects than codeine but is more expensive. It is unlikely to cause dependence.

PRESCRIBING POINTS FOR ANTIDIARRHOEAL DRUGS

- Antibiotics should not be given for acute diarrhoea with the exception of metronidazole where giardia infection is confirmed.
- Diarrhoea may require fluid and electrolyte replacement. This is particularly important in infants and in frail or elderly patients. For oral rehydration preparations.
- Patients with chronic diarrhoea need individualised treatment including dietary manipulation as well as drug treatment and maintenance of a liberal fluid intake. This will depend on underlying diagnosis.
- Antidiarrhoeal drugs which reduce gastrointestinal motility should not be used in children.
- Antidiarrhoeal drugs should not be given to patients with acute colitis as they may cause toxic megacolon.
- Bulk-forming drugs, such as ispaghula are useful in controlling faecal consistency in ileostomy and colostomy patients, and in controlling diarrhoea associated with diverticular disease.
- Co-phenotrope (*proprietary name, Lomotil*) is **not recommended**. The combination of diphenoxylate hydrochloride and atropine frequently cause side-effects. Overdosage is particularly dangerous in children.

PAEDIATRIC NOTES — ANTIDIARRHOEAL DRUGS

Oral rehydration is the first line treatment for dehydration in children.
Antidiarrhoeal drugs should not be used to treat acute diarrhoea. In cases of chronic diarrhoea, infection should be excluded before antidiarrhoeal drugs are prescribed.
Loperamide is preferable to codeine. It is not licensed for use in children under 4 years old. It should not be used for acute infectious diarrhoea, long-term use should be managed under close medical supervision.
Preparations containing absorbents, such as **kaolin**, are not recommended.

GERIATRIC NOTES — ANTIDIARRHOEAL DRUGS

Acute or prolonged diarrhoea may require fluid replacement in frail and elderly patients.
Faecal impaction in the frail elderly can give rise to 'overflow' diarrhoea, and soiling. This should be excluded before antidiarrhoeals are started.

Fig. 36.1 Example of formulary recommendations, illustrating style of presentation (From Grampian Joint Formulary 1999, reproduced with permission, copyright Grampian Medicines Committee.)

for whatever indications they are to be used, with minimal toxicity. Evidence of efficacy should be based on well-conducted clinical trials, rather than anecdotal reports. Generally, prescribers' personal preferences are not a sound basis for selection of a particular drug or product. This is especially true when the formulary is to be used by many prescribers, as each may have his own preference.

Occasionally there may be a range of similar drugs from which to select, but not all are licensed for all the indications the formulary is to cover. An example is beta-adrenoceptor antagonists, some of which have a range of licensed indications (Table 36.2). In this situation, selection of the drug which covers most indications may be appropriate. Alternatively, separate drugs could be selected for different

Table 36.2   Using factors to select drugs for a formulary.

Factor	Examples of information to be taken into account	Examples of possible selection
Licensed indications OR Evidence of efficacy	For hypertension there are many to select from For arrhythmias, few are licensed For secondary prevention of myocardial infarction For heart failure	Atenolol, propranolol, metoprolol, etc. Sotalol Atenolol injection, metoprolol, propranolol Bisoprolol, carvedilol
Toxicity	Water solubility results in less nightmares Intrinsic sympathomimetic activity causes less cold extremities	Atenolol, sotalol Oxprenolol, pindolol
Contraindications	Cardioselectivity is preferable in asthma and diabetes	Atenolol, bisoprolol, metoprolol
Pharmacokinetic profile	Long-acting drugs/products require fewer doses	Atenolol, modified-release propranolol
Generic availability	Usually reduces cost	Atenolol, propranolol, metoprolol
Acceptability to patients	Once-daily doses, combination products may be useful	Atenolol, modified-release propranolol with thiazide diuretics for hypertension
Cost	Cheapest preferable if all other factors equal	Atenolol, propranolol, metoprolol

indications. This option results in difficulties when auditing performance, as it is impossible to tell from looking at prescribing data only whether the drug is prescribed in line with the formulary recommendations.

If two drugs are equally efficacious, as is often the case within a group of pharmacologically similar drugs, the one which is least toxic is preferable. In this situation, any differences between the drugs in terms of their pharmacokinetics, contraindications, adverse effects and potential for interaction become important.

A knowledge of the pharmacokinetic profile of drugs is important to enable selection of a drug with an optimum half-life for its indications. It is also essential to know whether drugs undergo hepatic metabolism, to make recommendations for patients with hepatic dysfunction. Similarly it is important to know about the effect of renal impairment on a drug's elimination. It may be possible to select drugs which are minimally affected by either liver or renal impairment. Among the benzodiazepine group, for example, those with short half-lives and which have no active metabolites are preferred as hypnotics, as they have no hangover effect.

Differences in drug handling in children and the elderly may require different drugs to be recommended for use with these patients. A knowledge of the passage of drugs into the placenta and secretion into breast milk will enable selection of drugs to be used in pregnancy and breastfeeding.

The range of contraindications, precautions and adverse effects may differ for drugs within a group from which a selection is being made. Often these are a drug class effect, but this is not always the case. Beta-adrenoceptor antagonists are a good example of a situation where there are differences between the individual drugs in the class. Differences are most often found in the frequency and severity of adverse effects between drugs in a class. Where possible, drugs should be selected which have the lowest frequency of, and least severe, adverse effects.

If drugs are similar in terms of efficacy and toxicity, but have different potential for interaction, this could be a deciding factor. Drugs with fewer possibilities of interaction mean fewer problems in use.

Patient acceptability is an important factor, which will be affected by efficacy and toxicity. If drugs do not work, or if they cause side-effects, patients are less likely to accept the need to take them. For orally administered drugs, palatability and ease of swallowing will contribute to acceptability. Other considerations may also be important, such as the extent to which a dispersible preparation actually disperses, or not being able to break a modified-release tablet in half. Inhaled drugs are available in many different formulations and their selection will depend to a large extent on what patients will or can use properly, to achieve maximum efficacy. For topical products, such as creams and ointments, patient acceptability is particularly important.

A local formulary may simply list drugs which are recommended or it may specify particular dosage forms of those drugs. Patient acceptability is likely to influence the different formulations selected for inclusion in a formulary more than the drug entities. However, the range of formulations available, which will in turn affect patients' acceptance of drug therapy, may be a factor in deciding which drugs to include. If a drug is available in a wide range of formulations, it may be a better choice than one which has very few. It is simpler for the prescriber to remember one drug name when a particular class of drug is required, rather than to worry about which drug he should prescribe based on the formulation needed.

Many formularies exclude all combination products on classical clinical pharmacological grounds. A combination product includes two or more drugs in fixed ratio. It is impossible to increase the dose of one drug without also increasing the dose of the other(s). Some patients may receive higher doses of one of the constituents than they require as a result. However, combination products are particularly favoured in general practice, where they are considered to improve patient compliance. A further factor is the need for patients to pay only one prescription charge for a condition for which they may be prescribed two drugs. Combination products are often used unnecessarily for these reasons. The products may be useful if the pharmacokinetic characteristics of the components are compatible. They can be used appropriately if the patient has been shown to require, and to obtain benefit from, all the components individually, in the same ratio as the combination product. Unfortunately, very few combination products are used in this way. Their inclusion in a formulary will depend very much on local preferences and appropriate use will subsequently depend on individual prescribers.

Cost considerations are also important, since the aim of a formulary is to encourage rational and cost-effective prescribing, not primarily to save money. Cost-effective prescribing involves the use of the drug with the lowest costs which is also effective, has minimal toxicity and is acceptable to patients. The cheapest drugs may not be the most acceptable, or of adequate efficacy. For some groups of drugs, prescribing costs may actually rise as a result of using a local formulary, since the optimum drugs may be the most expensive. However, where efficacy, toxicity and patient acceptability are equal, cost should be the deciding factor in drug selection. As described above, both hospital and community costs of drugs should be considered when selecting drugs for a hospital formulary, as the bulk of the cost is likely to be borne by GPs. The purchase price of a drug may not be the only factor to be taken into account when considering costs. Pharmacoeconomic evaluations which take account of the costs of the consequences of treatments may also be necessary.

Drugs to be included in a formulary should be easily available, so 'specials', drugs available in hospital only, or on a named patient basis, should be avoided. Generic availability is a bonus, as it usually means costs are lower than for drugs which are only available as branded formulations. Most formularies specify that prescribing should be generic, where appropriate. The use of computer systems for prescribing, which automatically change prescriptions to the appropriate generic name, increases the proportion of generic prescriptions considerably. This should also reduce costs.

Pharmacists have a key role to play in providing unbiased information about any differences in efficacy, toxicity and cost between drugs. One useful source of such information is the National Prescribing Centre in Liverpool or the Scottish Medicines Resource Centre in Edinburgh. *Drug and Therapeutics Bulletin*, which is published monthly, also provides good short summaries of trials of new drugs and considers their place in relation to existing therapies.

Use of prescribing data

All the factors mentioned so far are also applicable to the selection of drugs for individual patients. A further factor which is often considered when selecting drugs to include in a formulary is current prescribing habits. The main reason for this is that it is much easier to encourage use of a formulary if it involves few changes of habit. However, if the drugs found to be commonly prescribed are not efficacious, or have a high incidence or severity of toxicity, it is better not to include them. Just because a drug is often prescribed, it is not necessarily an appropriate choice for a formulary. Information about the drugs currently prescribed is obtainable for either hospital or general practice prescribers. In hospital, these data may relate to wards or to directorates and can be obtained from computerized pharmacy supply systems. In UK general practice, data are available as Prescribing Analysis and CosT (PACT) in England, Practice Audit Reports and Catalogues (PARC) in Wales, as Scottish Prescribing Analysis (SPA) in Scotland and as COMPASS (COMputerised on-line Prescribing Analysis for Science and Stewardship) in Northern Ireland. Prescribing data are generated by the Prescription Pricing Authority in England, the Health Common Services Agency in Wales, the Information and Statistics Division of the Common Services Agency in Scotland and the Central Services Agency in Northern Ireland. The data can identify prescribing by an individual GP or by a practice. Prescribing is compared to the average for the health authority or health board. Detailed data which are useful in compiling a formulary are obtainable from the PACT catalogue in England and SPA Level 2 in Scotland. Examples of these types of data are shown in Figures 36.2 and 36.3.

Prescribing data provide information about the frequency with which different drug products are prescribed. From this it is usually possible to identify one or two drugs within each group which account for the bulk of prescriptions for that class. These should usually be considered for inclusion in a formulary, as little change in prescribing habits will be needed if they are selected. As already stated, they should be efficacious and have minimal toxicity. It may be possible to include only these drugs in a formulary, or there may be a need for others to be included on a more restricted basis. If the commonly prescribed drugs are inappropriate on therapeutic grounds, an alternative may be required.

FORMULARY MANAGEMENT SYSTEMS

A formulary needs to be flexible and dynamic. A system must be devised which allows this. This is known as the formulary management system and it covers many different aspects of formularies which have not yet been mentioned.

Production, distribution and revision

Producing a formulary is a very time-consuming task which involves collecting together the data on which the drug selection will be based (published evidence, prescribing data and expert or all group members' opinions). Once the selection is made, the format of the material and the design of the final document must be considered. Thought is required as to who will need to have a copy, to help in deciding how best it

should be produced. Photocopying is cheapest for small numbers and can still incorporate colour and be attractively bound for a professional appearance. However, if large numbers are required, printing becomes more economical.

The method of distribution must also be considered if the formulary is to be used by large numbers of people. Mailing may be easiest and will require a covering letter, but hand delivery, with verbal explanation, may help to encourage interest and therefore adherence to a formulary's recommendations. Launching of a new formulary (or indeed a revision) can usefully be accompanied by a meeting to explain its aims, describe how to use it and encourage discussion of its contents.

After all the effort which goes into producing a new formulary has resulted in the final document, the thought of revising it is likely to be far from popular. However, because of the time taken to produce a new formulary, it will soon go out of date. If this is allowed to happen, respect for its content will decline. Adherence to its recommendations may follow suit. Revision should therefore be considered even before the formulary is finished. The BNF is revised every 6 months, but most local formularies cannot hope to achieve a similar frequency, because of the amount of work involved. Annual or biennial revision should be aimed at. This should be included as one of the aims when launching a new formulary. As new drugs are coming onto the market all the time, even 6-monthly revision will not be adequate to keep a formulary right up to date. Some system, therefore, needs to be devised to allow new drugs to be considered for inclusion.

Responding to the needs of practice

Change is the norm in the world of drugs. New drugs are constantly becoming available, old drugs are removed from the market, new clinical trials provide evidence for efficacy of existing drugs in novel indications and postmarketing surveillance provides constantly changing data on adverse effect profiles. An awareness of all the facts this generates is essential, so that the formulary does not go out of date and can respond to the changes. In implementing a formulary, patients must not be deprived of the benefits of new information and drugs. There will also inevitably be an occasional need for patients to receive treatment outwith a formulary's recommendations, since a formulary cannot be expected to cover all possible situations. Methods are therefore needed to allow drugs to be considered for inclusion in the formulary, to allow drugs to be removed from the formulary and to supply non-formulary drugs when these are appropriate.

Dispensing Months: Mar 2002 - May 2002

Request Ref:

CHAPTER: 01 Gastro-Intestinal System

| This group represents of your prescribing costs: | 12.54 % |
| Scotland Average: | 12.00 % |

SECTION: 0101 Dyspep&Gastro-Oesophageal Reflux Disease

Total Items prescribed	Total Cost including Stock Orders	Stock Order Cost
2,699	£40,317.04	£6.25

Total Items Prescribed	Total Cost including Stock Orders	Stock Order Cost
239	£938.75	£0.00

ITEM DETAILS:

			Total Items Prescribed	Total Quantity	Total Cost including Stock Orders	Average Quantity	Average Cost	Stock Order Quantity	Stock Order Cost
CO-MAGALDROX	SUSP	SF 300/600mg in 5ml	4	2,000	£18.72	500	£4.68	0	£0.00
CO-MAGALDROX	TABS	300/600mg	1	100	£4.68	100	£4.68	0	£0.00
MAALOX	SUSP	195/220mg In 5ml SF	10	4,600	£23.80	460	£2.38	0	£0.00
MUCOGEL	SUSP	195/220mg In 5ml SF	2	1,000	£3.64	500	£1.82	0	£0.00
MAGNESIUM TRISILICATE	MIXT	SF	2	1,000	£2.44	500	£1.22	0	£0.00
MUCAINE	SUSP	SF	2	1,400	£5.32	700	£2.66	0	£0.00
SODIUM BICARBONATE	PDR		3	434	£0.75	145	£0.25	0	£0.00
GASTROCOTE	TABS		19	3,140	£100.24	165	£5.28	0	£0.00
GAVISCON	TABS	SF	32	3,657	£137.14	114	£4.29	0	£0.00
GAVISCON	LIQ	SF	28	16,340	£92.24	584	£3.29	0	£0.00
GAVISCON	LIQ	SF	118	78,940	£435.12	669	£3.69	0	£0.00
GAVISCON	TABS	SF	3	260	£9.75	87	£3.25	0	£0.00
GAVISCON ADVANCE	LIQ	SF	1	500	£5.40	500	£5.40	0	£0.00
GAVISCON ADVANCE	LIQ	SF	14	9,180	£99.51	656	£7.11	0	£0.00

Fig. 36.2 Example of SPA data. (Reproduced with permission from Information and Statistics Division Scotland.)

CATALOGUE OF PRESCRIBING (full)

2. Cardiovascular system

2.6.4 Peripheral & Cerebral Vasodilators	Quantity	No. of items	Quantity x items	Cost (£)
Naftidrofuryl Oxal Cap 100mg	84	3	252	22.47
		3	254	22.47
Sub-total Naftidrofuryl Oxal		3		22.47
Sub-total Chem. Sub. Naftidrofuryl Oxalate		3		**22.47**
Inositol Nicotinate Tab 500mg	50	2	100	20.44
	100	1	100	20.35
		3	200	40.79
Inositol Nicotinate Tab 750mg	224	4	896	272.16
		4	896	272.16
Sub-Total Nicotinate Acid Derivatives		7		312.95
Sub-Total Chem. Nicotinate Acid Derivatives		7		312.95
Sub total 2.6.4		10		335.42
SUB TOTAL 2.6		789		11,650.37

This report covers all prescribing attributed to DR WORKLOAD HA & Partners Practice

July 2001-September 2001 INCLUSIVE
BNF version Number 40

Fig. 36.3 Example of PACT data. (Reproduced with permission from the Prescription Pricing Authority.)

A method for allowing drugs to be considered for inclusion in a formulary should not be restricted to newly available drugs. It must allow any user of the formulary to propose a drug for consideration and should be able to provide an evaluated response within a reasonable time. Evidence of any advantages the proposed drug has over drugs already included, in terms of efficacy, reduced toxicity or cost, will be needed. This must be based on well-designed published clinical trials, the same basis as that used in the initial formulary development. Many hospital formulary management systems require a form to be completed; an example is given in Figure 36.4. The person making the request must be informed as to whether the drug will be included and, if so, whether any restrictions will be placed on its prescribing. Different categories of recommendation are shown in Box 36.2. One option is to have an appraisal period, during which prescribers can gain experience with a

> **Box 36.2 Categories of responses to requests for new drug inclusions in a formulary**
>
> 1 Recommended for general use (hospital and general practice)
>
> 2 Recommended for hospital use only (not general practice)
>
> 3 Recommended for shared care when suitable (hospital and general practice)
>
> 4 Not recommended for use at present as further evidence of clinical and/or cost-effectiveness required
>
> 5 Not recommended
>
> 6 Unable to categorize—more details required
>
> 7 Not categorized—item not a drug

newly recommended drug, after which its continuing recommendation can be reviewed; 6 months would seem to be a suitable time for such an appraisal period.

If a drug is accepted onto an existing formulary between revisions, it is essential to inform all users of the change.

One way of achieving this is to issue information bulletins. A similar method can be used to inform users of any changes in the indications or doses of drugs which may also occur during the life of a formulary. Similarly, if drugs are to be withdrawn from the formulary, users must be kept informed.

Request for inclusion of a new drug in a formulary

Drug name _____ Manufacturer _____

Formulations available _____

Indication(s) for which request is made _____

Usual dose and duration of treatment _____

Type of inclusion requested   ☐ recommendation for general use

                                               ☐ specialist use only

If specialist use, which specialist(s)?   _____

                                               ☐ restricted indications(s)

Reason for request   ☐ novel therapeutic advance

                                               ☐ benefits over existing drug

Will the new drug replace an existing drug?   Yes/No

If so, which? _____

Estimated number of patients per year who will receive drug _____

Estimated costs fo treatment _____

Evidence provided in support of request:

☐ Summary of Product Characteristics

☐ Copies of RCTs, meta-analyses, review articles

☐ Pharmaco-economic evaluation

This request is supported by: (signatures required)

Consultant   _____

Clinical Pharmacist   _____

Trust Clinical Director _____

Fig. 36.4 Example of a form which could be used to request new drugs to be considered for inclusion in a formulary.

Withdrawals may occur because of manufacturers ceasing production, product licences being withdrawn or changes in manufacturers' recommendations. However, it may also be useful to consider withdrawing drugs from the formulary if they have not been prescribed for a long time. Again, 6 months would be a suitable time to study the prescribing of most drugs, except those whose use is seasonal. This could be done on a regular basis between major revisions, but would require consultation with prescribers before the withdrawal was implemented. The advantage of a practice such as this is that it helps to keep the number of drugs in the formulary to a minimum.

As there will be situations when a non-formulary drug is requested for a patient, it is necessary to have a method of ensuring that the request is dealt with promptly. In general practice, there should be no problem in supplying a non-formulary drug, although there may be a delay if it is not stocked by local pharmacies owing to rare use. In hospital, however, pharmacies tend to stock only a limited range of drugs. Formulary drugs should always be easily available, but non-formulary drugs may need to be purchased specially. This will lead to delays in treatment. Some hospitals require completion of a form for every non-formulary drug which is prescribed. The purpose of this is twofold: it acts as a deterrent to prescribing non-formulary drugs and also allows monitoring to see whether any drugs are frequently requested. Consideration may be given to including frequently requested drugs in the formulary. Usually forms require a senior medical staff signature, but there is a possibility that this requirement may be abused. Once a form with the appropriate signature is received, pharmacists should not simply assume that the request should be complied with. If this occurs, all that has been achieved is an elaborate ordering system. For the formulary system to operate effectively, all prescribers requesting a non-formulary drug should be questioned to determine the reasons why a formulary drug is not suitable.

One of the most frequent reasons for requesting a non-formulary drug in hospital is that the patient was taking the drug prior to admission and prescribers are reluctant to change it. This can be viewed as an opportunity to review the medication, ensuring that it is appropriate for the individual patient. If it proves to be so, it may be possible to use the patient's own supply of the drug, if it has been brought into hospital. Further systems will then be necessary for ensuring that patients' medicines are those prescribed and are fit for use. It is possible to save money and prevent delays in treatment by using patients' own drugs.

If this is not an option, the decision must be made as to whether the requested drug will be supplied from the pharmacy. The systems in place must ensure that this is a rapid process, particularly if a special purchase is required.

In general practice too, the most common reason for using non-formulary drugs is that patients are already taking them and either they or their GPs are reluctant to change the prescription. Increasingly pharmacists are being called upon to provide regular medication reviews, which provides an opportunity to consider the appropriateness of any non-formulary drugs prescribed. Pharmacists also undertake regular review of repeat prescribing in many practices and can address non-formulary prescribing through this mechanism.

The promotional activities of drug manufacturers' representatives will need to be controlled to prevent them from undermining the principles of the formulary. Manufacturers can be an extremely useful source of information, but the inclusion of a drug in a formulary must be evidence based and unbiased.

GUIDELINE DEVELOPMENT AND USE

Guidelines may be developed by multidisciplinary groups who have expertise in a particular area of practice. ADTCs or smaller groups may derive local guidelines and prescribing policies from published clinical guidelines. This process allows the evidence-based guidelines to be adapted depending on local health needs and services available.

The criteria which should be used to appraise the quality of clinical guidelines have been agreed across Europe. (Box 36.3) It is most important that guidelines are based on scientific evidence and that, where expert judgment has to be made, this is secondary to scientific and clinical evidence. Guidelines are most useful where there is evidence of variation in treatment or there is potential to improve the quality of care. However there must be robust evidence of effective practice on which to base recommendations. This may not be available for every condition or for every aspect of treating a condition. It is in this situation that expert judgment is required.

Guideline developers often grade their recommendations. The purpose of this is to differentiate between those recommendations which are based on strong evidence and those which are based on weaker evidence. It provides an indication of the likelihood that the predicted outcome will be achieved if a recommendation is implemented. The grading is based on an assessment of the design and quality of the

---

Box 36.3   AGREE (Appraisal of Guidelines, Research and Evaluation for Europe) criteria for appraising clinical guideline (Reproduced with permission from Appraisal of Guidelines for Research and Evaluation Instrument. The AGREE Collaboration, September 2001)

Scope and purpose
1. The overall objective(s) of the guideline should be specifically described.
2. The clinical question(s) covered by the guideline should be specifically described.
3. The patients to whom the guideline is meant to apply should be specifically described.

Stakeholder involvement
4. The guideline development group should include individuals from all the relevant professional groups.
5. The patients' views and preferences should be sought.

Rigour of development
6. Systematic methods should be used to search for evidence.
7. The criteria for selecting the evidence should be clearly described.
8. The methods used for formulating the recommendations should be clearly described.
9. The health benefits, side-effects and risks should be considered in formulating the recommendations.
10. There should be an explicit link between the recommendations and the supporting evidence.
11. The guideline should be externally reviewed by experts prior to publication.
12. A procedure for updating the guideline should be provided.

Clarity and presentation
13. The recommendations should be specific and unambiguous.
14. The different options for diagnosis and/or treatment of the condition should be clearly presented.
15. Key recommendations should be easily identifiable.

Applicability
16. The target users of the guideline should be clearly defined.
17. The potential organizational barriers in applying the recommendations should be discussed.
18. The potential cost implications of applying the recommendations should be considered.
19. The guideline should be supported with tools for application.
20. The guideline should present key review criteria for monitoring and audit purposes.
21. The guideline should be piloted among end users.

Editorial independence
22. The guideline should be editorially independent from the funding body.
23. Conflicts of interest of guideline development members should be recorded.

---

studies which provide the evidence on which the recommendation is based (see Ch. 34).

Many of the factors which apply to formularies in relation to presentation also apply to guidelines. They must be made available to those who are expected to use them, clearly presented, portable or accessible electronically and consideration given to durability and format. Many offer a flow diagram or algorithm which is easy to follow, such as that shown in Figure 36.5.

Implementing guidelines

Guidelines are developed to help assure the highest standards of patient care and improved outcomes and minimize variation in practice. However local ownership of the implementation process is required in order to succeed in changing practice. As most guidelines are developed nationally and therefore everyone who is expected to use them cannot possibly be consulted, they need to be adapted to local use by development of treatment protocols. These usually include methods of identifying patients, diagnostic tests to be performed, recall procedures and documentation in addition to the drugs to be prescribed.

Methods of implementing guidelines which are known to be successful include visits to prescribers to provide education about the guideline, involving local opinion leaders in educational meetings and interactive educational workshops. Ideally a mixture of methods should be used,

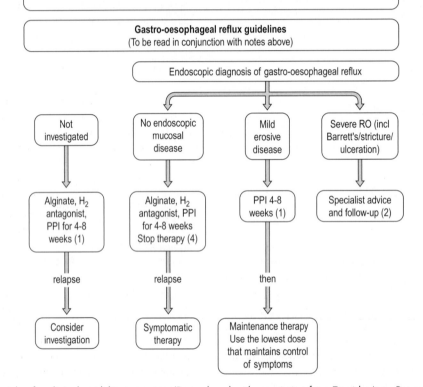

Gastro-oesophageal reflux

Gastro-oesophageal reflux disease (GORD) is a spectrum of disease caused by the reflux of gastric secretions into the oesophagus. It ranges in severity from symptoms without endoscopic abnormality, to erosive oesophagitis, to ulceration, to stricture formation and Barrett's oesophagitis.
1. Proton pump inhibitors (PPIs) are more effective in healing all grades of reflux oesophagitis (RO) and produce more rapid symptom relief than H_2 antagonists.
2. Patients with severe reflux oesophagitis may require specialist follow-up, and often require long-term maintenance therapy.
3. Use the lowest dose that maintains control of symptoms.
4. Patients with a normal endoscopy should stop drug therapy. If symptoms recur consider further anti-reflux therapy.
5. Surgery has a role in patients with severe oesophagitis and in some who require long-term maintenance therapy. Patients with reflux symptoms following upper GI surgery should be referred to a specialist.

Gastro-oesophageal reflux guidelines
(To be read in conjunction with notes above)

Endoscopic diagnosis of gastro-oesophageal reflux

| Not investigated | No endoscopic mucosal disease | Mild erosive disease | Severe RO (incl Barrett's/stricture/ulceration) |

| Alginate, H_2 antagonist, PPI for 4-8 weeks (1) | Alginate, H_2 antagonist, PPI for 4-8 weeks Stop therapy (4) | PPI 4-8 weeks (1) | Specialist advice and follow-up (2) |

relapse — relapse — then

| Consider investigation | Symptomatic therapy | Maintenance therapy Use the lowest dose that maintains control of symptoms |

Fig. 36.5 Example of a clinical guideline summary. (Reproduced with permission from Tayside Area Prescribing Guide, 2002)

because the more frequent the reminder, the more likely it is that practice will change. Involving users in developing a local treatment protocol from a clinical guideline is an extremely useful method of encouraging its use.

Clinical guidelines are increasingly important because of the possibility of litigation if they are not followed. Health care practitioners everywhere must be able to justify if necessary why the care they provide does not meet nationally agreed recommendations, when these exist. That is not to

say that it is compulsory to follow everything within a clinical guideline, but it is essential to be aware of the content of these and to ensure that they are followed when it is appropriate to do so.

Changing practice

Developing local formularies and treatment protocols encourages good relationships between prescribers and pharmacists. Building on this relationship is important to enable the changes to practice to be made which will be necessary in implementing these. Changing prescribing habits can be extremely difficult. Some prescribers dislike losing the freedom to prescribe as they choose and may reject a formulary and its concept. Often prescribers have developed personal drug preferences over the years and, even if they have no objection in principle to prescribing a different drug, may easily forget when actually writing prescriptions. Constant reminders may be necessary to maintain prescribing within the recommendations of a formulary or treatment protocol. If agreement on what drugs should be used has been difficult to achieve, the resultant formulary may contain a large number of drugs. This can be more easily adhered to, but is less likely to achieve rational prescribing or to reduce drug costs. Conversely a formulary which is too restrictive is more likely to be difficult to adhere to. Clearly where a treatment protocol has also been developed, it is important that it is based on formulary drugs so that a consistent message is seen.

When a formulary or protocol is introduced, some patients will be receiving medicines which are not included and they, too, may be resistant to change. The doctors who prescribe for these patients may also be unhappy about changing individual patients' drugs. This is especially likely if the patient is well stabilized on a particular drug, with little adverse effect. As drugs included in a formulary or protocol will have been selected on a sound basis, it could be more suitable for a patient than her current drug. Change may therefore be of benefit. Education of prescribers and patients may be necessary to convince them of potential benefits. Pharmacists are often those most actively involved in educating and persuading prescribers to carry out changes. Even without changing individual patients' drug therapy, if the drugs recommended in a local formulary or protocol are used for all patients starting new therapy, most prescriptions will in time be for formulary medicines.

Auditing performance

Providing feedback to prescribers on whether they follow formularies or guidelines is essential. Auditing practice against guidelines is described in more detail in Chapter 43. Because formularies encourage rational prescribing, the extent of their use can be used as an indicator of the quality of prescribing. The simplest way to gauge whether a formulary is being used is to look at prescribing data. Computerized data, such as PACT and SPA or their hospital equivalent, can easily be studied to assess whether

formulary drugs are being prescribed. However, this type of data provides no information about the patients for whom the drugs have been prescribed. It cannot, for example, identify why patients have received prescriptions for non-formulary drugs. Nor can it be used to determine whether the formulary drugs were prescribed appropriately or whether guidelines and treatment protocols are being followed. For this drug use review is required (see Ch. 34)

For data to be of any use, they must be easy to interpret, accurate and up to date. They must also be of direct relevance to the prescriber to whom they are given and may allow comparison either to earlier prescribing or to the prescribing of others. Comparing the prescribing of several GPs or hospital doctors to each other is known as peer review. Comparison to a 'norm' of prescribing practice, or to the practices of others in the same peer group, often increases the desire of prescribers to conform to the 'norm' or the peer group. However, it is important to ensure that the 'norm' is desirable.

Hospital data are often generated by the pharmacy computerized stock control system. As such they may refer to drugs issued to wards or directorates and care must be taken to determine whether this equates to drugs prescribed. Any drugs used on wards, which were not issued through the computer system, such as patients' own drugs, will not show up in these data. It is possible for drugs which are included in the formulary to be identified in the computer records, so that determination of formulary adherence is relatively simple. Care should, however, be taken to ensure that the quantities of the different drugs used are taken into account in some way.

For example, if a ward uses 180 tablets of a formulary drug and 20 tablets of a range of four other non-formulary drugs, adherence should be quantified as 90% (180 out of 200 tablets used in total). It could also be calculated that adherence was only 20%, if the range of drugs were used (one out of a range of five), but this would not be a reasonable representation of the overall prescribing on the ward.

Another source of data which can be valuable in hospital is the request forms for non-formulary drugs, if they are used. Review of these can indicate the extent of non-formulary prescribing. These also have the value of explaining the reasons why non-formulary drugs were used. Records of clinical pharmacists' interventions which have involved non-formulary prescribing can also be studied.

In primary care, PACT and SPA represent the number of prescriptions dispensed, so are a useful indicator of prescribing by medical practices. Only prescriptions which have not been presented to pharmacies and dispensed are excluded. They cannot, however, distinguish between formulary and non-formulary drugs. This must be done manually and a figure for adherence can then be calculated, again taking the quantities of each drug into account. Another source of data in primary care is the practice computer, which can be programmed to identify formulary drugs. If a practice does not generate or record all its prescriptions via the computer, the prescribing patterns obtained will not show the full picture.

Regular provision of information on performance is an essential part of formulary management. Any data which are presented to prescribers as a means of informing them of adherence to formulary recommendations will need to be attractive and easy to use, just like the formulary itself. Colour will add to their appearance and a simple highlighter pen can be used to emphasize parts of a table or figure which may be particularly important. Computer-generated graphics can also be a useful way of presenting data. Finally, evidence of cost savings, if they are made, may help to encourage use of the formulary. This is best expressed as actual expenditure compared to expected expenditure had the formulary not been used.

Feedback information such as this provides pharmacists with another opportunity to market a formulary, to promote relationships with prescribers and to discuss guidelines and treatment protocols.

Key Points

- A formulary is a list of drugs which are recommended and available for prescribing.
- A formulary may contain prescribing policies or treatment protocols, which detail the use of drugs in specific medical conditions.
- A clinical guideline is a series of systematically developed statements to assist practitioner and patient decisions about appropriate health care for specific clinical circumstances.
- Formularies, clinical guidelines and prescribing policies are tools used to promote rational and cost-effective prescribing.
- Compiling a formulary or guideline is a valuable educational exercise.
- Pharmacists should work with others to compile formularies and guidelines.
- Drugs are selected for inclusion in a formulary on the basis of efficacy, toxicity, patient acceptability and cost.

- Use of a formulary containing a restricted number of drugs may reduce the incidence of adverse drug reactions, interactions and lack of efficacy.
- For a formulary to be accepted, there should be widespread consultation on its content.
- A formulary should be easy to use and professionally presented and revised at least every 2 years.
- A formulary management system is required to provide systems for considering the inclusion of new drugs, deleting drugs and supplying non-formulary drugs.
- Information should be provided to prescribers on their adherence to a formulary to encourage its use.
- Prescribing data can be useful both in developing a formulary and feeding back on performance.
- Recommendations in clinical guidelines are often graded according to the strength of the evidence on which they are based.
- Ideally a mixture of methods should be used to encourage the use of formularies and guidelines.

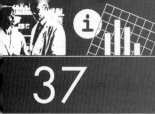

37

Responding to symptoms

C. Edwards and J. Krska

After studying this chapter you will know about:

The skills required to effectively respond to symptoms in the pharmacy, including observation, questioning and decision-making

The importance of structured questioning about signs and symptoms in order to collect all relevant information in a patient history

The principles involved in distinguishing between minor, self-limiting conditions and potentially more serious illnesses

Special considerations with children, the elderly, pregnant and breastfeeding women and patients with chronic conditions

Minor diseases which are suitable for over-the-counter management

Introduction

Responding to symptoms presented to them by patients has been an activity carried out by community pharmacists since the profession began. Pharmacists have always been in the frontline to the public who want accessible and informed advice about their symptoms and medicines. The process of responding to symptoms in the pharmacy implies firstly a screening or elementary diagnostic process to assess the presenting signs and symptoms. This will allow a decision to be made about whether the patient should be referred to a doctor or treat themselves. Secondly, if self-medication is appropriate the pharmacist can advise the patient about non-drug and over-the-counter (OTC) drug treatment.

Freedom of the individual and self-empowerment are important aspects of self-medication which are not only a reflection of changing attitudes to health but are also actively encouraged in the current political climate where increased accessibility to medicines and reducing health inequalities is paramount. Self-medication reduces some of the burden on constrained NHS budgets and is facilitated by the increasing re-regulation of more medicines to OTC status (from Prescription only Medicines (POM), to Pharmacy only (P) or general sales list (GSL) medicines) which has taken place in recent years. Easier access to medicines will also be complemented by increased affordability, brought about by the abolition of resale price maintenance in the UK. This however raises some questions about the appropriateness of such measures, since the public can now purchase many medicines without any professional supervision or advice.

A request for a medicine to be reclassified from the POM to P category is usually made by the manufacturer to the Medicines Control Agency in the UK. Several safeguards must be met for a medicine to be available over the counter without a prescription:

- Safety data should demonstrate, amongst other things, a wide therapeutic index and low toxicity profile.
- Efficacy data should provide evidence that the indications and dosage are suitable for self-medication and the indications should be capable of recognition by the lay public and not confused with serious disease.
- Product information must ensure safe consumer use and include warnings and advice on duration of treatment and when medical advice should be sought.

Further therapeutic classes which have been highlighted to contain potential candidates for re-regulation from POM to P status include drugs used in the treatment of chronic disease such as antihypertensives, lipid-lowering drugs, inhaled beta-2 agonists and corticosteroids, oral contraceptives and hormone replacement therapy. Thus the supply of medicines 'over the counter' may be seen, at least in part, from a new perspective of 'pharmacist prescribing'.

Surveys have found that the ailments which the lay public most commonly treat themselves are coughs and colds, gastrointestinal conditions, headaches, skin conditions and musculoskeletal symptoms. There are also a significant number of requests for advice about childhood ailments such as napkin dermatitis, eczema, coughs and colds and various public health issues like scabies and head lice treatment. The elderly are also a relatively large group of consumers of non-prescription medicines. Since a proportion of hospital admissions in this age group are due to an iatrogenic cause, the consumption of OTC medicines may be of some importance, due to misuse, overuse or duplication of prescription and non-prescription medicines.

Several options are available to people who suffer from symptoms. They may:

- Take no action
- Use a simple traditional home remedy, e.g. a hot water bottle and lemon and honey drink for a cold
- Use a prescription medicine already available at home
- Use a non-prescription medicine
- Consult a doctor.

Often a pharmacy assistant is the first person to be approached by a member of the public in the community pharmacy. Staff must be adequately trained to enable them to question patients and decide when the pharmacist should be directly involved in the consultation. All members of staff who are involved in the sale of medicines should have completed an accredited course. It may be useful to provide a list of medicines, requests for which should be referred directly to the pharmacist, such as medicines which have recently been re-regulated or which are liable to intentional misuse. Such measures should help to ensure that all medicines are sold safely and appropriately and that pharmacists will have more time to devote to transactions where their involvement is considered essential.

EVIDENCE BASE AND THE PLACEBO EFFECT

Evidence-based medicine, increasingly the standard by which health care professionals are expected to make decisions about treatment for individual patients, is described in Chapter 34.

Over many years, several therapeutic agents have fallen from favour and been blacklisted from the list of items prescribable on the NHS because of a lack of evidence of their efficacy.

Various trials and systematic reviews of the literature have revealed that many medicines, particularly OTC medicines, have little, if any, significant efficacy. Nevertheless the placebo effect is a powerful medicine and is part of the medication armamentarium which pharmacists and doctors have at their disposal.

In addition, effective marketing of medicines by pharmaceutical companies in the mass media has a dramatic effect on patients' expectations and outcomes. Both doctors and pharmacists can bear testimony to the number of patients who stride into their premises clutching newspaper cuttings bearing persuasive articles describing the latest drug launch or clinical trial with allegedly earth-shattering results.

Traditionally, doctors have used the prescription as a means of closing a consultation with a patient. The majority of patients who visit their doctor expect a sympathetic ear, an examination or laying on of hands, an explanation, reassurance and wise counsel, and finally a prescription as a tactile seal to the consultation. The therapeutic revolution of the latter half of the twentieth century has led to the belief by the public that there is 'a pill for every ill'. Although modern medicine is attempting to counter that philosophy by stressing preventative health measures, there is no doubt that this innate expectation exists in the minds of most patients who seek expert medical opinion and relief from symptoms. So it is also in the pharmacy—recommending an OTC medicine despite inadequate or counter evidence of its efficacy is justifiable because many patients have a desire to try something to give them symptomatic relief. A negative or dismissive response by the pharmacist to a request from a patient can be harmful in that such patients may in future bypass the pharmacist or even the pharmacy altogether and the future opportunity for the pharmacist to assess the patient's symptoms and give appropriate advice, will be lost.

Thus for patients who are judged to have minor self-limiting conditions and are otherwise well, a form of words can be used which will fall short of any exaggerated claim for an OTC product but will not deter a customer for whom the placebo effect will be of potential benefit. This approach will ensure that patients consult the pharmacist for advice and assessment, and at the same time retain some choice in how they manage their own illnesses.

THE PROCESS OF RESPONDING TO SYMPTOMS

Skills required by the pharmacist to respond to symptoms include knowledge of diseases and their treatment, astute observation, and communication and questioning skills to obtain all the information required to make a decision about whether to treat or refer. The pharmacist must select the most suitable treatment, explain its use, provide advice on related health care and inform the patient of the action to take if symptoms do not improve within an appropriate time scale.

General communication skills have been dealt with in Chapter 3. Other relevant skills and processes used in responding to symptoms are discussed here.

Diagnosis of exclusion

Before advising on any course of treatment, it is essential that the pharmacist has excluded any potentially serious condition which requires a medical opinion or urgent attention. This so-called diagnosis of exclusion is a screening process which is carried out at various levels of sophistication, not only by doctors but also by others in the primary health care team from general medical practice receptionists to nurses. It involves taking a history of the signs and symptoms presented by a patient and should be a process of careful structured questioning. The following format is one which will allow the pharmacist to take a full history and allow a decision to be made whether the patient is suffering from a minor, self-limiting illness or a more potentially serious condition requiring medical referral.

Knowledge of diseases

To perform a diagnosis at any level, the health professional must have a list of likely diseases and their characteristics so that a match can be made between the symptoms of which the patient complains and the generally accepted picture of a specific disease. As distinct from symptoms, there may be signs of disease, which will be noted by the observer but which may not be complained of by the sufferer, for example, paleness of the skin, abnormality of the pupils of the eyes, the shape of a rash, the speed of onset of a symptom or the spread of a pain from one site to a larger area of the body. These may all be important features which help to distinguish one condition from another which will be elicited only on questioning or by observation. Clearly there are limitations to the number of signs which can be elicited by observation and the doctor is in a much better position to detect signs of disease, for instance by using the stethoscope, sphygmomanometer or taking blood samples for laboratory tests to be carried out.

Early detection of abnormality

In making a decision about signs and symptoms, it is valuable to be able to detect any abnormality early on, rather than allowing some serious pathology to pass unnoticed until it may compromise the outcome of the illness. Though clearly, this is desirable, it is not always possible.

Labelling the condition

The pharmacist's diagnosis will, in most cases, be non-specific, at a level where she can simply reassure the patient that the symptoms are common and appear to represent nothing serious and are likely to be self-limiting. Sometimes it will be possible to attach a label to the condition such as a tension headache, migraine, an eczematous rash, a fungal infection or an allergic reaction. Such labelling is not always specific but it is obviously reassuring to the patient. Sometimes there may be doubts and this can occur when either there are too few symptoms to be confident enough to assess them or they do not match the picture of likely specific diseases which may require a referral.

Temporizing

Clearly if there is any doubt that a serious condition cannot be excluded, then depending on how ill the patient is or how dangerous it may be to delay referral, the pharmacist may wish to temporize. This involves either asking the patient to check his own progress over the next hours or days and report any new symptoms or alternatively asking the patient to return within a short time period to re-assess the situation. Clearly this requires some judgment to be made but provided that the pharmacist is aware of the most likely serious conditions and their signs and symptoms and makes the patient aware that the course of a disease can change and reveal new symptoms, then she will not be overstretching her competency. However the most important rule is that where there is any doubt about the nature of a condition which may be causing concern to the patient, the patient's carers or to the pharmacist, then a referral should be made for a medical opinion.

Treating the symptoms

Where the pharmacist is confident that the symptoms represent self-limiting disease, a recommendation can be made to the patient perhaps for some medication to provide symptomatic relief. If the medication does not have the desired effect within the time period suggested by the pharmacist or on the manufacturer's product pack or leaflet, the patient should be advised to either return for reassessment by the pharmacist or to consult the doctor. This allows the next step in the diagnostic process to occur. Thus if a patient obtains relief with any measures suggested by the pharmacist, then the working diagnosis of a self-limiting disease will have been proved correct. If, however, a referral to the doctor proves necessary, then appropriate examination and investigation may produce further information on which a diagnosis can be made.

PRINCIPLES FOR RESPONDING TO SYMPTOMS

As explained above, there are some ground rules which will enable the pharmacist to work at a comfortable and competent level in assessing signs and symptoms. There are some further principles which should also be taken into account.

Identifying the patient

Although it is almost too obvious to mention, it is important to establish whether the person relating the story or symptoms is the patient or his representative. It is far easier to question a patient than to obtain a history from a relative or neighbour, and in many instances this will compromise the pharmacist's judgment when assessing symptoms. If the patient is not present, the question has to be asked whether the severity of the illness is the reason for their absence. Parents however will usually give reasonable histories of their child's illness but it is more reassuring if the child is present so that the severity of the symptoms can be properly evaluated. If there is any uncertainty, in the absence of the patient, about the patient's condition, then the pharmacist must err on the side of caution and not make any recommendation.

Probability of disease

Although the process of matching the pattern of a patient's symptoms with the picture of a disease will give some confidence in being able to attach a label to a disease, the pharmacist must also consider the likelihood of specific diseases being encountered in the pharmacy. Thus purely for statistical reasons it is unlikely that rare conditions will present themselves in the pharmacy. A general medical practitioner is likely to be able to count on the fingers of one hand the

number of patients he has seen with a brain tumour, gastric cancer or leukaemia in the last 10 years. Hence a patient presenting to the pharmacist for the first time with a headache is very unlikely to have a brain tumour. Many patients will have a headache caused by stress or tension, a large proportion will have a self-limiting headache of unknown cause. A smaller percentage will have a migrainous headache, but it is extremely unlikely that a pharmacist will ever see a person in her pharmacy with a headache caused by a brain tumour. This is an important point of reassurance, especially if a patient suspects that there may be some sinister cause to his pain. Nevertheless, it is essential for the pharmacist to take the patient's history in a structured and systematic manner so that the relevant questions can be asked which will allow exclusion of such a serious diagnosis.

The general demeanour of the patient

Allowing the patient to tell his story in his own words can be helpful. To enable this it is useful to begin with a general question such as 'What is the problem?' or 'How do you feel?' More specific questions can then be used to follow up any clues given in the patient's general preamble. During this initial phase of the interview, the pharmacist can form an opinion about the patient's general demeanour and the severity of the illness. Sometimes a patient will be able to articulate this adequately but in some patients the body language and general appearance will be helpful. The basic question to be answered is simply 'Does the patient look ill?' A child who skips into the pharmacy is less likely to be as ill as one who is crying and clinging to its mother's skirt or behaving in some abnormal way.

Current state of health and medication

Questions on past medical history and detail of any current medication are required. This will allow the possibility of adverse drug reactions or possible drug interactions to be identified (see Ch. 32). Some symptoms may arise as a result of a current medical condition worsening. For example, coughing at night may be a sign that asthma is poorly controlled and requires referral for medical assessment.

Information on current medical conditions and medication taken will also be necessary. It allows the pharmacist to make an appropriate treatment recommendation that will not interact with existing medication or medical conditions. Information on any medicines that have been tried for the reported symptoms, successfully or otherwise, is also important. Many customers will have already tried something that is currently in their medicine cabinet, either a prescribed or an OTC medicine, or one that they have borrowed from a friend or relative. If the patient has used an apparently appropriate treatment already, then referral to the GP may be warranted.

Questions to confirm a diagnosis

Patients often make a self-diagnosis before seeking professional help. Confirmation of their symptoms should always be sought. For example, a patient may present stating that she wants a remedy for cystitis, but the symptoms of cystitis can easily be mistaken for vaginal thrush and vice versa. Patients do not always volunteer all the important information about symptoms, therefore asking about any other unusual symptoms will be an important prompt. If somebody is complaining of a cough, it would be significant to know whether he is coughing up blood or coloured sputum, as these are both signs for referral to a doctor. It will be useful to know about changes in lifestyle, such as a recent holiday or change in job, as some symptoms could be attributed to this.

It is important not to jump to conclusions about what the person may be suffering from early in the consultation and thereby omit asking vital questions. It is important to be able to ask key questions about the condition or symptoms that are being reported by the patient. An example of a key question for headache would be: 'Is there a possible trigger factor?' Some foods can trigger headaches, e.g. Chinese food (monosodium glutamate), cheese, chocolate and red wine. Reducing excess coffee intake has been known to cause caffeine-withdrawal headaches. Stress may precipitate tension headache and hypoglycaemic headaches can occur during dieting or fasting.

A structured approach to questioning

When doctors are trained to take medical histories, they follow a logical, step-by-step process which gathers all the useful information and allows them to include and exclude particular diagnoses as they proceed through the questions. Several mnemonics are available to prompt questioning when taking an initial history from a patient.

The use of mnemonics helps to minimize the risk of missing vital information, especially in a busy pharmacy where there are many potential distractions and interruptions. Care should be taken to follow the checklists of questions in an intelligent manner with particular application to the individual patient rather than in a thoughtless, robotic way. Attention must be paid to the responses given by the patient, following up any additional aspects as necessary. Examples of two popular mnemonics, SIT DOWN SIR and ASMETTHOD, are shown below.

S Site or location?
I Intensity or severity?
T Type or nature?
D Duration?
O Onset?
W With (other symptoms)?
N aNnoyed or aggravated by?
S Spread or radiation?
I Incidence or frequency pattern?
R Relieved by?

A Age and appearance of the patient?
S Self or for someone else?
M Medication the patient is taking?
E Exactly what does the patient mean by the symptoms?
T Time/duration of symptoms?
T Taken anything for it or seen the doctor?
H History of any disease or condition?
O Other symptoms being experienced?
D Doing anything to aggravate or alleviate the condition?

A worked example using one of the mnemonics is given in Case study 37.1 and more details can be found in the reference texts in Appendix 7.

A further mnemonic, WWHAM, was originally designed for use by counter assistants and is a useful starter for questioning, but is not adequate to gather all the essential information as described in the process above:

W Who is the patient?
W What are the symptoms?
H How long have the symptoms been present?
A Action already taken; what medicines have been tried?
M Medication being taken for other problems?

DISTINGUISHING BETWEEN MINOR ILLNESS AND MAJOR DISEASE

Pharmacists should be able to screen the many cases that they see each day, through observation and intelligent questioning, and identify those symptoms for which there may be a potentially serious cause. These latter patients should

CASE STUDY 37.1

This example shows the responses of two people who are complaining of similar symptoms and how structured questioning can assist the pharmacist in making a decision about how to advise the patient.

A woman is complaining of chest pain and asks for your advice.

The most obvious cause of chest pain which will be of greatest concern to the woman and which requires exclusion by the pharmacist is of cardiac origin. The following observations of two similar cases will assist in highlighting the pertinent parts of the history (the first woman's responses are indicated by 'Case A', the second woman's by 'Case B').

General demeanour of the patient—does she look and feel ill?
The first woman is known to be a previously fit person, is taking no medication and is a schoolteacher by profession. She appears to be in her twenties. She walks into the shop, appears apparently normal but grimaces a little as she describes her pain.

The second woman is middle aged and very anxious and comes in with her husband. She is having some pain at the time she comes into the pharmacy. She asks to sit down. [Note 1]

Site: 'Where is the pain?'
Case A: The woman rubs the tips of her fingers up and down over a small area of the central lower chest, just above and below the base of the breast bone.

Case B: The woman grips her fingers together to make a fist and places the fist centrally in the mid chest region. [Note 2]

Intensity: 'How severe is the pain?'
Case A: 'It hurts quite a bit'. She appears to obtain some relief by pressing on the area where the pain is felt and she continues the rubbing motion.

Case B: 'It is severe—it catches my breath.' [Note 3]

Type: What sort of pain is it?
Case A: 'It is a bad pain.'

The pharmacist asks a more focused question and gives some examples:

Pharmacist: 'Is it a sharp pain like being stabbed? Does it give a sense of tightness or pressure on the chest? Is it a gnawing background pain? Would it be described as a burning pain?'

Case A: 'It is a burning sensation'. There is no tightness.'

Case B: 'It is like a tightness in the chest.' [Note 4]

Duration: 'How long have you had it?'
Case A: 'On and off for two or three weeks.'

Pharmacist: 'How long does it last?'

Case A: 'It comes and goes and seems to last a few seconds at a time.'

Case B: 'I have just had it once before, a couple of weeks ago. It lasted a minute or two and then seemed to go away.' [Note 5]

Onset: 'Do you notice that the pain starts at a particular time, or after eating, exercise, or on bending down?'
Case A: 'I notice it sometimes when I am eating, I have to stop and take a deep breath when I have a twinge of pain. Sometimes I don't feel I can finish my meal.'

Pharmacist: 'What about when you bend down to pick something up, or lying down in bed?'

Case A: 'Yes bending over can make the pain come on.'

Case B: ' The last time I had it, it was a cold day and I had to run for a bus.' Eating does not seem to influence it.' [Note 6]

Accompanying symptoms: 'Is there anything else you feel when you have the pain?'
Case A: 'My food seems to stick sometimes when I am eating.'

Case B: 'I feel a bit breathless, I have to stop what I am doing and take some deep breaths and I feel that I want to be sick.'

Aggravating factors: 'What makes it worse?'
   Case A: 'As I have already said—eating, bending over.'

   Case B: 'As I have said—a cold wind or a frosty morning.' [Note 7]

Spread: Does the pain spread from your chest, for instance to your arms or neck?'
   Case A: 'No.'

   Case B: ' I get a tingling feeling in my neck and jaw.' [Note 8]

Frequency: 'How often do you have this pain?'
   Case A: 'Sometimes two or three times a day, and then sometimes I go for a day or two without it and then it comes back.'

   Case B: 'Just had it once before.' [Note 9]

Relieving factors: 'Does anything relieve it?'
   Case A: 'No not really.'

   Pharmacist: 'Have you taken anything for it?'

   Case A: 'Yes, I have taken some antacid and that seems to help a bit.'

   Case B: 'Just stopping and sitting down and having a rest.' [Note 10]

Notes
   1. The second woman comes in with her husband and seems more anxious than the first woman. This is easier to detect retrospectively and may not be apparent at the time, but is an indicator of the possible seriousness of the symptom and the anxiety it is provoking.
   2. The second woman's fist-like gesture is classic of patients who are describing an anginal pain. The feeling is often one of tightness.
   3. The second woman is describing here an unusually severe pain.
   4. See note 2.
   5. This is only the second time she has experienced this symptom—perhaps the fact that she is seeking help after only one episode may be a measure of its severity or the anxiety it has provoked.
   6. The factors which have brought on the pain are classic for a gastrointestinal origin in the first woman and a cardiac cause in the second.
   7. The second woman re-inforces her earlier statement.
   8. This is a typical description of the spread of cardiac pain.
   9. See note 5.
   10. Chest pain is classically relieved by rest in patients with angina.

The cases of the two people suffering with chest pain can thus be differentiated into:

- Acid reflux/indigestion—the first woman may benefit from a recommendation for a H_2 antagonist to see if the symptoms remit. If she does not obtain relief within 1 or 2 weeks, then she can be referred to see her doctor for a non-urgent appointment.
- Angina—the second woman has a classic history of angina and (providing the pain of this episode disappears within a few minutes) requires an appointment with her doctor within the next 12 or 24 hours for a medical opinion.

Often people do not present with textbook symptoms, but the above comparison of two women with similar presenting symptoms shows how simple questioning and a knowledge of the classic features of different conditions can help to differentiate a relatively minor condition from a potentially more serious one.

then be referred to a doctor for treatment. It is difficult to define a minor illness, although criteria which have been applied are the condition should be:

- Of limited duration
- Self-limiting and
- Perceived as non-threatening.

There are also conditions which are recurrent or persistent which can be managed by an individual following an initial consultation with a doctor, e.g. cold sores, eczema or allergies.

There are particular danger symptoms to be aware of which will always require referral of the patient to the doctor, as they may be a sign of a more serious disease. These are listed in Box 37.1, along with some common self-limiting conditions which can be safely managed by the pharmacist. Failed medication will often require a referral to the GP, if the medication was apparently appropriate for the patient's condition. Further investigation may be necessary, or a more potent medicine may be required.

Pharmacists should be alert to suspected adverse drug reactions as a causative factor of symptoms (see Ch. 32).

Box 37.1 Summary of some self-limiting conditions and symptoms requiring medical referral with some potentially relevant serious diseases which they may represent

Headache

Common self-limiting causes: idiosyncratic (cause unknown), premenstrual headache in women, sinusitis, tension headache, mild migraine, hangover

Referable symptoms: Adults—associated symptoms such as nausea, vomiting, drowsiness, irritable mood, slurred speech, loss of balance, pupils of eyes unequal in size or not reacting to light, visual disturbance, red eye, photophobia, rash, neck stiffness or pain on moving the neck, pain in the eye, pains over one side of the scalp or face, tenderness and pain over the temporal artery in the temple (in more elderly patients), sudden explosive onset, patient disabled by the pain or obviously unwell, recent history of a head injury
    Children—rash, fever, photophobia, pain on moving neck, not eating, (also see symptoms above)

Serious causes: glaucoma, meningitis, shingles, subarachnoid haemorrhage, temporal arteritis, head injury, tumour

Cough

Common, self-limiting causes: viral infection of the upper respiratory tract

Referable symptoms: difficulty in breathing, shortness of breath, wheeze, blood-stained sputum, chest tightness or pain, fever, night sweats, pain on inspiration, recurrent cough, weight loss, purulent sputum for 2 weeks with one other of these symptoms, patients taking ACE inhibitor drugs
    Children—persistent dry cough, especially at night, severe violent coughing, and noisy breathing

Serious causes: asthma, bronchitis, carcinomas, croup in children, emphysema, pneumonia, pneumothorax, pulmonary embolism, tuberculosis, whooping cough

Head cold and sore throat

Common self-limiting causes: allergic rhinitis, common cold, perennial rhinitis, sinusitis, viral sore throat

Referable symptoms : enlarged lymph nodes in the neck, difficulty in breathing, shortness of breath, fatigue or malaise for more than 1 week, white pus on tonsils, skin rash, history of artificial heart valves or endocarditis, persistent hoarseness, difficulty in swallowing for more than a few days, ear pain, patient taking drugs which may cause blood dyscrasias, e.g. carbimazole, phenothiazines, cytotoxic drugs, gold, immunosuppressants

Serious causes: glandular fever, laryngitis, tonsillitis, and influenza in susceptible patients such as the elderly, those with cardiovascular disease or diabetes.

Abdominal pain

Common self-limiting causes: non-ulcer dyspepsia, irritable bowel syndrome, mild oesophagitis

Referable symptoms: abdominal swelling, anaemia (paleness and fatigue), blood in the stool, blood in the vomit, difficulty in swallowing, dysuria and frequency, persistent diarrhoea, menstrual irregularities, signs of early pregnancy (e.g.

Box 37.1 *(cont'd)*

nausea or breast changes), jaundice, malaise, persistent vomiting, rash, recurrent pain or tenderness, swelling due to hernias, recent visit abroad, weight loss

  Children—projectile vomiting (in babies), screaming with pain, vomiting and diarrhoea in babies

Serious causes: acute abdomen, appendicitis, biliary colic, carcinoma, diverticular disease, dysmenorrhoea, endometriosis, gastroenteritis, inguinal or femoral hernia, hiatus hernia, inflammatory bowel disease, oesophagitis, pancreatitis, peptic ulcer, renal colic, salpingitis, urinary tract infection

Constipation

Common self-limiting causes: simple constipation, haemorrhoids, irritable bowel syndrome

Referable symptoms: constipation of more than 2 weeks' duration, abdominal pain, appetite loss, nausea and vomiting, postsurgical patients, blood in stool, weight loss, thirst, patients taking long-term, regular laxatives which are not pre-scribed by their doctor, constipation alternating with episodes of diarrhoea

  Children—babies under 1 year

Serious causes: bowel obstruction, carcinomas, diverticular disease, haemorrhoids (severe or previously undiagnosed)

Diarrhoea

Common self-limiting causes: gastroenteritis caused by suspected indiscretion in eating or drinking in last 24 hours, irritable bowel syndrome, viral gastroenteritis

Referable symptoms: persistent abdominal pain, blood in stool, mucus in stool, fever, persistent diarrhoea especially in patient of or beyond middle age, fatigue, loss of appetite, weight loss, persistent visits to the toilet at night, recent travel abroad

  Children (in babies)—dehydration, inadequate fluid intake, fever

Serious causes: carcinomas, diverticular disease, irritable bowel syndrome, bacterial or protozoal infection contracted abroad

---

Information on medicines that the patient is currently or has recently been taking is essential. The timing of commencement of any new medicine regimens will also be important in linking it to a suspected adverse drug reaction (ADR). If adverse drug reactions are suspected, then a referral to the GP should be made so that the patient's medication may be reviewed. Suspected ADRs to OTC or herbal medicines should be reported to the Committee on Safety of Medicines (see Ch. 32).

TREATMENT AND ADVICE

Once a full assessment of the symptoms has been made, and a decision made that the patient does not require referral, appropriate recommendations should be made by the pharmacist.

Selection of an appropriate treatment for a condition involves application of a knowledge of pharmacology, therapeutics and pharmaceutics. The first step will be to choose an appropriate therapeutic group to recommend. The next step would be to assist the customer in the choice of product within the therapeutic group. For many therapeutic groups there are a wide variety of products available, often supported by widespread advertising. Lists of some of the typical constituents of OTC products are shown in Box 37.2. It should be remembered that many of these drugs are available in various combinations in different products. The pharmacist should take into account the efficacy (both of the individual component drugs and of the combinations used), potential side effects, interactions, cautions and contraindications. The patient's needs should be borne in mind when selecting a product. Factors such as the ease of use of a formulation and dosage regimens should be considered. The purchaser will also be interested in value for money. There are many forms of OTC drugs available, from standard tablets and capsules to 'easy to swallow' caplets, effervescent tablets and liquids. The form which will suit the patient's needs best should be chosen. For example, antacids are available in both tablets and liquid form. Tablets are more convenient to carry around for occasional use, but it may be claimed that a liquid has a quicker onset of action

---

Box 37.2   Constituents of OTC medicines available to treat common conditions

---

Headache

Simple analgesics
Aspirin
Paracetamol
Ibuprofen

Combinations
Aspirin + codeine
Paracetamol + codeine
Aspirin + codeine + paracetamol,
Ibuprofen + codeine,
Paracetamol + dihydrocodeine

Others
Caffeine
Buclizine (antinauseant for migraine)

Cough

Suppressants
Codeine
Pholcodine
Dextromethorphan

Antihistamines
Brompheniramine
Chlorphenamine
    (chlorpheniramine)
Diphenhydramine
Promethazine
Triprolidine

Expectorants
Guaifenesin
Ammonium salts
Ipecacuanha
Squill, senega
Creosote, sodium citrate

Others
Ephedrine
Pseudoephedrine
Phenylpropanolamine
Theophylline
Glycerol, honey

Colds

Antihistamines
Triprolidine
Chlorphenamine
    (chlorpheniramine)
Brompheniramine
Pheniramine

Decongestants
Pseudoephedrine
Phenylpropanolamine
Phenylephrine
Topical agents: ephedrine,
oxymetazoline, phenylephrine,
xylometazoline

Analgesics
Aspirin
Paracetamol

Others
Ascorbic acid
Menthol
Eucalyptus oil

Indigestion

Alkaline antacids
Sodium bicarbonate
Calcium carbonate
Aluminium hydroxide
Magnesium salts
Bismuth salts

H_2-receptor antagonists
Cimetidine
Ranitidine
Famotidine

Others
Dicyclomine
Simethicone

Constipation

Bulk laxatives
Wheat bran
Ispaghula
Sterculia
Methylcellulose

Stimulant laxatives
Bisacodyl
Senna
Aloin
Frangula

Osmotic laxatives
Magnesium salts
Sodium sulphate
Lactulose, lactilol

Faecal softeners
Docusate

Diarrhoea

Electrolytes
Oral rehydration salts

Opioids
Loperamide
Codeine
Morphine

Adsorbents
Kaolin
Pectin
Attapulgite

Spasmolytics
Belladonna

Box 37.2 *(cont'd)*

Vaginal candidiasis

Antifungal creams and pessaries
Clotrimazole
Econazole
Miconazole

Oral antifungals
Fluconazole

Topical agents for skin conditions

(i) Allergic and irritant dermatitis, bites and stings

Steroids
Hydrocortisone

Antihistamines
Antazoline
Diphenhydramine
Mepyramine

Others
Crotamiton
Tetracaine (amethocaine), benzocaine
Calamine, zinc oxide

(ii) Atopic eczema

Steroids
Hydrocortisone
Clobetasone

Emollients
Mixtures of hard, soft and liquid paraffins

(iii) Acne

Keratolytics
Benzoyl peroxide
Salicylic acid
Sulphur
Resorcinol

Antimicrobials
Cetrimide
Chlorhexidine
Povidone-iodine
Triclosan

(iv) Topical fungal infections

Antifungals
Clotrimazole
Econazole
Miconazole
Tolnaftate
Undecanoic acid

(v) Head lice and scabies

Malathion
Permethrin
Phenothrin

---

and may be preferable if immediate relief from symptoms is required. Previous experience by customers of some products and repeat requests may also have an influence on the selection of a particular OTC medicine.

Patients should be advised on how to use the treatment that has been recommended, including the recommended dose, when to take it and for how long. Any other important advice, such as how to use the preparation, should also be offered, as for example with nasal sprays and eye drops. Advice on storage is also important, e.g. informing the customer that eye drops and ointments should be disposed of 28 days after opening.

Non-drug treatment should also be offered where appropriate. There are often non-drug suggestions which will help to manage a condition in addition to the use of OTC medicines. For example, for prevention of motion sickness, in addition to the use of medicines, visual mechanisms, such as focusing on distant objects or keeping eyes closed in a fixed position will help to reduce symptoms. Advice on increasing dietary fibre and fluids is an essential part of the management of conditions such as constipation and haemorrhoids. Lifestyle advice is crucial so that the patient may learn how to attempt to avoid recurrence of the symptoms (see Chs 38 and 39). Situations where pharmacists are being consulted by patients for advice on symptoms are ideal opportunities to promote health education. For example, someone who is asking for advice about a cough mixture should be asked about his smoking habits. Advice about smoking cessation may become an essential part of the management programme.

Outcomes

It is important that the pharmacist is aware of the timescales for treatment of conditions with OTC medication. This will allow the patient to be given a reasonable time period over which to try the treatment before seeking further advice from a GP. Timescales will vary considerably from condition to condition. The status of the patient may also have an effect. For example, a 2-year-old toddler suffering from diarrhoea will be referred to the GP in a shorter timescale than a teenager with the same symptoms. Patients should be encouraged to monitor outcomes of their therapy so that they can take further action if required. If there has been a long duration of symptoms, then the patient should be referred.

Counselling areas

It is important that pharmacists are sensitive to the needs of their patients when giving advice. A patient's body language may indicate that he wishes to speak privately, or in a quiet area, away from other customers. Every effort should be made to provide a quiet area for conversation with the customer, so that others cannot overhear. A counselling area is ideal for this purpose. Many community pharmacies are now being designed to allow for the inclusion of such an area. A counselling area is usually screened off from the main pharmacy counter area, or may be a separate room, although studies have shown that patients may feel inhibited in an enclosed space. If this is not possible, the pharmacist should take the patient to a quieter area of the shop, so that other customers cannot overhear them. The pharmacist should always seek to create an atmosphere of privacy and confidentiality in these circumstances.

Special considerations when responding to symptoms

Children

Special care and consideration are needed when responding to children's symptoms. Children in their first months of life are particularly susceptible to complications from certain conditions. For example, dehydration will result very quickly in a 1-month-old baby compared to an older child or adult. If there is any doubt about symptoms, then referral to the GP is the safest and most sensible course of action. Parents of young children will often consult the pharmacist to obtain reassurance that this is the best course of action.

There are more restrictions on the medicines available to recommend for children's symptoms. Pharmacists should be alert to the signs of childhood infections, especially those which can present with seemingly commonplace symptoms, e.g. meningitis. Children of primary school age are particularly susceptible to viral infections and other contagious conditions that are currently prevalent in the local schools. Local knowledge, and communication with the local doctor's surgery, will be invaluable to the pharmacist in recommending treatment for these conditions.

When selecting treatments to recommend for children, it is important to bear in mind that medicine consumption in children is very high and that sugar in medicines can contribute to increased levels of dental decay, especially when medicines are to be given at bedtime. This is the worst time to consume anything containing sugar, because the saliva flow is greatly reduced whilst sleeping and cannot, therefore, buffer the acid attack from plaque. Most manufacturers are aware of this, so, where there is a choice, sugar-free OTC medicines should always be offered for children in preference to equivalents that contain sugar.

Elderly patients

Elderly patients are more likely to be taking other medicines prescribed by their doctor and therefore extra caution is required to check that there are no drug–drug or drug–disease interactions with the medicine being recommended. Duplication of prescribed and non-prescribed medicines is possibly most likely to occur in this patient group. Some of the most common products where duplication can be a problem are listed in Table 37.1. The possibility of adverse effects from current drug regimens should also be considered to avoid the unnecessary addition of new medicines when a change in the existing regimen may lead to resolution of the symptoms.

Pregnant and breastfeeding mothers

Drugs may cause harmful effects to the fetus during pregnancy. The potential effect of OTC drugs should not be forgotten. The period of greatest risk of congenital malfor-

Table 37.1   Potential problems with duplication of some OTC and prescription products

Drug	OTC examples	Prescribed examples	Consequences of duplication
Paracetamol	Lemsip, Night Nurse	Co-proxamol, co-dydramol, co-codamol	Overdose leading to hepatic damage
Codeine	Panadol Ultra, Solpadeine	Co-codamol	Increased CNS side-effects, constipation
Dihydrocodeine	Paramol	Co-dydramol, dihydrocodeine	Increased CNS side-effects, constipation
Ibuprofen	Anadin Ultra, Nurofen	Any NSAID	Increased risk of GI bleeding
Histamine H_2 antagonists	Zantac, Tagamet, Pepcid AC	Any H_2 antagonist, Any proton pump inhibitor	Mask lack of efficacy or serious disease
Sedative	Piriton, Nytol	Drugs with sedative antimuscarinic effects, antihistamines, e.g. tricyclic antidepressants Prescribed hypnotics	Increased sedation and other CNS side-effects
Theophylline	Do-Do Chesteze, Franol	Theophylline, aminophylline	Increased risk of theophylline toxicity
Steroid nasal sprays	Beconase, budesonide	Any steroid nasal spray, inhaler or systemic steroid	Increased possibility of systemic steroid side-effects
Laxatives	Senna, lactulose	Reduced colonic function, hypokalaemia	Any laxatives
Chloroquine	Nivaquine, Paludrine/Avloclor	Mefloquine	Increased risk of convulsions

mations is from the third to the eleventh week of pregnancy. The effects of drugs during the second and third trimesters tend to be on growth and functional development. All drugs should be avoided if possible during the first trimester, although there is of course a risk–benefit situation with some conditions. There is a lack of information on the effects of OTC drugs in pregnancy and their use should be minimized. There are, however, some minor conditions which will be commonly suffered during pregnancy for which OTC medicine use is considered relatively safe, such as paracetamol for headaches, or low sodium content antacids for dyspepsia. Drugs which are known to cause definite adverse effects in pregnancy include aspirin, non-steroidal anti-inflammatory drugs, sympathomimetics and medicines with a high sodium content. These should, therefore, be avoided.

Some drugs may be excreted, in varying amounts, in the breast milk. This can potentially lead to toxicity in a baby who is being breastfed. Those that are excreted in significant amounts and which could have an effect include aspirin, sedating antihistamines, caffeine and vitamin A.

Sufferers of chronic medical conditions

Patients who suffer from some chronic medical conditions, such as diabetes mellitus, will be more likely to suffer from specific minor illnesses and will be more likely to be taking other medication.

Care will need to be taken when recommending medicines to diabetics, because many pharmaceutical preparations contain sugar. A list of sugar-free medicines is available from Diabetes UK and the National Pharmaceutical

Association. Sorbitol is often used as a sweetening agent in sugar-free medicines and excessive consumption of this agent can lead to an osmotic diarrhoea. Foot problems, particularly foot ulcers, may arise as one of the long-term complications of diabetes mellitus because of increased susceptibility to infection, neuropathy and vascular disease. Any lesions, including corns and calluses, in a diabetic patient should be treated by a chiropodist so that wound healing can be adequately monitored.

It is important to remember that some important drug–disease interactions will preclude certain medicines from being recommended. For example, oral cold remedies containing sympathomimetics, such as ephedrine and pseudo-ephedrine, are best avoided by patients with hypertension, hyperthyroidism, coronary heart disease and diabetes.

Some OTC medicines such as alcoholic head lice lotions may provoke bronchospasm and should be avoided by asthmatic patients. A small proportion of asthmatic patients are also sensitive to non-steroidal anti-inflammatory drugs, such as aspirin and ibuprofen, which should be avoided where sensitivity reactions have occurred, or if the patient has not used these painkillers before.

Interactions of OTC medicines with other drugs

Medicines that are available for sale to the public are relatively safe. However, there are some important drug–drug interactions to be aware of when recommending OTC medicines. Interactions may occur with prescribed medicines or other non-prescription medicines. Few are clinically significant, especially when associated with short-term use of OTC medicines. Some common and potentially clinically significant interactions are listed in Table 37.2. A more detailed table may be found in the *OTC Directory* produced annually by the Proprietary Association of Great Britain.

Table 37.2   Potentially common or important interactions involving OTC drugs

OTC drug	Interacting drugs	Potential consequences
Ibuprofen	• Anticoagulants	Enhanced anticoagulant effect, increased risk of GI bleed
	• Lithium	Reduced lithium excretion, toxicity
	• Methotrexate	Reduced methotrexate excretion, toxicity
Aspirin	• NSAIDs	Increased risk of GI bleeds
	• Anticoagulants	Increased risk of bleeding
	• Methotrexate	Reduced methotrexate excretion, toxicity
Cimetidine	• Antiarrhythmics, anticoagulants, valproate, carbamazepine, phenytoin, theophylline, ciclosporin	Inhibition of metabolism and enhanced effect of all drugs, potential toxicity
	Mebendazole	Increased mebendazole level
	Chloroquine	Increased chloroquine level
Antihistamines	• Erythromycin, ketoconazole, antivirals, cimetidine	Increased plasma concentration of loratidine
Theophylline	• Quinolones	Increased risk of convulsions
	• Erythromycin, clarithromycin, isoniazid, fluconazole, ketoconazole, fluvoxamine, ticlopidine, cimetidine, diltiazem, verapamil	Increased theophylline levels, toxicity
	• Rifampicin, St John's wort	Reduced theophylline levels

Table 37.2 (cont'd)

OTC drug	Interacting drugs	Potential consequences
St John's wort	• Anticoagulants • SSRIs, 5-HT$_1$ agonists • Phenytoin, phenobarbital, carbamazepine • Antivirals, ciclosporin, digoxin • Oral contraceptives	Reduced anticoagulant effect Potential serotonin syndrome Reduced antiepileptic serum level Reduced plasma concentrations Reduced efficacy of contraceptive
Fluconazole, miconazole gel	• Anticoagulants • Terfenadine, pimozide • Simvastatin, atorvastatin	Enhanced anticoagulant effect Increased risk of arrhythmias Possible increased risk of myopathy
Chloroquine	• Amiodarone • Digoxin • Ciclosporin	Increased risk of arrhythmias Increased digoxin level, toxicity Increased ciclosporin level, toxicity
Sympathomimetics	• MAOIs Some antihypertensives	Risk of hypertensive crisis Antagonism of antihypertensive effect
Paracetamol, used regularly	Warfarin	Enhanced anticoagulant effect
Dextromethorphan	MAOIs, SSRIs, sibutramine	Potential serotonin syndrome
Antacids	ACE inhibitors, angiotensin II antagonists, quinolones, tetracyclines, antifungals, antimalarials, bisphosphonates, penicillamine	Decreased absorption of all drugs if taken at same time
Kaolin	Chloroquine, digoxin, quinidine, tetracyclines, aspirin	Reduced absorption of all drugs if taken at same time
Sodium bicarbonate	Lithium	Reduced lithium level
Iron salts	Tetracyclines, quinolones, penicillamine	Reduced absorption of all drugs if taken at same time

• Indicates potentially hazardous interaction according to BNF 43rd edition 2002.

Misuse of non-prescription medicines

It is important to educate the general public that, although non-prescription medicines are perceived as being freely available and the pharmacist has been involved in their supply, there are still potential problems with their use. These will be minimized if the medicine is being used for its intended purpose and at the correct dose and dosage interval.

Overdosing has occurred with non-prescription medicines, particularly those that contain paracetamol. This most commonly occurs when patients take more than one paracetamol-containing product. Adverse reactions can also occur, but are rare. Medicines may also be used for indications which are not licensed when sold OTC, such as hydrocortisone cream used on the face. This may result in a delay in the patient seeking appropriate advice from a doctor. Inadequate storage of drugs in patients' homes can also lead

Table 37.3	OTC products liable to misuse
Product type	**Examples**
Solvents	Adhesive plaster remover, methylated and surgical spirit
Propellants	Pain-relieving sprays
Chemicals	Citric acid
Opioids	Codeine, morphine
Antihistamines	Diphenhydramine, cyclizine
Laxatives	Senna
Sympathomimetics	Ephedrine, phenylpropanolamine

to problems, especially if they are accessible to young children.

Pharmacists should therefore ensure that advice and information are available on the safe and effective use of medicines. There is also a vast array of information available to the consumer about health issues. This has led to members of the public being better informed and wanting to know more about the medicines that they take.

Some products that are available for sale in community pharmacies may also be subject to intentional misuse by some people (see Ch. 42). It is important that pharmacists are aware of the products that have the potential for misuse which can arise either through frequent use over a long period of time or by taking substantially higher doses than are recommended. Pharmacists should be able to exercise professional judgment to prevent the sale or supply of any product that they suspect is not being used for a genuine medicinal purpose. Commonly abused products are listed in Table 37.3.

CONDITIONS TREATABLE BY THE PHARMACIST

There are a wide range of symptoms and ailments which can be treated using OTC medicines. A summary of some of the most common conditions appears in Box 37.1, along with symptoms requiring referral and a potential list of more serious illnesses which these symptoms may represent. Further reading will be required for details on symptoms, key questions, referral points and treatment and advice to give.

The pharmacist is also in an ideal position to give advice to travellers, including how to avoid suffering from symptoms or a simple first aid kit to treat common ailments suf-

fered when holidaying or travelling abroad. Advice on the recommended regimen for prophylaxis against malaria and travel vaccinations can be given in the pharmacy. The provision of advice on prevention of skin cancer is another important area in relation to travel abroad.

Requests around issues such as smoking and diet can also be opportunities to provide advice on lifestyle and OTC products. Indeed there are many areas where the pharmacist needs to be proactive, rather than simply reacting to requests. While responding to symptoms is a major and increasing role for community pharmacists with the wider availability of OTC products, their role in prevention of disease is equally important (see also Ch. 39).

Key Points

- Pharmacists are recognized and used as sources of advice on patient's symptoms and medicines.
- Medicines are increasingly being re-regulated to allow pharmacy sale, thus encouraging self-medication.
- A wide mix of skills is required by the pharmacist to respond competently to symptoms presented by patients.
- Open questions are best in the early stages of finding out about symptoms, using closed questions to seek clarification of specific aspects.
- A process of structured questioning should be used to ensure adequate collection of available information from the patient to construct an appropriate history and determine whether a patient's symptoms represent a self-limiting condition or the possibility of a more serious illness which requires a medical opinion and referral to a doctor.
- Various mnemonics are useful to assist the questioning process.
- Patients may require professional assistance in the choice of OTC medicines.
- Non-drug treatment should be offered where appropriate, including lifestyle advice.
- A quiet area where privacy and confidentiality can be provided should be available.
- Particular care is required when dealing with symptoms in young children, pregnant women, the elderly and patients with some chronic diseases.
- Duplication of OTC and prescribed medicines can sometimes have serious consequences.
- There are a number of clinically significant drug interactions involving OTC medicines.
- Pharmacists must be alert to the possibility of misuse of OTC medicines.

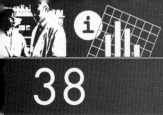

Counselling

J. A. Rees

After studying this chapter you will know about:

The rationale and need for counselling
What is counselling
Assessing the need for counselling
How to decide on the content and method of counselling
Aids to counselling

Introduction

Traditionally, pharmacists have always given advice on the use of medicines. In 1986, the Nuffield Report recognized that there were 'some categories of individuals who certainly will need advice, help and encouragement in the handling of their medicines' and that 'anyone ... who has to rely on a continuous drug regime, should be a candidate for additional support and help from pharmacies'. These statements highlight the importance placed on patient counselling in the Nuffield Report.

Since the Nuffield Report there have been developments in the research, production and packaging of medicines together with changes in society's attitudes towards patient/professional relationships, which have led to advice/counselling becoming an even greater part of the role of the pharmacist.

Medicines research has led to the production of new powerful, effective drugs formulated in many specialized dosage forms, e.g. modified-release formulations, aerosols, patches, etc., which utilize different absorption routes such as percutaneous, nasal, vaginal, buccal, as well as more conventional routes. Additionally many medicines are packaged in specialized containers, e.g. self-administered injections, rectal foams, inhalers, etc., and often with complicated dosage methods, e.g. small-volume pipettes, times of administration. Patients prescribed or purchasing these newer dosage formulations will almost certainly require some information from pharmacists on their method of use and the dosage regimen.

Additionally, many modern medicines have side-effects. Some of these side-effects will be relatively insignificant, others inconvenient, whilst others may be serious and as an extreme threaten the life of the patient (see Ch. 32). Clearly it is essential that patients are provided with the knowledge of these side-effects and what to do if they occur. In addition many medicines interact with other drugs (both over-the-counter (OTC) and prescribed medicines) and/or with food and drink. Thus, if patients/consumers are to get the best out of their medicines, then they need to know how to correctly use/administer these medicines in as safe a manner as possible, with knowledge about side-effects, interactions, etc. Pharmacists are in an excellent position to provide such advice/counselling to patients/consumers. It has been suggested that the advent of providing all medicines in original packs should release time for the pharmacist and thus enable the pharmacist to spend more time on individualized patient advice/counselling.

Against this background of technological and pharmaceutical advances in the delivery of medicines, attitudes within society have also changed. The 1980s and 1990s saw a rapid rise in the consumer movement, with consumers questioning and demanding better products, safer products, ecologically friendly products, etc., as well as more information on the products. Alongside and in response to these challenges by consumers, there has been the development of legislation giving consumers more rights and hence more power. Medicines have not been isolated from this consumer movement and patients and purchasers of medicines have become more demanding in their quest for knowledge about the medicines that they consume. Such patients have also become more questioning about their illness, its treatment and the need for specific medicines, their dosage regimens, alternative medicines, alternative formulations, etc. The introduction of the Internet has provided consumers with a readily available and extensive source of information about medicines, although the quality of some of the information may be dubious and the ability of the general public to understand the information questionable. All the above has led to patients acting more like consumers and becoming empowered and much more autonomous, resulting in them wanting more choice in the selection of their medicines/dosage regimens and questioning the justification for the prescribing and use of medicines. Thus patient advice/counselling on such issues is one way in which pharmacists can address the concerns of the patient.

Within the health care professions, there has been a move towards the accommodation of the consumer movement and a commitment to patient autonomy and choice. This has led to the acceptance that patients have the right to be involved in decisions about their health care. However in order to make an informed decision patients need the information surrounding the issues to make that decision. One of the first documents to accept that patients have the right to choose and the right to be involved in decision making about their medicines was published in 1997. 'From compliance to concordance' outlined the move towards developing patient/professional relationships which represent a negotiation between the patient and the professional and allow the patient to take an active part in decision making about their medicines (see Ch. 40).

The NHS Plan 2000 outlined the need for pharmacists to become more involved in helping patients to get the best from their medicines. The NHS Plan accepts that many patients are receiving less than optimum care because they find their medicines difficult to take or hard to remember, because they don't have anyone to talk to about their medicines, or because they have complicated medication regimens. According to the NHS Plan, by 2004, pharmacists will be giving extra help to patients who have difficulty in using their medicines correctly. Additionally the NHS Plan aims to 'Give patients the confidence that they are getting good advice when they consult a pharmacist'. In other words, the NHS Plan is advocating a greater role for pharmacists in counselling and advice giving to patients. Furthermore, the NHS Plan emphasizes the need for medicines management services, the aims of which are to prevent, detect and address medicines-related problems to achieve optimum use of medicines. Pharmacists are already providing many of the elements of medicines management informally. However, medicines management implies a coordination and formalization of these elements. The element of relevance to this chapter is the 'provision of support on medicines taking, which includes the identification of an individual's pharmaceutical needs, provision of an opportunity for patients to discuss their medicines and the development of patient–professional partnerships to provide improvements in medicine taking'. Such support could in

part be provided in the form of counselling by pharmacists, when handing out prescription medicines or selling OTC medicines. Other opportunities for such counselling exist on hospital discharge of patients, during medication reviews and with residential and nursing home staff and clients.

National Service Frameworks (NSF) have been introduced in recent years to define standards for the treatment, health and social services necessary to ensure high-quality care of individuals with specific diseases or conditions, e.g. diabetes, mental health, or groups of individuals with special needs, e.g. older people. The use of medicines is a fundamental component of NSF standards. Emphasis is placed on achieving a greater partnership in medicine taking between patients and health professionals, improving choice and addressing information needs. For example, the NSF for older people sets out its aims as ensuring that older people:

- Gain the maximum benefit from their medication to maintain or increase their quality and duration of life.
- Do not suffer unnecessarily from illness caused by excessive, inappropriate or inadequate consumption of medicines.

Both these aims encompass the need for pharmacists to advise/counsel older people (and their carers) about their medicines. Underlying all the above government documents is an acceptance that individuals need help with using their medicines.

Recently it has been acknowledged that some individuals with chronic conditions are very capable and competent in using their medicines to manage their condition(s). Such individuals have been termed 'expert patients'. At the same time there is an increasing awareness of the importance of self-care and active patient involvement in making decisions about preventing and treating minor and major conditions/illness. Successful self-management programmes for chronic conditions such as arthritis have been developed and have been facilitated by lay individuals with patient experience of the condition. The identification of such 'expert patients' could lead to more user-led self-management programmes. It has been suggested that expert patients could help to 'educate' professionals about the self-management of illness. Health professionals could pass on this 'education' to other patients with chronic conditions via counselling techniques. However, the self-care of minor ailments will probably require a different approach. Pharmacists will need to facilitate the development of self-care and support the development of competencies by individuals to enable them to use appropriate medicines correctly and effectively. In other words, counselling skills will be required by pharmacists to help in the empowerment of patients, so that they will be capable of making informed decisions about self-treatment with medicines for minor ailments.

WHAT IS COUNSELLING?

The term counselling is widely used in pharmaceutical literature but the definition of the term is less readily available. The British Association for Counselling (BAC) describes counselling as 'giving clients the opportunity to explore, discover and clarify ways of living more resourcefully and towards greater well being'. Whilst this definition encompasses some aspects of patient counselling, patient counselling is more about giving information and guidance on medicines to patients and allowing the patient to make informed decisions but with the interests of the patient uppermost. Another description of patient counselling is 'the sympathetic interaction between pharmacists and patients, which may go beyond conveyance of straightforward information about the medicine and how and when to use it'.

The Service Specifications of the Code of Ethics provides some guidance on the content of the counselling role of pharmacists. The specification on the supply of dispensed medicines states 'Pharmacists must ensure that the patient receives sufficient information and advice to enable the safe and effective use of the medicine'. Furthermore, it states 'the dispensed medicines should normally be supplied directly to the patient or their carer in the pharmacy, where there is opportunity for face to face contact … '. Similarly, in the case of on-line supplies of dispensed medicines, the Service Specification requires that the pharmacist 'must ensure the patient receives sufficient information to enable the safe and effective use of the medicine'.

The sale of OTC pharmacy medicines is similarly covered by the Service Specifications and the pharmacist is required to provide 'advice relevant to the product and the intended customer'. In the case of on-line supply 'the pharmacist must ensure that … they have the opportunity to provide appropriate counselling or advice'.

The *British National Formulary* (BNF) 'expects pharmacists will counsel when necessary' and is a little more explicit in defining counselling. It states that:

> *Counselling needs to be related to the age, experience, background, and understanding of the individual patient. The pharmacist should ensure that the patient understands how to take or use the medicine and how to follow the correct dosage schedule. Any effects of the medicine on driving or work, any foods or medicines to be avoided, and what to do if a dose is missed should also be explained. Other matters, such as the possibility of staining of the clothes or skin by a medicine should also be mentioned. For some preparations there is a special need for counselling, such as an unusual method or time of administration or a potential interaction with a common food or domestic remedy.*

The need for counselling

It is generally accepted that some patients have difficulty taking/using their medicines and complying with the dosage regimens. Evidence comes from compliance and wastage studies.

It has been estimated that up to 50% of older people do not take their medicines as intended. The scope of this problem can be seen when some facts are considered. It is estimated that 80% of over 75 year olds in the UK take at least one prescribed medicine and 36% take four or more medicines. Additionally, research has shown that 50% of patients (not necessarily older people) with hypertension failed to take their medicines correctly and one in ten deaths were attributable to stroke. It has been suggested that counselling by pharmacists could lead to better compliance and hence less therapeutic failure and possible death.

The cost of unused medicines returned by patients to pharmacies has been estimated to be in excess of £100million each year. Many of these unused and hence wasted medicines are because patients do not understand why their medicine(s) has been prescribed or how to take/use it. Although many medicines are supplied with a patient information leaflet, many patients do not always understand the contents and require further explanation from the pharmacist. Pharmacists are in an ideal situation to provide additional information and counselling when prescription medicines are handed out and when OTC medicines are sold.

The aims of counselling

There is a lack of evidence that the provision of information alone is sufficient to enable patients to correctly take medicines or to change their existing behaviours and attitudes. Counselling as the definition from the BAC states enables clients to explore their beliefs and to develop plans for behaviour change. Pharmacists in their patient counselling roles may adapt and make use of the problem-solving model of counselling developed by Egan (1990).

Thus, the aims of patient counselling in addition to the provision of advice from the pharmacist could be to:

- Encourage patients to identify any problems they perceive with medicines and also any solutions to these problems.
- Encourage patients to develop their own action plan for taking/using medicines correctly.
- Gain an understanding of the patient's perspective.
- Respect the patient's beliefs and be non-judgmental of their use (or non-use) of medicines.

OPPORTUNITIES FOR COUNSELLING

The pharmacist is often the last health care professional whom a patient sees before starting drug therapy. It is at this stage that patient counselling should take place. Pharmacists should take a prominent and proactive role in counselling, especially since some patients do not expect it. The opportunities for patient counselling are many, but the main opportunity is at the end of the dispensing process or the sale of a medicine.

In community pharmacy, patient counselling should be an integral part of the dispensing of a prescription. No patient should receive a dispensed medicine without the pharmacist making an assessment of the counselling needs of the patient. The availability of prescription medication records and the information contained within will underpin the extent and type of counselling provided to an individual patient. Some pharmaceutical companies have developed computer-aided counselling systems associated with their products, which offer guidelines to pharmacists to assist with counselling, after dispensing the product. Such computerized systems provide an audit trail on counselling and can verify when counselling took place.

Another opportunity in community pharmacy for counselling is the provision of Prescription Only Medicines via patient group directions (PGD). All PGD require that the patient is counselled during the initial assessment of the appropriateness of the medicine for the patient and immediately on supply of the medicine.

The sale of medicines from a community pharmacy is another opportunity for patient counselling. The sale of medicines can be the result of: (i) a direct request for a named medicine by a customer and (ii) a request for advice on the treatment of a symptom or minor ailment by a patient. The amount and content of the patient counselling will vary with the type of initial request, the medicine sold and the patient

The introduction of self-care programmes for patients with chronic disease or presenting with minor ailments will involve the community pharmacist becoming actively engaged and using their counselling skills with patients.

Community pharmacists may provide diagnostic testing and health screening services to the public. In such situations the Service Specifications to the Code of Ethics requires pharmacists to provide patients with 'any necessary counselling and available information'. Thus the opportunities for community pharmacists to become involved in patient counselling are wide ranging.

Similarly there are many opportunities for hospital pharmacists to counsel patients. Hospital pharmacists, unlike their community counterparts, have the advantage of access to a considerable amount of information about the patient. This information can include details of disease state, current therapy and home circumstances, all of which can be useful in providing counselling. Patients in hospital often have their medication changed during their stay and so should be made fully aware of any alterations on discharge. Outpatients and inpatients at discharge receiving dispensed medicines will require the same sort of advice and counselling as patients receiving dispensed medicines from community pharmacies. Additionally, inpatients may require counselling on their medicines during admission.

Both community and hospital pharmacists may be involved in providing medication to patients in long-term residential homes. Such patients are often on multiple therapies. In such situations it may be necessary to counsel the patient or their carers if the medicines are to be used effectively (see Ch. 31).

HOW TO COUNSEL

Counselling, wherever it occurs, should take place in a thoughtful, structured way. The pharmacist must possess not only a sound knowledge of the drugs and appliances being dispensed or sold, but also excellent communication skills. Pharmacists must have the ability to explain information clearly and unambiguously and in language the recipient can understand. They must know which questions to ask and how to ask them. The counselling process should not be a monologue by the pharmacist giving a long list of information points. To be successful, it must be a two-way process.

There should be ample opportunity for the patient to ask questions. Importantly the pharmacist should know how to listen. Rapport is built up between the pharmacist and the patient and a much more meaningful dialogue can take place. The pharmacist should introduce aids to comprehension, if this is felt to be necessary, e.g. an explanatory leaflet or diagram, a placebo device. The communication skills needed have been discussed in detail in Chapter 3.

Privacy and confidentiality

Trying to give patients advice about their medication in a busy pharmacy can be difficult. Information on a patient's medicines is both private and confidential to them. Some pharmacies have a room or a special area set aside for counselling so that a private discussion can take place. If neither of these is available then the pharmacist must try to take the patient to an area in the pharmacy where they will not be overheard and a private discussion can be carried on. Constant interruptions and customers milling around nearby are a major distraction and are barriers to good communication.

What information to include in counselling

Each situation and each patient will have different information needs, but as a general summary no patient who has been given medication should leave a community or hospital pharmacy without knowing:

- How to take or use the medicine
- When to take or use the medicine
- How much to take or use
- How long to continue to take or use
- What to expect, e.g. immediate relief, no effect for several days
- Why the medicine is being taken or used
- What to do if something goes wrong, e.g. if a dose is missed
- How to recognize side-effects and minimize their incidence
- Lifestyle changes which need to be made
- Dietary changes which need to be made.

Who to counsel

Not every patient will require extensive counselling and advice, but it is important that pharmacists can correctly identify those who do. In deciding who to counsel it is important to consider both the patient and the medicine.

Consideration of the medicine

The medicine can be prescribed or bought. If prescribed the prescription may contain one or several items. A multiple item prescription may present more problems to the patient in terms of different drugs, different dosage forms and regimens, etc. and so patients presenting such a prescription may require more counselling than patients presenting single-item prescriptions. Additionally, the individual medicine on any prescription, due to their characteristics, e.g. complex dosage regimen, special delivery methods, novel packaging etc., may require explanation to ensure the patient has a clear understanding of how to use them.

Other reasons for considering counselling will be if the drug has:

- A narrow therapeutic index. The need for strict adherence to dosing should be emphasized. Drugs such as lithium or theophylline are common examples.
- The potential for interaction with another drug or food. Appendix 1 in the BNF lists drug–drug interactions and Appendix 9 lists any interactions with food. See Examples 38.2 and 38.3.
- The potential to cause side-effects. In these instances the patient should be told not only how to recognize the side-effects but also how to reduce the incidence or severity of them. See Example 38.4.
- Any drug in the BNF, which has a recommendation that counselling is advised. See Example 38.3.
- New drugs under intensive surveillance by the Committee on Safety of Medicines.
- Those medicines which require special storage conditions. See Example 38.6
- A recommendation in the BNF (see Appendix 9) that a cautionary and advisory label should be used. The information on these labels should always be reinforced. See Example 38.3.

Many pharmacists are unsure how much information about side-effects should be given to patients. There is concern that the patient may be put off taking the medicine to avoid suffering these unwanted effects. No two situations or patients are alike and it is difficult to make a definite statement about this. However, it has been shown that if patients are informed of commonly occurring side-effects, how to recognize them and how to deal with them, they are less likely to be anxious. Therefore, pharmacists should select

> **Box 38.1   Some drugs and the type of side-effects that can occur**
>
> **Some drugs cause side-effects which can be minimized by good management**
>
> | Drug | Side-effect | Precaution |
> | --- | --- | --- |
> | Chlorpromazine | Photosensitivity | Use sunscreen |
> | NSAIDs | GI disturbances | Take with food |
> | Tamoxifen | Nausea | Take at bedtime |
>
> **Some drugs have side-effects which require the patient to be warned for their information and benefit**
>
> | Drug | Side-effect |
> | --- | --- |
> | CNS drugs | Drowsiness |
> | Co-beneldopa | Colours urine |
>
> **Some drugs have side-effects that need monitoring**
>
> | Drug | Side-effect |
> | --- | --- |
> | Penicillamine | Blood and urine tests |
> | Chloroquine | Ocular tests |
>
> **Some drugs have side-effects that require immediate reporting to the prescriber**
>
> | Drug | Side-effect |
> | --- | --- |
> | Gold therapy | Sore throat, breathlessness, rashes |
> | Aminosalicylates | Bleeding, bruising |

the side-effects that are most likely to occur and advise on them. Box 38.1 details some drugs and the type of side-effects.

Consideration of the patient

It is part of the pharmacist's role to decide which patients require counselling and advice. The level and type of information given and how it is given will depend on a variety of factors.

- Is the patient known at the pharmacy and has the patient been previously identified as having problems with drug therapy?
- What counselling has the patient previously received?
- What are the patient's comprehension levels?
- What level of support does the patient need or have?
- The age of the patient. In general all patients who are elderly should be offered counselling and advice. If the prescription is for a child, the parent or guardian should be given advice.

- Is the patient pregnant or breastfeeding? Such patients may require reassurance that the therapy is safe to take. Similarly a breastfeeding mother may require advice on when to take the medication so that it least affects the child.
- Does the patient have physical disabilities? These could include mobility problems, causing problems in opening containers, blindness or deafness. A sight-impaired patient may not benefit from a patient information leaflet, while this may be the best way of providing information for someone who is hearing impaired.
- Does the patient have mental disabilities? These could include states of confusion, anxiety or forgetfulness. Limited intellectual capacity could lead to patients being unable to read labels, etc. or understand instructions.
- Known poor compliance.

Other instances which should alert the pharmacist to the need for counselling would be:

- The purchase by a patient of an OTC product which is incompatible with the prescribed medication, e.g. a patient with hypertension who is taking atenolol and wishes to purchase Sudafed for nasal congestion.
- A patient asking for a prescription item not to be dispensed. This could indicate that the patient is non-compliant with that medication.
- A patient asking to buy an OTC medicine, which is to relieve the side-effects of a prescribed medicine. An example of this would be a patient who is being prescribed NSAIDs asking for an indigestion remedy. This should be investigated. The pharmacist will want to make sure that the indigestion is not due to side-effects of the drug.

Aids to counselling

Patient information leaflets, warning cards and placebo devices are all useful aids when giving advice to patients. Many medicines are available in manufacturers' original packs complete with a patient information leaflet (PIL). These PILs should be used during counselling where appropriate and important points highlighted. Placebo devices, e.g., inhalers, epipens, patches, etc., can be used to demonstrate a particular technique and also to check a patient's ability to use a device. The NPA is a useful source of information leaflets and warning cards. Leaflets on how to use ear drops, eye drops, eye ointment, pessaries, suppositories, a nebulizer, malaria tablets and head louse lotions are available. These, along with warning cards recommended by the

BNF for anticoagulant therapy, lithium and steroid treatment, should be available in all pharmacies, hospitals and any other areas where counselling patients on drug therapy takes place. Whether commercially produced or prepared by individual pharmacists, it is important to ensure that the quality of any information leaflet is of the highest standard and is comprehensible to the patient.

STAGES IN THE COUNSELLING PROCESS

If counselling is approached in a structured manner, then time will be used efficiently and the counselling has a greater likelihood of success. The following stages in the counselling process have been adapted from the guidelines on Counselling and Advice on Medicines and Appliances in Community Pharmacy Practice produced in 1996 by the Scottish Office Clinical Research and Audit Group:

- Recognizing the need for counselling
- Assessing and prioritizing the needs
- Specifying the assessment methods to be used
- Implementation
- Assessing the success of the process.

Recognizing the need for counselling

The need for counselling based on a consideration of the characteristics of the patient and the drug has been discussed earlier. In addition the pharmacist will need to consider the content of the prescription.

Has the medicine been prescribed before for the patient? A review of the patient medication record (PMR) can often provide the answer (see Ch. 31). However, the PMR may be incomplete or not available, in which case, it is important to find out this information from the patient.

Are the instructions clear? It is the pharmacist's responsibility to make sure that the patient knows what instructions such as 'when necessary' or 'as directed' mean. An open question should be used here, e.g. 'Tell me how you take this medicine'. If the patient does not know, then the necessary information can be provided. In some cases patients may be taking the medication incorrectly. The pharmacist is then in a position to rectify any misconceptions. Checking an imprecise dosage instruction can also pre-empt possible errors, as in the following example.

EXAMPLE 38.1

A prescription for 56 Chorpropamide 100 mg tablets was received. The instructions read 'm.d.u.'

The prescription was dispensed as written and handed over to the patient without any dialogue taking place. Approximately 2 hours later the patient returned saying that the tablets had a different name and appearance from the ones dispensed previously. On checking with the prescriber the pharmacist found out that an error in entering the drug details into the surgery computer had occurred. The patient should have been prescribed chlorpromazine 100 mg tablets. The dose to be taken was 'three tablets daily'. If the pharmacist had asked the patient how she was taking her medication he would have realized something was wrong, the patient's usual dose for chlorpropamide being 'two tablets at breakfast'. Fortunately in this instance no harm was done to the patient, but it illustrates very clearly how important is the pharmacist's involvement.

Is the prescription for drugs that have a complicated or unusual regimen? In some instances, with a little thought, the pharmacist can simplify matters. The following example is an illustration.

EXAMPLE 38.2

A prescription for Questran sachets, 1 t.i.d., penicillin V tablets 250 mg, 2 q.i.d., and captopril tablets, 25 mg b.d. was received.

Because Questran interferes with the absorption of drugs it must be given either 1 hour before, or 4–6 hours after other drugs. A considerable amount of organization is needed to get this regimen right. Trying to fit three doses of Questran around the other drug therapy could cause the patient considerable problems. Fortunately, Questran can be given as a single dose, instead of divided doses. This would considerably simplify the regimen.

Assessing and prioritizing the needs

Although all individuals should be considered for counselling, there will be some for whom little or none is required. For example a customer who asks for an OTC by name and has used it successfully on several previous occasions or an 'expert patient' receiving a dispensed medicine may require minimal counselling. Counselling is time consuming and so pharmacists should concentrate their time and efforts on those patients requiring counselling. This entails assessing the needs of the patient and prioritizing so that counselling is directed at the most needy patients. In addition the pharmacist may have to be selective in what advice is given to a patient. The average number of facts which can be retained at any one time by most individuals is three. Example 38.3 illustrates this point.

Some patients may be offered advice at certain time intervals rather than each time that a prescription is dispensed. Such patients include those with asthma, diabetes, mental illness and epilepsy. These patients are on long-term therapy and may only need reminding or asking if they require any information at time intervals or when they have a change in medication.

EXAMPLE 38.3

A prescription for vibramycin 100 mg capsules is received.

The BNF suggests four additional cautionary labels and counselling on posture for vibramycin. These additional cautionary labels are:

'Take at regular intervals. Complete the prescribed course unless otherwise directed.' Because of the antimicrobial effect of vibramycin, blood levels must be maintained and therapy must be continued for a minimum time period to prevent bacterial resistance developing.

'Do not take indigestion remedies or medicines containing iron or zinc at the same time of day as these medicines.' The effect of vibramycin is limited by such medicines. Many patients regularly use indigestions remedies and both iron and zinc are found in vitamin/mineral supplements available over the counter.

'Avoid exposure of skin to direct sunlight or sun lamps.' Such exposure will result in the patient developing reddening and itching of the skin resembling sunburn. Patients should be advised to avoid the sun. Patients may be counselled to use high skin protection factor sunscreens on exposed skin, e.g. the face and hands, if they are likely to be exposed to the sun and to keep the remaining skin covered by clothing and wear a hat.

'Take with plenty of water.' The capsules may become sticky and if not taken with a reasonable draught of water can stick in the oesophagus. The drug will be released and could cause irritation to this, least protected, area of the GI tract.

The counselling advised by the BNF emphasizes the above and the need for an upright posture when taking the capsules: *'Capsules should be swallowed whole with plenty of fluid during meals while sitting or standing'*. This counselling should be verbally imparted to the patient.

Counselling on cautionary labels should always include the reason why the precaution should be taken. Obviously, in this instance, to go into a detailed explanation for each caution could take a considerable amount of time. The large amount of information required might confuse the patient and the whole process becomes self-defeating. In instances like this the most important points should be selected for emphasis. But remember, the dispensed medicine will be labelled with all the additional cautionary labels. Any other points may have to be left to another counselling session. If only two points could be selected for this prescription they would differ for different patients, but all patients should be given the verbal counselling. For a patient who works outside, then it is essential to give them appropriate counselling on protecting themselves from the sun and using sunscreen products. Similarly a patient who regularly buys OTC mineral/vitamin supplements should be advised about their possible interaction with the prescribed medicine.

Specifying assessment methods

It cannot be assumed that because the counselling and advice has been given that the patient understands or is able to adhere to that advice. It is therefore important that, before embarking on any counselling process, the pharmacist has an idea how the success of the process can be measured.

This assessment could consist of checking that the patient can read the label, use an inhaler device or open a container with a child-resistant cap. Checking on understanding may require follow-up, such as an enquiry, the next time the patient visits the pharmacy, to ensure that no problems have occurred and the response to the therapy is as expected.

Implementation

The appearance of the pharmacy is an important factor. The environment should have a professional appearance and it should be apparent that counselling and advice is offered as a professional service. The service can be advertised in practice leaflets and within the pharmacy.

How the pharmacist appears is also of importance. An organized, calm person is more likely to instil confidence in the patient than a pharmacist who appears distracted, harassed and unsure of themselves.

Over the last decade or so, through the National Pharmaceutical Association's 'Ask Your Pharmacist' campaign, the public have been made more aware of the pharmacist's role in the provision of health care advice. It is important that patients are made aware that pharmacies are sources of information about drug therapy and that information is available. If patients expect to be given information about their drug therapy then they will become more receptive to it.

Patients should be given an indication of why you wish to speak to them and you should always check that they have the time to listen. A patient with time constraints is unlikely to give undivided attention.

If the patient is unknown to the pharmacist, it is important at the beginning of the conversation to try to gauge not just the amount of information that is needed but also the patient's level of comprehension. The type of language used is very important, particularly guarding against being patronizing by oversimplification. However, the use of medical terminology must be considered carefully.

Assessing the success of the process

Having given the information it is then of major importance to check if the counselling has been successful. What does the patient understand, can they use the device, and do they have any problems? The ideal, where possible, is to assess compliance through follow-up.

During the counselling process the pharmacist should be checking if the patient understands the information. Watching the patient's body language and maintaining eye contact can give useful clues as to whether the message is being understood and whether compliance is likely.

SOME EXAMPLES

In the following examples details of a prescription and some biographical details of the patient are given. Various counselling points are identified and information which could be given to the patient detailed. These examples illustrate the wide variety of issues which have to be dealt with in the counselling process. They are not intended to be comprehensive, as different situations and different patients will produce a variety of problems and issues.

EXAMPLE 38.4

Mrs Good, an elderly lady of about 75 years, presents a prescription for diclofenac 50 mg tablets. She has lived alone since the death of her husband, 2 years ago. When she is signing the back of her prescription she has difficulty holding the pen and complains that her hands and fingers are rather sore and stiff and hopes that the prescription will help. This is the first time she has presented a prescription for these tablets.

Recognize the need for counselling
Mrs Good has never been prescribed the tablets before, therefore basic information about the drug name and dose timings need to be given.

Diclofenac is an NSAID and can cause GI irritation if not taken with or after food. The appropriate warning label will need to be reinforced.

Mrs Good appears to have problems with her hands. Will she be able to cope with a blister pack? She lives alone so does not have anyone to help her.

She has not been to the doctor previously for a prescription for her hands but has she been buying anything OTC to try to alleviate the pain? Many of the OTC products available for relief of arthritic pain contain ibuprofen, another NSAID.

Will she have any problems swallowing the tablets? Diclofenac is available as a dispersible tablet or a suppository.

There are a variety of issues here that will need to be checked.

Assessing and prioritizing the counselling and advice needs
Compliance problems. It is important to ensure that Mrs Good can access the tablets and that she will have no difficulty swallowing the tablets.
Side-effects. It is vitally important to alert Mrs Good to the fact that the tablets may irritate her stomach and how she can avoid this.
OTC purchases. To avoid any duplication of drug therapy it is very important to find out if Mrs Good is taking any OTC medicines, what they are and make sure they are not going to cause any problems.
Timing of doses and duration of treatment. Mrs Good should be told that the tablets are not simply painkillers, to be taken infrequently. NSAIDs should give pain relief reasonably quickly and successful anti-inflammatory action should be seen within 3 weeks. To achieve these benefits the drug must be taken at regular intervals. This should be explained to Mrs Good.

There is obviously a considerable amount of information that needs to be given to Mrs Good. However, none of it is too complex so it should be possible to deal with all of it.

Showing her the tablets will also provide a clue as to whether she will be able to swallow them. Patients with swallowing difficulties can rarely conceal a look of horror when presented with tablets they know they cannot cope with. If swallowing is identified as a problem she can be reassured that alternative therapy is available as a dispersible tablet or as a suppository. It may then be necessary to contact the prescriber to alert him to this.

It is preferable to give the patient all the drug details, if possible. However, if it is felt this will be counterproductive, dosing in relation to food is one that should have high priority.

Mrs Good should be invited to let you know how she is getting on with her tablets and to contact you if she has any queries.

EXAMPLE 38.5

You receive the following prescription:

Beclometasone 200 microgram inhaler
Mitte 1
Sig. 1 puff m. et n.

Ventolin Accuhaler
Mitte 1
Sig. Use m.d.u.

The patient, Mr Charles Ferrier, is a patient of long standing. He has been on the steroid (beclometasone) inhaler for several months and was also prescribed salbutamol as a metered dose inhaler. He seemed to be well controlled and did not need to use his bronchodilator (salbutamol) very frequently. He tells you that recently he has had one or two frightening wheezing attacks where his ability to inhale was severely impaired. For that reason, the doctor has given him a new type of inhaler (Accuhaler).

The need for counselling
Mr Ferrier has not had the Accuhaler before. The different type of device and its method of use will need to be explained. The method of replacing the disk containing the blisters will need to be shown. Also the patient will need to be told that the device is a dry powder inhalation and not an aerosol as previously.

He will need to be told that the Accuhaler is the same drug as his salbutamol metered-dose inhaler and that he must not use them both.

The maximum dose of one puff up to four times daily will need to be reinforced, as this is different from the metered-dose inhaler dose. This advice is recommended by BNF.

During the counselling session it is probably worth checking Mr Ferrier's inhaler technique. The deterioration in his condition may be caused by insufficient steroid being inhaled. This could lead to ineffective prophylaxis.

Although asthmatic patients are normally on long-term treatment, it is dangerous to assume that they have good inhaler technique or are knowledgeable about their drug therapy. There should be regular checking of how devices are used and how frequently they are inhaled. Further information on this is found in Chapter 24.

EXAMPLE 38.6

The following prescription is received:

Propanolol tablets 40 mg one tablet b.d.

Chloramphenicol eye drops
m.d.u.

Chloramphenicol eye ointment
Use nocte

You notice from your PMR that, other than the propranolol tablets, which had previously been prescribed as the proprietary brand, Inderal, the other two items are new to the patient. A number of issues need to be dealt with here.

An explanation needs to be given that, although the appearance and name have changed, propranolol and Inderal are the same drug. If the patient has any left at home they should be finished and the generic then started. Unfortunately, cases are reported of patients who end up taking double doses of drugs owing to a generic being prescribed in place of the branded preparation.

Information about shelf life and storage of the eye drops should be given, i.e. the eye drops must be discarded 4 weeks after being opened and should preferably be stored in a fridge. In addition the patient should be informed of the usual dose for chloramphenicol eye drops, which is one drop every 2 hours, and given details of how to instil them.

If the patient has any difficulty with hand movements, etc. that would make the application of eye drops difficult, then a compliance aid may be suggested.

The patient should be advised to use the eye drops during the day and the eye ointment at night. The method of applying the eye ointment should be fully explained.

EXAMPLE 38.7

A hospital pharmacist has to dispense a discharge prescription for a patient (male, about 45 years old and smartly dressed) who was admitted, a few days ago, suffering from a mild cardiac event. On receiving the prescribed medication, the patient says that he has been told to give up smoking. He says that he wants to give up and has tried several times but unsuccessfully. He mutters something about not wanting to 'act like a teenager, although his mates had been successful in quitting smoking by that method'. It is fairly clear that the patient would like some help from you.

In such a scenario, it is important that the pharmacist uses good communication skills to find out the patient's concerns and then works through the possible actions with the patient, enabling the patient to choose and decide for himself. Clearly the patient wants to stop smoking and this is a very positive decision and helpful for somebody wanting to stop smoking (see Ch. 39).

On talking with the patient, it becomes clear that the patient does not want to use a nicotine replacement gum, as his 'mates had done' because he does not like chewing gum and considers it unsuitable for his job. The pharmacist is now in an ideal position to discuss the alternative products (e.g. nicotine-containing sublingual tablets, lozenges, patches and inhalators) available to the patient and the advantages and disadvantages of each preparation. By counselling the patient in this way and providing information and alternatives, it is possible to enable the patient to choose and make an informed decision for himself.

EXAMPLE 38.8

Patient counselling may involve enabling patients/customers to make a decision about their choice of treatment. In the following example a young mother asks the pharmacist for advice on treatments for insect bites for herself and her 5-year-old daughter. The young mother explains that she is going on holiday and would like to buy something 'just in case one of the family gets an insect bite, whilst on holiday'. The young woman says that her mother used to apply some pink powdery fluid—cala... something—on her insect bites, when she was a child, but her friend had suggested a spray. Another friend had suggested antihistamine tablets and an article in a magazine had suggested hydrocortisone cream. She asks you which would be best. In this situation the pharmacist needs to explain the advantages and disadvantages of the various products available for insect bites so that the customer can make an informed choice. The pharmacist also needs to explain the suitable doses of antihistamine tablets for a child and whether a liquid formulation would be preferable to tablets for a 5-year-old; also that hydrocortisone cream should not be used on young children and is not suitable for bites on the face. There are a number of issues, which need to be clearly explained to this customer. It is also important that the conversation is two way and that the patient feels she can asks questions if she does not understand. It is essential that the pharmacist makes sure that the customer has understood all the information and options available before making a decision. In this type of example the pharmacist assists the patient to make a decision about the type of treatment that is best for her situation.

CONCLUSION

Develop the habit of thinking about medicines from the patients' point of view. What do they need to know? What are their concerns about taking the medicine? What can be done to help patients resolve their concerns? Identifying counselling points from the information at your disposal is fundamental to good pharmacy practice. It is important to remember, however, that asking questions and listening carefully to the information provided by patients is critical to the success of the process. Approximately 16% of hospital admissions are directly due to adverse drug reactions. How many of these could have been avoided if the patient had received appropriate counselling and advice from the pharmacist?

Key Points

- Counselling is an important part of the role of the pharmacist and there are many opportunities for counselling.
- Counselling is for the benefit of patients and purchasers of medicines.
- The importance of counselling is recognized in many official documents.
- Counselling must be structured and deal with the key information in an easily understood form.
- The prescription is a useful guide to possible counselling needs.
- The extent to which patients should be told about side-effects will vary from one patient to another.

- Counselling should be used to reinforce the label and compliance and warn against the potential for interactions.
- Some groups can be identified as requiring special counselling—the elderly, where there have been previous problems, parents of ill children.
- It may be necessary to limit the amount of information given during counselling to avoid confusion and meet patients' needs.
- Checking is important in ensuring the effectiveness of counselling.
- A busy setting is a barrier to effective communication.
- Patients are becoming more aware that pharmacists can give valuable advice.
- Counselling is not a lecture—patients must be given the opportunity to ask questions.

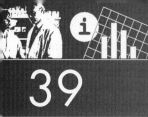

Health promotion

J. A. Rees

After studying this chapter you will know about:

What is meant by health promotion, health development and health education?
The approaches to health promotion and stages in changing health behaviour
The support for health promotion from government and the profession
Opportunities and involvement of pharmacists in health promotion

What is health promotion?

Health promotion at its simplest involves improving people's health and keeping them healthy. It is an integral part of pharmaceutical care and a recognized role for the pharmacist.

Health promotion has been defined in the Ottawa Charter for Health Promotion (1986) as 'the process of enabling people to increase control over, and to improve, their health'. This is a very broad definition, which focuses on the individual taking control over and responsibility for his own health. However, it gives no indication of the methods to be used to 'enable' people, the amount of improvement expected or the individuals involved in the process of health promotion.

More recently the WHO Health Promotion Glossary (1998) gave a definition of the term health development: 'Health development is the process of continuous, progressive improvement of the health status of individuals and groups in the population'. This definition implies that health development is a process which has no end point. In a similar way to the definition of health promotion it does not state who is involved in promoting the health development or what methods should be used. However it does include groups and individuals rather than just concentrating on individuals. Much of the definition of health development encompasses and describes the health promotion activities currently carried out by pharmacists.

A major criticism of both the above definitions is that they are dependent on what is meant by the term health. Health has been defined in many ways and may mean different things to different people (see Ch. 2). It is not the intention in this chapter to discuss the meaning of the term health but in order to progress with the subject of health promotion, it is necessary to accept that there may be many different understandings of the term 'health'.

Health promotion or education?

Health promotion is a broad umbrella term that encompasses, for example, political action to change social policies, responsibilities of employers towards the health of employees, environmental issues that influence health, etc. as well as health education. Health education is a part of health promotion and is essentially about giving information and working towards individual attitude and behaviour change. Research suggests that most people do know at least some of the basics about what keeps them healthy, but their reasons for continuing their unhealthy lifestyles are complex and not clearly understood. Health education involves providing differing levels of information for different individuals or groups, e.g. young people/elderly people, heavy drinkers/occasional drinkers. It has an essential role to play in the health of communities and is an integral part of health promotion.

Health education has been classified into three types:

Type 1—education about the body and how to look after it.
Type 2—provision of information about access to, and the most appropriate use of, health services.
Type 3—education about national, regional and local policies and structures and processes in the wider environment which are detrimental to health.

Thus, health education has a wide remit with the aim of providing information and education on issues affecting the health of individuals.

Health education isn't just about unhealthy people. Health education programmes have been classified into three classes depending on the health status of the group of people to which the education is aimed:

- Primary health education is directed at healthy people and aims to prevent ill health arising and to positively improve the quality of health, and hence life. Examples of this type of health education, conducted by pharmacists, include smoking cessation, preconceptual care and pregnancy, sun awareness, immunization.
- Secondary health education is directed at people who are ill. It has the aim of preventing ill health moving to a chronic or irreversible stage and to restore individuals to their former state. Restoring good health may involve the patient in a behaviour change, e.g. stopping smoking, changing eating habits if the patient is overweight or has a high cholesterol level. Secondary health education also includes ensuring patients comply with a medication regimen; can they use an inhaler or other medication devices or do they simply need to learn about the self-care of their ailment?
- Tertiary health education is concerned with educating patients and their relatives or carers about how to make the most of the remaining potential for healthy living. Pharmaceutical examples include providing patients with advice on the side-effects of medicines and how to manage them, the prevention of complications of diabetes, prevention of falls in the elderly due to the adverse effects of medicines and providing information on disability aids.

Some health education topics may span primary, secondary and tertiary health education but the content of the education will differ depending on the aim and recipient. For example, dietary advice can be given, firstly, with the aim of keeping a person healthy or preventing ill health, such as maturity onset diabetes (primary health education). Secondly, it can be given to help individuals adjust their eating habits and so reduce their cholesterol levels or to overweight patients to reduce their hypertension (secondary health education). Finally, it can be given to stoma patients to enable them to lead a less restrictive life or given to diabetic patients to prevent the development of complications (tertiary health education).

With all these types of health education the emphasis is on the provision of education and information with the aim of changing behaviour. But there is also a need to respect people who, for their own reasons, do not wish to change their behaviour. Therefore, there is a need to educate people

to make informed decisions about their health and to acquire the skills to enable voluntary behaviour change to take place, if that is what the individual decides. Thus whilst health education is a component of health promotion, it is not the whole. The aims of health promotion should be to:

- Give people appropriate education and information to make choices
- Enable people to examine these informed choices
- Help people to develop the skills to analyse and recognize alternative choices
- Empower people to be able to make informed decisions about their health.

Stages in changing health behaviour

As stated above, health promotion is about providing information to enable an individual to make an informed decision with the possibility of behaviour change. However, behaviour change is not a simple one-step process. Prochaska and Di Clemente (1986) studied the process of behaviour change and proposed a cyclical model consisting of several stages. An understanding of this model by health promotion facilitators is useful if an individual is to be supported through the process of behaviour change. The model describes the stages and accepts that the process is not usually linear and that many individuals go through the stages on more than one occasion. Thus the process can be considered as cyclical with individuals entering the cycle and going round, often several times, before emerging to a permanently changed state of behaviour. This model fits the actions of many smokers who 'give up' several times before eventually becoming a non-smoker. Indeed this model underpinned a very successful smoking cessation programme, which was conducted in community pharmacies. The stages in the model are as follows:

Precontemplation stage

At this stage an individual can either have no awareness that they need to change their behaviour or they do not accept that a behaviour change is necessary. Individuals at this stage have either never been the recipient of any form of health education on the topic concerned or they did not understand or comprehend the message or were unprepared to accept the message. At this stage the individual is not interested in changing their behaviour.

Contemplation stage

As the name suggests, during this stage individuals may be contemplating, thinking about or becoming positively motivated towards a behaviour change. They are starting to make a decision about a behaviour change. For example an individual may be thinking about 'starting to loose weight' or 'giving up smoking' or 'cutting down on drinking'. It is at this stage that the cycle of stages of change is entered.

Commitment stage

This is the stage when an individual has a serious determination to change their behaviour. At this stage an individual is 'ready to change', their motivation is high and they are in the 'I am going to … ' frame of mind. The decision is made and this may be the time when family and friends are told.

Action stage

At this stage an individual starts to make changes to their behaviour. For example if trying to stop smoking, they may throw away all their cigarettes and smoking equipment and buy and apply nicotine replacement patches. This stage is the time of action and it is a natural progression from the commitment stage.

Maintenance stage

During this stage an individual will need to continue with the actions commenced in the previous stage. At this time an individual may struggle with their self-imposed changes and may need to adapt the changes to suit their lifestyle or to try various coping strategies. The support of friends and family and/or health promotion facilitator is important at this stage. If an individual can continue with their behaviour changes for a considerable time, then they may emerge to the exit stage. However, most individuals will loose motivation during the maintenance stage and will find it becoming harder and harder to maintain their new behaviour style and eventually proceed to the relapse stage. The maintenance stage may last for a very short time or it may be considerably longer.

Relapse stage

Many individuals go from the maintenance to the relapse stage. Thus, individuals go back to their previous behaviour, for example they start to smoke again. But this isn't usually

the end point. Many individuals, in time, will re-enter the contemplative stage and may progress into the other stages. This is the cyclical nature of the process of behaviour change. For some individuals it may take several revolutions of the cycle before they progress to the exit stage.

Exit stage

When this stage is reached, the individual has changed their behaviour in such a way that they will not relapse. The changed behaviour becomes permanent.

Identifying the stage at which an individual presents, can help a health promoter adapt the interventions to the needs of the individual. For example, a person at the precontemplative stage requires their awareness of the topic to be raised. It would not be helpful at this stage to suggest to a smoker that they bought chewing gum containing nicotine because they have not accepted that there is a need to stop smoking, whereas a smoker in the contemplative or commitment stage may welcome a pharmacist explaining the range of smoking cessation products available for purchase. A pharmacist providing encouragement, asking 'how the patient is getting on with their … ?,' would be helpful to an individual in the maintenance stage.

HEALTH PROMOTION AND PHARMACY

In the context of pharmacy, health promotion is not just about changing people's lifestyle, nor is it limited to providing information. It is also about providing services that improve the health of individuals and communities. In addition, it is about empowering individuals so that they have increased control over their own health (Andersen 1998).

Health promotion activities conducted by pharmacists have been divided into four separate and distinct categories:

- Promoting health and well being (e.g. nutrition, physical activity)
- Preventing illness (e.g. smoking cessation, immunization, travel health)
- Identifying illness (e.g. screening and detection of disease)
- The maintenance of health for those with chronic or potentially long-term conditions (e.g. asthma, hypertension).

It should be noted that one of these categories, namely identifying illness, has not been mentioned previously and whilst not unique to pharmacy, is a very definite role for the community pharmacist. Indeed, a service specification for diagnostic testing and health screening is included in the Code of Ethics of the Royal Pharmaceutical Society of Great Britain (RPSGB).

Approaches to health promotion

Compliance or concordance

Whilst all pharmacists involved in health promotion will want to do their best for the patient, it must be accepted that we cannot impose our own values on other people or force them to do something against their will. Thus we have to accept that our health promotion activities may result in total compliance of an individual at one end of the spectrum to total non-compliance at the other, with varying degrees of compliance in the middle. We may have to accept that the aims of our health promotion activities may present us with ethical dilemmas. Do we aim and expect complete compliance from our patients or do we accept that, if the individual has made an informed choice, non-compliance is acceptable, even if the non-compliance goes against the best interests of the patient? This aspect of health promotion extends the compliance–concordance issue discussed in Chapter 40. For example, if a pharmacist is advising a patient with a high cholesterol level about healthy eating and reducing fat intake then, if the aim is compliance, the pharmacist will be persuasive, stress the risks and consider the session a failure if the patient does not comply with the advice. On the other hand, if the aim of the pharmacist is to enable and give the patient the confidence and skills to make an informed choice, then an outcome in which the patient did not change their behaviour would not be considered a failure.

Thus, there is no one 'right' aim for health promotion and therefore there is no one 'right' way of providing health promotion. Different health professionals may tackle health promotion activities using different approaches depending on the needs of the clients, as perceived by that professional, and the values and skills possessed by that professional.

Models of health promotion

Five models of health promotion have been identified; each model having different aims and implicit values. Pharmacists can use all these models in different ways to tackle health promotion issues.

Medical approach. This approach aims for freedom from medically defined disease and disability, such as diabetes, cancer and cardiac disease. Medical intervention techniques include immunization, screening, contraceptive advice and supply, dietary advice or prescribed medication. Patient compliance is the expectation of this approach.

Behaviour change. This approach aims to change an individual's attitudes and behaviour such that the changed behaviour is conducive to freedom from disease and/or a healthy lifestyle is adopted. Examples of this approach include advising and encouraging individuals to eat healthily, consume alcohol sensibly, stop smoking, practise safe sex, take more exercise, comply with medication regimens, etc. Pharmacists using this approach must be convinced that a healthy lifestyle is in the interests of the individual and that behaviour change is possible and beneficial.

Educational approach. As the name suggests this approach aims to give information so that individuals have knowledge and understanding about health issues. In addition individuals are helped to explore their own values and attitudes and so are able to make informed decisions. This approach may use health promotion leaflets, educational programmes, and national campaigns, e.g. no smoking day. Individuals using this approach will value the educational process, seek to provide the 'best' educational methods and techniques and respect the right of the individual to make their own decisions about their health.

Patient-centred approach. This approach aims to work with individuals to help them to identify what they want to know and what they want to do about a health issue. It includes allowing individuals to make their own decisions taking into account their own values. A major aim of this approach is self-empowerment of the individual and treating them as an equal, who has an absolute right to control over their health destinies. This approach assumes a fully autonomous patient. Using this approach a pharmacist would only discuss a health promotion issue, e.g. healthy eating, smoking cessation, if the patient expressed their own concerns about the topic.

Societal change. As the name suggests this approach is concerned with changing society, not the behaviour of individuals. Thus the approach is to effect change in society and to make the environment a better and healthier place. However changing the environment will impinge on the rights of the individual. Examples of societal change would be making smoking socially unacceptable or making the use of condoms socially acceptable to sexually active teenagers. Thus, in the case of smoking, the result of this approach to health promotion would be that smoking would be forbidden in all work, social and public places. However this approach takes away the rights of individuals to make their own decisions, but is regarded by most people as being democratic.

SUPPORT FOR HEALTH PROMOTION

Support from government

In the UK, government support for health promotion has been on going for many years. The advantages of successful health promotion to the UK and any other society is the reduction of health inequalities and the improvement in the quality of life of individuals, leading to less illness and longer life expectancy. Concomitant with these gains is a reduction in total health care costs. Thus the relatively low costs incurred in providing health promotion measures are far outweighed by the benefits to the individual and the nation.

A White Paper, 'Saving Lives: Our Healthier Nation' (1999), was a comprehensive document describing public health policy. It had two goals:

- To improve health
- To reduce the health gap (inequalities).

In particular it set four national targets in the following areas:

- Cancer
- Coronary heart disease and stroke
- Accidents
- Mental health.

Within each of these targets there are aspects of health promotion. The White Paper required each local area to address these targets and also to set additional local targets, including health inequalities. By setting local targets the White Paper accepts that local needs may differ from national needs. These local needs will be met by the development of Health Improvement Programmes.

The Health Development Agency (announced in the White Paper) was set up as a national body with the aim of improving the health of everyone. Its role in achieving this aim is to:

- Gather evidence of what works
- Advise on good practice
- Support all those working to improve the public's health.

One of its tasks, of particular relevance to pharmacy, is the development and implementation of National Service Frameworks (NSFs). The aims of the implementation of NSFs are to raise quality and decrease variations in service. NSFs set national standards and defined models for a defined service or care group. Performance milestones will be set to establish whether NSFs are achieving the set standards. A rolling programme of NSFs was introduced. The first NSF was mental health in 1999 followed, at almost yearly intervals, by coronary heart disease (CHD), older people and diabetes. In its broadest sense health promotion is included in all the NSFs. For example, the NSF on mental health defines mental health promotion, whilst the NSF for older people has one of its standards as 'promoting an active healthy life' and one of its aims is to ensure that older people 'gain the maximum benefit from their medications to maintain or increase their quality and duration of life'. The latter aim is transferable to other NSF covering people with chronic conditions requiring medication. The NSF for CHD, similarly, covers 'reducing heart diseases' 'preventing CHD' and 'structuring and funding health promotion activities' amongst its remit: all a part of health promotion. Pharmacists have a role to play in all aspects of health promotion included in the NSFs.

In addition, Health Action Zones (HAZs) have been set up in the most deprived areas to tackle health inequalities. HAZs are partnerships between the NHS, the local authority and the local community. To date all the HAZs have initiated smoking cessation programmes with the involvement of community pharmacists. Other community pharmacy-based health promotion programmes initiated with the involvement of the HAZ include head lice treatment and prevention and healthy heart campaigns.

More recently, a major theme in The NHS Plan (2000) was improving health and reducing inequality. Included in the plans for investment and reform were: reducing smoking, improving diet and nutrition, tackling drugs- and alcohol-related crime and ensuring children have a healthy start in life. There is a role for pharmacists as health promoters in all these areas.

'Pharmacy in the future', the government's programme for pharmacy, will result in local pharmaceutical services, which will allow pharmaceutical services to be provided under locally tailored arrangement. These arrangements will cover health promotion, focused on the needs of the local population.

Thus it can be seen that there is support at governmental level for health promotion and a need for pharmacists to be actively involved in helping to tackle health improvement in the population.

Pharmacy support for health promotion

Alongside government initiatives for improving the health of the population, bodies within pharmacy have also supported and contributed to the move for more health promotion activities by pharmacists. The 'Pharmacy in a New Age' documents published by the Royal Pharmaceutical Society (see Ch. 1) in 1996 supported the pharmacists' role, both in the present and future, as that of health promoter and health screener. This role, one of promoting and supporting healthy lifestyles, was given further support in a strategy document published in 1997 and resulted in a document entitled 'Guidance for the Development of Health Promotion by Community Pharmacists'. This document outlined the levels and types of activity in which pharmacists should be involved in health promotion, health screening and the use of consultation areas, as well as providing guidance to other stakeholders.

The Royal Pharmaceutical Society has given its support in other ways. The Audit Unit has produced audit templates many of which are concerned with the promotion and support of healthy lifestyles. Examples include accident prevention (such as driving and CNS-acting medicines, storage of medicines, falls in the elderly), oral health, travel health, preconceptual care and pregnancy and smoking cessation. In addition, practice guides for community pharmacists have been produced and these include health promotion activities. Examples include the care of people with diabetes and the care of people with asthma and chronic obstructive pulmonary disease.

More recently, a report based on the systematic assessment of the contribution of the evidence of pharmacy services to public health in Britain has suggested that community pharmacists should have a greater role in health improvement. In particular the report says that there is sufficient evidence to support the implementation through community pharmacies of smoking cessation, lipid management, emergency contraception and immunization services, while involvement in diabetes and anticoagulation monitoring and weight reduction programmes show promise.

Alongside all these activities sits the Pharmacy Healthcare Scheme. This Scheme is an independent charity set up to develop the contribution of pharmacy to public health through research, training and education. One of its main contributions to the support of health promotion is the

Box 39.1 Examples of topics included in health information leaflets
Dental health
Sensible drinking
Meningitis C
Folic acid
Smoking cessation

provision of free health information leaflets, which are distributed to the public through community pharmacies. Examples of the topics included in the health information leaflets are shown in Box 39.1. In addition, the Pharmacy Healthcare Scheme provides booklets, fact sheets and packs for community pharmacists to encourage and educate them about their potential role in health education.

WHY SHOULD PHARMACISTS BE INVOLVED IN HEALTH PROMOTION?

Pharmacists should be involved in health promotion for a number of reasons including upholding their Code of Ethics, accessibility to the general public, their knowledge base, their place in the primary care team and because government initiatives include them. These reasons are expanded below.

The Code of Ethics of the Royal Pharmaceutical Society states that 'pharmacists' prime concern … must be for the well being of patients and the public' and it recognizes in the Service Specifications the role of the pharmacist in 'health care information and advice' and 'diagnostic testing and health screening'. Thus health promotion is an expected role of the pharmacist.

At a practical level, it is estimated that 6 million visits are made to community pharmacies per day in the UK. Many of these visits will be for health-related matters and thus there is the opportunity for pharmacists to encourage healthy lifestyles and advise on other relevant aspects of health promotion. Many of these encounters can be personalized one-to-one sessions based on the opportunities presented by patients presenting prescriptions or asking for advice or wishing to purchase an over-the-counter medicine. Thus, the health promotion activity can be tailored to the needs of the individual and will be seen as relevant and more likely to be effective and acted upon.

Additionally, the public perceives pharmacists as being knowledgeable about health and medicines and, thus, health promotion activities by pharmacists will be seen as a credible activity alongside their other roles.

One important facet of community pharmacy is that due to its neighbourhood setting, accessibility and long opening hours there is no social exclusion. All members of the public have access irrespective of their social class, sex, ethnic origin or religion, and thus pharmacists have an important role to play in delivering health promotion activities to many people that are often excluded, for a variety of reasons, from other forms of health promotion. The informal and non-threatening atmosphere of a community pharmacy makes it an ideal place for heath promotion activities, especially for the more vulnerable members of society. The informality may encourage people to actively seek advice on their health. Additionally, pharmacies do not run an appointment system (unlike other health care professionals) and so individuals can approach pharmacists for advice or information at any time convenient to themselves.

Some community pharmacies will be situated in a HAZ and be part of the overall plan to improve the health of the local area. Also, all pharmacies will be included in local health improvement programmes and become part of a local pharmaceutical service. Thus it is expected that pharmacists will contribute to health promotion activities in their local area.

HEALTH PROMOTION ACTIVITIES IN PHARMACY

Whatever activities or materials are provided in pharmacies, the main aim should be to raise the public's awareness to the pharmacist as a source of professional advice on health promotion. However, provision of materials alone is not considered to be sufficient.

Provision of health promotion materials

Pharmacies are a source of health promotion materials (often free) for the general public.

Leaflets. Leaflets are the major provision. These are available from the Pharmacy Healthcare Scheme, local health promotion units and commercial sources and should be displayed appropriately so that the public has easy access, yet the pharmacist is sufficiently close to be available to explain anything that is not understood by the reader or to supplement the information. Alternatively, leaflets can be displayed near to relevant products, e.g. leaflets about sun awareness close to sunscreen products. It is essential that pharmacists are familiar with the contents of leaflets and carefully select the leaflets so that a suitable choice is available for the needs of the surrounding population. Thus, pharmacists need to consider including leaflets printed in minority languages if that is appropriate to the area or to target specific health issues that are prevalent in the neighbourhood or are the subject of local health promotion campaigns. Leaflets should also be used to support any national health promotion campaign and any national campaign days, e.g. no smoking day, national osteoporosis awareness day.

The quality of leaflets has improved over a number of years but pharmacists should critically consider any new leaflet to ensure that it is suitable for the target population. Ideally, leaflets should be individualized and tailored to the needs of individuals for the most effect. New information technology systems are becoming available to support the production of such individualized leaflets.

Books and pamphlets. Books and pamphlets on health issues may be sold or loaned by pharmacies to their clients. Several community pharmacists have set up libraries of such books, pamphlets and videos for use by the local population.

Non-written health promotion materials. Such materials include audiotapes, videos, touch-screen computer programmes, CD-ROMs and the Internet. All these different materials, some more developed than others, have their place in health promotion. Some materials are developed for the specific needs of people with disabilities, e.g. audio tapes for the blind or illiterate, others are being developed to test the use of new technology to inform and educate people, e.g. a touch screen programme on CHD has been used successfully in community pharmacies.

Health promotion displays

These can include window displays, in-store displays and noticeboards, or at its simplest just a poster displayed in an appropriate space. All displays are a form of communication and provide information to the viewer. The displays should have a clear message and provide information in a friendly but professional manner. Displays can be linked to local or national campaigns, e.g. a display on smoking cessation can be synchronized with national no smoking day. All displays should encourage the viewer to speak to the pharmacist for further explanation or information. Window displays make effective use of window space. One study reported the use of window displays in pharmacies to raise the awareness of emergency hormonal contraception and resulted in an increased demand for emergency contraception, pregnancy tests and informational leaflets. Window displays may also enable some people to access information that in their normal lives may be relatively inaccessible or of a sensitive nature, e.g. displays on men's health. Depending on the neighbourhood of the pharmacy it may be helpful to the local community to make the display multilingual and/or to use symbols in addition to text.

Products

If pharmacists are to be seen to be health promoters then it is incumbent on them to provide healthy lifestyle products. Examples include sugar-free medicines and drinks, a good range of dental hygiene materials (dental floss, dental cleaning materials, fluoride supplements, mouthwashes, etc.), folic acid supplements, nicotine replacement therapy products, low sodium salt, etc. In addition, some pharmacies may stock disability aids or display notices to announce that disability aids may be ordered.

No smoking policy

If pharmacies are to be seen as a source of information on health promotion, it is important that the pharmacy is seen as a good role model. Thus all pharmacies should have a no smoking policy and be seen as an environment which supports healthy living.

Social inclusion policy

Health and health promotion is for everyone, irrespective of gender, age, ethnicity, social class, disabilities and health status, etc. Thus pharmacies and their services should be available to all. Ideally all pharmacies should have easy access for the physically disabled, mothers with prams, the less mobile and the blind. Similarly pharmacies may be fitted with 'Loop' systems for the hard of hearing. Notices and directional boards should be in English with other languages and symbols if this is appropriate to the neighbourhood.

Consultation areas/room

The discussion of health promotion topics with an individual may raise sensitive issues that need to be conducted in private or in such a way that the conversation is not overheard by other people. Additionally the privacy of all individuals should be respected. Thus it is essential that an area or room is set aside within a pharmacy for

consultations with individuals. Nowadays the use of a designated 'consultation area' is seen to be preferable to a separate room, since it is less formal and hence less threatening than a separate room. The consultation area should be designed so that a conversation can be held without others overhearing and without distraction or interruption. If a consultation room is used, then it should be appropriately decorated with health promotion materials freely on display and available.

Topics for health promotion activities

Evidence shows that pharmacists are more likely to engage in health promotion activities that are related to the use of medicines. However, some health promotion activities in pharmacies are not related to medicines, e.g. men's health. Box 39.2 (although not totally inclusive) lists some of the health promotion topics that are dealt with in community pharmacy.

Box 39.2   List of health promotion topics dealt with in community pharmacy

Accident prevention
Alcohol consumption
Asthma
Aspirin for prevention of CHD
CHD
Contraception
Diabetes
Drug misuse
Emergency hormonal contraception
Folic acid and pregnancy
Head lice and other infestations
Immunization
Lipid management
Men's health
Mental health awareness
Nutrition
Physical activity
Obesity and weight reduction
Oral health
Safe sex
Skin cancers/sun awareness
Smoking cessation
Women's health

ROLE OF THE PHARMACIST IN HEALTH PROMOTION

All pharmacists should encourage healthy behaviours and respond to those seeking advice on health issues. However, in the future pharmacists will need to seek opportunities and proactively develop health promotion activities. Pharmacists will be part of an integrated health promotion effort that works at a local level to implement both local and national targets. In order to provide health promotion advice, pharmacists will need to have good communications skills (this topic is discussed in Ch. 3) and, ideally, be able to assess at what stage in the 'cycle of change' the individual presents, so that any health promotion activity can be individualized to help the recipient.

Opportunistic and patient-driven opportunities

Many of the current health promotion activities of pharmacists are opportunistic and patient driven. These can be conveniently categorized as follows:

Sale of goods other than medicines

Community pharmacies sell many goods, which are not medicines but may be related directly or indirectly to health issues. For many such sales, it is possible for the pharmacist to engage in verbal health advice with the purchaser or provide health promotion leaflets on related topics. Examples are provided in Table 39.1.

Table 39.1 Some examples of health promotion opportunities when sales are made	
Sale	**Health promotion activity**
Sunglasses	Leaflet on sun awareness
Children's toothpaste	Leaflet on oral health
Slimming foods	Discussion on healthy eating and leaflet on weight control
Nit comb	Discussion and leaflet on head lice
Diabetic chocolate	Healthy eating leaflets, advocate membership of Diabetes UK or similar
Ovulation testing kit	Leaflet on folic acid

Sale of medicines

Sales of over-the-counter medicines provide the opportunity for pharmacists to relate the purchase to some health promotion activity. This activity can be advice on the use of the medicines or the condition it is bought to treat or some related topic. For example, the purchase of a medicine for cystitis or vaginal thrush could be accompanied by a leaflet on women's health in general or specific leaflets on cystitis or vaginal thrush. A customer buying a laxative could be provided with information on healthy eating. Similarly a customer, known to smoke, purchasing a cough mixture could be given advice on smoking cessation or the associated risks of CHD. All purchasers of nicotine replacement therapies should be encouraged in their attempt at smoking cessation. Some pharmacists may feel that such activities are intrusive on the individual, but the aim is always to help an individual live a more healthy life.

Prescription medicines

The presentation of a prescription may provide the pharmacist with the opportunity for some health promotion activity since the medicines prescribed may give an indication of the illness suffered by the patient or the side-effects of the medicine may necessitate giving advice. For example, some medicines have the potential to cause a patient to fall. Falling can be serious especially in the elderly and so advice on avoiding falls should always be given (see later). Similarly, car drivers should always be warned about the dangers of driving whilst taking certain medicines that may cause drowsiness. Any person receiving a prescription for a number of medicines should be informed about safe storage of medicines and the need to keep them away from young children. Foot care advice and information is important for all diabetic patients as well as healthy eating, physical activity and smoking cessation. Patients receiving medicines for hypertension and cardiac conditions should be encouraged to eat healthily, stop smoking and reduce sodium intake. These examples illustrate the wide range of opportunities for health promotion activities by pharmacists with regard to dispensed medicines.

Responding to symptoms or requests for advice

As part of their daily work life, pharmacists are asked for their advice on symptoms or choice of treatment for various minor and sometimes major illnesses. These requests provide many opportunities for pharmacists to engage in health promotion activities and because the request is made to the pharmacist, it is often easier for the pharmacist to provide or discuss a healthy lifestyle or other health promotion issues without feeling intrusive. There are many examples including the detection of major illness from presenting symptoms. For example any individual suffering from thirst, passing large amounts of urine, blurred vision, tiredness and weight loss or requesting treatments for fungal infections may be suspected of undiagnosed diabetes and referred to a GP. Customers requesting advice on the choice of medicines for potential travellers' diarrhoea during foreign travel could be given advice on malarial prevention, immunization, sun awareness, etc. A customer requesting 'something for toothache' could be given advice on oral health, whilst a request for advice on the treatment of constipation could be accompanied by healthy eating information.

Patient Group Directions (PGD)

Emergency hormonal contraception was the first example of a PGD and this provides an excellent example of the role of the pharmacist in health promotion. As part of the PGD, the pharmacist is required to discuss safe sex and contraception with the customer. Another PGD is for the supply of nicotine replacement therapy through pharmacies. In this PGD, pharmacists are expected to provide specialist advice and support to the client. Thus the role of a pharmacist as health promotion adviser is implicitly accepted in these PGD.

Proactive health promotion activities

Besides patient-driven opportunities for health promotion, pharmacists may also be proactive in their health promotion activities. These activities can be conveniently categorized into educational interventions and pharmacy-based programmes or structured interventions

Educational interventions

There are many examples in which pharmacists provide educational interventions to groups of individuals. For example, in two separate studies involving patients and primary school children, their knowledge about asthma was shown to be improved by an educational intervention conducted by pharmacists. Some pharmacists' present education/information-based talks to specific patient groups, e.g. pharmacy-based group education for diabetic patients was shown to be successful by significantly improved metabolic control after 6 months. Many hospital pharmacists routinely provide educational interventions on medicine management for patients with specific conditions, e.g. patients with high cholesterol levels, cardiac bypass, diabetes, arthritis, chronic respiratory disease. Other pharmacists give regular talks to schoolchildren, women's groups and local self-help groups on health promotion issues.

Pharmacy-based programmes or structured interventions

Pharmacy-based programmes or structured interventions are proactive attempts by pharmacists to engage in health promotion activities. These pharmacy-based programmes may be led by pharmacists, or may involve multidisciplinary teamwork. The aim of these programmes is to show that pharmacists are effective in providing health promotion and that pharmacies are suitable places for dissemination. An example of one such programme is the reduction in falls among older people (referred to earlier). This programme showed that pharmacists can reduce the risk of falls by:

* Identifying, from prescription medication records and prescriptions, older people at risk of falls
* Ensuring medicines are prescribed appropriately and used effectively
* Providing a home safety checklist to identify potential hazards for falls
* Referring those at high risk of falls to physical exercise classes
* Promoting falls prevention programmes as part of a multidisciplinary team.

Another successful programme on the provision of smoking cessation services by community pharmacists was based on the 'stages of change' model of behaviour. Community pharmacists trained in the model to provide structured behavioural support were shown to be much more effective at providing smoking cessation services. Because these pharmacists were knowledgeable about smoking cessation products and services, they were more proactive about raising the issues with potential non-smokers.

Another pharmacy-based programme concerns head lice management. Patients are counselled on how to detect head lice and supplied with a free detection comb and given a contact trace sheet. After checking all people living in the same household, any lice that are found are stuck to paper and taken to the pharmacy. Infected patients are supplied with the appropriate head lice eradication product and counselled by the pharmacist on its use.

The role of pharmacists in health promotion also includes training their staff on the provision of health promotion advice and information and themselves becoming involved in teamwork in the community. Thus pharmacists should liaise with other health care professionals and local health promotion units, which will provide support for pharmacy-based health promotion activities.

From all of the above it can be seen that pharmacists have an important role to play in health promotion and, hence, the health of the public, both now and in the future.

Key points

- Health education can be education about health, how to access health services or about policies, processes and structures amongst other things.
- Primary health education is directed at healthy people, secondary at those who are ill and tertiary to patients and carers to optimize healthy living.
- The 'stages of change' model can be a good guide on how to approach health promotion for an individual patient.
- There are various models of health promotion which pharmacists can use.
- The role of pharmacists in health promotion is supported by the UK government through White Papers, the NHS Plan, setting up Health Action Zones and the development of National Service Frameworks.
- The RPSGB has produced templates to assist pharmacists to meet their obligations under the Code of Ethics.
- Pharmacists may provide materials, have displays and products as well as other methods to promote health amongst patients and customers.
- There can be opportunistic and patient-driven health promotion during sales of medicines and other goods, supplying prescription medicines and in responding to queries.

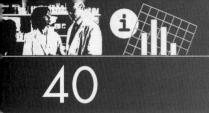

Concordance and compliance

A. J. Winfield and C. M. Bond

After studying this chapter you should know about:

Definitions of concordance, compliance and non-compliance
The relationship between concordance and compliance
The methods used to measure compliance
Some of the causes of non-compliance
Techniques for improving compliance

Introduction

For many years health professionals have expected patients to take their medicines as directed. The extent to which they do this is referred to as compliance, coming from the dictionary definition 'an action in accordance with a request or command'. It has also long been recognized that many patients may not comply with their recommended treatment for a variety of intentional, and non-intentional, reasons. This may lead to ineffective therapy, if the level of compliance means that therapeutic blood levels are either not reached, or not maintained long enough. It will also almost certainly lead to a waste of NHS resources as unused medicines are thrown away. One estimate suggests that, in the UK, more than 25% of medicines are not used at an annual cost of about £500 million. Because of both these intentional, and non-intentional reasons, there have been many initiatives to improve compliance involving different health care professionals (e.g. nurses, pharmacists, general practitioners) and different media (e.g. mechanical devices, patient prompts, incentives). These are discussed later in the chapter. However, despite all of them having some limited benefit, it is generally recognized that, unless reinforced regularly, their effect is short lived. We will only be able to improve compliance in the longer term if we take time to consider the complex psychological and sociological interactions which are involved.

When patients do not comply it is called non-compliance or non-adherence and it may be intentional or non-intentional. Non-compliance is usually thought of as not taking a dose, but it could be taking it at the wrong time, or taking too much. It is also necessary to decide the level of deviation from the instructions that will be called non-compliance. There is no clear answer, although many who study the problem regard taking 80% of doses correctly as being compliance.

Some studies indicate a wide spread in the levels of compliance with an average in the range of 40–60% compliant; yet non-compliance is not a new phenomenon. Hippocrates, around 400 BC, warned of patients who 'lie about taking their medicines and refuse to confess when things go wrong'. Without accurate information it is very difficult for clinicians to make appropriate decisions about future treatment. For example if a patient on antihypertensive medication appears to have uncontrolled blood pressure, the obvious solution could be to increase the dose of the antihypertensive. However if the patient, for whatever reason, had not been taking the original medication as intended then this further prescribing decision will have been based on a false premise and is doomed to fail. Assessing and understanding medicine taking is therefore an important clinical skill, and one which has been the topic of much recent debate and change in attitude. A new paradigm, concordance, has evolved encapsulating these issues. It is discussed in this chapter, together with its implications for explaining intentional non-compliance, and improving compliance. Non-intentional non-compliance is similarly considered, and addressed.

CONCORDANCE

The background

Chapter 2 discusses some of the social concepts of health and illness and people's responses to ill health. Although psychologists and sociologists have been interested in these

Table 40.1   Psychosocial models applicable to medicine taking

Model	Description
Health behaviour model (Janz & Becker 1984)	Balances the threat of a health problem (perceived vulnerability or susceptibility, and perceived seriousness of ill health) against the advantages and disadvantages of taking the medicine (the perceived benefits and the perceived barriers)
Illness representation model (Myer, Levanthal & Gutman 1985)	Balances a cognitive representation of the illness (what is wrong) with action (a plan to deal with the problem) and appraisal (evaluation of the success of the action)
Theory of planned behaviour (Ajzen 1991)	States behaviour is affected by the attitudes to the particular behaviour (which depend on the likely outcome of that behaviour, and the value placed on that outcome), and the subjective norms (i.e. perceptions of what we might be expected to do) associated with the behaviour
Beliefs about medicines (Horne 2000)	Balances and quantifies strengths of general beliefs about medicine taking (overuse and harm) with specific beliefs about one's own treatment (necessity to take and concerns about taking)

theories for some time, it is only recently that health care professionals have become generally aware of them, and realized the implications they have for their practice. This has in part contributed to the shift away from the traditional authoritarian doctor role to a more patient-centred role, which has benefits such as improved diagnoses and treatment. In addition this shift to a patient-centred role reflects social and cultural norms of today which emphasize patient autonomy, shared decision making, patient centredness, patient partnerships, informed choices, patient empowerment and holistic care. The 'expert' patient is now recognized as a genuine partner in health care as is exemplified by the following quote from a recent government document: 'the era of the patient as the passive recipient of care is changing and being replaced with one in which health professionals and patients are genuine partners seeking together the best solution to each patient's problem, one in which patients are empowered with information and contribute to their treatment and care'.

For many patients medicines are a required commodity, yet unlike many other commodities, they are often denied direct access to them, and have to have their wishes interpreted by an intermediary, namely a health care professional. This is most often a doctor for prescribed medicines, and a pharmacist for over-the-counter medicines, but increasingly nurses, pharmacists and health care professionals will be involved in the supply of prescribed medicines.

A satisfied customer is one who gets what they want not what the supplier thinks they wanted. It is therefore incumbent on health care professionals to understand the patient's agenda and the theoretical frameworks which govern patients' actions. Their decision to purchase or request a medicine is a complex result of balancing perceived benefits and risks of medicine taking. These have been described by various models, the most important and relevant of which are summarized in Table 40.1. These models explain the relationship between the patient's internal (intrinsic), and external (formed by personal experience and information) beliefs.

The 'beliefs about the medicines' model is further illustrated in Figure 40.1, which includes an indication of how this affects compliance.

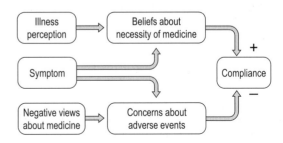

Fig. 40.1   Beliefs about medicines and the implications for compliance.

These models translate practically into a need to find out from the patient about their:

- Beliefs (medicines natural/unnatural, efficacy)
- Expectations (relief of pain, return to normality)
- Concerns (side-effects, addiction, tolerance)
- Fears (about the diagnosis and the future)
- Main problem (symptoms, effect on family, work).

These may be volunteered or they may be elicited during the consultation, and it is up to the professional to facilitate this. Research has shown that patients are most likely to voice information about symptoms, requests for diagnoses and requests for a prescription. They are least likely to voice worries about the diagnosis or the future, their own idea of what is wrong, side-effects, not wanting a prescription or social issues. When issues are not voiced this leads to misunderstandings, unwanted prescriptions, non-use of medicines and non-compliance, which is not surprising as 'patients have many needs and when these are not voiced they cannot be addressed'.

Concordance in the patient encounter

A concordant consultation is a term now used to describe one in which the health care professional facilitates and empowers the patient to contribute all the information described in the previous section, so that the prescribing decision is made in the light of all the necessary facts, and taking into account the patient's agenda. It may be that the decision is one not to prescribe a particular treatment, although in theory this may be the only recommended action. A definition of concordance is given below (http://www.concordance.org):

> Concordance is a new approach to the prescribing and taking of medicines. It is an agreement reached after negotiation between a patient and a health care professional that respects the beliefs and wishes of the patient in determining whether, when and how the medicine is to be taken. Although reciprocal this is an alliance in which the health care professional recognizes the primacy of the patient's decision about taking the recommended medicine.

It must be noted that compliance is not another word for concordance, but that concordant consultations are more likely to lead to compliance with treatment and better outcomes.

Concordance is still a relatively new concept and there is still much to be understood. There are, for example, ethical issues and concerns for professional liability if the agreement with the patient is not to follow current best practice. There is also a recognition that not all patients respond to this approach, and that some patients still just want to be told what to do. How does the practitioner decide what style of consultation is required? Embedded within the concordance approach is also a need to give the patient better information—at one time all that was seen to be necessary—but also to explore what information sources they themselves have already accessed in this information age. The central place of information in the interchange between patient and professional is clear in the following, original, definition of concordance:

> The clinical encounter is concerned with two sets of contrasted but equally cogent health beliefs—that of the patient and that of the doctor. The task of the patient is to convey her or his health beliefs to the doctor; and of the doctor to enable this to happen. The task of the doctor (prescriber) is to convey his or her (professionally informed) health beliefs to the patient; and of the patient to entertain these. The intention is to assist the patient to make as informed a choice as possible about the diagnosis and treatment, about benefit and risk, and to take full part in a therapeutic alliance. Although reciprocal this is an alliance in which the most important determinations are agreed to be those that are made by the patient.

COMPLIANCE

Whilst we believe that a concordant consultation will result in greater compliance, the evidence for this is still being identified. We therefore need accurate methods to measure compliance; these are discussed in the next section.

Measurement of compliance

A number of different methods for measuring compliance have been devised (Table 40.2), but none is accurate. Some rely on the honesty of patients in reporting their own compliance, whilst others are intrusive and thereby alter the level of compliance which is being measured. They are also only of value in experimental circumstances, such as clinical trials, and cannot readily be used to inform daily practice. Some of the methods are briefly discussed below.

Table 40.2 Methods of measuring compliance by patients with their prescribed medicines

Method	Comments
Experimental methods	
Mechanical devices	Do not indicate taking of medicine. Indicate timing
Body fluid tests	Only indicate short-term compliance, individual kinetics varies. Very invasive
Patient reports	No observation, relies on patient. As reliable as any other method
Pill and bottle counts	No proof of consumption or timing
Methods for routine practice	
Direct observation	Useful for checking technique. Impractical for routine use
Outcome measurement	Insensitive and makes assumptions. Clinical judgment is not reliable
Discussion	Talking to patients—may be best
GP computing systems	Only readily accessible by pharmacists working in GP practice
Community pharmacy PMRs	Useful for check of compliance at point of dispensing. Good time to counsel patient

Experimental methods

Mechanical devices. These were first used with eye drops. A chip was built into the cap that recorded each inversion of the bottle, which was taken to indicate use. However, the bottle could have been deliberately inverted, accidentally inverted or a genuine attempt made to instil a drop which failed. Similar technology can be adapted to show the opening of bottle tops, but with similar reservations about interpretation.

Blood and urine tests. Concentrations of drug in blood or urine can be measured. The drug can be the therapeutic drug in question or can be a subtherapeutic dose of a marker drug (e.g. low-dose phenobarbital), added to the formulation for experimental purposes. With knowledge of drug kinetics, an estimate of dosing can be made. There are a number of problems with this approach, not least being the invasion needed to obtain the samples for analysis. Usually samples are obtained on visits to clinics. However, it is well recognized that patients tend to become more compliant just prior to such visits. A second problem is that the half-life of drugs means that drug-taking behaviour can only be assessed over the last 48 hours at best. The one exception at present is the measurement of haemoglobin A1c (glycosylated haemoglobin) which gives a 2- to 3-month history of insulin compliance. There is also interest in the possibility that drug laid down in hair could provide a record over a longer time span once analytical techniques are sufficiently sensitive. A third problem is that, because individual kinetics varies, answers can only be approximate.

Patient reports. The method relies on patients reporting their own compliance, and may be conducted using prospective diaries or retrospectively by questionnaire or at interview. It is important that the questions are asked in a non-judgmental way. Despite care with the use of words, there is a tendency for patients to exaggerate their compliance. However, some patients will deliberately indicate a poor level of compliance. This is called social non-compliance and can arise with, for example, lonely people in receipt of home visits. The patient report method assumes that patients know how to take their medicine. Thus, they may think they are complying, but actually be misusing their medicine. Patient diaries may give more information on this aspect; they also reduce any implied criticism and enable an assessment of compliance to the regimen to be made. It is, however, difficult to sustain diary keeping for long periods of time.

Pill and bottle counts. The principle here is that a spot check is made to count the number of doses which have been removed from the container since the last check. It is widely used in the clinical trial situation when patients are requested to bring their current bottle of medication back at each visit to the clinic. Alert patients could ensure that the correct number of doses are missing. No information about the timing of doses, or whether the dose was actually taken is obtained. The method may also be used in clinical practice but would involve prearranged domiciliary visits with, again, the possibility of 'cheating' by the alert patient. It is invasive of a patient's privacy and time consuming.

Methods for routine practice

Direct observation. Medicine administration in residential homes (see Ch. 31) and in hospitals could involve observing that the patient actually takes the medicine. It has been argued that in the care situation, the patient is being coerced into taking the medicine, rather than being allowed freedom of choice. However, direct observation is a useful tool when a level of skill is required in order to use a medicine successfully. This will arise with, for example, eye drops, various inhaler devices and use of buccal tablets. Here the method is being used to help give patients the skill to comply, rather than to measure their level of compliance. In the domiciliary situation, the method is impractical other than for special groups of patients. This supervised administration of medicines is a role commonly undertaken by community pharmacists. Patient groups include drug misusers being treated on a maintenance or reducing schedule with prescribed substitute drugs, psychiatric patients who may otherwise forget to take essential medication, and patients on long-term treatments which require constant therapeutic blood levels to be maintained. A well-documented example of this is the long-term treatment of tuberculosis with antibiotics.

Outcome measurement and clinical judgment. In theory, if an effective drug is being taken correctly, there should be an observable improvement in the condition, which would not occur if there were poor compliance. There are a number of objections to this hypothesis. Firstly, the diagnosis may not be correct, secondly the drug may not be effective, thirdly the outcome may not be sensitive to small changes in compliance, and fourthly there may be other factors involved, such as socioeconomic pressures. Likewise, reliance on the clinical judgment of a doctor is unreliable. Studies have shown that, whilst doctors thought their patients had no problems with compliance, up to 70% of the same patients admitted non-compliance. Apart from these formal methods, an impression of compliance may be formed from comments made by patients.

Records of prescriptions ordered and cashed. A final method which is of great practical value is the frequency with which repeat prescriptions are presented. This can be assessed by pharmacists working within the general practice setting and accessing GP computer systems, or by individual community pharmacists reviewing their own patient medication records (see Ch. 31). It is a relatively simple procedure to either mentally calculate the period of return based on the dose and quantity of the drug previously supplied, or to chart this over a longer period to take account of, for example, early and late presentations due to illness, or absence from home.

CAUSES OF NON-COMPLIANCE

There is an almost endless list of reasons why patients fail to comply, and as mentioned earlier these may be intentional or non-intentional. Box 40.1 lists the main groups of reasons classified under these two headings. However, under each

---

Box 40.1   A summary of the main factors contributing to patient non-compliance

Unintentional
Understanding:
Inability to read
Intellectual ability
Poor instructions
Misunderstanding
Confusion

Medicine management:
Number of medicines
Times of day to be taken
Lifestyle issues
Forgetfulness and confusion

Disease-related factors:
Physical effects
Vomiting and diarrhoea
Progress of disease
Asymptomatic diseases
Prophylaxis
Mental state
Health beliefs

Physical limitations:
Obtaining medicines
Physical dexterity
Dysphagia

Drug-related factors:
Organoleptic properties
Side-effects
Generic variations
Religious factors

Intentional
Social and psychological:
Confidence in the doctor and medicine
Beliefs about medicines
Expectations of treatment
Cost of prescriptions
Religious observances
Help seeking

---

subheading there are many complex reasons, and often there is cross over between the intentional and non-intentional categories. Where an individual fails to comply, there may be several simultaneous factors. Some of the main reasons for non-compliance will be discussed in more detail.

Understanding

Poor understanding appears to be one of the most important reasons for non-compliance, but there are many aspects to it, some of which are linked to issues of concordance already discussed in theory.

The patient may be unable to understand the instructions. Some people cannot read, others have poor eyesight, the writing may be too small, or the ink too faint. Understanding is impaired by the choice of language. If it is vague, confusion may arise. Instructions may be ambiguous, such as 'two tablets a day'. When patients are counselled, they may not be listening, may have a hearing difficulty, and may have a problem with their educational level or their level of consciousness. They could also be suffering from mental confusion. With frail elderly patients, it may be a carer who collects the prescription, so that the pharmacist does not see the patient, and therefore cannot provide direct counselling or reinforcement of the presciber's directions. Another difficulty is a failure to appreciate the need for, use of, or rationale for particular medicines. Such situations are common with asthma sufferers who are prescribed inhalers for both prophylaxis and relief.

Medicine management

Some people are well organized. Such people will probably be able to manage their medicines. However, those who are less well organized may have difficulties with their medicines. The more different medicines the patient has, the more the problems increase. Likewise, the more complex the regimen, the worse will be compliance. Thus if all medicines are to be taken at the same time of day, compliance will be higher than if several different times throughout the day are used. Confusion can also arise over which medicine is which. These problems are increased where the patient is either confused or forgetful, both of which tend to increase with age. Since, in general, it is the elderly who require most medication, the incidence of non-compliance is higher in this group. However, problems are not confined to the elderly. Those in work may also have problems, for instance where tablets are expected to be taken regularly through the day with food, but the patient has very irregular meal times, or with dose administration in a working environment. Another problem is remembering whether a dose has been taken. Calendar packs are designed to help this process. However, they too can be confusing, depending on their layout, how they label the doses and how they accommodate differing starting days.

Disease-related problems

Various aspects of a patient's state of health can influence compliance. The disease may simply interfere with the patient's ability to comply. Thus a patient with arthritis may have problems opening a container, a skin condition may require application of a cream to a part of the body which the person cannot reach. A patient may be suffering from vomiting or diarrhoea, so that, despite taking a tablet, he may only gain a small benefit from it. A patient in pain is more likely to comply with analgesia because of the relief which it brings.

The attitude of the patient to the disease is important, as discussed earlier. The more 'serious' and life threatening the patient regards it, the more likely he is to comply with its treatment. This is not universal. Some studies have shown, for example, that a high proportion of transplant patients fail to take the drugs used to prevent tissue rejection. Compliance is more critical in conditions such as diabetes and epilepsy, where accurate drug plasma concentration is required for effective control.

The reaction of patients to the progress of their disease is also important. A common example is of patients prescribed a 1-week or 10-day course of antibiotics who stop taking their medicine after a few days because they feel better. Patients may also stop because they do not perceive any improvement in their condition. This is a particular problem with asymptomatic conditions such as glaucoma and high blood pressure. The patient does not feel unwell at the start and so sees no improvement, and may even feel worse. A similar situation arises with prophylactic medication, e.g. with antimalarials, where the individual may see no advantage in taking a medicine with its associated risks. Some patients may overuse a medicine to 'complete' a cure, such as using topical corticosteroids in some skin conditions.

The state of mind of the patient will also have an impact on compliance. The psychological state of an individual can markedly affect his compliance, although the effect is not necessarily predictable. Depression, distress, tension and aggression can reduce people's motivation towards taking their medicines. However, the effect may be reversed, with the patient coming to rely on medicines almost as a ritual.

Some of the factors which affect patients' reactions to disease and treatment are relevant here (see Ch. 2). Anything about their beliefs or perceptions which supports medicine taking will improve compliance, as has been discussed in the sections on concordance. On the contrary, factors which undermine people's confidence or belief in the medical service in general, will increase their non-compliance. Thus attitudes to the 'sick role' and health beliefs are going to be important in compliance.

Physical limitations

A number of factors are important under this heading. One aspect is how easy the patient finds it to either obtain a repeat prescription or have it dispensed. Distance, particularly where the patient has limited access to transport or lives in a rural area, can be a major problem. Walking up hills can also be difficult for some elderly people. Access to surgeries and pharmacies may be a problem for people working long hours or difficult shift patterns.

Physical dexterity is required for administering some medicines. Eye drops are the most obvious, where the patient needs to tilt the head, squeeze on a small bottle and aim accurately a short distance from the eye in order to successfully instil a drop. Many find this very difficult or impossible. Inhaler devices, especially pressurized aerosols, require coordination between fingers and breathing which many either find difficult or require training in order to achieve. Other dosage forms may also present some problems, including injections, ointments and creams, suppositories and pessaries, skin 'patches', buccal tablets. Very small tablets can present handling problems for people with arthritic fingers, because they have lost the fineness of movement required to pick them up. Gaining access to the medicine is not always easy, e.g. with child-resistant closures, blister packs or sachets.

Dysphagia, a difficulty in swallowing, is often overlooked, but is a problem for many, not just in certain medical conditions (such as stroke and parkinsonism) where it is recognized. Many people will indicate a problem in swallowing large tablets. There also appears to be a minimum size of tablet, below which swallowing also becomes difficult. In severe dysphagia, swallowing thin liquids will be a problem, often leading to aspiration of the liquid into the lungs.

Drug-related problems

The medicines themselves can also create compliance problems. Side-effects of a drug, particularly if unpleasant, may deter patients, although the effect is minor if patients believe that the medicine is helping them. Some have argued that non-compliance is an advantage in that it protects patients from adverse effects. In the past, taste, smell and colour were problems which could reduce compliance. With improved technology, most medicines can be flavoured and coloured to avoid these problems. However, a related problem arises with colour, size and shape, where generic products are being used. Since there is no standardization on colour, size and shape, patients may be given tablets which are different in appearance each time a prescription is dispensed. This can produce uncertainty, confusion, even a rejection of the tablets, with a consequent effect on compliance.

Religious beliefs can also affect compliance because of materials used in medicines. Examples include the use of alcohol in medicines for Muslims, porcine insulin for Jews and gelatin for Hindus. In addition people of some cultures may associate disease with spiritual causes and not see the relevance of physical treatments. Finally under this heading, the impact of religious observance must be remembered. Perhaps the most significant is the Muslim observation of Ramadan, where medicine should not be taken between dawn and dusk throughout the month. Less significant in its impact may be short-term fasting or an unwillingness to ingest anything in a morning before a ritual has been completed.

Financial considerations

Another factor, most often quoted over recent years, has been the impact of prescription charges. Since each item incurs a substantial charge, there are many reports of patients asking the pharmacist which is the more important item. A less obvious consequence of this is that patients may try to make a medicine last longer by 'rationing' their doses, say to one or two per day instead of the three prescribed.

Other factors

Social and psychological influences on patients will be important (see Ch. 2, and the section 'Concordance' above). Of particular importance is the level of confidence which patients have in the doctor. If confidence is low, they are less likely to comply, because they will also doubt the effectiveness of the treatment. Conversely, if they have a very high level of confidence, they may tend to overcomply if there is no improvement. Related to this is the confidence of patients in the drug which has been prescribed. From their own experience or, more commonly, from neighbours or publicity, they form an impression of the efficacy of a drug. In some situations, doctors can come under extreme pressure to prescribe particular drugs because of magazine articles or the neighbourhood 'grapevine'. If these influences are positive, compliance will be enhanced. If they are unfavourable, it can become a self-fulfilling prophecy, where the patient 'knows' it will not work, has poor compliance and so does not improve.

People have different beliefs about medicines. Many see them as beneficial and helpful. Others regard them as poisons to be used as a last resort. This latter attitude has led, amongst other influences, to the present interest in alternative therapies such as homoeopathy (see Ch. 41). People with such attitudes will take conventional medicines reluctantly, often with poor compliance.

Some patients feel that they are being used as guinea pigs when they are prescribed a medicine. They are, therefore, sceptical about the medicine and its potential benefit to them. As a result, compliance is reduced, particularly if there is no immediate improvement.

There can be situations when people quite deliberately do not comply because of the effect non-compliance will have. One example was mentioned earlier, where people living on their own come to rely on a visit by a member of the health care team for their only social contact. An improvement in their condition could result in their loss of that visit. Another example can arise with mentally ill people who prefer to live in a hospital rather than the community. If they do not comply, their condition will be assessed as being unsuitable for community living.

IMPROVING COMPLIANCE

The foregoing section has reviewed briefly some of the main factors which influence the compliance of an individual patient. The point has already been made that, ultimately, the patient has the right not to comply. However, it may be regarded as a professional responsibility to try to persuade the patient of the benefit of compliance, before accepting the situation. The following section considers some of the many techniques which the pharmacist can use to achieve this.

Understanding

The aim is to ensure as a high a level of understanding by the patient as possible. This means that optimum communication skills must be used. Orally, this will come from counselling patients (see Chs 3 and 38). This may simply involve passing on relevant information to the patient. However, the pharmacist needs to be alert to indications of the patient's health beliefs, their own objectives of the treatment and any information they may already have acquired from other sources. If these are at variance with fact, an attempt may be required to correct the error.

Apart from routine counselling, it may be necessary to give additional information to fill in gaps in understanding following the patient's consultation with the doctor. Alternatively, it could be providing information about the disease, the drug, lifestyle advice or giving training in using the medicine (see Ch. 39). Where a patient relies on a carer, it is advisable to involve the carer in any counselling or other advice which is being given.

Along with verbal communication, written information is supplied. Labels must be clear, easy to read and unambiguous (see Ch. 11). Where necessary, some computers can produce large-print labels, and Braille labels are available for a limited range of instructions. Other written information must be in non-technical language to make it readily understood.

Compliance charts may also be useful and are discussed below.

Medicine management

When compliance aids are discussed, it is usually those designed to assist medicine management which are thought of first. The aim of any actions taken is to assist patients to manage their medicine taking. There are three main approaches which can be tried. A diary of the day, indicating on it the times at which each medicine should be taken is the simplest form of compliance chart. Colour coding may be used to link the medicine bottle and chart. Computers can assist in producing these charts. Marking the chart as each dose is taken assists in preventing readministration.

Devices designed as compliance aids can be used. There is a wide range of different designs of memory aid devices for tablets and capsules. Monitored dosage systems can be used as an alternative. The principle on which they all operate is that compartments are used to hold doses, each compartment corresponding to a time of day. The patient works through the device as the day progresses, removal of the medicine indicating that it has been remembered. Audible devices are also available. There can be some problems. Errors may be made in filling the aid, there are questions about the stability of some medicines in these devices and some patients may have difficulty getting the tablets or capsules out of the compartments. Liquids are much more

---

> **Box 40.2   Some compliance aids and monitored dosage systems which will assist patients to remember to take their medicines**
>
> **Compliance aids**
> 7-day pill organizer
> Automatic pill timer
> Daily Pillminder
> Day planner
> Dosett
> Medidos
> Medimax
> Mediset Mini
> Mediwheel (and week pack)
> MedTime Minder (audible)
> Redidose
>
> **Monitored dosage systems**
> Nomad
> W + W Medsystems (including various 'planners')

difficult to handle using these aids. Box 40.2 lists some of the compliance aids and monitored dosage systems available, but there are many similar aids and new ones are being introduced continually.

The third possibility is to review the medicines to see if the regimen can be simplified to make it easier to manage. Thus the use of sustained-release dosage forms reduces dosage frequency and combination dosage forms reduce the total number to be remembered. It is known that going from three or four times daily dosing to twice daily improves compliance, but there seems to be no further advantage with once daily dosing.

Disease-related problems

Careful counselling can answer many of the problems which arise from a lack of understanding about the disease and its treatment. This can be particularly important with asymptomatic conditions or prophylactic treatments. Where the disease has reduced the manipulative ability of the patient, some compliance aids or other simple measures may be useful. The simplest is to suggest non-child-resistant closures for some elderly patients. Larger bottles can be used to make handling easier. Devices are available to get tablets from blister packs, which many people with arthritis find particularly difficult. A long-armed roller is available to assist applying ointments and creams to parts of the skin that are difficult to reach.

Physical limitations

Many compliance aids have been developed to assist people use their medicines. Some of these are shown in Box 40.3. Different aids can contribute in different ways, so selection needs to be made to meet the specific needs of the patient. For example, there are different types of aids to help with eye drops. Some help with aim only, others with aim and squeezing. For pressurized inhalers the Haleraid helps squeeze and various spacer devices are available, or it may be more appropriate to change to a breath-activated delivery device (see Ch. 24). Small tablets are a problem for those with limited movement in their fingers, but the Tiltab tablet shape can help.

Where dysphagia is a problem, an alternative dosage form or route of administration may be the best option. When tablets must be used, they may need to be crushed and suspended in liquid or semi-solid. This cannot be used if the tablet is designed to give a modified release. In all cases, very thin liquids are best avoided to reduce the danger of aspiration. Adopting an upright position is advisable and small changes in head and neck position can be of considerable help.

> **Box 40.3   Compliance aids available to help patients overcome specific problems of medicine use or administration**
>
> **External preparations**
> Mediderm applicator
>
> **Eye drops**
> Autodrop and Autosqueeze
> Easidrop
> Opticare and Opticare Arthro
>
> **Medicine bottle opener**
> Grip-it bottle opener
> Medigrip
>
> **Inhalers**
> Haleraid
> Spacers
>
> **Liquids**
> Ezydose and other non-spill spoons
> Oral syringes
> Rotadose (liquid dispenser)
>
> **Tablets**
> Pill-out (foil and blister pack tablet remover)
> Tablet crushers
> Tablet splitters

Drug-related problems

Many community pharmacists find it difficult to obtain generics for dispensing which are always consistent in appearance. Thus it may not be possible to reduce the problems that arise from changes of colour, shape and size, other than by reassuring the patient. Where some control is possible, the use of the patient medication record (PMR) to record the source of tablets dispensed for an individual will reduce these variations to a minimum. Control of side-effects may require a change in prescription. However, it is sometimes possible to modify the method of taking a medicine to reduce the problems, such as avoiding tablets on an empty stomach to reduce the incidence of nausea. Where ingredients would be unacceptable to some patients, it is necessary for the pharmacist to be aware of the problem and to be in a position to suggest alternative products where possible.

Financial considerations

Pharmacists cannot alter the cost of NHS prescriptions. However, they can ensure that all those who are exempt charges are claiming exemption, and they should be alert to situations where it is cheaper to purchase a non-POM medicine. Where patients are not having all their medicines dispensed, a discussion with the doctor might be useful to see if rational priorities can be established.

Other problems

There are no simple answers to many of the other sociological and psychological factors which affect compliance. The correct prescribing decision for the patient will be more likely if a concordant approach is adopted to the consultation and compliance should increase as the goals of treatment are the patient's. However in order that the pharmacist can provide counselling consistent with the decision of the prescriber, mechanisms will need to be developed for the sharing of this information. Future integration of community pharmacy into the NHSnet and shared patient records will facilitate this, although issues of patient confidentiality and sharing of data need to be resolved.

Depending on the nature of the problem, effective counselling by the pharmacist may assist with improving compliance. In other situations it may require a concerted effort by the whole health care team to help patients understand their treatment and the personal value of compliance for them.

Compliance can be a very difficult problem which may go undetected. When non-compliance is recognized, the pharmacist is in a good position to offer support to the patient. The approach should be to attempt to remove obvious barriers to compliance first, e.g. by suggesting compliance aids, drawing up compliance charts or instructing in the method of administration. For many, this will be adequate. Others will have remaining problems where a range of techniques may be required. Some patients will always be poor compliers, but many can be helped towards effective use of their medicines.

Key Points

- Concordance recognizes the rights of the patient to have their own beliefs.
- It is up to the health care professional to elicit the patients' beliefs and use them in their decision making.
- Concordance may increase compliance.
- There may be ethical issues to consider if the patient's agenda does not match the professional agenda.
- Non-compliance may be intentional or non-intentional.
- Untaken medicine costs the NHS a large amount of money each year.
- No method for measuring compliance is accurate, although many have been devised.
- There is an almost limitless list of reasons for non-compliance, reflecting a complex interplay of factors.
- One of the main reasons for non-compliance is a lack of understanding or comprehension about the medicine and how to use it.
- Poor medicine management is a problem with many, especially when they are on complex regimens.
- The disease may affect compliance levels.
- Physical limitations can have a marked effect on compliance in some situations.
- Increasing understanding and comprehension can increase compliance.
- It may be necessary to counsel a carer rather than the patients about medicine taking.
- Compliance charts and aids may help some patients who are trying but failing to comply.
- Whilst useful for some, compliance aids must be selected to meet the specific needs of the patient.
- Pharmacists must be alert to problems which may arise from the cost of medicine and take appropriate action.
- Some patients will always be poor compliers.

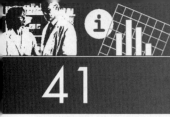

41

Complementary/alternative medicine

J. Barnes

After studying this chapter you will know about:

Types of complementary medicines and complementary therapies
Extent and reasons for use of complementary/alternative medicine (CAM)
Regulation of CAM practitioners and complementary medicines
The overlap of pharmacy and CAM

INTRODUCTION

Complementary/alternative medicine, originally referred to as 'fringe', 'holistic' or 'natural' medicine, was known as 'alternative' medicine in the 1970s and 1980s and, today, increasingly is called 'integrated' or 'integrative' medicine. Generally, it is referred to as complementary/alternative medicine, abbreviated to CAM, although the terms complementary medicine, alternative medicine and complementary therapies are used interchangeably. Zollman and Vickers' (1999) definition of CAM, which has been adopted by the Cochrane Collaboration (see Ch. 33), is given in Box 41.1.

Box 41.1   Definition of complementary and alternative medicine (Zollman & Vickers 1999)

Complementary and alternative medicine (CAM) is a broad domain of healing resources that encompasses all health systems, modalities and practices and their accompanying theories and beliefs, other than those intrinsic to the politically dominant health system of a particular society or culture in a given historical period. CAM includes all such practices and ideas self-defined by their users as preventing or treating illness or promoting health and well being. Boundaries within CAM and between the CAM domain and that of the dominant system are not always sharp or fixed.

In essence, CAM is an umbrella term for a collection of different approaches to diagnosis and treatment. Over 50 diverse complementary therapies have been listed, from homoeopathy (which involves the use of infinitely dilute preparations) to herbal medicine (the use of chemically rich plant material), and from acupuncture (which involves the insertion of needles into specific points on the body) to therapeutic touch and spiritual healing (including 'distant' healing, which does not require the laying on of hands). Some of the most well known complementary therapies are described in Box 41.2.

Box 41.2   Descriptions of complementary therapies common in the UK

Acupuncture
The insertion of needles into a specific point or set of points on the body for the treatment of specific conditions. Various forms exist, such as auriculoacupuncture (needling of specific points on the ear) and electroacupuncture (electrical stimulation of inserted needles). The two main types practised in the UK are described below.

Medical acupuncture: usually practised by doctors who have trained in acupuncture and who use the therapy alongside conventional medicine. Insertion of needles is given as far as possible according to the principles of neurophysiology and anatomy (i.e. directed at stimulating nerve endings).

Traditional Chinese acupuncture: part of the broader system of traditional Chinese medicine (TCM). Uses concepts of 'yin-yang' and the 'five elements' to explain the physiological functioning of the human body and the development of medical disorders in order to guide diagnosis and treatment. Traditional Chinese acupuncturists aim to restore the balance of energy in the body by 'unblocking meridians' (pathways along which life energy is believed to flow) by inserting needles strategically in specific points along meridians.

Anthroposophical medicine

A philosophical vision of health and disease based on the work of Rudolf Steiner who explored how man's soul and spiritual nature relate to the health and function of the body. Steiner viewed each person as having four 'bodies' or 'forces': physical; etheric; astral; spiritual. Practitioners of anthroposophy aim to understand illness in terms of how these four elements interact; the aim of treatment is to stimulate the natural healing forces of the body. The anthroposophic approach is a holistic one; practitioners may use a range of therapies including diet, therapeutic movement (eurhythmy) and artistic therapies as well as anthroposophic medicines in an integrated therapeutic programme.

Aromatherapy

The therapeutic use of aromatic substances, largely essential oils, extracted from plants. Aromatherapists believe that essential oils can be used not only for the prevention and treatment of disease, but also for their effects on mood, emotion and well being. Aromatherapy is claimed to be a holistic therapy in that practitioners will select an essential oil or combination of essential oils to suit each client's symptoms, personality and emotional state. The most common method used for application of essential oils is massage using a carrier oil; other methods include the addition of essential oils to baths and footbaths, inhalations, compresses and use in aromatherapy equipment, e.g. burners and vaporizers.

Ayurvedic medicine

The traditional system of medicine of India. Its essence is to achieve and maintain balance between the 'elements' and 'energies'; illness is believed to result from imbalance. Ayurvedic diagnosis is based on physical observation and questioning. Treatment usually involves Ayurvedic herbal remedies as well as dietary modifications, meditation, exercise, massage.

Chiropractic

Chiropractors believe that misaligned or maladjusted vertebrae ('subluxations'), caused by accidents, strains, poor posture, innate skeletal distortions, etc., affect the spine and surrounding muscles, nerves and ligaments. This is believed to result in local or radiating pain, affecting joint movement, and causing swelling or weakening of muscle groups, thereby contributing to the disease process. There is, as yet, no clear explanation from current knowledge of spinal mechanics and neurophysiology how this might happen.

Chiropractic diagnosis includes physical examination, palpation of the vertebral column, assessment of posture, etc. and often the use of X-rays to examine bone alignment and to detect conditions such as osteoporosis which would contraindicate manipulative treatment. The principal technique used in chiropractic is a series of short sharp thrusts aimed at restoring normal joint motion, correcting subluxations, improving posture and/or removing painful stimulation to the nerves. Generally, chiropractors manipulate the neck and spine, but may also use techniques such as massage and even dietary and lifestyle advice as part of a holistic approach. McTimoney chiropractic uses lighter movements than does standard chiropractic.

Flower remedies and essences

Developed in the UK by Dr Edward Bach who believed that physical disease was the result of being at odds with one's spiritual purpose, i.e. negative states of mind induce illness. His approach to health focused only on the mental state of the patient. He identified 38 negative psychological states of mind (e.g. jealousy, guilt, hopelessness) and developed a remedy designed to be used for each of these emotional states. Many other countries have their own collection of flower remedies/essences based on native plants/trees, e.g. Australian Bush Essences.

Healing

A transmission of 'therapeutic energy' between healer and patient, which may or may not be associated with particular religious beliefs. Can be performed at a distance ('distant healing') or by laying on of hands ('therapeutic touch').

Herbalism

Traditional herbalism had an historical basis, party based on the galenical model of the four 'humours' and the belief that an excess of any of the humours leads to disease. Today treatment is aimed at 'restoring balance' and 'strengthening bodily systems'. Herbalists aim to treat patients in a holistic way by selecting a herb or combination of herbs to treat a particular person and his/her unique set of symptoms. One of the principal tenets is that the whole plant extract, and not an isolated constituent, is responsible for the clinical effect. It is claimed that herbal constituents, and even combinations of herbs, work synergistically to achieve benefit and reduce the possibility of adverse effects.

Rational phytotherapy/phytomedicine (science-based herbal medicine) has an entirely different approach to that of traditional herbalism. It involves the use of specific plant (or plant part) extracts standardized to specific constituents (where possible) with documented pharmacological activity for the treatment of specific clinical conditions. In this regard, phytotherapy has a similar approach to that of conventional medicine.

Homoeopathy

The use of highly dilute, succussed substances to stimulate the body's own healing activity (the 'vital force'). One of the key principles is 'like cures like'—a substance which in large doses causes a set of symptoms in a healthy person can be used to treat such symptoms in an ill person, e.g. homoeopathic preparations of coffee (Coffea) are used to treat insomnia. Treatment is holistic—two patients with the same set of symptoms may be given different remedies depending on their personal characteristics, physical appearance, mental and emotional state, etc. Although there are several hypotheses, there is not yet a plausible explanation for the mechanism of action of homoeopathy. Furthermore, on balance, rigorous clinical trials do not show an effect for homoeopathy over that of placebo.

Osteopathy

Osteopaths believe that a wide variety of disorders can be traced to disorders of the musculoskeletal system, particularly the spinal vertebrae, but also to dysfunction in certain muscle groups. Manipulative techniques are used to correct these joint and tissue disturbances to restore normal bodily function. Osteopaths use a detailed medical history, physical examination, assessment of posture, observation of patient movement, etc. and, occasionally, X-rays in diagnosis. Direct techniques (soft tissue and joint movement, and high-velocity thrusts) and indirect techniques (positioning-type techniques where the joints are moved without force) are used in treatment. Generally osteopaths use more rhythmical and gentler pressure on the whole body, including the spine, whereas chiropractors tend to use more sharp, short, thrusting pressure on the spine (see Chiropractic).

Reflexology (also known as reflex therapy)

A form of treatment and diagnosis which involves massage of specific points on the feet (mainly on the soles but also on the tops and sides—maps of the areas of the feet corresponding to different areas/organs of the body have been drawn up). It is based on the belief that there are reflexes in the feet for all parts of the body. Reflexologists claim to be able to identify sites of tenderness and 'lumps' or granules of crystalline material, which, in reflexology, are taken to represent remote organ disease. Manual stimulation of the reflex points is believed to break down the deposits so that they can be eliminated, and to increase the flow of 'healing energy' through 'channels'. At present, these theories are unsubstantiated.

Traditional Chinese Medicine (TCM)

An ancient Chinese method of health care which coexists alongside orthodox medicine today. TCM includes a range of therapies, such as Chinese massage, but is best known for the practices of traditional Chinese acupuncture (see Acupuncture) and traditional Chinese herbal medicine (CHM). The basic concepts of TCM ('yin-yang' and the 'five elements') apply to CHM. The fundamental principle of treatment is to restore 'balance and harmony'. Medicinal substances are classified as having particular attributes, e.g. hot, cold, tonifying, moistening, and it is the consideration and combining of these attributes during therapy that is thought to bring about balance to patterns of clinical dysfunction. For example, 'cooling' herbs would be used to treat a patient whose pattern of illness is described as 'hot'. Usually, herbal formulae comprising around 4 to 12 different medicinal substances are used to treat specific clinical patterns.

Several complementary therapies, such as herbalism, homoeopathy, aromatherapy and others, involve the administration of pharmaceutical-type remedies, e.g. herbal medicines, homoeopathic remedies and essential oils (Box 41.3). These are collectively referred to as complementary (or 'alternative') medicines. As well as being used by some CAM practitioners in their practice, these types of products are widely available for purchase for self-treatment from pharmacies, health-food stores, supermarkets, by mail order, via the Internet and from other outlets. In the UK, patients, the public, the media and many other groups consider the use of herbal medicines, (whether prescribed by a herbalist or purchased over the counter), to be part of CAM. However, there is a view that herbal medicinal products with documented pharmacological activity and clinical efficacy lie alongside conventional medicines. Indeed, some herbal medicines, such as senna preparations, are conventional medicines.

This chapter discusses CAM, mainly from a UK perspective. In particular, the extent of use, and regulatory aspects of CAM are considered, as well as issues of importance to pharmacy and pharmacists. There is a particular emphasis on complementary medicines, as these are widely available in pharmacies, and especially on 'European' herbal medicines, as these are among the most widely used 'complementary medicines' in the UK. Also, from a biomedical perspective, herbal medicines (rather than for example homoeopathic remedies) are likely to have the greatest potential in terms of both benefits and risks.

Box 41.3 Examples and descriptions of types of complementary medicines

Anthroposophic medicines

Used as part of the anthroposophical approach to the treatment of illness. They are derived mainly from plant and mineral sources; many are combinations of herbal ingredients. Particular attention is paid to the source and methods of farming used in growing raw plant materials for preparing anthroposophic medicines (e.g. organic only).

Ayurvedic medicines

Used in Ayurveda, the traditional system of medicine of India. They are herbal/mineral preparations; heavy metals (e.g. lead, arsenic) are sometimes used in the manufacturing process.

Dietary/food supplements

Preparations of substances commonly found in the diet, such as fish oils, or occurring naturally in the body, e.g. co-enzyme Q_{10}. In the UK, many herbal products, e.g. garlic tablets, are sold as dietary/food supplements.

Essential oils

Aromatic substances extracted from plant material and which typically contain numerous chemical constituents. Used mainly in aromatherapy, most commonly applied in a carrier oil during massage.

Flower remedies/essences

Flower remedies/essences are used to treat emotional and psychological symptoms, e.g. jealousy, indecision. The Bach collection comprises 39 remedies, 37 of which originate from flowers/trees, one from natural spring water, and 'Rescue Remedy', a combination of five of the other 38 remedies. Flower remedies are extremely dilute preparations, but are not homoeopathic remedies.

Herbal medicines

Preparations made from plants or plant parts. In some instances (e.g. use by herbalists) a crude drug (e.g. dried leaf) is used. Manufactured products use extracts of plants or plant parts, formulated as, for example, tablets, capsules, creams and tinctures. They may contain a single or multiple herbal ingredients.

Homoeopathic medicines

Highly dilute preparations which may be of plant, animal, mineral, insect, biological, drug/chemical or other origin. Formulations include pillules, tablets, creams/ointments, liquids and injections.

Traditional Chinese medicines

Substances used as part of traditional Chinese medicine. Preparations may include animal as well as herbal material.

Vitamins and minerals

Single or multi-ingredient preparations of vitamins and/or minerals, sometimes in combination with other ingredients, e.g. herbal drugs. It is a matter of debate whether vitamins and minerals should be considered to be complementary medicines.

CLASSIFICATION OF CAM THERAPIES

Attempts have been made to classify complementary therapies into certain groups. For example, the House of Lords Select Committee on Science and Technology's Subcommittee on Complementary and Alternative Medicine, which scrutinized CAM during 1999 and 2000 (House of Lords, 2000), proposed that CAM therapies could be divided into three groups (Table 41.1).

- Group 1 comprises the 'principal disciplines', namely the major CAM therapies in the UK.
- Group 2 includes 'therapies which are most often used to complement conventional medicine and do not purport to embrace diagnostic skills'.
- Group 3 includes 'those other disciplines which purport to offer diagnostic information as well as treatment and which, in general, favour a philosophical approach and are indifferent to the scientific principles of conventional medicine, and through which various and disparate frameworks of disease causation and its management are proposed'.

Group 3 therapies are further categorized as 'long-established and traditional systems of health care' and 'other alternative disciplines which lack any credible evidence base'. This classification can, however, be criticized. For example, it could be argued that homoeopathy is indifferent to the scientific principles of conventional medicine, and that flower remedies lack any credible evidence base.

EXTENT OF USE OF CAM

The use of CAM is a popular health care approach in developed countries, and there is evidence that use of complementary therapies and complementary medicines is increasing.

Table 41.1 **Classification of complementary/alternative therapies. (From House of Lords Select Committee on Science and Technology, Report on complementary/alternative medicine, 2000)**

Group	Therapy
Group 1: Professionally organized alternative therapies	Acupuncture, chiropractic, herbal medicine, homoeopathy, osteopathy
Group 2: Complementary therapies	Alexander technique, aromatherapy, Bach and other flower remedies, bodywork therapies including massage, counselling stress therapy, hypnotherapy, meditation, reflexology, shiatsu, healing, Maharishi Ayurvedic medicine, nutritional medicine, yoga
Group 3: Alternative disciplines Group 3a: Long-established and traditional systems of health care	Anthroposophical medicine, Ayurvedic medicine, Chinese herbal medicine,
Group 3b: Other alternative disciplines	Eastern medicine, naturopathy, traditional Chinese medicine Crystal therapy, dowsing, iridology, kinesiology, radionics

Data from nationwide surveys involving US adults indicated that the use of CAM is increasing (Eisenberg et al 1998). Use of at least one of 16 complementary therapies in the previous year had risen significantly from 33.8% of the sample in 1990 to 42.1% in 1997. Self-treatment with herbal medicines was one of the therapies showing the greatest increase over this period (2.5% of sample in 1990 compared with 12.5% in 1997).

Reliable estimates of CAM use among adults in England come from a postal questionnaire survey involving 5010 adults (response rate = 59%) carried out in 1998 by Thomas et al (2001). The study found that within the previous 12 months, approximately 10% of the sample had used at least one of six complementary therapies (acupuncture, chiropractic, homoeopathy, medical herbalism, hypnotherapy or osteopathy), and that approximately 22% had purchased over-the-counter (OTC) homoeopathic or herbal medicines in the previous year.

Market research carried out by Mintel International Ltd (2001) estimated that retail sales of complementary medicines (herbal medicines, homoeopathic remedies and essential oils) were worth £115 million in 2000, representing growth of 23% since 1998. Around 49% of sales of herbal medicines and homoeopathic remedies are made in pharmacies, although this figure has decreased by 2% since 1998 in favour of health-food stores and supermarkets.

The use of CAM is not limited to the private sector—in some cases, the NHS funds access. For example, there are five NHS homoeopathic hospitals in the UK, to which GPs can refer their patients. Also, GPs can prescribe homoeo-

pathic preparations on NHS prescriptions. In 1998, over 150 000 homoeopathic items were dispensed against NHS prescriptions; data from the Prescription Pricing Authority show that the net ingredient cost for these was £927 600. Furthermore, a survey reported by Thomas et al (2001) estimated that in 1998 there were over 2 million visits to complementary therapists funded by the NHS, and that the annual NHS expenditure on CAM was £52.8 million.

REASONS FOR USE OF CAM

Symptoms and conditions

Complementary medicines are used by the general public and by patients both for general health maintenance and for the relief of minor, self-limiting conditions. For example, studies involving pharmacists and consumers have suggested that herbal products to help relieve stress and sleep problems are those most frequently requested by pharmacy customers and 'recommended' by pharmacists to consumers following consultations regarding symptoms.

Use of complementary medicines is not necessarily limited to symptoms or conditions suitable for OTC treatment. Indeed, many patients use complementary medicines and complementary therapies for symptom relief in, or treatment of, serious chronic illnesses, such as cancer, HIV/AIDS, multiple sclerosis, rheumatological conditions, asthma, depression, gastroenterological disorders, skin conditions and so on. Use of CAM is usually (but not always) to supplement conventional health care, rather than to replace it. Special patient groups also use CAM, including the elderly and women who are pregnant or breastfeeding. It is also used by some parents/guardians for children in their care.

Beliefs, perceptions and attitudes

There are numerous reasons why people choose to use complementary medicines and therapies. They include dissatisfaction with conventional medicine in terms of effectiveness and/or safety, satisfaction with CAM, and the perception that it is 'safe', as well as more complex reasons that are associated with cultural and personal beliefs, views on life and health, and experiences with conventional health care professionals and CAM practitioners.

An individual's choice to use CAM approaches is tied in with 'health care pluralism'—people may use any of several treatment options, such as taking advice from family and friends, consulting a CAM practitioner and consulting a pharmacist, GP or other health care professional. Related issues include whether individuals disclose CAM use to conventional health care professionals, and whether there is better compliance with CAM treatment regimens than with conventional drug regimens.

REGULATION OF CAM

CAM practitioners

There are around 40 000 CAM practitioners in the UK, according to a 1997 survey of CAM organizations, commissioned by the Department of Health (Mills & Peacock 1997).

With the exception of osteopaths and chiropractors (the General Osteopathic Council and the General Chiropractic Council were established by acts of parliament to regulate their respective disciplines), CAM practitioners are not legally required to undertake any training before practising. While most CAM practitioners will have trained in their chosen therapy, others may not, or may have trained in one complementary therapy, but practise several. Furthermore, there is wide variation in the level of training and methods of assessment. For the major therapies—acupuncture, homoeopathy, herbal medicine, osteopathy and chiropractic—training is generally highly developed, with many institutions having university affiliation and offering courses at degree level. However, training for other complementary therapies is less intensive and more disparate.

The estimate of numbers of CAM practitioners given above is based on membership of CAM organizations, but cannot be precise as some practitioners are registered with more than one organization and some are not registered at all. Generally, practitioners are members of a registering or accrediting body, although criteria for membership vary widely. Also, many complementary therapies have several registering organizations, although some disciplines are taking steps to become unified under one regulatory body.

The practice of complementary therapies is not limited to CAM practitioners—some conventional health care professionals including pharmacists practise CAM. Some institutions offer specialized courses for conventional health care professionals, and there are registering organizations which represent state-registered health care professionals who have undertaken training in and practise certain complementary therapies. For example, the British Medical Acupuncture Society represents medically qualified individuals with training in acupuncture.

Against this background, the House of Lords (2000) report on CAM included several recommendations regarding training and regulation of CAM practitioners, including conventional health care professionals who practise CAM. In summary, these recommendations were:

- Regulatory bodies of health care professionals should develop guidelines on competence and training in CAM
- Statutory regulation of CAM practitioners, particularly acupuncture and herbal medicine, and possibly non-medical homoeopathy; a Herbal Medicines Regulation Working Group has been set up to take the process forward for Herbal Medicines.
- Training for CAM practitioners should be standardized, independently accredited and include basic biomedical science.

The issue of training also relates to staff employed in retail outlets, e.g. health-food stores which sell a vast range of complementary medicines, who sell or advise on complementary medicines. A small study has suggested that information and advice given by health-food store staff may not always be appropriate.

Complementary medicines

The majority of complementary health products are not licensed as medicines and, therefore, evidence of their quality, efficacy and safety has not been assessed by the competent authority which, in the UK, is the Medicines Control Agency (MCA).

Herbal medicines

Herbal products are available on the UK market as licensed herbal medicines, herbal medicines exempt from licensing and unlicensed herbal products sold as food supplements (Barnes et al 2002). In several cases, the same herb is available in all three categories. Potentially hazardous plants are controlled as Prescription Only Medicines (POM) and certain others are subject to dose (but not duration of treatment) and route of administration restrictions, or can only be supplied via a pharmacy and by, or under the supervision of, a pharmacist.

Most licensed herbal products were initially granted a product licence of right (PLR) because they were already on the market when the licensing system was introduced in the 1970s. When PLRs were reviewed, manufacturers of herbal products intended for use in minor self-limiting conditions were permitted to rely on bibliographic evidence to support efficacy and safety, rather than being required to carry out new controlled clinical trials, so, many licensed herbal medicinal products have not necessarily undergone stringent testing.

Herbal products exempt from licensing are those compounded and supplied by herbalists on their own recommendation, those consisting solely of dried, crushed or comminuted (fragmented) plants (i.e. they must not contain any non-herbal 'active' ingredients) sold under their botanical name and with no written recommendations for use, and those made by the holder of a specials manufacturing licence. This category was initially intended to give herbalists the flexibility to prepare remedies for their patients. However, manufacturers can legally sell products under this exemption. Furthermore, at present, there is no statutory regulation of herbalists in the UK, although this is under review.

The majority of herbal products are sold as food supplements without making medical claims and are regulated under food, not pharmaceutical, legislation. In the UK, the MCA has the statutory power to decide whether a specific product satisfies the definition of a relevant 'medicinal product' and, therefore, is subject to the provisions of regulations relating to Medicines for Human Use Regulations (1994, 2000). If a product is determined to be a relevant medicinal product, and if it does not meet criteria for exemption, then the manufacturer is required to submit an application for a full product licence and/or remove the product from the market. The procedure allows for the company to request a review of the decision. In this case, the views of an independent panel, the Independent Review Panel on Borderline Products, are taken into consideration.

Manufacturers of licensed medicines, including licensed herbal products, are required to satisfy the MCA that their products are made according to the principles of good manufacturing practice (GMP). While some established manufacturers of unlicensed herbal products also manufacture their products to GMP standards, others do not, and there is no guarantee that such products are of suitable pharmaceutical quality. The quality of plant raw materials can be affected by several factors and, therefore, it is important that finished (marketed) herbal products are of suitable quality. The *European Pharmacopoeia* now contains over 120 monographs on herbal drugs, and a similar number are in preparation.

'Ethnic' medicines available in the UK include traditional Chinese medicines (TCM) and Ayurvedic medicines (Box 41.3). Such products are subject to the same legislation as 'Western' complementary medicines. In the UK, there are further restrictions on certain toxic herbal ingredients, namely *Aristolochia* species, found in some TCM products, and on other herbal ingredients that may be confused with toxic herbal ingredients. In addition to containing non-herbal ingredients such as animal parts and/or minerals, some manufactured ('patent') TCM products have been found to contain conventional drugs as listed ingredients, some of which (e.g. glibenclamide) may have POM status in the UK. Non-herbal active ingredients of any type cannot legally be included in unlicensed herbal remedies, and inclusion of drugs with POM status represents an additional infringement of UK medicines legislation. For some ingredients, such as certain animal parts, restrictions under the Convention on International Trade in Endangered Species of Wild Fauna and Flora (CITES) also apply.

There is a widely held opinion that the current system of licensing for herbal medicines does not give consumers adequate protection against poor quality and unsafe unlicensed products, nor does it allow manufacturers to provide appropriate information to inform consumers' choice of products. Against this background, a new European Union (EU) directive (Commission of the European Communities 2002) has been proposed which aims to establish a harmonized legislative framework for authorizing the marketing of traditional herbal medicinal products by 2005. The directive will require EU member states to set up a specified simplified registration procedure for traditional herbal medicinal products which could not fulfil medicines licensing criteria. Some of the main features of this are that manufacturers will be required to provide:

- Evidence that the herb has been used traditionally in the EU for at least 30 years (15 years' non-EU use will be taken into account)

- Bibliographic data on safety with an expert report
- Quality dossier demonstrating manufacture according to principles of good manufacturing practice (GMP).

The new directive is not a route to licensing for herbal POMs or for traditional herbal medicines that can be licensed by the conventional route. As it stands, the proposed directive would accommodate ethnic medicines that have been used in the UK (or any other member state) for at least 15 years.

Homoeopathic remedies

In the UK, homoeopathic remedies are subject to medicines legislation. A simplified registration scheme exists in the UK (and the rest of the EU) for homoeopathic medicinal products which:

- Are intended for oral or external use
- Are sufficiently dilute (usually a minimum dilution of 1 in 10 000) and
- No medical claims are made.

For such products, manufacturers are required to demonstrate quality and safety, but not efficacy. Manufacturers of homoeopathic medicinal products which are administered parenterally, are below the minimum dilution, or make efficacy claims are required to substantiate this in the same manner as is required for conventional drugs.

Other complementary medicines

Products marketed as food or dietary supplements include non-herbal substances, such as glucosamine, vitamins, minerals and fish oils. These products are sold under food legislation and are marketed without medical claims. Such products may be deemed by the MCA to be a relevant medicinal product (see 'Herbal medicines' above). Some 'supplements' are subject to stringent restrictions on their use. Melatonin is a prescription-only medicine, available on a 'named patient' basis only as there are no licensed melatonin products in the UK. However, in the USA, melatonin is sold as a food supplement. A new draft EU directive is aimed at harmonizing the marketing of food supplements in member states.

Essential oils used by aromatherapists in their practice for medicinal purposes are considered to be medicinal products, but are exempt from licensing provided they meet certain criteria (see 'Herbal medicines' above). Aromatherapy products sold through retail outlets are not subject to licensing regulations unless they are marketed as medicinal products. Some essential oils are available as licensed medicinal products, e.g. peppermint oil capsules, although such products are conventional medicines, not aromatherapy products.

PHARMACY AND CAM

Provision of CAM

Pharmacies and pharmacists have several roles in the provision of CAM. Community pharmacies are a major source of complementary medicines for people who purchase and self-treat with these products, and pharmacists may be asked for information and advice on self-treatment with complementary medicines. In addition, community pharmacists may be presented with NHS (FP10) prescriptions for homoeopathic medicines. Some independent pharmacies provide consulting rooms that are available for use on a sessional basis by CAM practitioners, and a similar initiative was recently adopted by some branches of a large multiple, which offered consultations with practitioners of several CAM therapies, including homoeopathy, herbalism and osteopathy. Also, there are several community pharmacies which specialize in CAM, e.g. homoeopathic pharmacies which offer professional homoeopathic pharmaceutical services.

Pharmacists' involvement with CAM is not limited to the community. Pharmacists employed in NHS homoeopathic hospitals provide pharmaceutical services in the pharmacy and on the wards. Pharmacists employed in conventional NHS hospitals may be involved with the supply of certain complementary medicines.

Pharmacists' training in CAM

In September 1999, the Science Committee of the Royal Pharmaceutical Society of Great Britain set up a working group on complementary and alternative medicine to examine issues in this area of importance to pharmacy and pharmacists.

Pharmacists' involvement in the provision of CAM at any level raises several issues, particularly with regard to pharmacists' knowledge of and training in CAM, their professional accountability, and the quality, safety and efficacy of complementary medicines sold or supplied. The Royal Pharmaceutical Society of Great Britain's (RPSGB) Code of Ethics states that pharmacists providing homoeopathic or herbal medicines or other complementary therapies have a professional responsibility:

- To ensure that stocks of homoeopathic or herbal medicines or other complementary therapies are obtained from a reputable source of supply
- Not to recommend any remedy where they have any reason to doubt its safety or quality
- Only to offer advice on homoeopathic or herbal medicines or other complementary therapies or medicines if they have undertaken suitable training or have specialized knowledge.

Almost all pharmacies sell complementary medicines, particularly herbal medicines and homoeopathic remedies, and the majority of pharmacists are asked for and 'recommend' specific complementary medicines. However, the extent of teaching on pharmacognosy (the scientific discipline which covers the chemistry, biological and clinical effects of natural products, particularly plants) and herbal and complementary medicines in the MPharm programme is limited and varies between schools pharmacy. Furthermore, the majority of practising pharmacists have not undertaken or received training in areas of CAM.

Pharmacists' training in CAM should not be limited to complementary medicines. It should include an awareness of the background to, evidence for and safety concerns with regard to complementary therapies, such as acupuncture. This is because patients' use of such treatments may have implications for pharmaceutical care. For example, research involving community pharmacists in the USA has suggested that some patients with chronic conditions temporarily or permanently use complementary therapies instead of their prescribed medicines.

Pharmacists' professional practice

At present, pharmacists' professional practice with regard to complementary medicines is not optimal—many pharmacists do not routinely ask customers and patients specifically about their use of complementary medicines, nor record such use on patient medication records. Pharmacists are encouraged to apply principles of good professional practice with regard to complementary medicines, and to be aware that patients' use of complementary medicines may have implications for pharmaceutical care. For example, it is possible that patients may use complementary medicines in addition to, or instead of, conventional medicines, without telling their doctor or pharmacist. The concurrent use of complementary medicines, particularly herbal medicines,

and conventional drugs is of concern as there is a potential for interactions to occur. For example, important interactions have been documented between St John's wort and certain prescribed medicines, including warfarin, digoxin, theophylline, ciclosporin, HIV protease inhibitors, anticonvulsants and oral contraceptives.

The role of the pharmacist in reporting suspected adverse drug reactions (ADRs) associated with herbal medicines has been recognized by the Committee on Safety of Medicines (CSM) and the Medicines Control Agency (MCA). In November 1999, the CSMs' Yellow Card scheme for ADR reporting was extended to include reporting by all community pharmacists (hospital pharmacists were granted reporter status in April 1997) (see Ch. 32). Community pharmacists are asked by the CSM/MCA to concentrate on areas of limited reporting by doctors, namely conventional OTC medicines and herbal products. The Yellow Card scheme also applies to unlicensed herbal products and, whilst the CSM/MCA do not formally request reports of suspected ADRs associated with other types of unlicensed products, it is unlikely that CSM/MCA would ignore a genuine report of a serious suspected ADR associated with a non-herbal unlicensed product.

EFFICACY AND SAFETY OF CAM APPROACHES

It is beyond the scope of this chapter to consider evidence for the efficacy and safety of individual complementary medicines and complementary therapies. In very general terms, evidence from randomized controlled trials for the efficacy of complementary therapies for specific conditions is lacking. This is not to say that such approaches are not efficacious, but that for many, rigorous research has not been carried out. There are several reasons for this, including a lack of research funding for and research infrastructure in CAM.

Similarly, CAM is often assumed to be 'safe', but this assumption is not based on appropriate studies. In fact, some complementary therapies have been associated with serious adverse effects. In addition, formal spontaneous reporting schemes (i.e. similar to the CSMs' Yellow Card scheme for adverse drug reaction reporting) do not exist for 'manual' complementary therapies, such as acupuncture, chiropractic and osteopathy.

The relative lack of research in CAM means that there is also a lack of evidence-based information on which to base treatment decisions for specific patients. Nevertheless, there are several sources of information in CAM, including specialist databases and specialist fields within established databases, as well as several reference texts written by pharmacists which have summarized and critiqued the available evidence in areas of CAM (see further reading suggestions).

THE FUTURE FOR COMPLEMENTARY MEDICINES

On the basis of current trends in market research data, it has been predicted that sales of complementary medicines will continue to increase (Mintel 2001). Longitudinal data on the utilization of complementary therapists are not available for the UK, although increasing numbers of such practitioners may suggest increasing public demand for treatment with these therapies.

With the EU directive on traditional herbal medicinal products, the future is set to bring improved quality standards for these preparations—manufacturers will need to meet standards for GMP, or remove their products from the market. Initiatives involving ethnic medicines are also aimed at improving quality standards for these preparations. However, as this sector is less developed in the UK, it is likely that improvements in the quality of ethnic medicines will be seen over a longer time period.

Improvements in quality standards, together with other requirements in the traditional herbal medicinal products directive, will put an increased emphasis on manufacturers to provide evidence supporting the safety of their products. At the same time, the increasing use of herbal medicines, particularly by patients using conventional drugs and those with serious chronic illness, may result in the emergence of new safety concerns, such as indications of uncommon ADRs, those occurring with long-term use and interactions with conventional medicines.

Against a background of widespread and increasing use of CAM, it is recognized that CAM practitioners need to be regulated, and that conventional health care professionals need to be knowledgeable about complementary medicines and therapies. The House of Lords' Select Committee on Science and Technology's report on CAM made several recommendations with regard to statutory regulation of those who practise CAM (see above), and these recommendations were accepted by the government (Department of Health 2001). Thus, in the future, conventional health care professionals should have a basic knowledge of complementary medicines and therapies, and doctors, pharmacists, and others may have interactions with state-registered CAM practitioners.

In its response to the House of Lords' report, the government stated that if a therapy gains a critical mass of evidence, the NHS and the medical profession should ensure that the public has access to that therapy. Thus, in addition to homoeopathic treatment, which is already available through the NHS, certain complementary therapies and licensed complementary medicines with a sound evidence base may also be available on NHS prescriptions.

In the long term, the future for 'complementary medicines', particularly herbal medicines, may lie with pharmacogenetics and pharmacogenomics. These relatively new fields of research are widely held to be central to the discovery of new drugs and to the future of therapeutics, yet the pharmacogenetics of ADRs, and optimizing treatment on the basis of a patient's genotype, has not been discussed in the context of herbal medicines. It is reasonable to assume that individuals with a different genetic profile will have different responses to herbal medicines as well as to conventional drugs.

Key points

- The use of complementary/alternative therapies, particularly herbal medicines, is widespread and appears to be increasing.
- Most community pharmacies sell complementary medicines, particularly herbal medicines, and many pharmacists are asked for advice on such products.
- Hospital pharmacists may also encounter patients who use complementary medicines and complementary therapies.
- The use of complementary medicines and complementary therapies may have implications for pharmaceutical care, e.g. drug–herb interactions can occur.
- Most complementary medicines currently are sold as unlicensed products, so evidence of their quality, safety and efficacy has not been assessed by the Medicines Control Agency.
- Other than for osteopaths and chiropractors, there is at present no statutory regulation of practitioners of complementary therapies.

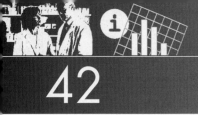
Substance use and misuse

J. Scott

After studying this chapter you should be able to:

List the main psychoactive substances that are taken for non-medicinal purposes

List the range of professional interventions used in the field of substance misuse and state their aims

Explain the role of the pharmacist in substance misuse

State the aim of pharmaceutical interventions and describe their operation

Explain key factors to consider when providing pharmaceutical care to people with drug misuse problems

Introduction

This chapter will begin with some background information before it summarizes current thinking on drug misuse and drug dependence. It will then look at treatment provision in the UK and the range of interventions used, focusing on the practical provision of the two main pharmaceutical interventions—needle exchange and pharmacotherapy provision.

Terminology

Terminology used in the field of drug misuse can be confusing, even for those who work in the area. There are political and philosophical differences behind the use of various terms, a discussion of which is outside the scope of this work. However it is important to be aware that a variety of terms essentially refer to the same things.

'Drug use' in the context of this chapter is the term commonly used to refer to the consumption of psychoactive substances without medical or health care instruction. The term 'drug misuse' refers to drug use that is problematical and

incurs a significant risk of harm. These two terms are often used interchangeably. 'Drug abuse' essentially refers to the same thing but its use is less common in recent publications. 'Substance' is sometimes used in place of 'drug' to include non-medicinal chemicals such as solvents, alcohol and nicotine.

'Dependence' or 'addiction' refers to the compulsion to continue administration of psychoactive substance(s) in order to avoid physical and/or psychological withdrawal effects. Drug dependence is defined by the World Health Organization (WHO) as:

> ... a cluster of psychological, behavioural and cognitive phenomena of variable intensity, in which the use of a psychoactive drug (or drugs) takes on a high priority. The necessary descriptive characteristics are preoccupation with a desire to obtain and take the drug and persistent drug seeking behaviour' (World Health Organization 1993).

Dependence can be classified in more detail, as found in the *Oxford Textbook of Psychiatry*.

'Drug user' is commonly used to refer to someone who participates in drug/substance use. The term 'drug misuser' refers to someone undertaking drug use in such a way that it is problematical and presents a significant risk of harm. Again the two terms tend to be used interchangeably. Terms such as 'drug addict' and 'drug abuser' are less used in recent literature.

Historical note

Historical works on psychoactive drug consumption make interesting reading and help us to understand how current drug policy came to be formulated. They indicate that psychoactive drug use is not a new phenomenon in society—psychoactive drug use has been recorded as part of some societies more than 7000 years ago. More information is given by Berridge (1998).

SUBSTANCES THAT ARE USED AND THEIR EFFECTS

Table 42.1 lists some commonly used psychoactive substances in Western societies and summarizes their effects. Nicotine is included for completeness, but the role of the pharmacist in smoking cessation is covered in Chapter 39. The unwanted and harmful effects of some drugs relate to prolonged and excessive use whereas others occur with single doses of smaller amounts. The method of administration also influences the extent of the risks, e.g. injecting opiates presents greater health risks than taking them by vaporization ('Chasing the dragon'). This table is presented as a guide, it is not comprehensive. The books *Drugs of Abuse* (Wills 1997) and *Living with Drugs* (Gossop 2000) and the Drugscope website (http://www.drugscope.org.uk/) provide extensive information and the common street names of various drugs. Drugscope is a UK charity that provides information on drugs and support mainly for policy makers and service providers.

WHY DO PEOPLE USE PSYCHOACTIVE DRUGS?

Benefits

'Why do people use psychoactive drugs?' is a multifaceted question to which there is no simple answer. As a crude summary, people who use psychoactive drugs do so because they expect to experience a benefit in some way. They may be aware of risks too, but these are weighed up against the perceived benefits and the decision to take the drug prevails. The extent of the benefits and risks will of course vary depending on the drug, the circumstances and how it is used.

The expected or perceived benefits may include the attainment of pleasurable feelings (e.g. relaxation), increased social interaction (e.g. reduced inhibitions), alteration of the person's psychological condition to a more desirable state (e.g. escapism), physical change (e.g. anabolic steroids taken by bodybuilders) or avoidance of withdrawal symptoms in someone who is dependent on a drug.

The reasons for use may change over time with the same user; e.g. opiate use may been commenced to escape from reality but then continued to avoid the withdrawal effects.

Choice of drug used

The decision to use a drug may be influenced by many things, including:

- Availability and opportunity to try
- Legal status of the drug
- Perceived desired effects
- Perceived risks
- Specifically the desirability of the effects versus the risks
- Acceptability of the drug and/or method of administration to the individual, the individual's peer group and society.

Risks

The risks from various drugs are not equivalent. Their incidence and nature vary with the drug and how it is used, the individual concerned and the circumstances. Examples of such variables include the drug substance, the presence of impurities, the dose, the frequency of use, the route of administration, the legal status of the drug, related social and financial circumstances, the personality of the individual drug user and the interaction between drug use and lifestyle.

Weighing up benefits vs. risks

If the benefits from drug use are experienced before the harm, or to a greater perceived extent than the harm, positive endorsement of drug taking occurs. Following positive endorsement drug use may, but does not necessarily, continue.

Control and dependence

A lack of specific types of neurological control is sometimes given as the reason why some people develop addictions to specific psychoactive drug(s) whereas others do not. Published studies can be criticized as the models of behaviour are largely shown in animals not humans, making the assumption that the two findings are transferable.

The level of control a drug user has over his use will influence the balance between the benefits and harms experienced. With controlled use harms can be prevented or contained, e.g. the quantity of alcohol consumed may be controlled to avoid unwanted effects. In uncontrolled use, harms can escalate. Uncontrolled use is a characteristic of drug dependence.

When a person looses control over his drug consumption, or rather drug consumption controls the person, this may be described as dependence. Drug dependence can present a significant amount of risk and harm to the individual and to society. There is a clear association between drug dependence and social deprivation. In areas where social

Table 42.1 Some common psychoactive drugs used/misused and selected information on their effects

Common name	Active/main psychoactive component	Most common method(s) of administration	Effect on central nervous system	Examples of desired effects (e.g. reasons for taking)	Examples of unwanted effects/harm from use
Acid/LSD	Lysergic acid diethylamine	Orally dissolved on the tongue	Hallucinogenic	Altered sensory perceptions e.g. visual hallucinations, time distortion, detachment from reality	Panic attacks, frightening altered perceptions, dysphoria, delusions, psychosis, tachycardia. After-effects include 'flashbacks'
Alcohol	Ethanol	Orally in drinks e.g. wines, spirits, beers etc.	CNS depressant	Relaxation, disinhibition, promotes social interaction,	Aggressive mood, diuresis, dehydration, hypoglycaemia, sedation, vomiting, depression, anxiety, liver cirrhosis, acute hepatitis, gastric cancer
Caffeine	Caffeine	Orally in drinks e.g. tea, coffee, and some soft drinks	CNS stimulation	Increased alertness, combats fatigue, promotes stamina	Diuresis, insomnia, restlessness, anxiety, poor concentration, tremor, headaches
Cannabis	Delta-9-tetrahydrocannabinol (THC) plus other cannabinoids	Hashish (resin) or marijuana (dried flower heads and leaves) both of which are smoked often with tobacco in hand-rolled cigarettes	CNS depressant	Relaxation, enhances mood, disinhibition, sociability.	Anxiety, panic reactions, sedation, tachycardia, coughing, lung disorders, loss of motivation
Ecstasy	3,4-methylenedioxy-methamphetamine (MDMA) (Other similar amphetamine derivatives also used).	Oral ingestion in tablet form often in association with attendance at dance music event	CNS stimulation, hallucinogenic	Physical and mental stimulation, confidence, sociability, happy, elevated mood, increased energy	Sweating, tachycardia, headache, dry mouth, rhabdomyolysis, hyperpyrexia, hyponatremia, renal failure. After-effects include depression, insomnia, anxiety, lethargy

Table 42.1 (cont'd)

Common name	Active/main psychoactive component	Most common method(s) of administration	Effect on central nervous system	Examples of desired effects (e.g. reasons for taking)	Examples of unwanted effects/harm from use
Heroin	Diamorphine	Inhalation of vapour produced when heated on tin foil, intravenous injection	CNS depressant	Intense pleasure including euphoria, warmth, relaxation, mood elevation, detachment from emotional distress	Initially nausea and vomiting, constipation, drowsiness, confusion, dry mouth, sweating, in overdose—respiratory depression, pulmonary oedema, hypoxia, arrhythmias
Tobacco	Nicotine	Cigarette smoking, chewing tobacco	CNS stimulation	Social activity, mood elevation, increases concentration, promote relaxation,	Various cancers, cardiac disease, chronic obstructive airways disease, cough, halitosis
Cocaine	Cocaine hydrochloride (cocaine powder), cocaine free base ('crack')	Nasal administration though snorting, injecting, smoking (free base)	CNS stimulation	Euphoria, alertness, increased confidence, excitement, mental and physical stimulation. Intense exhilaration (injection and crack)	Cardiac toxicity, tachycardia, palpitations, hypertension, chest pain, sweating, tremor, anxiety, psychosis. After-effects include dysphoria, depression, fatigue, intense craving
Speed	Amfetamine	Nasal administration through snorting, orally, intravenous injecting	CNS stimulation	Physical and mental stimulation, confidence, increased energy	Sweating, tachycardia, hypertension, anxiety, paranoia and psychosis. After-effects include fatigue and depression

deprivation is high there tends to be a greater incidence of drug problems. However drug problems are not exclusive to deprived areas and can be found in most parts of the UK, in both urban and rural environments. Please remember at this stage that drug **use** and drug **dependence** do not refer to the same things.

Withdrawal

When a person stops using a substance they are dependent on they often experience withdrawal. Withdrawal can be described in two forms:

Physical withdrawal effects. These are physical signs and symptoms experienced when the drug is removed. Examples include seizures in alcohol withdrawal, stomach cramps and severe influenza-type symptoms experienced in opiate withdrawal, palpitations and anxiety in cocaine withdrawal, insomnia in nicotine withdrawal. Physical withdrawal effects can be quite severe and tend to be of shorter duration than psychological withdrawal effects. For example the acute physical withdrawal stage from heroin lasts about 7 days.

Psychological withdrawal effects. These are psychological disturbances experienced when a drug is removed. These cannot be so easily observed in the way that many physical withdrawal effects usually can, but they must not be underestimated. Psychological withdrawal includes intense emotional experiences such as unmasking of grief, inability to cope, intense craving, altered mood and depression. It tends to be of long duration and contributes markedly to relapse back to drug use.

THE HARMS RELATING TO PSYCHOACTIVE DRUG USE AND DEPENDENCE

The risks and harms that drug use and dependence can present to the individual and society vary with the drug taken, the individual and the circumstances in which the drugs are taken. It is not possible to list all possible consequences from drug use/misuse in this chapter, but these are dealt with in the 'Key references and further reading' section. The risks are categorized below.

Health problems

These affect the individual drug user and include physical and psychological health problems, which can be large and complex. As well as being caused by the individual substances concerned, health problems may relate to the method of administration. For example, injecting drug use is associated with damage to the circulatory system and infection (e.g. with HIV, hepatitis B and hepatitis C) is associated with the sharing of injecting equipment. Pharmacists are largely involved in preventing or reducing the harm from drug dependence, benefiting both the individual and society. Hence the role of the pharmacist in drug dependence is about contributing towards individual and public health and safety.

Social problems

The social problems that relate to drug dependence must not be underestimated. It is often these that drive people to seek treatment. Social problems may include poverty (e.g. social deprivation, exclusion or failure in education, inability to obtain or sustain employment, spending of income on drugs), damage to family relationships, difficulties forming relationships, exclusion from society and homelessness.

Drug-related crime

Drug-related crime includes not only the criminal activities committed against the Misuse of Drugs Act (see below) for which the individual is punished, but also crime that impacts on communities and society at large. The latter may relate to the acquisition of drugs or the effects of drugs, e.g. burglary to obtain money to buy drugs, robbery, violence associated with drunkenness, drunk/drug driving. Drug-related crime is of concern to society and is one of the reasons why treatment of drug problems and drug dependence is a key public health issue. Additionally there is evidence that treatment of drug dependence contributes towards a very marked reduction in drug-related crime. Hence treatment benefits not only the individual in terms of improved health but also society by making communities safer.

Drug users are often at greater risk than non-drug users of being victims of crime, e.g. violence associated with debt to drug dealers, prostitution, robbery and mugging if homeless or intoxicated.

Legislation

Misuse of Drugs Act

Pharmacists are often concerned with the Misuse of Drugs Regulations (1985) as these relate to the legal supply of

Table 42.2   Classification of some commonly misused substances according to the Misuse of Drugs Act (1971)

Class	Drugs	Maximum penalties
A	Cocaine including crack cocaine, diamorphine (heroin), dipipanone Ecstasy, LSD, methadone, morphine, opium, pethidine	Seven years imprisonment and/or unlimited fine for possession Life imprisonment and/or fine for supply*
B[†]	Most amphetamines, cannabis[‡],codeine, dihydrocodeine, methylphenidate	Five years imprisonment and/or fine for possession Fourteen years imprisonment and a fine for supply
C	Benzodiazepines, anabolic steroids and growth hormones	Two years imprisonment and/or fine for possession Five years imprisonment and/or fine for supply

* The term 'supply' includes drug trafficking and unauthorized production.
† If Class B drugs are prepared for injection they become Class A.
‡ Pure cannabinoids are Class A drugs. The UK government has proposed reclassifying cannabis to Class C, at the time of writing (July 2002). This proposal awaits parliamentary approval.

many drugs liable to non-medicinal use (see Appendix 1). The Misuse of Drugs Act (1971) classifies drugs into Class A, Class B and Class C. The purpose of this legislation is to define the penalties imposed for the illegal undertaking of various activities, e.g. possession, supply, import, export. These are summarized in Table 42.2.

Road Traffic Act

This 1988 act makes it is illegal to be in charge of a motor vehicle if 'unfit to drive through drink or drugs'. This includes both illicit substances and prescribed medicines. Drivers are required by law to notify the Driving and Vehicle Licensing Agency (DVLA) if there is any reason that the safety of their driving may be impaired, e.g. disability, the misuse of drugs, the need for drugs that impair reactions or cause sedation. The responsibility for notification lies with the patient not health care professionals (see the publication *At a Glance Guide to Medical Aspects of Fitness to Drive* (DVLA 1998), which is also available on the Internet at http://www.dvla.gov.uk/at_a_glance/what_is.htm).

THE MANAGEMENT OF DRUG USE AND DEPENDENCE

This chapter will focus on problematical drug use and specifically on drug dependence. The reason for this is that

pharmacists are primarily involved with the treatment of dependence rather than interventions aimed at recreational and non-problematic drug use. Drug dependence must however be kept in perspective as not everyone who tries drugs or uses drugs will become dependent on them. The prevalence of drug dependence on a population basis is relatively small compared to national statistics that estimate numbers of people who have ever tried drug(s). However, the extent of harm from drug dependence can be large and affect not only the individual but their families and communities, hence the need for effective strategies to support people change their drug use is great.

A range of strategies is used to prevent, limit the extent of and address the problems associated with drug use and dependence. These will be summarized in order to illustrate the contribution made by pharmacists. Figure 42.1 illustrates the range of strategies used in preventing, reducing and controlling drug use and dependence and managing the adverse consequences. These will be briefly reviewed.

Primary prevention

Primary prevention is concerned with preventing people from starting to use drugs. Target groups include vulnerable groups such as school children and young people who have left education. It includes warning of the harm that can result from drug use and dependence using health promotion and education campaigns. Primary prevention also includes legislation,

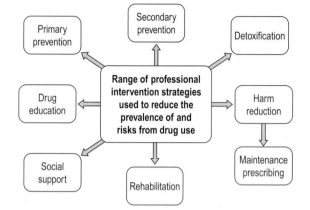

Fig. 42.1 The range of professional intervention strategies used to reduce or manage drug use and dependence.

as the illegal nature of many drugs may prevent some people from using them. It is difficult to evaluate the impact of primary prevention activities as so many factors may influence the person's decision to use or not to use drugs. This does not mean that primary prevention activities should not be used. They are very important for informing children and young people about drugs and their effects. Such activities should not be scaremongering but need to be factually accurate to give young people an informed knowledge base about drugs which reflects what they may see within society.

Secondary prevention

Secondary prevention is aimed at people who use drugs by discouraging further use. Examples of secondary prevention are giving advice to prevent problems such as overheating and dehydration to Ecstasy users and the use of CNS depressant drugs (such as heroin and methadone) by stimulant users (such as Ecstasy and amfetamine) to assist with the 'come down' following CNS stimulation.

Drug education

Drug education is a tool used in primary and secondary prevention campaigns and includes leaflets, booklets, videos and posters. People who are dependent on drugs may also benefit from drug education as they may not be fully informed on the drugs they use or may consider using, e.g. long-term risks and overdose prevention. Drug education is also a key part of harm reduction, giving people information to assist them in minimizing risks from drug taking, e.g. safer injecting information. Drug education may be pro-

vided by a range of people, e.g. teachers, youth workers, health promotion workers, medical and nursing staff and police officers. Pharmacists may be asked to provide talks and should only deliver such talks if they feel competent to do so and capable of answering questions. Before such talks are given it is advisable to get advice and information from a credible source such as publications by drug charities and health promotion units. Inaccurate advice can be harmful.

Social support

Social support refers loosely to non-medical/pharmacological interventions that can be made. These may include practical advice and assistance (e.g. seeking housing, benefits advice, provision of hostel accommodation) and use of psychological tools such as motivational interviewing. Motivational interviewing aims to assist people in examining their drug use and the impact it has on their lives and those of others to move people towards a psychological state where they are motivated to change their behaviour and attempt to change their drug use (see Ch. 39). There are many psychological tools that are used by clinical psychologists and counsellors in the treatment and support of people with drug problems. Pharmacists should be aware of the need for a holistic approach to care, using not only pharmacological therapies where appropriate, but non-drug treatments too.

Detoxification

Detoxification refers to the provision of treatment to help someone who is dependent on a drug to stop using it. Examples include the use of methadone at gradually reducing doses and the use of nicotine replacement therapy. The aim of detoxification is for the person to become abstinent from the drug on which they are dependent.

Rehabilitation

Rehabilitation may include a detoxification process followed by a period of social support and intensive psychotherapy to facilitate sustained change. Alternatively it may comprise the social support and intensive psychotherapy phase only, with successful detoxification being a requirement for entry on the programme. Rehabilitation is usually provided within a therapeutic community—participants live in the environment where treatment is given, often for several months. Often people who enter rehabilitation programmes have serious, complex and chronic drug dependency problems and may previously have experienced community-based treatment. The outcomes from various drug rehabilitation programmes were studied as part of the National Treatment Outcomes Research Study (NTORS), undertaken in the UK. Improvements were seen in drug use, physical health, psychological health and involvement in crime. At 4–5 year follow-up, 47% of people who had previously been dependent on opiates were abstinent with reductions in frequency of opiate use seen in a significant number of the remainder (Gossop et al 2001).

Harm reduction

Harm reduction is a generic term to describe the range of interventions used to reduce the adverse consequences of drug dependence experienced by both individual drug users and society. Strategies prioritize goals in treatment recognizing that, whereas abstinence from drug use may be the end goal, in some cases and for some drugs it is not always immediately achievable. Instead the risks and harm to the individual and others is reduced.

Examples of harm reduction interventions include the provision of sterile injecting equipment and information to drug injectors to prevent the sharing of injecting equipment (to prevent the transmission of viruses such as HIV, hepatitis B and C). Minimizing the prevalence of such diseases also protects the non-injecting community.

Harm reduction also includes the provision of substitute therapies with the aim of reducing illicit drug use and reducing drug-related crime, hence benefiting communities. This is often done by providing substitute therapy either at an adequate maintenance dose or as a detoxification agent. Pharmacists are frequently involved in the provision of harm reduction services (see later).

SERVICE PROVIDERS

Drug and alcohol services in the UK can be broadly grouped according to their different sources of funding. The three main groups are described below.

Statutory sector

The statutory sector comprises NHS and local authority services and includes prevention interventions, harm reduction services and abstinence-directed care. A large amount of NHS drug treatment is provided in GP surgeries, either by GPs alone or in partnership with GP liaison workers from specialist drugs services, who advise the GP on prescribing and offer patient counselling and support. Community drug teams (CDTs) are attached to secondary care NHS trusts often managed by psychiatrists. CDTs also provide primary care drug treatment, either through GP liaison work or with their own doctors running special clinics, similar to outpatient clinics. CDT services are typically provided by specialist registrars and psychiatric nurses but some employ pharmacists to advise on prescribing and undertake on-site dispensing. Statutory sector needle exchanges also exist, often staffed by specialist nurses.

NHS services also include secondary care, where treatment such as inpatient detoxification from alcohol and other drugs is provided, typically over a short time period such as 2 weeks.

Voluntary sector

Voluntary services are particularly prevalent in the substance misuse field because they developed quickly in response to the threat of HIV in the mid 1980s. The voluntary sector services receive funding from a range of sources (e.g. NHS, criminal justice money, local authorities and donations) and are usually registered charities, with paid workers and/or volunteers operating under a management committee structure. Workers may come from a range of backgrounds, e.g. nursing, social work and community work. Some projects employ current or ex drug users. Services may include:

- Support and/or counselling
- Information and advice including harm reduction information
- Needle exchange
- Preparation for rehabilitation or inpatient detoxification and aftercare
- Client advocacy
- Complementary therapies
- Support to and liaison with GPs
- Specialist services such as women-only sessions
- Outreach and detached street-based work
- Prescribing services
- Input into multidisciplinary groups funded by the statutory service such as pregnancy clinics for drug-using women.

Other voluntary sector services offer spiritual and practical support, e.g. hostel accommodation and self-help groups. The voluntary sector also may represent drug users' views in policy and service planning (e.g. The Methadone Alliance).

Private sector

The private sector includes ultra-rapid detoxification units, inpatient detoxification clinics, private primary care doctors and residential rehabilitation providers, private psychotherapists and alternative therapy providers. Funding for some of these treatments may come through the statutory sector but is most often paid for by the patients or their families. Some pharmacists work in private sector treatment facilities advising on prescribing and dispensing. Private services offer a wide range of choice to patients but access is obviously limited by ability to pay.

PHARMACEUTICAL CARE

This section focuses on pharmaceutical care of drug users, specifically looking at aspects of good pharmacy practice.

The role of the pharmacist in drug dependence

Community pharmacists

Community pharmacists are ideally placed to contribute to the care of drug users. In addition to the health gains, there are several advantages for drug users, the community and pharmacists from providing care:

- Extended opening hours: most pharmacies are open at least part of the weekend and some evenings, when specialist drugs services may be closed.
- Accessibility: pharmacies tend to be based within communities, making them near to need. No appointment is needed so people can access care with little prior planning and at their convenience, which can encourage use.
- Expert advice: pharmacies give access to a trained health care practitioner and free advice. Advice may be sought by needle exchange users, people receiving substitute therapies or their families. Alternatively the pharmacist may give advice proactively when an opportunity arises (see Ch. 39).
- Discretion: pharmacies provide a confidential service. Service users tend to see pharmacies as separate from the 'health care system' and are encouraged to use them because no personal data is requested.
- Network of service: through widespread provision of services by many pharmacies, the workload can be shared and a network of good practice developed. Joint training with other pharmacists and GPs can develop professional relationships.

- Job satisfaction: the pharmacist may be the only health care professional with whom some drug users have regular contact. Over time and with an approachable, non-judgmental service a strong therapeutic relationship can develop between the pharmacist and the service user. The pharmacist may then be approached for advice or be in a position to offer risk-reduction information. Trust in the pharmacist can allow the pharmacist to encourage the person to access drugs services. Over time improvements in health can often be seen in people receiving substitute therapies, bringing job satisfaction.

The two most common services provided by community pharmacists to prevent and reduce harm are needle exchange and dispensing services. These are discussed later.

Hospital pharmacists

Hospitals should have guidelines for the admission and discharge of drug users to ensure that any ongoing prescribing is continued. This is especially important for cases when people are admitted to general medical or surgical wards for matters not relating to their drug use. The teams on these wards may not be familiar with substance misuse prescribing. Hospital pharmacists may contribute to the formulation of such guidelines. Issues to include are:

- Admissions: how to ensure the safe and prompt continuation of substitute prescribing when someone comes into secondary care from the community, with attention paid to acute and out of hours admissions. Methadone is a controlled drug, unlikely to be kept routinely on wards, so the pharmacy department must establish procedures to supply methadone out of hours.
- Discharge: how to ensure safe continuation of substitute prescribing on discharge without a break in care or doubling up of prescribing. Contact with GPs and community drug teams is vital. Liaison with the patient's nominated community pharmacist is also important to ensure sufficient supplies and to communicate any changes made to treatment whilst in hospital.
- Appropriate referral: there are opportunities for identification of drug users not in contact with service providers especially by accident and emergency staff. Knowledge of local service providers and opening hours, including needle exchanges, is important and written details should be available on wards. Development of formal rapid access/referral systems should be undertaken in partnership with community-based services. At present many specialist services have waiting lists for care. Guidance

on identifying patients at particular risk and rapid referral from hospital to primary care services is recommended.

Hospital pharmacists also play a key role in advising on co-prescribing for people on substitute therapies such as methadone. Many drug interactions can occur and changes in doses may be necessary if methadone is co-administered with enzyme-inhibiting or enzyme-inducing drugs. Treatments for epilepsy and HIV/AIDS in particular must be carefully considered. Clinical issues of co-prescribing cannot be covered here, instead reference to appropriate texts on drug interactions is advised.

Specialist pharmacists

There are pharmacists who specialize in drug dependency. Some are based in drugs services, where they support clinical colleagues, e.g. by advising on prescribing or providing drug information. They may also oversee dispensing and liaise with community pharmacists. Others undertake strategic roles such as coordinating local pharmacy needle exchange services or overseeing the pharmacy contribution to shared-care (see below).

NEEDLE AND SYRINGE EXCHANGE

Background

Needle and syringe exchange (NSE) began in the UK in the mid 1980s in response to the threat from HIV. Prior to this, availability of clean injecting equipment was limited due to the belief that this would prevent people injecting. There was grave concern in the mid 1980s regarding the threat to public health that HIV presented and fears of an epidemic unless something was done to reduce its spread. Large health education campaigns were aimed at those at high risk, e.g. gay men, people having casual unprotected heterosexual sex and injecting drug users. In order to enable injecting drug users to follow the advice not to share needles and syringes, NSE programmes were started in many countries. These programmes were studied in several research projects which found that NSE programmes were effective in reducing the transmission of HIV without causing an increase in injecting drug use. A comparative study of 12 cities was conducted by Stimson et al for the World Health Organization (WHO); this is described in the text *Drug Injecting and HIV Infection* (Stimson et al 1998).

In the early 1990s hepatitis C was identified. This blood-borne virus appears to be highly transmissible amongst injectors and there is as yet no vaccine. It is thought to be spread through the sharing of injecting paraphernalia, not only needles and syringes, but also other items used in the preparation of illicit injections, for example, the spoon or metal container in which the drug is mixed with water, the makeshift filter used to remove insoluble materials and adulterants and items such as swabs used to clean injecting sites. The exact method of transmission is unclear and research is ongoing. It is important that NSE is widely available in order to limit the spread of blood-borne viruses. Community pharmacies contribute to the network of needle exchanges. They provide access to sterile injecting equipment, especially for those reluctant to access specialist agencies, at times when agencies are closed (such as weekends) and in areas where no such agencies exists. Privacy may be limited in community pharmacies, so there are limits to the extent of dialogue and examination that can take place. Additionally drug users may not perceive the pharmacist to be knowledgeable about drug misuse so pharmacists need to be proactive.

Practical issues in NSE provision

Training

Before any pharmacist begins to provide any new service it is important that they are adequately trained and competent to provide the service. NSE is no exception. Therefore pharmacists and their staff should undertake training on issues relating to needle exchange. Specialist agencies may be able to offer training for pharmacists and their staff.

Hepatitis B vaccination

Although pharmacists and their staff do not handle loose needles during the needle exchange process, it is a wise health and safety precaution for all staff to be vaccinated against hepatitis B. There are no vaccines for hepatitis C or HIV. In areas where pharmacy needle exchange schemes are coordinated by a specialist pharmacist, vaccination arrangements against hepatitis B should be in place. In other areas the community pharmacist must make provision for all staff to be vaccinated following the advice of the local public health consultant.

Needle exchange procedure

NSE involves supplying clean, sterile injecting equipment in exchange for used equipment, which is returned in a sealed sharps container. As well as supplying equipment, NSE services should provide advice and check injecting sites, with referral to medical services when problems such as abscesses are identified.

The guidance given by the Royal Pharmaceutical Society of Great Britain (RPSGB) on needle exchange in *Medicine, Ethics and Practice* should be followed. Needle exchange schemes are usually coordinated within the health locality, so local policies may exist and support and guidance should be available to pharmacists. Failing this policies and procedures for needle exchange need to be drafted in order to minimize risk. Guidance from public health departments and needle exchange agencies can assist. Adequate storage facilities are essential. Used equipment returned to the pharmacy should be placed in a larger bin by the client, stored in a separate area from clean equipment and away from medicines. These bins are sealed when full and collected for incineration by clinical waste disposal companies.

To maximize the public health benefits, injecting drug users need to be able to use a clean set of equipment for each injection and every set of equipment supplied should be returned for incineration. In order to try to meet this aim, adequate amounts of injecting equipment should be supplied, bearing in mind that some crack cocaine injectors may be injecting very frequently (e.g. 15 times per day or more). The number of needles and syringes that can be supplied in any one visit may be dictated locally by scheme coordinators. It is wise to discuss supply quantities with local needle exchange agencies to ensure continuity in service provision. In Scotland the Lord Advocate's Guidance dictates the number of sets that can be supplied. A sharps bin should be supplied with every exchange. Bins range from pocket size to large clinical waste tubs. The return of equipment should be strongly encouraged. Written advice on safe disposal accompanied by verbal emphasis is important. However if a person requests needle exchange but has no used equipment to return, it is advocated that supply of clean needles and syringes is made, as the health risks of not supplying are large. Pharmacy staff should not open disposal bins to count the number of sets of returned. Instead estimates of returned numbers should be made based on the number of returns reported by the service user and the size and estimated fullness of the returned disposal bin.

Record keeping and audit

Records need to be kept in order to audit the pharmacy NSE service. In order to encourage use, pharmacy NSE should be provided on an anonymous basis (no names recorded).

Attractions of pharmacy-based NSE are the anonymity and low threshold access. Too many obstacles will discourage use. In some schemes, pharmacies issue cards which give the service user an identification number or code. This can be used to record service usage but it also allows discreet service provision, as the person only needs to show the card to indicate that they require needle exchange. This can be helpful in a crowded pharmacy. The advantage of having a record for each service user is that it can quickly be seen if someone returns used equipment. Those who do not can be targeted with information and firm requests to return equipment. The disadvantage is that in a busy pharmacy this system can be too time consuming. Additionally some people do not want to carry a card that identifies them as an injector. As a basic requirement, the daily number of sets of injecting equipment supplied and the approximate number returned should be recorded and data compiled for weekly or monthly audit purposes. Data should be returned to the scheme coordinator where one exists. Pharmacies with poor return rates should seek the advice of specialist drugs agencies and the scheme coordinator on strategies to increase return rates and be proactive in encouraging returns.

Risk management

A written procedure for needle exchange should be in place and followed. Body fluid spillage kits should be kept in all pharmacies as a matter of routine, irrespective of whether the pharmacy is part of a NSE scheme, and staff should be trained in their use. In the event of an incident (e.g. a patient bleeds or vomits on the floor), the kit should be used. It should be noted that use of the kit is dictated by the situation and not the perceived risk presented by the patient, i.e. use of the kit does not depend on whether the patient is a known injector or not.

Chain mail gloves should be kept in needle exchange pharmacies for use in the event of loose used injecting equipment requiring disposal. However this is only a precaution, as the needle exchange scheme procedure should be such that it minimizes the risk of such events. If any such events occur they should be documented as part of the pharmacy's critical incident scheme. Procedures should then be reviewed to see if anything could be done to avoid such an incident in the future.

Links with specialist services

Pharmacy NSE providers should have links with local drugs agencies and know what services they provide. Often younger and newer injectors use pharmacy needle exchanges because of the low threshold and discretion. These people may also not want to stop injecting and consider agencies to be for people with drug 'problems' or people who want to stop using. Women may also prefer the anonymity of using pharmacy services. Female drug users are often extremely stigmatized, especially if they are also mothers. The pharmacist may be the only health care professional their service users have contact with. Knowledge of other local services means that the pharmacist can advise when a need is identified or an opportunity arises. The pharmacy should consider itself a gateway to specialist services. Some specialist agencies may be able to supply pharmacists with targeted written information for drug injectors, such as safer injecting leaflets, and with free condoms to reduce sexually transmitted diseases. Safer injecting leaflets should not be available for self-selection but should be targeted at injectors.

USE OF PHARMACOTHERAPIES IN DRUG DEPENDENCE

The term pharmacotherapy in this context refers to any drug treatment used to assist in the management of drug dependence or symptoms of withdrawal. Substitute therapy refers to drug treatment that replaces an illegal drug with a legal one of the same or similar pharmacological class. For example methadone is a substitute for opiates such as heroin. Non-substitute drugs may also be used to control withdrawal symptoms (e.g. lofexidine to manage opiate withdrawal) and to manage symptoms secondary to withdrawal (e.g. loperamide to manage diarrhoea associated with opiate withdrawal).

Role of pharmacotherapy

Pharmacotherapy can be mistaken both by patients and professionals as an all-encompassing solution but it is one of several tools used in the care of drug dependence. Alone it cannot stop someone using drugs but it can facilitate change in motivated people by providing what many describe as 'breathing space'. For example substitute therapy can prevent withdrawal symptoms thus giving the person a chance to sever links with illicit drug suppliers. Substitute therapy also removes the need to commit crime to obtain money for drugs. Pharmacotherapy therefore has benefits for both the individual and society. Substitute therapy, from a risk-reduction point of view, is also preferable to illicit drugs because the quality and dose of the product is assured.

The psychoactive and non-psychoactive effects of substitute therapies are not usually the same as the illicit drugs they replace and an awareness of this in the patient at the start of treatment is important. For example, methadone is used as a long-acting substitute in opiate dependence. When taken orally it does not produce euphoria and it can cause lethargy and a feeling of 'heaviness' not associated with heroin use.

All who receive pharmacotherapy, especially in the early stages of treatment, may not achieve complete abstinence from illicit drug use. It is a common misconception that substitute treatment should be given at a reducing dose leading in a short time period to abstinence from illicit drug use. Whereas in a minority of patients this will produce sustained benefits, for many, rapid detoxification has been shown not to produce long-term abstinence from illicit drugs.

Methadone

Methadone is used as a substitute drug in opiate dependence. Its long half-life (24–48 hours) makes it suitable for once-daily dosing in the majority of cases, although a few patients prefer to divide the dose. Providing it is given in adequate doses and for a satisfactory length of time, there is substantial evidence to suggest that methadone treatment has several benefits:

- Improved physical health
- Improved psychological health
- Reduced illicit drug consumption
- Reduced incidence and frequency of injecting episodes.
- Reduced drug-related crime.

As can be seen, the benefits extend beyond the individual patient into the community. Less injecting will reduce the risks of blood-borne virus transmission. The reductions seen in drug-related crime have been large. These findings have been reported in a range of publications including in the UK those from the National Treatment Outcomes Research Study (NTORS) (Gossop et al 2001).

Failure to reduce or prevent illicit drug consumption is associated with maintenance doses of methadone less than 60 mg per day and premature pressure to abstain from methadone (Ward et al 1999). Before detoxification can be considered, treatment may need to be given at maintenance dose level for prolonged periods of time, with some people remaining on maintenance doses indefinitely. Withdrawal of treatment should begin only when the patient is willing to attempt this, as motivation is the key to success. Regular review of patients on maintenance doses and on detoxification schemes is necessary. In detoxification, the speed of dose reduction largely depends on how well the patient is coping. Reductions should be calculated as a percentage of the dose, hence towards the smaller end of the scale dosing will be reduced by smaller quantities. For some people the small doses can be the hardest to reduce and some people remain on doses of as little as 1 mg and 2 mg per day for several months until they feel capable of stopping treatment completely. Psychological adjustment is very important at this stage, especially if drug use has been used as a coping mechanism. Withdrawal can take several months, even years. If the dose needs to be increased at any point during detoxification, emotional support and reassurance may be necessary as some people can regard such increases as failure.

It is important to discuss with patients potential overdose risks from combining CNS depressants, including alcohol. Health care teams need to understand that some illicit drug use may continue, especially at the early stages of treatment. This can be a time when there is a greater risk of overdose, so the patient must be advised of this and monitored closely. Several information leaflets are available which explain this to patients, e.g. the 'Methadone Briefing' from Exchange Health Information. If illicit drug use continues at a similar frequency as it was before methadone therapy was introduced it is important to review the dose and treatment goals with the patient. Methadone treatment may be suboptimal or the person is not ready to change their drug use. In this case methadone may be compounding the risks and other harm reduction strategies may be more appropriate.

Pharmacists should have a good understanding of the clinical aspects relating to methadone treatment before they begin providing methadone dispensing services. This should be gained as part of a continuous professional development plan if needed.

Safe storage in the home

If take-home doses are dispensed, pharmacists should discuss safe storage of methadone and other drugs in the home with patients, especially those with children. As little as 5 mg of methadone can kill a small child. Parents on methadone prescriptions should store take-home doses in overhead cupboards, which should be locked to prevent access by children. In addition parents should be advised not to consume medicines in front of children to prevent copying behaviours.

Other treatments

Buprenorphine, lofexidine and naltrexone are also used in the management of opiate withdrawal. There are also recognized regimens to assist withdrawal for those with stimulant, benzodiazepine and alcohol dependence. When a person is dependent on more than one drug, withdrawal should be done one drug at a time. Further reading regarding these treatments is advised.

Urine screening and responding to symptoms

People receiving treatment for drug dependence may have their urine screened. This is done to check for evidence of compliance with prescribed regimens or to confirm for the consumption of illicit drugs. In some areas urine screen results may be used to make a decision on whether treatment is continued or not. Pharmacists should undertake training in this area of toxicology, as some OTC and prescribed medicines can interfere with urine screens, giving false results. It is important to have an understanding of what medicines to avoid in people receiving treatment for dependence, so that patients and prescribers can be advised. This is also relevant to athletes subject to urine screens for banned substances.

PHARMACEUTICAL DISPENSING SERVICES

Shared care

Shared care with regard to substance misuse is GPs, pharmacists, drugs services and the patient being in partnership to manage dependence within a formalized, structured scheme. Pharmacists participating in such schemes receive additional remuneration. Examples of schemes in the UK include those in Glasgow and Berkshire (Roberts & Bryson 1999, Walker 2001). Daily dispensing of controlled drugs is often advocated by prescribers, especially at the start of treatment, as it is believed to prevent leakage onto illegal markets. This means that the pharmacist is likely to be the health care professional with the most frequent contact with the patient as they see the patient daily, whilst the prescribing team may see them weekly or fortnightly. Pharmacists can play an important role in monitoring the patient's health.

One of the benefits of shared care is that the workload of providing care is distributed locally. This prevents one or two pharmacies becoming overburdened and allows patients access to care within their communities. Participation of all or the majority of community pharmacies in the area is therefore vital for the scheme to succeed. To date this has not always been the case as some pharmacies have refused to provide services to drug users.

Before joining a shared-care scheme pharmacists should consider any changes within the pharmacy that may be necessary. These should be discussed with the scheme coordinator who may be able to source financial assistance for such changes. For example is there enough space in the CD cabinet to store dispensed controlled drugs waiting for collection? Consider the layout of the premises. What can be done to ensure an appropriate area is available to allow a respectful service to be provided? Is there a private area for methadone consumption? A private room is not usually desired by patients but a discrete area can be very welcome.

Supervised consumption

The development of shared-care schemes for the management of drug dependence has lead to an increased involvement of pharmacists, especially community pharmacists, in providing care to drug users. Many shared-care schemes require daily dispensing and supervision of consumption of all or most doses of substitute therapy, at least for the first 3–6 months of treatment. Supervised consumption was introduced because of leakage of methadone and other drugs to the illicit market contributing to overdoses in people who had not been prescribed the drugs.

Supervised consumption is a contentious area. Some patients view it as a useful part of treatment whereas others dislike it (Neale 1999). Supervised consumption can cause the patient much embarrassment. In a busy shop it may be very humiliating for a person if a pharmacist presents them with a measure of green liquid to drink or some tablets to take in front of other customers. As it is not 'normal' to take medicines in front of the pharmacist, people can quickly be identified as drug users. Much can be done by the pharmacist to show respect and consideration for someone when they are required to consume their treatment in the pharmacy, e.g. ask if they wish to wait until the shop is free of other customers before their dose is given. Pharmacists should also ask patients whether they wish to use a private area, if one is available. Patients appreciate such respect.

To assist with organization, it is suggested that pharmacists prepare all daily dispensed prescriptions the day before or early in the day required. Doses should be packaged appropriately in individually labelled containers and stored in the CD cupboard, or as legislation dictates, with the prescription attached. When the patient presents for supervised consumption, the pharmacist should recheck the dispensed item. The patient should then be given the substance to be consumed together with a drink of water. The water helps take the taste of the medicine away, rinses the mouth (methadone has a high sugar content and is acidic, which could damage tooth enamel) and helps ensure the dose has been swallowed. Disposable cups should be used. Under no circumstances should patients be expected to share the same cup for water in case this presents a risk of infection transmission. The pharmacist should take the opportunity for discussion with the patient to assess their well being and offer any advice as the opportunity arises. Over time a good rapport and therapeutic relationship can develop with patients.

When instalment dispensing is required, the instalment can only be collected on the date specified on the prescription. This should be explained to patients at the start of treatment.

Confidentiality

Communication between health care professionals is key in shared care. However patient confidentiality must be borne in mind. Information should not be shared without consent. The patient should be involved in negotiations about care and treatment changes. When discussion with another service provider about a patient is necessary this should be discussed with the patient. They should be informed of what the other service provider is to be told and their permission sought. Patient's wishes should only be breached when a severe risk to health or well being is considered to exist if confidentiality is not broken. All matters relating to the upholding or breaching of confidentiality should be documented.

Contracts

Some shared-care schemes advocate the use of contracts, which clearly state what is expected of the patient and what the patient can expect from the service. Often they dictate standards of behaviour and include clauses requiring the patient to fulfil certain criteria, including restricting the times when patients can collect prescriptions. It is debated whether contracts should be used specifically for patients with drug problems. They imply that it is expected that the person will not behave appropriately and as such stereotypes patients. Contracts are not routinely used within health care for other patients and it can be argued that using one for drug users is unfair and discriminatory. Pharmacies should have practice leaflets as a matter of routine which are available to all pharmacy users. These may include a statement that all pharmacy customers have a right to privacy and respect and all pharmacy staff have a right to be treated with courtesy. If individuals present any problems the pharmacist should deal with these individually. This applies to any customers who cause difficulty within the pharmacy. Many pharmacies have a documented complaints procedure which can be useful for reviewing response to such incidents.

When pharmacists are asked to use contracts as part of the shared-care scheme, the pharmacist should review the contract before agreeing. Pharmacists should ask themselves whether they, as a patient, would consider it fair to sign such terms. The contract should not imply that it is expected that the person cannot behave or will cause problems.

Restricted collection hours for drug users should also be considered with caution. Pharmacists are required to dispense prescriptions with 'reasonable promptness'. Refusing to dispense a prescription during opening hours because a person has not arrived within a designated collection time may be considered discriminatory.

Locums

All standard operating procedures for pharmacy services should be documented and available for locums to use. This includes needle exchange and supervised consumption. It is important that all locums are aware of all the services provided, including those to drug users, and are briefed on the completion of any necessary documentation such as needle exchange usage.

Key points

- Pharmacists can make an important contribution to the care and support of people with drug misuse problems.
- Treatment of substance misuse benefits not only the patient but the community as well by reducing blood-borne virus transmission and drug-related crime.
- Pharmacists should seek adequate continuous professional development to increase their competence in providing services to drug users. This should include clinical and therapeutic knowledge of treatment in this area as well as service provision skills.
- Pharmacists should seek to be informed on local specialist services for drug users and have good professional links with such treatment providers.
- Pharmacists should treat all pharmacy users with respect. This includes not discriminating on the basis of a person's disease state or drug dependence.
- Local pharmacy scheme coordinators can be of great benefit in supporting pharmacists who provide services to drug users.

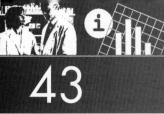

43

Clinical governance

J. Krska

After studying this chapter you will know about:

Mechanisms for ensuring quality of care
Audit—definitions and types of audit
What is measured in audit
The audit cycle:
  Standard setting
  Data collection
  Comparison with standards
  Identifying problems
  Implementing change
  Re-audit
Continuous professional development
Practice research, practice development and audit
Competency and clinical governance

MECHANISMS FOR ENSURING QUALITY OF CARE

Quality of care is of essential importance in health services. This applies to pharmacists just as much as to doctors, nurses and all other health care professionals. Within the NHS, the term used to describe the responsibility for quality of clinical care is 'clinical governance'. Clinical governance makes sure that NHS organizations are accountable for continuously improving the quality of their service. It means that professionals, including pharmacists, now have to prove that their performance is acceptable. The main implications of clinical governance for pharmacists are given in Box 43.1.

Previous chapters have provided some information on clinical guidelines, drug use review and evaluation. This chapter explains what is meant by clinical audit and describes how pharmacists can use it to help improve the quality of care. Continuous professional development (CPD) is also essential for maintaining standards of patient care and improving practice. This chapter also explains what is meant by CPD and how it and audit are important in clinical governance.

Audit—definitions

Audit is about quality—the quality of professional activities and services. Those who carry out audit seek to determine whether best practice is being delivered and, equally importantly, to improve practice. A useful definition of audit is 'the process of reviewing the delivery of health care to identify deficiencies so that they may be remedied'.

Box 43.1   Implications of clinical governance for pharmacists

Superintendent or proprietor pharmacist is responsible for quality of clinical care in community pharmacies

Primary care trust or local health care cooperative pharmacist is responsible for quality of clinical care provided by employee pharmacists in their organizations

Chief pharmacists in hospital NHS trusts are responsible for quality of clinical care provided by employee pharmacists in their organizations

Pharmacists should participate in implementing clinical guidelines, clinical audit, drug use review and evaluation

Pharmacists must undertake continuing professional development and continually develop their practice

Pharmacists must develop and implement policies to manage risks associated with medicines use

Procedures must be in place to identify and remedy poor performance by pharmacists

Pharmacists must integrate their work with that of other health care professionals

Pharmacists should document their work to enable its quality to be assessed and document their CPD

As a profession, pharmacists are involved in the creation of standards, e.g. registration procedures and standards of professional practice. The hallmark of a professional is the maintenance of these standards, which exist to protect the public from poor quality services.

Any of the health care professions may carry out audit of services provided by their own peer group. This is professional audit. Some aspects of pharmacy are concerned with professionalism per se, such as standards of medicines storage or of pharmacy premises. Audit of these aspects may, therefore, be termed pharmaceutical audit.

Most of the activities of health professionals, however, have an impact on patients, either directly or indirectly. Any service which has an effect on the outcome of a patient's care may be deemed to be a clinical service. Audit of these services may be called clinical audit. Clinical audit is defined as the systematic and critical appraisal of the quality of clinical care.

There are few instances where pharmacists provide a service to patients in isolation from other health care professionals. Even the provision of advice and sale of non-prescription medicines may involve referral to a GP or conversely a GP may have advised patients to seek help from a pharmacist. Dispensing prescriptions always involves some sort of review of prescribing by another professional. Pharmacists' counselling of patients does not stand alone as a service, since the patient will usually have had some instruction from others as well. Thus clinical services are in the main multidisciplinary and the audit of these clinical services must also be multidisciplinary.

Audit provides a method of accountability, both to the public and to government. It is also essential that managers have information about the quality of the services their staff are providing. Although this may seem to be a somewhat threatening situation, ultimately the aim of audit is to improve the efficiency and effectiveness of services, to promote higher standards and, in the case of clinical audit, to improve the outcome for patients. It also allows changes in practice to be evaluated. Therefore it is an essential component of any professional's work and should be seen as an integral part of day-to-day practice.

TYPES OF AUDIT

Audit may be of three types, classified according to who undertakes it. These are:

- Self-audit
- Peer or group audit
- External audit.

Self-audit is undertaken by individuals and may be seen as the development of a professional attitude to work, in which critical appraisal of actions taken and of their results is constantly being made. It is most commonly undertaken by those who work in isolation from others, such as single-handed community pharmacists. There are many self-audits which community pharmacists can undertake. Many have been developed by Glasgow pharmacy audit programme and the relevant checklists can be obtained from the following web site: http://www.show.nhs.uk/gghbpharmacy/.

Peer audit is undertaken by people within the same peer group, which is usually the same profession. This means that there is joint setting of standards and the other group members assess the activities of everyone in the group. For example, pharmacists from several hospitals could get together and audit a service being provided by each hospital. Pharmacists from one hospital would look at the services provided from other hospitals, while their own service would be open to the scrutiny of pharmacists from these hospitals.

Multidisciplinary audit is the most common type of group audit. It is usually required for clinical services audits. In this type of audit, it is essential to ensure that one subgroup is not auditing the activities of another subgroup. This would lead to tensions and be counterproductive. An example of how this could occur is an audit of prescribing errors detected by pharmacists. The pharmacists may consider there are too many errors, without the prescribers being involved in deciding what constitutes an error or what is an acceptable frequency of errors. If the prescribers are not part of the team responsible for designing the audit, there is also little chance of any improvement.

External audit is carried out by people other than those actually providing the service. and because of this is perceived as threatening by those whose services are being audited. It may be more objective in its criticisms than self- or peer audit, but there may be less enthusiasm for corrective action to improve services.

Externally organized audits may be particularly suitable for services which are difficult for individuals to audit, such as responding to symptoms in community pharmacies. However, it is still possible to involve those whose services are to be audited in deciding what best practice should be and in making improvements. This is not the same as external audit in which the standard of best practice is imposed and where there is a perceived threat if an individual's performance is not of the standard required.

WHAT IS MEASURED IN AUDIT?

There are three aspects of any professional activity which may be audited:

- The structures or resources involved
- The processes used
- The outcomes of the activity.

Structures are the resources available to help deliver services or carry out activities; examples are the staff, their expertise and knowledge, books, learning materials or training courses, drug stocks, equipment and layout of premises.

Processes are the systems and procedures which take place when carrying out an activity and may include quality assurance procedures and policies and protocols of all types. An example of this could be a written procedure to be followed in a hospital when patients bring their own medicines into hospital. Prescribing policies and disease management protocols can also be considered as processes which can be audited.

Outcomes are the results of the activity and are arguably the most important aspect of any activity. In clinical audit involving patients, outcomes which involve a change in health status, attitude or behaviour may be very difficult to measure. Other clinical outcomes are relatively easily measured, such as changes in physiological and other parameters such as blood pressure, INR (International Normalized Ratio) control and serum biochemistry. Changes in the behaviour of other health professionals may be another outcome measure, e.g. changes in prescribing. In pharmaceutical audits which look at drug procurement or distribution or standards of premises, outcomes will be much easier to measure.

Any individual audit can examine structures, processes and outcomes individually or together.

THE AUDIT CYCLE

The audit of any activity is a continuous process, which follows a cycle of measurement, evaluation and improvement. This cycle is shown in Figure 43.1. It incorporates:

- The setting of standards for practice
- Measuring actual practice
- Comparing the two
- Finding out any reasons why best practice is not being achieved
- Changing what is done to improve this.

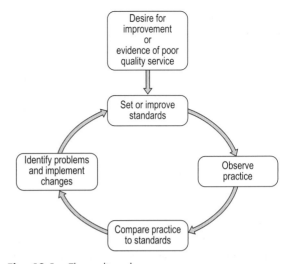

Fig. 43.1 The audit cycle.

Although the process is continuous, it is not practicable to audit all activities or services all the time. It is often appropriate to have intervals between periods when actual practice is measured, to allow for changes to take effect. It is also important to select topics for audit carefully, because of the time involved in doing the audit. In choosing which activities should be audited, two of the main criteria to be considered are whether or not there is a problem and whether there is a realistic possibility of improvement. If this is the case and an audit is planned, then the first stage is to set standards against which practice will be measured.

Setting standards

All audit should be based on standards which are widely accepted in terms of what should be done (i.e. best practice). There are many guidelines covering individual aspects of pharmacy practice published by the Royal Pharmaceutical Society of Great Britain in *Medicines, Ethics and Practice*. In addition, many other organizations have produced materials which pharmacists can use for audit. Examples include good practice guidelines, counselling, clinical pharmacy practice, or the many clinical guidelines for the treatment of individual medical conditions. These will need modification to form criteria and measurable standards which can be used for audit. Several standards are usually set for any individual audit. These may concern resources, processes or outcomes.

Because audit is about comparing actual practice to standards of best practice, numerical values need to be added which will allow this. A guideline may suggest a criterion, e.g. that patients receiving warfarin should be counselled about avoiding aspirin. For this to be useful in audit, it needs to be clarified whether this applies to all patients, i.e. 100%. This numerical value is the target which together with the criterion forms the standard. It then becomes easy to measure whether this is the case in actual practice.

This is termed an ideal standard, since it is ideally what should happen. However, the level of standard set may need to be a compromise between what is desirable and what is possible, since resources may be limited. In this case, an optimal standard may be set. Using the previous example, it may be considered that there were insufficient staff to ensure that 100% of patients receiving warfarin could be counselled about avoiding aspirin. A useful compromise could be that 100% of patients prescribed warfarin for the first time are counselled. Another type of standard is the minimal standard, which, as its name implies, is the minimum level of service which is acceptable. This type of standard is often that used in external audits.

For some of the services or activities that are to be audited, there may be no published guidelines or standards to help, in which case it will be necessary to devise them. This may involve searching the literature, e.g. recent journals, standard textbooks or perhaps educational material to provide criteria. It can be useful to undertake a baseline survey to find out what current practice is before setting targets. Whatever approach is used, it is important that everybody involved in providing the service is also involved in deciding what the standard will be. For much of clinical audit, this will include other health professionals and is most likely to involve at least medical practitioners. However, nurses, health visitors, technical staff and non-medical staff, such as receptionists, practice managers or porters, may also need to be involved. It may also be appropriate to include patients or their carers as recipients of services.

By involving everyone who plays a part in a health care service in deciding standards, the audit is clearly a peer or group audit. This avoids the potential feeling of threat which may be created by excluding individuals. To anyone excluded at this stage, it appears that the audit is external. This could result in the whole exercise being a waste of time, since these individuals may refuse to help in raising performance later. Once standards have been set, the next stage of audit involves finding out what actually happens.

Observing practice

Finding out what is actual practice involves collecting data of some sort. Usually a simple form needs to be designed, onto which data from other sources are transferred. In audits involving structures, checklists are often most useful, those involving processes may use checklists or may need space for other types of data, while auditing outcomes often involves questionnaires. As with any data collection, it is important that the information obtained is able to answer the questions asked. In the case of an audit the question(s) may be relatively simple, such as 'What is the percentage of patients receiving warfarin who are counselled?' As in research, finding out whether a similar audit has been done before and by adapting or modifying the data collection procedures used can save time and effort. Some useful starting points for audits are available from the Royal Pharmaceutical Society of Great Britain website. If a new procedure is required, the same basic requirements as for any data collection must be considered (Box 43.2).

In addition, because audit is about improvement of services, it is often necessary to find out why best practice is not followed. Again using warfarin counselling described above as an example, the data may show that only 75% of patients were counselled. If no reasons have been found to explain why the remainder were not counselled, it may not be clear what needs to be done to improve practice. One reason may be that the 25% who were not counselled already knew about avoiding aspirin. On the other hand it may be that one particular member of staff, who had insufficient knowledge, handed out all these prescriptions. Another cause could be that the prescriptions were all given out when the pharmacy was particularly busy and staff felt that they had no time for counselling. Each of these different reasons for best practice not being delivered would need different solutions, so it is essential to determine the reasons as part of the audit. This shows that the data collection procedures need to anticipate, to some extent at least, potential causes for failing to provide best practice.

Box 43.2 Requirements for data collection procedures

Provide information required
Validity
Reliability
Controlled for bias
Adequate sampling technique
Feasible
Quantitative or qualitative
Retrospective or prospective
Routinely or specially collected
Pilot study

The method of data collection must be valid and reliable. If sampling procedures are used, they too must be appropriate, avoiding bias, and equally importantly it must be feasible to carry them out.

Validity is the extent to which what is measured is actually what is supposed to be measured. To use the warfarin counselling example again, the standard was about advice concerning aspirin. If the only data collected were the number of patients who were counselled and not what advice they were given about aspirin, these data would be invalid, since they did not measure what they set out to measure.

Reliability is a measure of the consistency or reproducibility of the data collection procedure. Good reliability can be difficult to achieve when trying to measure outcomes in health care. It is therefore important to use recognized measures wherever possible. Reliability may also vary among individuals collecting data, despite their using the same data collection tool. It is important to check this and ensure that they agree how they will use the tools before they start to collect data which will be used for audit.

Sampling is important in collecting data for audit, because the data should be unbiased and representative of actual practice. It may be that the numbers and time involved are small enough that all examples of the activity are included in data collection procedures. In the case of large numbers, it may be easier to include just a proportion in the audit. If so, a plan is needed which ensures that those selected are representative. Many different sampling methods could be used, including random (using number tables) or systematic (such as every tenth patient presenting a prescription for warfarin). Another way is to decide in advance that a certain percentage of the total population (a quota) will be sampled, usually ensuring that they will be typical of the population. These techniques require that the total population size within the audit period is known. A large population may also need to be stratified into subgroups first before using these techniques.

Sampling, or even large numbers, may not always be necessary. Since audit is about a particular service or activity carried out by one or more particular individual professionals, an audit can be carried out on a service provided to one patient. It still involves determining whether actual practice equates to best practice.

Feasibility of data collection is very important. It must be possible to collect the data which are required to answer the question. It is often necessary to incorporate data collection for audit into routine work, so the time taken is an important consideration.

Some of the data which will answer audit questions may already be collected on a routine basis. Data kept on computerized patient medication records or on patient profiles may be useful for some types of audit. Some pharmacies routinely log the time when prescriptions are handed in and given out, so an audit of turnaround time could easily be carried out using these data. Hospitals routinely collect data on length of stay and number of admissions, discharges and deaths, which may be useful outcome measures. Often data have to be specially collected for the audit, which needs a specifically designed data collection tool.

Data for audit can be either quantitative or qualitative in nature. Qualitative data are often useful in obtaining opinions about services or for measuring outcomes in patients. Large numbers are not required for producing qualitative data. It may be useful to undertake qualitative work, which can then be used to help design a good data collection tool to be used in a quantitative way, using larger numbers. Quantitative audit almost always generates large amounts of data, which require subsequent analysis, usually using statistics. These may be purely descriptive or simple comparative statistics.

Whether the data collected are retrospective or prospective depends to a large extent on the topic of the audit and the data available. Retrospective audit can only be undertaken if good records of activities have been kept. Prospective audits should ensure that the data required are recorded, even if only for the audit period. The possibility of practice changing during the audit period simply because the audit is being undertaken is a real one. This may not always be a problem if practice is better than usual and if audit is continuous, since the ultimate aim is to improve services. It is more important to be aware of this effect if practice is measured periodically, although it is very difficult to control for.

In large audits, as in most practice research, piloting the data collection tool which will be used is a valuable way of finding out if it is suitable. It is always worth spending time undertaking a small pilot study, using a sample similar to those to be included in the audit. This should avoid the discovery that there were difficulties in interpretation or that vital information has not been recorded after acquiring large amounts of data.

Comparing practice to standards

This is the evaluation stage of audit, in which actual practice is compared to best practice. This involves the analysis and presentation of the data obtained. Most audit data require only descriptive analysis, such as percentages, means or medians, along with ranges and standard deviations to show the spread of the data. Comparative statistical tests are useful for looking at one or more subgroups of quantitative data. This could be for different data collection periods (audit cycles) or for subgroups within one audit. Examples where comparison may be useful are three different pharmacies' prescription turnaround times or the counselling frequencies for patients presenting prescriptions for warfarin for the first time compared to those who have taken it before. The statistical test must be appropriate for the type of data. Chi-square is used for non-parametric data, such as frequencies. For parametric data which are normally distributed, t-tests can be used.

In audit, as in any use of statistics, it is important to consider the practical significance of the data. An improvement which is statistically significant may not always be of practical significance and vice versa.

Data collected for audit purposes relate to the activities of individual professionals and to their effects on patients. It is therefore essential to maintain confidentiality. Permission is required before any information about one individual's practice is given to other members of the audit team. Managers who may need this sort of information should be part of the audit team anyway. The general results of an audit should, however, be made available to others, after ensuring that no individual practitioner or patient can be identified. This is essential if the audit is to improve services, as it will help others to learn and allow comparisons to be made.

When comparing the results of audits between centres, there will most probably be differences, perhaps in staffing levels, population served, case mix and so on, which could account for differences in apparent performance. The results of any audit should not be extrapolated beyond the sample audited. Audit applies to a particular activity, carried out by particular individuals and involving particular patients.

In presenting data collected during audit, as with any other data, graphics can be particularly useful, as tables can be discouraging to many people. This is particularly important in a group audit, where everyone needs to see the results. Simple graphics should be adequate, such as pie charts or bar charts.

Providing the standards for the audit have been set appropriately, it should be relatively easy to determine whether they have been achieved. Often the most difficult part of audit is finding out why best practice is not being delivered and ensuring that improvement occurs.

Identifying problems

It is important in any audit to find out not only what is wrong with a service, but also why it is wrong. The underlying causes of failure need to be established. Thus the data collected during measurement of practice should have attempted to identify them. Suboptimal practice can arise because of inadequate skills or knowledge, poor systems of work or patient attitudes and behaviour. Each should be examined as a possible contributory factor to disappointing results of an audit. In most audits, health care professionals' lack of knowledge is not a problem, although lack of awareness, for example about guidelines for disease management, can contribute to reduced performance against standards. Lack of skill may be related to infrequency of carrying out a particular activity. Both are relatively easily remedied. Both behaviour and the way in which work is organized are more difficult to change. The strategies adopted for effecting change will need to differ depending on which of these underlying causes is present.

Implementing changes

Achieving an improvement in practice requires a change in behaviour. Change can be threatening simply because of its novelty. It may also involve increased work and is often resisted. For these reasons all those whose work pattern may need to change should be active members of the audit team from the start. Change must be seen as leading to improvement in performance and ultimately benefits to the patient. The changes proposed to improve practice must be closely tailored to the underlying cause of the suboptimal results. They should be specific to the situation which has been audited, rather than general. They should be non-threatening and may need to be introduced gradually. Change may require resources, including time. It may also have other knock-on effects which need to be anticipated. The effect of changes must be monitored, to see whether they have been successful. This can be done by re-audit.

Re-audit

In some audits it may be appropriate to reconsider the standards before undertaking a further period of data collection. Standards which involved targets set too high may always be unattainable, although this may not have been apparent before practice was measured. It is equally possible to have used low standards and to have found they were surpassed. In this case it may be appropriate to raise them, which is a good way of improving practice. Whether or not the standards remain the same, a second period of measuring practice is needed if changes have been implemented, so that the effectiveness of these changes can be determined.

It is always difficult to change behaviour and improvements in practice may be short lived. It may therefore be necessary to repeat audits at regular intervals to reinforce the desired practice and maintain the improvement in service.

CONTINUOUS PROFESSIONAL DEVELOPMENT

The need for continuous improvements to practice to maintain the highest quality health care services is the purpose of audit. One finding of an audit may be lack of knowledge or awareness of information. Another may be the need to change practice or develop new ways of delivering services. In undertaking audit, drug use review or evaluation, pharmacists may identify areas where their knowledge or expertise is lacking. This awareness may also arise through many other mechanisms, such as being asked questions by patients or colleagues to which they do not know the answers. Delivery of high quality health care depends on the competence of those involved in providing services to patients. New medicines, formulations, indications and evidence of benefits or harm are being discovered daily. Keeping up to date with these developments is a requirement for pharmacists. This requires continuous professional development (CPD). However CPD is much more than just keeping abreast of new drug developments. It is a process of ensuring fitness to practice and encompasses skills and expertise required for delivering all aspects of a pharmaceutical service.

CPD is defined as a systematic, ongoing, cyclical process of self-directed learning. It should enable pharmacists to do their job more effectively and involves employers as well as individuals.

Like audit, CPD follows a cyclical process. The cycle is shown in Figure 43.2 and involves:

- Reflection
- Planning
- Implementing the plan
- Evaluation.

Reflection involves thinking about how you have carried out daily tasks, the areas in which you feel your knowledge or skills are weak or events which have happened. Sometimes

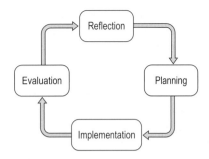

Fig. 43.2 The CPD cycle.

a particular situation or event will draw to attention a weakness in knowledge, ability or systems of work which, if left as they are, could cause further problems. This is called a critical event. Asking colleagues for feedback on your performance is another useful way of finding out whether there are any gaps in knowledge or skills. Of course the results of an audit may also identify gaps in knowledge. The process of reflecting on what you do not know or are unable to do results in identification of training needs.

Planning involves setting out what is needed to ensure that the gaps in knowledge or skills are overcome and the ways in which these gaps can be filled. It may be necessary to identify courses, training events, reading or people to seek assistance from to enable the training needs to be fulfilled.

Action is simply carrying out the plan. While it sounds simple, the time taken to undertake the learning needs to be built into the plan and the timetable adhered to. In some cases, the most effective way of learning new skills is to learn from colleagues or simply to start teaching oneself, using whatever resources are available. This is called learning by doing and is just as important as attending formal training courses.

Evaluation involves assessing whether the learning undertaken has been effective. This requires asking the question: 'Can practice now be shown to have improved as a result of the learning experience or is further learning required?'

This process should be documented to demonstrate that learning is being undertaken which meets the needs of the individuals and the organizations in which they work. One way in which this can be done is to use a portfolio, specially designed for documenting CPD. These are available from the RPSGB or the College of Pharmacy Practice.

CPD, like audit, is a cyclical process. For everyone, the need for updating of knowledge and skills is a continuous one. Pharmacists moving from one post to another may need new skills, job descriptions may change over time and new developments in practice need to be implemented, which may also require new skills and knowledge. Learning does not stop after the first degree course is completed, or after pre-registration or after completing a higher degree. Learning continues throughout life. What CPD does is to focus that learning on the needs of individuals and the organizations which employ them.

PRACTICE RESEARCH, PRACTICE DEVELOPMENT AND AUDIT

It is important for pharmacists to have a clear understanding of the relationship between these three facets of pharmaceutical practice. Practice research is designed to establish what is best practice. An example of this would be a randomized, controlled trial of pharmacists undertaking a new service, compared to normal care: e.g. medication

review. In a controlled trial, such as this, patients are often carefully selected, using inclusion and exclusion criteria, special documentation and outcome measures must be used, which would not necessarily form part of routine practice and care must be taken to ensure uniformity of all aspects of the practice.

When this service is implemented into routine practice, further development is likely to be required. This may involve provision of staff training, development of documentation which is easily incorporated into routine practice, mechanisms for patient selection, referral and follow-up care. These aspects which may differ from those used in a research situation, may need to be specific to every individual setting. The whole process in the individual setting then requires to be evaluated. This involves determining for example whether the pharmacists are carrying out effective reviews, whether referral mechanisms work or whether patients are happy with the service. Changes to a service may be necessary if problems are identified in its evaluation. All this constitutes practice development.

Box 43.3	Key elements of a core competency framework for pharmacists working in primary care		
Working as a pharmacist	**The NHS and its partners** Understands primary care in the context of the NHS as a whole	**Clinical/pharmaceutical knowledge** Uses clinical and pharmaceutical knowledge to optimize the balance between effectiveness, safety and cost of medicines	**Professional issues** Works within professional and organizational standards and takes responsibility for continuing professional development
Working with information	**Gathering information** Knows where to get relevant, up-to-date information	**Analysing information** Cuts through irrelevant and poor information. Identifies key points	**Applying information** Applies results of analysis to individual practice
Working with people	**Leadership** Leads individuals and teams, giving a clear focus, motivation and support	**Team working** Understands the importance of, and works to develop and maintain, team and pan-professional relationships	**Communication** Influences individuals and organizations using a variety of techniques
Personal contribution	**How you are** Takes responsibility for self-developments and own actions	**How you work** Has a disciplined approach to setting and achieving objectives, identifies new roles	**How you think** Sees opportunities for change and development

Once a service is running smoothly it should be subject to audit. This will of course involve setting standards for the service and measuring practice against these standards. Research findings can contribute to standard setting in audit. For a medication review service, this may include the type of patients who receive a review, the timescale between reviews, what is included in the reviews. One useful standard could be taken from the National Service Framework for older people, which, based on research findings, states that 'people aged 75 or over should have their medication reviewed annually and if taking four or more medicines, review should be every six months.'

Although there are many similarities in the methods used to obtain data for research and for audit, there are important differences. In research, it is important to have controlled studies, to be able to extrapolate the results and to have large enough samples to demonstrate statistical significance of any differences between groups. None of these applies to audit. Audit compares actual practice to a predetermined level of best practice, not to a control. The results of audit apply to a particular situation and should not be extrapolated. Audit can be applied to a single case; large numbers are not required.

COMPETENCY AND CLINICAL GOVERNANCE

Demonstrating competency to practice is an essential component of clinical governance. A competency is a quality of characteristic of a person which is related to effective or superior performance. Competencies can be described as knowledge, skills, motives and personal traits. The competencies required for pharmacists carrying out medication review are suggested in the document 'Competencies for pharmacists working in primary care' (NHS Executive and National Prescribing Centre 2000). The basic requirements included in the Core Competency Framework for pharmacists working in primary care are shown in Box 43.3. Identifying the competencies required to perform a specific role, such as medication review, enable training needs to be identified. This feeds into the CPD cycle. Competencies could also be adapted to form standards for audit. Documenting CPD, evaluating practice development and

carrying out audit of routine services are some ways which can contribute to demonstrating competency. All are important to demonstrate the quality of care provided to patients.

Key points

- Clinical governance is the term used to describe the responsibility for quality of clinical care.
- Clinical audit and continuous professional development (CPD) contribute to clinical governance.
- Pharmacists are involved in setting standards of practice and need to audit their practice to show that they meet these standards.
- Audit may be of professional activity or clinical service.
- The main aim of audit must be to improve standards of service and outcome for patients.
- The three main types of audit are self, peer and external audit.
- Audit may measure structures, processes or outcomes.
- Standard setting should involve at least all those involved in delivering the service being audited.
- Data collection must answer the audit question and have the potential to give reasons for failure to meet the standard.
- Confidentiality must be respected, but outcomes should be shared with all the audit team.
- Implementing change may feel threatening, but is an essential part of audit.
- Re-audit is a way of testing whether changes have achieved their objective.
- CPD is a systematic, ongoing, cyclical process of self-directed learning.
- The results of audit, feedback from colleagues and critical events can all help to identify CPD needs.
- Documenting CPD is essential to demonstrate a professional approach to practice.
- Practice research answers questions about how best to provide a service, practice development is the process of putting a service in place and audit examines the quality of services.
- Documenting CPD, evaluating practice development and carrying out audit of routine services are some ways which can contribute to demonstrating pharmacists' competency to practice.

PART 5

APPENDICES

Current UK pharmaceutical legislation

C. M. Bond (original author M. M. Moody)

Introduction

When dealing with the supply of medicines, poisons and related substances, pharmacists must comply with a wide range of legal requirements. It is not the purpose of this appendix to reiterate many of these legal requirements, but rather to give some reasoning to the various legal procedures. Additionally, it is hoped that some commonly held misconceptions might be clarified. The legal procedures referred to are found in a variety of comprehensive reference sources, e.g. *Medicines, Ethics and Practice* (RPSGB), *Dale and Appelbe's Pharmacy Law and Ethics* (Appelbe & Wingfield 2001), *Pharmacy Law and Practice* (Merrills & Fisher 2001). All practising pharmacists, pre-registration students and pharmacy undergraduates should consult these volumes extensively. Only the most recent editions should be consulted as pharmaceutical law is constantly being updated to deal with the ever-changing requirements of medicines and medication. In addition, the Law and Ethics Department of the Royal Pharmaceutical Society of Great Britain (RPSGB) should be consulted regarding matters too recent to appear in any of the aforementioned publications. Changes in pharmaceutical law are published in *The Pharmaceutical Journal* and again it is every practising pharmacist's professional responsibility to keep up to date. The Royal Pharmaceutical Society website (http://www.rspgb.org) is also a good resource for the most up-to-date legislation.

CONSUMER PROTECTION ACT

Although this Act does not immediately appear to have a direct link with drug therapy it is of considerable relevance to pharmacists. It deals with products the quality of which are lower than the consumer should expect. Prior to this Act it was the consumer's responsibility to prove that the producer of a particular product was guilty of negligence. The emphasis has now shifted and it is the producer's responsibility to prove that negligence has not occurred. This obviously makes it a more realistic option for the average consumer to bring a genuine complaint against a producer who may be a multinational company with considerable resources and legal expertise at its disposal.

Why should this have a bearing on practising pharmacists? When community pharmacists supply medicines against prescriptions they are identified as the supplier because the medicine will have attached to it a label bearing the name and address of the issuing pharmacy. This in itself does not indicate that the pharmacist is the producer of the medication, but it does put the onus on the pharmacist to be able to identify who the producer is. There are four main areas which have direct relevance to pharmacists.

1. Generic prescribing

Pharmacists should always be able to provide evidence of their source of supply for generic drugs. It is advisable to use only a very limited number of generic suppliers and preferably use manufacturers who produce a product which bears a means of identification, e.g. a company trademark. A pharmacist who is unable to identify the source of a preparation will be held liable for any problems caused by the preparation.

2. Extemporaneous dispensing

When preparing an extemporaneous preparation, full records of the ingredients used, their batch numbers and who supplied them should be kept by the pharmacist. If a fault is identified, e.g. an ingredient used in good faith but supplied incorrectly labelled by the manufacturer, the pharmacist must be able to identify the supplier or manufacturer or he will be held liable for any problems caused by the product.

3. 'Own label' products

A pharmacist who has 'own label' products manufactured by an outside agency must ensure that full records and details of all supplies are available. This ensures that the manufacturer is liable for any product defects, not the pharmacist.

4. The provision of advice

The Consumer Protection Act requires the supplier of goods to ensure that the consumer is provided with comprehensive instructions on the safe use of the goods. This has obvious implications when supplying medicines. Although this requirement may be satisfied by the provision of a patient information leaflet, a patient may not receive one on every occasion. It is therefore essential that products are clearly labelled with instructions regarding safe use and pharmacists should satisfy themselves that appropriate information has been provided.

THE MEDICINES ACT

This is the major piece of legislation which governs the professional activities of pharmacists and, in particular, community pharmacists. The major thrust of this Act is to ensure the protection of the general public in respect of medicines. It ensures the quality, safety and efficacy of medicines and controls the level of access which the general public have to them.

The Act classifies medicinal products into three groups.

1. General sales list (GSL)

The products in this category have been deemed to be relatively safe and can be sold without any pharmaceutical or medical input.

2. Pharmacy medicines (P)

These preparations require some control and, apart from a few exceptions, are only allowed to be sold from a registered retail pharmacy. A pharmacist must supervise the sale. This ensures that the sale of any inappropriate medicine should be avoided. The reality of this situation is less clear cut. In many instances, after questioning the purchaser, pharmacists will refuse a sale. It can often be very difficult to persuade customers that a particular product is not suitable for their needs. In some instances the customer may merely go to another pharmacy where the pharmacist and staff are less vigilant and the purchase is made. The introduction of protocols for the sale of medicines in pharmacies has helped to make the general public more aware that a degree of control is required on the sale of medicines.

3. Prescription-only medicines (POM)

These are medicines which can only be obtained by the general public if they are in possession of a valid prescription. All the preparations in this category have been identified as drugs which are to be used for conditions where appropriate diagnosis and treatment should be carried out by a properly qualified practitioner. Medical practitioners, dentists and vets may all prescribe POM drugs. Recently, suitably qualified and trained nurses have been allowed to write prescriptions for specified POM classified preparations.

Current proposals will soon permit prescription-only medicines to be prescribed by a supplementary prescriber, as part of an agreed clinical management plan for an individual patient. Nurses and pharmacists are specified as the two professional groups who will be accorded supplementary prescribing status after they have completed approved training. This means that once a diagnosis and management have been agreed between a doctor and patient, and with the consent of the patient, continuation of treatment by repeat prescribing of POMs could be delegated to a nurse or pharmacist.

Emergency supply procedures

There are certain other situations when a pharmacist may supply a POM to a member of the public who is not in possession of a prescription. This is known as an emergency supply.

Prior to this being made legal, community pharmacists often found themselves facing major moral dilemmas. A customer would present herself at the pharmacy in desperate need of a POM but with no prescription. No doctor was available to write one and the pharmacist knew that without appropriate medication the customer's state of health would be compromised. However, if the POM were supplied the pharmacist would be in breach of the law. To overcome these very difficult situations the procedures for emergency supply of a POM were devised and became part of the Act. Used in appropriate situations they are a welcome addition to the Act. However, there are still some pharmacists who have difficulty interpreting this piece of legislation and for that reason details of correct procedures are given.

1. The person requiring the POM must be present and be interviewed by the pharmacist.
2. The pharmacist must satisfy himself that a genuine emergency exists, i.e. there is no possibility of obtaining a prescription (for this reason the majority of emergency supplies occur at the weekend, on public holidays or when the patient is on holiday). The emergency supply procedure should not be used just because a patient cannot be bothered to visit the surgery.
3. The pharmacist should consider the consequences of not making the supply. For instance, how seriously will the patient's health suffer if the required medication is not available?
4. The pharmacist must ensure that the medicine being requested has previously been prescribed for the patient. The emergency supply procedure is not a situation where the pharmacist can initiate new drug therapy. The normal requirement is that the drug should have been prescribed within the last 6 months; however, this requirement is waived when the condition being treated occurs intermittently, e.g. hay fever or urinary tract infection. Many emergency supplies are given for medication which the patient is currently taking, e.g. antihypertensive therapy. This has led to a misconception among some pharmacists that only medication being currently taken by the patient is allowed on an emergency supply. This is incorrect. As long as it has previously been prescribed and the pharmacist considers it appropriate, it can be supplied.
5. Unless the medication requested is supplied in a complete container such as a tube of ointment, an aerosol or a course of contraceptive tablets, a maximum of 5 days' supply only may be given. During the interview with the patient the pharmacist must find out when a prescription can be obtained. Some patients may have adequate supplies of medication at home but have forgotten to bring them with them on holiday. Information on when they are going home should be sought. In many cases the maximum 5-day supply will not be required and should not be issued.
6. The supply should be appropriately documented in the prescription book.
7. Drugs which are either Controlled Drugs Schedule 2 or Schedule 3 of the Misuse of Drugs Act may not be supplied as an emergency supply. The only exception to this rule is when phenobarbital or its salts are required for the treatment of epilepsy.

In addition to making an Emergency Supply at the request of the patient, an emergency supply may also be made at the request of the doctor. In this case the following conditions apply:

1. The pharmacist must be satisfied that the request is from a UK doctor and that there is no other way of immediately providing a prescription.
2. The prescription must be made available within 72 hours.
3. The supply must be made, and labelled, as directed by the doctor.
4. An appropriate record must be made in the prescription book.
5. Drugs which are either Controlled Drugs Schedule 2 or Schedule 3 of the Misuse of Drugs Act may not be supplied as an emergency supply. The only exception to this rule is when phenobarbital or its salts are required for the treatment of epilepsy

For further details of Medicine Act legislation and the procedures to be followed to comply with the Act, the current edition of *Medicines, Ethics and Practice* should be consulted.

THE MISUSE OF DRUGS ACT

This Act deals with all the drugs which have been identified as drugs of dependence or have the potential for dependence (see Ch. 42). The primary purpose of the Act is to prevent misuse, by imposing total prohibition on the possession, supply, manufacture, import or export, except as allowed by the regulations. The Misuse of Drugs Act 2001 permits the use of Controlled Drugs in medicine. The drugs are classified into five schedules, each schedule having varying degrees of control.

Schedule 1 drugs include the hallucinogenic drugs, Ecstasy and cannabis, which have little therapeutic use, although recent successful clinical trials of cannabis in the treatment of multiple sclerosis may require this to be reviewed. However at the current time pharmacists would only be involved with these drugs for the purposes of destruction.

Most pharmacists will be involved with prescriptions for drugs which are categorized in Schedules 2 or 3. These require the greatest degree of scrutiny and highest level of vigilance. With one or two exceptions, all prescriptions for Schedule 2 (includes opiates, major stimulants and secobarbital) and Schedule 3 (includes minor stimulants such as benzamfetamine and other drugs less likely to be misused) drugs must be written in the prescriber's own hand (handwriting requirements) and satisfy certain prescription requirements, e.g. the form of the drug must be stated, the quantity prescribed must be stated in words and figures and the dose to be taken indicated. The frequency of dose does not need to be stated but the dose taken at any one time does. Therefore, 'as directed' is not acceptable but 'one as directed' is.

Schedule 4 drugs include most of the benzodiazepines and anabolic and androgenic steroids. The restrictions are more relaxed than for Schedule 3 drugs, and in particular do not include the stringent prescription writing or storage requirements. Schedule 5 drugs include preparations of certain controlled drugs such as codeine, or morphine, at low strengths which render the preparations exempt from the full controls. The main impact on a community pharmacist is that the invoices for the supply of these preparations have to be kept for 2 years.

Private prescriptions for Schedule 2 and Schedule 3 drugs

Private prescriptions for POM drugs can be repeated if this is indicated on the prescription by the prescriber. However, this facility is not allowed if the prescription is for a Schedule 2 or 3 drug. If a prescription is received which has a repeat indication on it the pharmacist may have two courses of action:

1. If the prescription has not previously been dispensed and is in date, i.e. not older than 13 weeks, it may be legally dispensed. The repeat indication however must not be complied with. The pharmacist should explain to the patient that the prescription must be retained and a courtesy call made to the prescriber explaining the situation.
2. If the prescription has previously been dispensed and the patient has returned for a repeat supply, this may not be given. Another prescription must be obtained from the prescriber. In these situations it is more appropriate for the pharmacist to contact the prescriber and explain the situation. The prescription should be retained if the previous dispensing was carried out in that pharmacy. If the dispensing was carried out in different premises, it should theoretically be returned to those premises.

The situation above may arise if a drug is reclassified into a schedule with a greater number of controls. An example of this was the reclassification of Equagesic from POM to POM Schedule 3, and temazepam from POM Schedule 4 to POM Schedule 3. Prescriptions were legal at the time of writing but immediately the reclassification came into force

the appropriate controls were applied and the repeat facility disallowed.

Record keeping for Schedule 2 drugs

It is a legal requirement that both receipts and supplies of Schedule 2 drugs are recorded in a Controlled Drug Register. Full information of the details to be kept can be found in *Medicines, Ethics and Practice*. The law states that, if possible, the records should be entered at the time of receipt or supply but in any case within 24 hours of the transaction. However, pharmacists should make every effort to make entries at the time of the transaction, as it is all too easy, in a busy pharmacy, to forget. The Register will then be incomplete and give the appearance of discrepancies in the stock held.

Destruction of Schedule 2 drugs

Drugs returned to the pharmacy by a patient or the patient's representative

The pharmacist may destroy Schedule 2 drugs which have been dispensed for a patient and are returned because they are no longer required. A controlled drug denaturing kit can be used. No record of the destruction need be made nor does the destruction need to be witnessed. A pharmacist accepts returned drugs from a patient on the legal understanding that they are destroyed. On no account must these preparations be put back into stock.

Destruction of stocks of Schedule 2 drugs held in the pharmacy

Out-of-date stocks or drugs which are no longer required can be destroyed but their destruction must be witnessed and an entry regarding the destruction must be made in the Controlled Drug Register.

Witnesses. The witness can be a police officer. Some pharmacies have regular visits from police officers who are chemist liaison officers. If there is no regular visit then a phone call to the local police station should be made to arrange for an officer to witness the destruction. In addition, a RPSGB inspector or a Home Office inspector can also witness controlled drug destruction.

Records. A record of the destruction should be made in the Controlled Drug Register. Details should be entered in the appropriate 'supplied' section of the Register and should include:

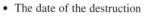

- The date of the destruction
- The name and quantity of the drug destroyed
- The signature of the witness.

Because of stricter waste disposal legislation which does not allow medicines to be disposed of into the water or sewage system, pharmacists may use a denaturing kit, which can then be put with other waste for disposal. If destruction does not need to be witnessed, the drugs can be handed to an authorized waste disposal carrier who is authorized to handle controlled drugs.

Dispensing for drug misusers

With the rise in the number of registered drug misusers in the UK there has been a proportionate increase in the number of prescriptions issued for drug misusers. There are certain procedures which should be adhered to when dispensing prescriptions for controlled drugs for misusers (see also Ch. 42).

Ideally, the misuser should be introduced to the pharmacy by drug clinic staff or the prescriber issuing the prescriptions. Pharmacists have the right to refuse to take on a drug misuser for supervised self-administration. Some pharmacists feel that they can only cope with a certain number of misusers, while others have concerns about the effect the presence of misusers in the pharmacy may have on their other customers. Many pharmacists operate a written contract system with the misusers under their care. The misusers are often required to sign a contract in which they guarantee to abide by certain rules, usually involving their behaviour and demeanour within the pharmacy. If a misuser breaches the terms of the contract the pharmacist reserves the right to withdraw dispensing services.

Only the registered misuser may collect the dispensed items. If, for any reason, this is not possible, the pharmacist must receive a written instruction from the misuser naming the representative who will collect the drugs.

If the prescription has to be dispensed in instalments, the instalment must be collected at the appropriate time or the supply is forfeited.

Dispensing by instalments

Where a drug is to be dispensed in instalments the prescription must satisfy certain criteria. The number of instalments, the intervals between the instalments and the

quantity in each instalment must be stated. These three criteria may be written in a variety of ways but must be present for the prescription to be legal. Some prescribers may indicate a starting date. If present, this must be complied with. If no starting date is indicated then the prescription may be started any time within the legal time limits of the prescription, e.g. 13 weeks for a Schedule 2 or 3 drug. The timing of the instalments must be strictly adhered to. They may not be dispensed ahead of time and if a patient is late in coming to collect a supply it is forfeited.

The prescription must be endorsed with the date of dispensing and the quantity dispensed, each time an instalment is dispensed. If an instalment is not collected the prescription should be dated and the words 'not dispensed' added.

Records for instalment dispensing

When the prescription is for a Schedule 2 drug a record of each instalment must be made in the Controlled Drug Register. This should not be done prior to the instalment being collected. If for some reason the instalment is not uplifted an incorrect entry would then have been made in the Register.

POISONS ACT 1972 AND POISONS RULES

A 'non-medicinal' poison or simply a 'poison' is a substance included in the poisons list made under the Poisons Act. A reference to a poison includes substances containing that poison. Substances which are listed in the Poisons List but which also have medicinal uses are controlled by the Medicines Act 1968 when sold for such purposes.

Classification of poisons

Poisons are either classified as Part 1 or Part 2 poisons.

Part 1 poisons, in general, may only be sold by retail from a registered retail pharmacy under the supervision of a pharmacist.

Part 2 poisons can be sold from either registered retail pharmacies or from a listed seller, i.e. a person whose name appears in a list of sellers maintained by a local authority.

The classification of a substance into Part 1 or Part 2 has nothing to do with the level of toxicity of the poison but is governed by the extent to which the substance is required for use by the general public.

Poisons Rules

The Poisons Rules either cause additional restrictions to be applied to the poison or cause the regulations to be relaxed. The Rules classify certain, but not all, poisons into schedules. The two which pharmacists are most likely to have to deal with are Schedule 1 and Schedule 12.

Schedule 1

Sales of Schedule 1 poisons are strictly controlled. The person purchasing the poison must be personally known to the seller as a person fit to be in possession of the poison. If the seller does not know the purchaser she must provide documentation, endorsed by the police, before the sale can be made. Full details of the documents required are found in *Medicines, Ethics and Practice*.

The seller must make a record of the sale in the Poisons Register. The details required are:

- The date of the sale
- The name and address of the purchaser
- Details of any documentation required
- The name and quantity of the poison
- The purpose for which the poison is to be used
- The signature of the purchaser or, if appropriate, details of a signed order.

Point to note. Unlike entries for controlled drugs, the Poisons Register must be completed before the poison is handed over to the purchaser.

Schedule 12

This schedule indicates the restrictions which apply to the supply of strychnine and other substances which are used to eliminate certain verminous animals. Full details of all the requirements are found in *Medicines, Ethics and Practice*.

Labelling of poisons

All substances classified as poisons are subject to Chemicals (Hazard Information and Packaging) Regulations (CHIP).

CHIP Regulations

These regulations are a major piece of Health and Safety legislation. They ensure that all chemicals which have potentially damaging or dangerous properties are clearly labelled.

The basic labelling requirements are:

- The name of the substance
- The name, address and telephone number of the supplier
- An indication of the general nature of the risk, e.g. toxic, corrosive, teratogenic
- The symbols specified for the above risks, e.g. skull and crossbones
- Risk phrases—these are general statements of the properties of the substance, e.g. 'Causes severe burns'
- Safety phrases—these contain advice on what to do to avoid problems, e.g. 'Wear suitable protective clothing', 'Do not breathe vapour'.

Because of the complex nature of these labelling requirements it is generally recommended that pharmacists should supply substances which are controlled by the CHIP regulations in the original container. The pharmacist must, of course, ensure that the labelling on the container complies with current legislation.

Further information in the form of a safety data sheet should also be supplied to the purchaser. This applies when the chemical is being used for business, but is not a requirement when being used for domestic purposes. As long as the domestic purchaser is supplied with 'sufficient information' for the safe use of the chemical the regulations are satisfied. This does however put additional responsibility on the pharmacist. It is unlikely that the label alone will provide sufficient detailed information. It may therefore be appropriate, although not required by law, to provide all purchasers with a safety data sheet. Pharmacists should ensure that domestic users, in particular, understand the procedures required for the safe use of the substance.

METHYLATED SPIRITS LEGISLATION

The Alcoholic Liquor Duties Act 1979 gives the power to Customs and Excise to make regulations regarding the manufacture, sale, supply and use of methylated spirits.

There are several forms of methylated spirits but the two of main interest to the pharmacist are Mineralized Methylated Spirits (MMS) used for household purposes such as cleaning and lighting and Industrial Methylated Spirits (IMS) which is used for medical purposes. Substances containing IMS such as surgical spirit are also controlled by the legislation.

Industrial Methylated Spirits

Pharmacists who wish to use or supply IMS must first apply to Customs and Excise for authority to receive IMS. On receipt of this authority a statement to that effect must be issued to the wholesaler from whom the pharmacist wishes to purchase the IMS. The statement must be renewed annually. Full details of the content and format of these two documents are found in *Medicines, Ethics and Practice*.

Supply of IMS from a community pharmacy

IMS can be supplied:

- On receipt of a legally written prescription or order from a medical practitioner
- On receipt of a signed order addressed to the pharmacist and signed by a medical practitioner, the quantity not to exceed 3 L.

Note that the definition of 'medical practitioner' in this legislation differs from the definition in the Medicines Act. In the Methylated Spirits Regulations the definition is 'any doctor, dentist, nurse, chiropodist, veterinary surgeon or any other person entitled by law to provide medical or veterinary services in the UK'.

Mineralized Methylated Spirits

England and Wales

Authority to purchase MMS is not required by pharmacists and it can be sold, subject to certain conditions, to the general public. No sales may be made between 10 p.m. on Saturday and 8 a.m. on the following Monday, and this also applies to supplies on prescription and written orders. There are, however, additional procedures to be followed in Scotland, and Northern Ireland.

Scotland

In addition to the above, a record of the sale of either MMS or surgical spirit must be made. Details required to be kept are:

- Date of the sale
- Name and address of the purchaser
- Name of substance and quantity supplied
- Purpose for use
- Signature of purchaser or details of any signed order.

The maximum quantity which can be sold, if not for resale, is 4 gallons (18 L). The purchaser must be over the age of 14 years.

Northern Ireland

Similar time restrictions apply, no records need to be kept but the minimum age of the purchaser must be 18 years.

For further information on the legislation governing methylated spirits consult *Medicines, Ethics and Practice*.

DATA PROTECTION ACT 1998

This Act is of relevance to pharmacists because it deals with the storage of information on computers. Any pharmacist who uses a computer for the maintenance of patient medication records must ensure that they are registered with the Data Protection Registrar. It is an offence to keep such records otherwise. Patient consent is also required.

To comply with the Data Protection Act pharmacists should ensure that only essential information is held on computer, the information is kept up to date, security systems are in place to prevent unauthorized access and the pharmacy has a procedure for dealing with a request for computer-held data.

Unauthorized access

- All systems should be protected by a password.
- Computer screens should not be on view to the general public.
- Computers should not be left running in an unattended dispensary.
- Staff should be informed of the necessity for total confidentiality.

Requests for information

Pharmacists may receive requests from members of the general public for details of information held about them on computer. Except in instances where the physical or mental health of the person could suffer, the information must be supplied. The pharmacist must supply the information, in an understandable form, within 40 days of the request. Any pharmacist receiving such a request should not, however, immediately access the information. Details of who is requesting the information and the date on which the request was made should be taken. The pharmacist should then check on what information is held, consult with the patient's doctor if necessary, and then if it is deemed appropriate, send a copy of the information to the patient.

HUMAN RIGHTS ACT 1998

The aim in introducing the Human Rights Act was to allow cases concerning the rights of individuals under the European Convention to be brought in the UK courts. It was intended that it would 'create a society in which the rights and responsibilities of individuals are properly balanced and in which an awareness of the Convention rights permeates our governmental and legal systems at all levels'. It is increasingly recognized that the Act will have an impact on the NHS with respect to patient's rights to information, to confidentiality and to life.

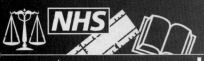

National Health Service dispensing

C. M. Bond (original author M. M. Moody)

Introduction

The provision of medicines ordered on National Health Service (NHS) prescriptions is the major activity in most community pharmacies in the UK. The NHS is administered separately in England and Wales from Scotland and Northern Ireland. This means that there are variations both in the requirements of the contract which community pharmacies have with the government and in the levels of remuneration.

In England and Wales each pharmacy should have a contract with their local health authority. The terms of the contract are negotiated annually with the Department of Health. The negotiating body, on behalf of the chemist contractors in England and Wales, is the Pharmaceutical Services Negotiating Committee (PSNC). In Scotland the contract is with the local primary care trust, is negotiated with the Scottish Executive Health Department, and the negotiating body is the Scottish Pharmaceutical General Council (SPGC). In Northern Ireland the Department of Health and Social Services is responsible for providing an integrated health service. There are four health and social services boards who are in contract with the contractors in their particular area.

Because the contracts are negotiated separately and there are differences in some of the terms and conditions, it is important that pharmacists working in community pharmacy who move from one country in the UK to another are aware of the different requirements and procedures. The terms and conditions of the contract are printed in the current edition of the *Drug Tariff*, which is published monthly in England and Wales and quarterly in Scotland. The Northern Ireland *Drug Tariff* is presented in a loose-leaf format and is updated quarterly.

THE *DRUG TARIFF*

This publication contains details of all the requirements which have to be met when providing an NHS dispensing service. It includes information on allowances paid to contractors, medicines, dressings, hosiery and appliances permitted to be prescribed on an NHS prescription form, prescription endorsement requirements, amounts payable, exempt categories of patients and details of charges made for prescriptions. It also identifies core services for which fees are negotiated locally, such as methadone dispensing fees, oxygen delivery and disposal of pharmaceutical waste.

OTHER PROFESSIONAL SERVICES

Over and above the provision of dispensing services the terms of service require pharmacists to provide a range of professional services. These are the subject of negotiation with government and requirements change from one period of negotiation to another, and from home country to home country. Examples which have occurred in the last few years are:

- Ensuring the availability in the pharmacy of appropriate health education leaflets
- The provision of a practice leaflet indicating the services provided by the pharmacy
- The provision, where appropriate, of counselling and advice on prescription medicines and appliances (currently Scotland only)
- Participation in clinical audit (currently Scotland only)
- Maintaining patient medication records.

Pharmacists should consult a current edition of the *Drug Tariff* for information on the conditions which apply and the allowances payable.

PRESCRIPTION FORMS

NHS prescription forms can be issued by GPs and dispensing doctors, hospital doctors, nurses, dentists and sampling officers of the Drug Testing scheme. For each of these prescribers there is a specific colour-coded form which is identifiable by a unique code number. These colours and identifying codes differ between the home countries; e.g. the English forms are prefixed by 'FP', the Scottish forms by GP (or HB for their hospitals or clinics) and the Northern Ireland forms by HS. Thus the English form used by GPs is white and is an FP10 whereas the Scottish equivalent, also white, is a GP10 (see Ch. 15). In addition all the prescribers are identifiable by a unique cipher number. With a few highly specialized exceptions, despite the differences in form, they are all valid across the UK. Thus, a form written in England by an English GP could be dispensed in London, Belfast, Cardiff or Edinburgh.

PAYMENT FOR PRESCRIPTIONS

On presentation of a valid NHS prescription at a pharmacy, pharmacists, under the terms of their contract, are required to dispense the prescription without undue delay. The prescription is then submitted to the relevant pricing bureau (the Prescription Pricing Authority (PPA) in England, the Prescription Pricing Division (PPD) in Wales or the Practitioner Services (Pharmacy) Division (PPD) in Scotland). The contractor is then reimbursed for the cost of the drugs or appliances and paid the appropriate dispensing fee. Details of appropriate costs and fees are published in the *Drug Tariff*. There are differences of detail between the home countries, but the principles of payment are broadly similar. There is a basic item fee which may be enhanced by additional payments to recognize extra workload, such as extemporaneous dispensing, or responsibility, such as the dispensing of a controlled drug. The need for the introduction of a new contract for the profession is now widely recognized. It is anticipated that this will give more financial recognition to non-dispensing pharmaceutical services, and it is likely that the differences across the UK, between the home countries, will be further increased.

Currently, submission of prescriptions for payment is a paper-based, time-consuming exercise. Trials are presently being carried out on the electronic transfer of prescription information. This will provide a quicker and less labour-intensive method of submitting prescriptions for pricing. Pharmacy plans for both England and Wales, and Scotland, indicate that this may be fully implemented across the UK by 2005.

Prescription endorsement

To ensure accurate pricing of the prescriptions they must be endorsed before submission. If omissions or errors occur in the endorsing process, the prescription is returned to the pharmacy for clarification, thereby causing a delay in the pharmacist's remuneration. Endorsement requirements are clearly stated in the *Drug Tariff* which should be consulted. The National Pharmaceutical Association (NPA) publishes a guide to the *Drug Tariff* and NHS dispensing which also provides much useful information.

In general, the prescription should state, clearly and unambiguously, a description of the drugs dispensed, the strength and the quantity. If these are present the need for further endorsement is unlikely. Some common reasons why prescriptions are referred back to the submitting pharmacy are:

- Failure to endorse 'illegible' prescriptions
- Failure to endorse the prescription with details of the manufacturer or supplier, when required to do so
- Failure to endorse the prescription with pack size details, when required to do so
- Failure to endorse prescriptions which have vital details omitted by the prescriber, e.g. strength, when there is more than one
- Dispensing a prescription which has not been signed or dated by the prescriber.

Disallowed payments

In addition, certain prescriptions will be disallowed for payment. There is a variety of reasons for this and the following list gives some examples.

- The item dispensed is blacklisted, i.e. an item which is not available on the NHS.
- The prescription is either written by a dentist or a nurse on the appropriate form and the item is not allowed to be prescribed by these practitioners.
- The prescribed item is a chemical reagent or appliance which is not allowed to be prescribed on an NHS form.

Neither of these lists is comprehensive and further information can be obtained from the PPA or PPD.

PRESCRIPTION CHARGES

The government currently levies a flat rate prescription charge on each prescription item. Community pharmacists must collect this as part of their contractual agreement. There are several categories of people who are exempt from charges and a declaration to that effect and an indication of why they are claiming exemption must be completed on the reverse of the prescription form. A full list of exemption categories can be found in the *Drug Tariff* and there are some minor differences between the home countries. In England, exemptions include groups such as: men and women over 60 years old; children under 16 years; women who are pregnant or within one year of the birth of their child; people suffering from specified medical conditions (e.g. diabetes, hypothyroidism, epilepsy needing continuous anticonvulsant therapy); or on grounds of income (as evidenced, for example by receipt of income support or the working Family Tax Credit). Some categories are automatically exempt while others must apply for exemption. As part of their contract, pharmacists are required to check claims for exemption against documentary proof which patients and/or their representatives are required to provide if asked. Figures vary from area to area, but approximately 70% of prescription items dispensed are for people who are exempt from prescription charges.

Pharmacists must ensure that the declaration on the reverse of the prescription form is accurately completed. Failure to do this could lead to contractors having prescription charges incorrectly deducted from their remuneration.

Charges payable

Whilst, as stated above, there is a flat rate per item, the definition of an item is not as simple as it might seem. This is an area where confusion can occur for both patients and pharmacists. It can cause financial loss to the contractor and also irritation to the patient. A complete list of criteria on how many prescription charges should be made is found in the *Drug Tariff*. The following is a list of commonly occurring situations, with examples.

Unless the patient is exempt, one charge is payable if:

- Different strengths of the same drug, in the same formulation, are prescribed at the same time, e.g. warfarin tablets 1 mg and 5 mg.
- One appliance of the same type (other than hosiery) is supplied at the same time, e.g. six open-wove bandages 2.5 cm and six open-wove bandages 5 cm. Although the bandages are two different sizes and more than one of each is supplied, only one charge should be made for this prescription.
- A drug is supplied with a throat brush, dropper or vaginal applicator, e.g. Ortho Dienestrol cream with applicator.
- Different flavours of the same preparation are prescribed at the same time, e.g. 60 Fybogel sachets (plain) and 60 Fybogel sachets (orange).

Conversely, unless the patient is exempt, multiple prescription charges are made if:

- Different drugs, types of dressings or appliances are supplied.
- Different formulations or presentations of the same preparation are supplied.
- Additional parts are supplied together with a complete set of apparatus or additional dressings together with a dressing pack.
- More than one piece of elastic hosiery is supplied.

The area where probably the greatest number of errors occurs is with combination packs. Patients think they are only receiving one item but in fact the pack may contain two or more. Examples of these are Canesten Combi which includes a pessary and a tube of cream. Two charges must therefore be made. A pack of Menophase tablets consists of six different types of tablet. Strictly speaking, this is six items, two of which incur charges, and four of which have been exempted by the government .

More examples of single and multiple charges are found in the *Drug Tariff*. In cases of uncertainty the PPA or the PPD is an extremely helpful and useful source of advice.

THE BLACK LIST

In 1985 the Government issued a list of preparations which would no longer be prescribable on NHS prescriptions.

Various criteria were used in selecting which items would be 'blacklisted'. These included products which were deemed to be of limited therapeutic value, e.g. certain cough preparations, products which were too expensive and products for which there was considerable duplication. The Black List may, therefore, contain a particular brand of a drug but the generic equivalent is allowable, e.g. generic diazepam may be prescribed on an NHS prescription but may not be written as the branded form, Valium, which is disallowed. A patient who wishes the proprietary brand must obtain a private prescription. The Black List is continuously updated with products being added or removed from the list. Practising pharmacists should ensure that they keep up to date with any alterations.

When presented with a prescription for a blacklisted item the pharmacist always has one option, and the possibility of another three, if appropriate:

- The patient can always be referred back to the prescriber to obtain a private prescription for the blacklisted item.
- If the preparation is available in an allowable generic form, an NHS prescription for the generic could be requested, if this is acceptable to the patient and the prescriber.
- If the item can be legally purchased without a prescription, i.e. is not a prescription-only medicine (POM), then this option can be offered to the patient.

- In exceptional circumstances, e.g. where it is impossible to contact the prescriber, it may be possible to use the emergency supply procedures, if requested by the patient.

PRIVATE PRESCRIPTIONS

NHS prescription forms may not be used or treated as private prescriptions. The form is considered to be the property of the Secretary of State for Health and, as such, may only be used for the provision of drugs and appliances on the NHS. The two situations when problems might arise are:

- A blacklisted item, which is a POM, is written on an NHS prescription. If the patient wants this particular item he must return to the prescriber and obtain a private prescription. The pharmacist must not treat the NHS form as a private prescription, i.e. charge the patient for the item and retain the prescription in the pharmacy.
- The cost of the item prescribed is less than the prescription charge. It is against the NHS terms of service to dispense NHS prescriptions as private prescriptions in order to save patients' money.

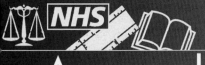

Medical abbreviations

M. R. Thomas

INTRODUCTION

Abbreviations are widely used throughout all areas of life. While some abbreviations are so well known as to be accepted as part of everyday conversation, other abbreviations are very specific to a particular profession or even a speciality within a profession. This can easily lead to confusion, as the meaning of the abbreviation may not be immediately clear to the reader or listener. Indeed some abbreviations have a number of different interpretations and it is important to take them within context. For instance, 'aka' is widely understood to mean 'also known as', but can also stand for above knee amputation. While NPA might immediately suggest the National Pharmaceutical Association to the majority of the readers of this book, found in a set of medical records it is more likely to refer to nasopharyngeal aspirate. Perhaps more confusingly BM can be used for bone marrow, bowel movement or blood sugar level (in reference to the type of reagent strip used to measure the blood sugar). It would be easy to recommend that abbreviations were never used but with the sheer volume of information that requires recording and the often linguistically challenging terminology, their use is inevitable. Listed below are some of the more widely used terms adopted by the medical profession in the UK, including a separate section on the abbreviations commonly used to document physical examination findings. There will be many others you will come across, specific to a particular speciality or area of the country. It is best as with all things in life, never to assume.

COMMON MEDICAL ABBREVIATIONS

Abbreviation	Term
AAA	abdominal aortic aneurysm
Ab	antibody, abortion

Abbreviation	Term
Abd	Abdomen
ABG	arterial blood gas
ABO	blood group classification
ABX	antibiotic
ACTH	adrenocorticotrophic hormone
AD(H)D	attention deficit (hyperactivity) disorder
ADH	antidiuretic hormone
ADL	activities of daily living
ADR	adverse drug reaction
A&E	accident and emergency
AF	anterior fontanelle, atrial fibrillation
AFB	acid fast bacilli
AFL	atrial flutter
AFP	alpha fetoprotein
A/G	albumin/globulin ratio
Ag	antigen
AIDS	acquired immunodeficiency syndrome
aka	also known as
AKA	above knee amputation
ALL	acute lymphocytic leukaemia
ALT	alanine aminotransferase
ALTEs	acute life threatening episodes
AMA	against medical advice
AML	acute myeloid leukaemia
amnio	amniocentesis
ANA	antinuclear antibody
ANF	antinuclear factor
AOB	alcohol on breath
AP	anteroposterior
A&P	anterior and posterior
APLS	advanced paediatric life support
appt	appointment
AR	aortic regurgitation
A–R	apical–radial pulse
ARDS	adult respiratory distress syndrome
ARF	acute renal failure
AS	aortic stenosis

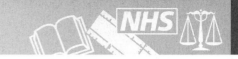

Abbreviation	Term	Abbreviation	Term
ASCVD	arteriosclerotic cardiovascular disease	C(A)T	computed (axial) tomography
ASD	atrial septal defect	cath	catheter
ASHD	atherosclerotic heart disease	CBC	complete blood count
ASO(T)	antistreptolysin O (titre)	CBG	capillary blood gas
AV	arteriovenous, atrioventricular	CC	chief complaint
A&W	alive and well	CCF	congestive cardiac failure
AXR	abdominal X-ray	CCU	coronary care unit, clean catch urine
Ba	barium	CDs	controlled drugs
Bact	bacteriology	CDH	congenital diaphragmatic hernia, congenital dislocation of the hips
BaE	barium enema		
BBA	born before arrival	CF	cystic fibrosis
BBB	bundle branch block, blood–brain barrier	CHD	congenital heart disease
BCC	basal cell carcinoma	CHF	congestive heart failure
BCG	bacillus Calmette–Guérin vaccine (against tubercullosis)	chroms	chromosomes
		CIBD	chronic inflammatory bowel disease
BEAM	brain electrical activity mapping	CK	creatinine kinase
beta HCG	human chorionic gonadotrophin	Cl	chloride
BID	brought in dead	CLL	chronic lymphocytic leukaemia
bil	bilateral	CMV	cytomegalovirus
bili	bilirubin	CN	cranial nerves
BKA	below knee amputation	CNS	central nervous system
BLS	basic life support	CO	carbon monoxide, cardiac output
BM	bowel movement, bone marrow, blood sugar	c/o	complains of
		COAD	chronic obstructive airway disease
BMR	basal metabolic rate	co-arct	coarctation of the aorta
BNO	bowels not open	COLD	chronic obstructive lung disease
BOM	bilateral otitis media	COPD	chronic obstructive pulmonary disease
BOR	bowels open regularly	CP	chest pain, cerebral palsy
BP	blood pressure	CPAP	continuous positive airways pressure
BPD	bipolar disorder, borderline personality disorder, bronchopulmonary dysplasia	CPK	creatinine phosphokinase
		CPR	cardiopulmonary resuscitation
BPH	benign prostatic hypertrophy	CRF	chronic renal failure
BPLS	basic paediatric life support	CRP	C-reactive protein
bpm	beats per minute	C&S	culture and sensitivity
BS	bowel sounds, breath sounds, blood sugar	CSF	cerebrospinal fluid
BSA	body surface area	C section	caesarean section
BSER	brain stem evoked response	CTS	carpal tunnel syndrome
BTL	bilateral tubal ligation	CVA	cerebrovascular accident
BUN	blood urea nitrogen	CVP	central venous pressure
BW	birth weight	CVS	cardiovascular system, chorionic villus sampling
Bx	biopsy		
c	cum (with)	Cx	cervix, cervical
C1	first cervical vertebra, etc.	CXR	chest X-ray
Ca	calcium	D(x)	diagnosis
CA,Ca,ca	cancer, carcinoma	D&C	dilatation and curettage
CAB(G)	coronary artery bypass (graft)	DH	drug history
CAD	coronary artery disease	DIC	disseminated intravascular coagulation
CAPD	continuous ambulatory peritoneal dialysis	diff	differential blood count

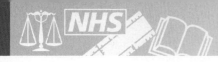

Abbreviation	Term
DIP	distal interphalangeal joint
DM	diabetes mellitus
DNA	did not attend (outpatient)
DNR	do not resuscitate
DOA	dead on arrival
DOB	date of birth
DOE	dyspnoea on exertion
DPL	diagnostic peritoneal lavage
DPT	diphtheria, pertussis, tetanus vaccine
DSA	digital subtraction angiography
DTR	deep tendon reflexes
DTs	delirium tremens
DU	duodenal ulcer
D&V	diarrhoea and vomiting
DVT	deep vein thrombosis
D/W	discussed with
DXT	deep X-ray treatment
ECF	extracellular fluid
ECG	electrocardiogram
ECMO	extracorporeal membrane oxygenation
ECT	electroconvulsive therapy
EDD	expected date of delivery (baby)
EEG	electroencephalogram
ELBW	extremely low birth weight
EMG	electromyogram
EMU	early morning urine
ENT	ear, nose and throat
EOM	extraocular muscles
Ep	epilepsy
ERCP	endoscopic retrograde cholangiopancreatography
ERG	electroretinogram
ESM	ejection systolic murmur
ESR	erythrocyte sedimentation rate
ET	endotracheal
ETA	expected time of arrival
EUA	examination under anaesthetic
exc	excision
FB	finger breadths, foreign body
FBC	full blood count
FBS	fasting blood sugar
FDPs	fibrin degradation products
FEV_1	forced expiratory volume (in 1 second)
FFA	free fatty acids
FFP	fresh frozen plasma
FH	family history
FISH	fluorescent in situ hybridization
FOB	faecal occult blood, foot of the bed

Abbreviation	Term
FraX	fragile X syndrome
FROM	full range of movement
FSH	follicle stimulating hormone
FTNVD	full term normal vaginal delivery
FTT	failure to thrive
FU	follow-up
FUO	fever of unknown origin
FVC	forced vital capacity
Fx	fracture
GA	general anaesthetic
GCS	Glasgow Coma Scale
GFR	glomerular filtration rate
GI(T)	gastrointestinal (tract)
GN	glomerulonephritis
G6PD	glucose-6-phosphate dehydrogenase
G&S	group and save
GSW	gun shot wound
GTN	glyceryl trinitrate
GTT	glucose tolerance test
GU	genitourinary, gastric ulcer
GYN, gyn	gynaecology
Hb, Hgb	haemoglobin
HC	head circumference
Hct	haematocrit
HCVD	hypertensive cardiovascular disease
HDL	high density lipoprotein
HDN	haemolytic disease of the newborn
HDU	high dependency unit
Hep	hepatitis
HFO	high frequency oscillation
HH	hiatus hernia
HI	haemaglutination inhibition, head injury
HIE	hypoxic ischaemic encephalopathy
HIV	human immunodeficiency virus
HL	Hodgkin's lymphoma
HLA	human leukocyte antigen
HMD	hyaline membrane disease
HO	house officer
HOCM	hypertrophic obstructive cardiomyopathy
H&P	history and physical
HPI	history of presenting illness
HR	heart rate
HRT	hormone replacement therapy
HSM	hepatosplenomegaly
HSP	Henoch–Schönlein purpura
HT	hypertension
ht	height
HUS	haemolytic uraemic syndrome

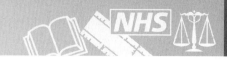

Abbreviation	Term	Abbreviation	Term
HVS	high vaginal swab	KO'd	knocked out
Hx	history	KUB	kidneys, ureters, bladder
IA	intra-arterial	L1	first lumbar vertebra, etc.
IABP	intra-aortic balloon pump	LA	local anaesthetic, left atrium
IBS	irritable bowel syndrome	Lab	laboratory
ICF	intracellular fluid	labs	results of tests
ICM	intracostal margin	lac	laceration
ICP	intracranial pressure	LAD	left anterior descending (coronary artery), left axis deviation
ICS	intercostal space		
ICU	intensive care unit	lat	lateral
ID	intradermal, initial dose	LBBB	left bundle branch block
I&D	incision and drainage	LBW	low birth weight
IDD	insulin dependent diabetic	LD	lethal dose
IDM	infant of a diabetic mother	LDH	lactate dehydrogenase
Ig	immunoglobulin	LDL	low density lipoprotein
IG	immune globulin	LE	lupus erythematosus
IHD	ischaemic heart disease	LFTs	liver function tests
IHSS	idiopathic hypertrophic subaortic stenosis	LH	luteinizing hormone
IM	intramuscular	LIH	left inguinal hernia
imp	impression	LMN	lower motor neurone
IMV	intermittent mandatory ventilation	LMP	last menstrual period
inf	inferior	LN	lymph node
inj	injury, injection	LOC	loss of consciousness
INR	International Normalized Ratio (prothrombin time)	LP	light perception, lumbar puncture
		LSCS	lower segment caesarean section
I&O	intake and output	LSE	left sternal edge
IO	intraosseous	Lt	left
IOP	intraoccular pressure	LUQ	left upper quadrant
IP	intraperitoneal, inpatient	LV	left ventricle
IPPV	intermittent positive pressure ventilation	LVF	left ventricular failure
IRDS	idiopathic respiratory distress syndrome	LVH	left ventricular hypertrophy
ISQ	no change (in status quo)	LVOT	left ventricular outflow tract
ITP	idiopathic thrombocytopenic purpura	LWBS	left without being seen
ITU	intensive therapy unit	MAOI's	monoamine oxidase inhibitors
IUD	intrauterine device, intrauterine death	MAP	mean arterial pressure
IUGR	intrauterine growth retardation	MCH	mean corpuscular haemoglobin
IV	intravenous	MCHC	mean corpuscular haemoglobin concentration
IVH	intraventricular haemorrhage		
IVI	intravenous infusion	MCT	medium chain triglyceride
IVP	intravenous pyelogram	MCU	micturating cystourethrogram
IVU	intravenous urography	MCV	mean corpuscular volume
Ix	investigations	MD	muscular dystrophy
J	jaundice	mets	metastasis
JRA	juvenile rheumatoid arthritis	Mg	magnesium
jt	joint	MI	mitral incompetence or insufficiency, myocardial infarction
JVP	jugular venous pulse		
K	potassium	MMR	mumps, measles, rubella vaccine
KO	keep open	MR	mitral regurgitation

Abbreviation	Term
MRI	magnetic resonance imaging
MRSA	methicillin resistant *Staphylococcus aureus*
MS	mitral stenosis, morphine sulphate, multiple sclerosis
MSU	midstream urine
MVA	motor vehicle accident
N	normal
Na	sodium
NAD	nothing abnormal detected, no active disease, no acute distress
NAI	non-accidental injury
NBI	no bony injury
NBM	nil by mouth
NCPAP	nasal continuous positive airways pressure
Neb	nebulizer
NEC	narcotizing enterocolitis
Neuro	neurology
NF	neurofibromatosis
NFR	not for resuscitation
NG	new growth
NG(T)	nasogastric (tube)
NHL	non-Hodgkin's lymphoma
NICU	neonatal intensive care unit
NIDDM	non-insulin dependent diabetes mellitus
NKA	no known allergies
NMR	nuclear magnetic resonance
NPA	nasopharyngeal aspirate
NPN	non-protein nitrogen
NPO	nothing orally
NSR	normal sinus rhythm, no sign of recurrence
NTD	neural tube defect
N&V	nausea and vomiting
NWB	non weight bearing
O	oedema
O/A	on admission
OA	osteoarthritis
Obs-Gyn	obstetrics and gynaecology
OD	overdose, right eye
OGD	oesophagogastroduodenoscopy
OOB	out of bed
op	operation
OP	outpatient
OPA	outpatient appointment
OPD	outpatient department
open + shut	inoperable case

Abbreviation	Term
OPV	oral polio vaccine
OR	operating room
ortho	orthopaedics
OS	left eye
O_2 sat	oxygen concentration
OT	occupational therapy
OTC	over the counter (medicine)
OU	both eyes
P	pulse
PA	posteroanterior, pulmonary artery
$Paco_2$	partial pressure of carbon dioxide in arterial blood
Paeds	paediatrics
Pao_2	partial pressure of oxygen in arterial blood
Pap	Papanicolaou smear
path	pathology
PBI	protein bound iodine
PC	presenting complaint
PCA	patient controlled analgesia
Pco_2	partial pressure of carbon dioxide
PCR	polymerase chain reaction
PCV	packed cell volume
PD	peritoneal dialysis
PDA	persistent ductus arteriosus
PE	physical examination, pulmonary embolus
PEEP	positive end expiratory pressure
PEFR	peak expiratory flow rate
PERRLA	pupils equal, round, react to light and accommodation
PET	positron emission tomography
PF(R)	peak flow (rate)
PFO	persistent foramen ovale
PFT	pulmonary function tests
PG	prostaglandin
PH	past history
PHT	pulmonary hypertension
PID	pelvic inflammatory disease, prolapsed intervertebral disc
PIP	proximal interphalangeal joint
PKU	phenylketonuria
Plt	platelets
PM	post mortem
PMA	post menstrual age
PMD	post micturition dribbling
PMH	past medical history
PMS	premenstrual syndrome
PND	paroxysmal nocturnal dyspnoea

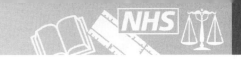

Abbreviation	Term	Abbreviation	Term
PO	per oral	RN	registered nurse
PO$_2$	partial pressure of oxygen	R/O	rule out
POD	post operative day	ROM	range of movement, ruptured membranes
post op	after operation	ROP	retinopathy of prematurity
PP	private patient	ROS	review of systems
PPD	purified protein derivative (of tuberculin)	RR	respiratory rate
PPHN	persistent pulmonary hypertension of the newborn	RS	respiratory system
		RSV	respiratory syncytial virus
PR	per rectum, pulmonary regurgitation	rt	right
pre op	before operation	RT	radiotherapy
prep	prepare for surgery	RTA	road traffic accident
prn	as required	RUQ	right upper quadrant
PROM	premature rupture of membranes	RV	residual volume, right ventricle
PS	pulmonary stenosis	RVH	right ventricular hypertrophy
PSM	pansystolic murmur	RVT	renal vein thrombosis
Psych	psychiatry	Rx	prescription
Pt	patient	s	without
PT	physiotherapy, prothrombin time	SA	sino-atrial
PTA	prior to admission	Sab	spontaneous abortion
PTC	percutaneous transhepatic cholangiogram	SAH	subarachnoid haemorrhage
PTCA	percutaneous transluminal coronary angioplasty	SB	stillbirth, short of breath
		S/B	seen by
PTH	parathyroid hormone	SBE	subacute bacterial endocarditis
PTT	partial thromboplastin time	SBFT	small bowel follow through
PUO	pyrexia (fever) of unknown origin	SBO	small bowel obstruction
PV	per vagina	SBS	short bowel syndrome
PVC	premature ventricular contraction	SC	subcutaneous
PVD	peripheral vascular disease	SCC	sickle cell crisis, squamous cell carcinoma
PVL	periventricular leukomalacia	SCBU	special care baby unit
PVR	pulmonary vascular resistance	SCID	severe combined immunodeficiency
RA	rheumatoid arthritis, right atrium	SGA	small for gestational age
RAIU	radioactive iodine uptake	SH	social history, serum hepatitis
RBBB	right bundle branch block	SHO	senior house officer
RBC	red blood cell, red blood count	SIADH	syndrome of inappropriate antidiuretic hormone
RBS	random blood sugar		
RCA	right coronary artery	SIDS	sudden infant death syndrome
RCC	red cell count	SL	sublingual
RDS	respiratory distress syndrome	SLE	systemic lupus erythematosus
rehab	rehabilitation	SOA	swelling of the ankles
REM	rapid eye movement	SOB(OE)	short of breath (on exertion)
RF	renal failure, rheumatic fever, rheumatoid factor	SOL	space occupying lesion
		SOS	swelling of the sacrum
RHD	rheumatic heart disease	spec	specimen
Rh	rhesus blood factor	SPECT	single photon emission computed tomography
Rh neg. (Rh–)	Rhesus factor negative		
Rh pos. (Rh+)	Rhesus factor positive	SR	sinus rhythm
RLF	retrolental fibroplasia	S&S	signs and symptoms
RLQ	right lower quadrant	SSS	sick sinus syndrome

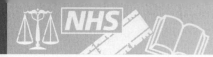

Abbreviation	Term
stat	immediately
STD	sexually transmitted disease
STOP	suction termination of pregnancy
SVC	superior vena cava
SVD	spontaneous vaginal delivery
SVT	supraventricular tachycardia
SW	social worker
Sx	symptoms
SXR	skull X- ray
T	temperature
T1	first thoracic vertebra, etc.
T_3	tri-idothyronine
T_4	levothyroxine (thyroxine)
T&A	tonsillectomy and adenoidectomy
Tabs	tablets
TAPVD	total anomalous pulmonary venous drainage
TB	tuberculosis
TBA	to be arranged, to be administered
TBI	total body involvement
T&C	type and crossmatch
TCI	to come in
TED stocking	thromboembolic deterrent stocking
temp	temperature
TFT's	thyroid function tests
TGA	transposition of great arteries
THR	total hip replacement
TIA	transient ischaemic attack
tib and fib	tibula and fibula
TIBC	total iron binding capacity
TKVO	to keep vein open
TL	tubal ligation
TLC	tender loving care, total lung capacity
TLE	temporal lobe epilepsy
TMJ	temperomandibular joint
TOF	tetralogy of Fallot, tracheo-oesophogeal fistula
TOP	termination of pregnancy
TORCH screen	toxoplasma, rubella, cytomegalovirus, herpes simplex infection
TPN	total parenteral nutrition
TPR	temperature, pulse, respirations
TR	tricuspid regurgitation
Trachy	tracheostomy
TS	tricuspid stenosis
TSH	thyroid stimulating hormone
TTAs	to take away (discharge medicines)
TTN	transient tachypnoea of the newborn

Abbreviation	Term
TTOs	to take out (discharge medicines)
TURP	transurethral resection of prostate
TVH	total vaginal hysterectomy
Tx	treatment
UA	uric acid, urinalysis
UC	ulcerative colitis
U&Es	urea and electrolytes
UMN	upper motor neurone
UR(T)I	upper respiratory (tract) infection
U/S	ultrasound
UTA	unable to attend (outpatient appointment)
UTI	urinary tract infection
VA	visual acuity
VD	venereal disease
VDRL	venereal disease research laboratory
VE	vaginal examination
vent	ventilator
VEP	visual evoked potential
VF(ib)	ventricular fibrillation
VF	visual fields
VLBW	very low birth weight
VMA	vanilmandelic acid
VMI	very much improved
VP	venous pressure, ventriculoperitoneal
VPB	ventricular premature beats
VQ scan	ventilation perfusion scan
VS	vital signs
VSD	ventricular septal defect
VT	ventricular tachycardia
VZIG	varicella zoster immune globulin
WBC	white blood count
WBS	whole body scan
WC	wheelchair
WNL	within normal limits
WPW	Wolff Parkinson White
WR	ward round, Wasserman reaction
wt	weight
X-match	crossmatch
XR	X-ray
y.o.	year old
ZIG	zoster immune globulin

Common abbreviations used to document physical examination findings

AAL	anterior axillary line
AB	apex beat
HO	hernial orifices

Abbreviation	Term	Abbreviation	Term
HS	heart sounds	∵	because
ICS	intercostal space	↑BP	high blood pressure
MAL	midaxillary line	Δ	diagnosis
MCL	midclavicular line	†	died
N/P	not palpable	ΔΔ	differential diagnosis
^{0}	absent	#	fracture
^{0}JAClCyL	no jaundice, anaemia, clubbing, cyanosis or lymphadenopathy	−ve	negative
		+ve	positive
^{0}LKKS	no liver, kidney, kidney, spleen palpable	↔	no change
O/E	on examination	1^0	primary
PAL	posterior axillary line	2^0	secondary
S_1	first heart sound	Σ	sigmoidoscopy
S_2	second heart sound	∴	therefore
TGR	tenderness, guarding and rebound	1/7	one day
VF	vocal fremitus	2/52	2 weeks
VR	vocal resonance	3/12	3 months

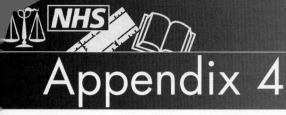

Appendix 4

Latin terms and abbreviations

D. M. Collett

Introduction

Prescriptions written in the UK should be written in English and the use of Latin is strongly discouraged. However, the use of some Latin terms persists and abbreviations are often used, especially to indicate the frequency of dosing. Abbreviations may have different meanings in different countries. Great care is required to avoid errors arising through misunderstanding.

The following lists include terms which may be encountered in current practice. For more comprehensive lists see previous editions of this book (Carter 1975) and the *Pharmaceutical Handbook* (Wade 1980).

DOSAGE FORMS

Latin name	Abbreviation	English name
Auristillae	aurist.	ear drops
Capsula	caps.	capsule
Cataplasma	cataplasm.	poultice
Collunarium	collun.	nosewash
Collutorium	collut.	mouthwash
Collyrium	collyr.	eye lotion
Cremor	crem.	cream
Guttae	gtt.	drops
Haustus	ht.	draught
Liquor	liq.	solution
Lotio	lot.	lotion
Mistura	mist.	mixture
Naristillae	narist.	nose drops
Nebula	neb.	spray solution
Oculentum	oculent.	eye oinment
Pasta	past.	paste
Pigmentum	pig.	paint
Pulvis	pulv.	powder
Pulvis conspersus	pulv. consp.	dusting powder
Trochiscus	troch.	lozenge
Unguentum	ung.	ointment

Latin name	Abbreviation	English name
Vapor	vap.	inhalation
Vitrella	vitrell.	glass capsule (crushable)

TERMS USED IN PRESCRIPTIONS

Latin	Abbreviation	English
ante cibum	a.c.	before food
ante meridiem	a.m.	before noon
ana	aa.	of each
ad	ad	to
ad libitum	ad lib.	as much as desired
alternus	alt.	alternate
ante	ante	before
applicandus	applic.	to be applied
aqua	aq.	water
bis	b.	twice
bis die	b.d.	twice daily
bis in die	b.i.d.	twice daily
calidus	calid.	warm
cibus	cib.	food
compositus	co.	compound
concentratus	conc.	concentrated
cum	c.	with
dies	d.	a day
destillatus	dest.	distilled
dilutus	dil.	diluted
duplex	dup.	double
ex aqua	ex aq.	in water
fiat	ft.	let it be made
fortis	fort.	strong
hora	h.	at the hour of
hora somni	h.s.	at bedtime
inter cibos	i.c.	between meals
inter	int.	between
mane	m.	in the morning
more dicto	m.d.	as directed

Latin	Abbreviation	English
more dicto utendus	m.d.u.	to be used as directed
mitte	mitt.	send
nocte	n.	at night
nocte et mane	n. et m.	night and morning
nocte maneque	n.m.	night and morning
nomen proprium	n.p.	the proper name
nocte	noct.	at night
omnibus alternis horis	o.alt.hor	every other hour
omni die	o.d.	every day
omni mane	o.m.	every morning
omni nocte	o.n.	every night
parti affectae	p.a.	to the affected part
parti affectae applicandus	part. affect.	to be applied to the affected part
partes aequales	p.aeq.	equal parts
post cibum	p.c.	after food
post meridiem	p.m.	afternoon
partes	pp.	parts
pro re nata	p.r.n.	when required
parti dolenti	part. dolent.	to the painful part
quarter die	q.d.	four times daily
quarter die sumendus	q.d.s.	to be taken four times daily
quarter in die	q.i.d.	four times daily
quaque	qq.	every
quaque hora	qq.h.	every hour
quarta quaque hora	q.qq.h.	every fourth hour
	q.q.h.	every fourth hour

Latin	Abbreviation	English
quantum sufficiat	q.s.	sufficient
recipe	℞	take
secundum artem	sec. art.	with pharmaceutical skill
semisse	ss.	half
si opus sit	s.o.s.	if necessary
signa	sig.	label
statim	stat.	immediately
sumendus ter	sum. t.	to be taken thrice
ter de die	t.d.d.	three times daily
ter die sumendus	t.d.s.	to be taken three times daily
ter in die	t.i.d.	three times daily
tussis	tuss.	a cough
tussi urgente	tuss. urg.	when the cough troubles
ut antea	u.a.	as before
ut dictum	ut. dict.	as directed
ut directum	ut. direct.	as directed
utendus	utend.	to be used

Numerals

The *cardinals* in Table A4.1 refer to number and thus are translated, one, two, three, etc.

The *ordinals* refer to position and thus are translated first, second, third, etc.

The *adverbs* qualify verbs and thus are translated once, twice, three times, etc.

Table A4.1 Roman numerals: Roman symbol and corresponding Latin names for the cardinal and ordinal numbers and their adverbs

Arabic number	Roman symbol	Cardinals	Ordinals	Adverbs
1	I	unus	primus, -a, -um	semel (once)
2	II	duo	secundus or alter	bis (twice)
3	III	tres, tria(n.)	tertius	ter (three times)
4	IV	quattuor	quartus	quater (four times)
5	V	quinque	quintus	quinquies
6	VI	sex	sextus	sexies
7	VII	septem	septimus	septies
8	VIII	octo	octavus	octies
9	IX	novem	nonus	novies
10	X	decem	decimus	decies
11	XI	undecim	undecimus	undecies
12	XII	duodecim	duodecimus	duodecies

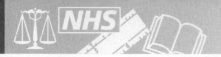

Table A4.1 *(cont'd)*

Arabic number	Roman symbol	Cardinals	Ordinals	Adverbs
14	XIV	quattuordecim	quartis decimus	quattuor-decies
15	XV	quindecim	quintus decimus	quindecies
20	XX	viginti	vicesimus	vicies
50	L	quinquaginta	quinquagesimus	quinquagies
100	C	centum	centesimus	centies

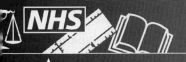

Appendix 5

Systems of weights and measures

A. J. Winfield

Introduction

In 1960 the Système International d'Unités (SI system), based on the metric system, was adopted as the standard. Since 1969 all prescriptions in the UK have been dispensed in this system. The older Imperial and Apothecary systems are still found in older books and formularies. This appendix outlines the three systems for weight and volume.

General

When expressing quantity, it is important to avoid the risk of error or misinterpretation. To reduce this it is best to avoid decimal fractions where possible. Thus, it is better to use 50 mg rather than 0.05 g. Where a decimal point is used, it should be preceded by a 0, thus it should be 0.1 g rather than .1 g.

UNITS OF WEIGHT

Metric (SI) system

The basic unit is the kilogram (kg), which is the mass of the International Prototype Kilogram.

Name of unit	Abbreviation	Relationship
Kilogram	kg	
Gram	g	1/1000 (0.001) kg
Milligram	mg	1/1000 (0.001) g
Microgram	μg (or mcg)	1/1000 (0.001) mg
Nanogram	ng	1/1000 (0.001) μg
Picogram	pg	1/1000 (0.001) ng

To avoid confusion between mg, mcg and ng it is advisable not to use these abbreviations in dispensing.

Imperial system

The pound (avoirdupois) (lb) is the basic unit.

Name of unit	Abbreviation	Relationship
Pound	lb	
Ounce	oz	1/16 lb
Grain	gr	1/7000 1b
		1/437.5 oz

Apothecary system

The grain is the basic standard and is the same as the Imperial grain (gr).

Name of unit	Abbreviation	Relationship
Grain	gr	
Scruple		20 gr
Drachm		60 gr
Ounce (Apoth.)		480 gr
		8 drachms

Note: the Imperial and Apothecary ounce are not the same weight.

VOLUME

Metric (SI) system

The basic unit is the litre (L) which is defined as 1 cubic decimetre.

Name of unit	Abbreviation	Relationship
Litre	L	
Millilitre	mL	1/1000 (0.001) L
Microlitre	μL	1/1000 (0.001) mL

Imperial system

The basic unit is the pint (pt).

Name of unit	Abbreviation	Relationship
Pint	pt	
Fluid ounce	fl. oz.	1/20 pt

Apothecary system

The minim (m) is the basic unit.

Name of unit	Abbreviation	Relationship
Minim	m	
Fluid drachm	fl. dr.	60 m
Fluid ounce	fl. oz.	8 fl dr
		480 m

AMOUNT OF SUBSTANCE

The basic unit is the mole which is the amount of substance containing as many formula units as there are in 12 g of carbon-12. The formula units may be atoms, molecules, ions, etc.

Name of unit	Abbreviation	Relationship
Mole	mol	
Millimole	mmol	1/1000 (0.001) mol
Micromole	μmol	1/1000 (0.001) mmol

CONCENTRATION

Concentration can be expressed as g per L (g per dm³) or mol per L. In dispensing, the former is normally used for drug concentration. Electrolyte concentration may be expressed as amount of substance (mol per L). In medical records and literature, mol per L is normally used.

LENGTH

The metre (m) is the basic unit.

Name of unit	Abbreviation	Relationship
Metre	m	
Centimetre	cm	1/100 (0.01) m
Millimetre	mm	1/1000 (0.001) m
Micrometre	μm	1/1000 (0.001) mm
Nanometre	nm	1/1000 (0.001) μm

Appendix 6

Presentation skills

R. M. E. Richards

Introduction

Short presentations by students, often known as 'giving a seminar', have become an integral part of most academic courses. Although you may regard it as a bit of an ordeal at first it does in fact have many benefits. You will gain confidence at putting across your ideas and answering questions. This will be very beneficial for you in interview situations. It is also likely that you will be expected to make presentations all through your future career and so the skills you develop in making presentations as a student will have life-long benefits. Pharmacy students may expect to present short reviews of academic material or research findings and also present case studies. Case studies are not dealt with specifically in this appendix but many of the skills needed are similar. Basically a good presentation is a form of effective communication between two or more individuals. As such making a good presentation is something which can be learnt. The good news is that every pharmacy student is capable of making a good presentation provided they make adequate preparation. This appendix provides information on the basic skills needed for helping with that preparation. These basic skills are concerned with:

- Preparation
- Visual aids
- Communication
- Delivery.

There is considerable overlap between these areas and this is obvious from a study of Figure A6.1. Nevertheless for the purpose of this appendix each area will be discussed separately.

PREPARATION

Subject material

Once the subject for the presentation is known the initial preparation is to ensure a thorough grasp of the relevant material which will provide the basis of the presentation. This knowledge may be gained as the result of some form of literature survey or as the result of carrying out a research project plus a literature study. The material given here follows the general outline of the 'preparation' section of the spidergram given in Figure A6.1.

The study of the original material, literature or research findings, will involve a critical assessment and interpretation of the material in order to assemble the relevant and valid information. Through a process of integration, synthesis and refinement the body of knowledge thus obtained will be applied to compose the draft outline of the text. Before this is done, however, it would be wise to take a step back and consider the level of knowledge and the expectations of the intended audience. For the undergraduate preparing a presentation for his peers this is fairly straightforward. Should it be a postgraduate or multidisciplinary audience the situation would need careful consideration. It is very discouraging for an audience to be talked down to by assuming that they did not have the most basic knowledge of the subject. On the other hand it is equally discouraging for the presenter to assume knowledge which the audience in general did not possess. It is also important to understand the expectations the audience have of the presentation. Do they wish to have a broad overview of a subject or are they expecting to have considerable detail on

535

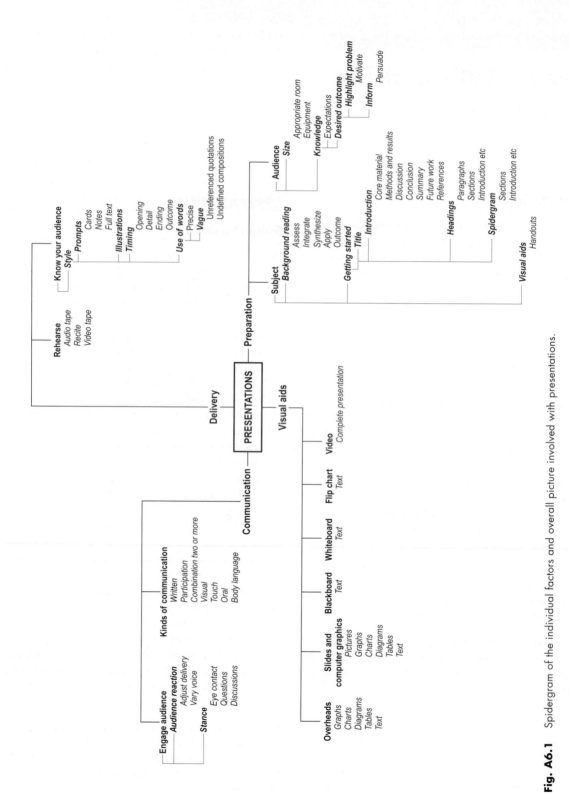

Fig. A6.1 Spidergram of the individual factors and overall picture involved with presentations.

part of the subject which is of particular interest to them at that point in time? The other side of this coin is that you may have been given a brief of what you were expected to achieve with the presentation; that is, the purpose it was intended that the presentation would achieve. In the student situation the main purpose of the presentation is likely to be to provide accurate and reliable information on a particular subject. It could also be to highlight a problem. In other situations it could be to motivate, involve, persuade or encourage creativity.

Having assembled the required information on the subject, the level of knowledge and expectations of the audience and the purpose of the presentation, the draft outline of the text can be prepared. There are several ways this may be done. If the presentation is to follow an accepted scientific communication format the structure has already been decided; it will follow the sequence:

- Title
- Introduction
- Core material (methods and results)
- Discussion, conclusions
- Suggestions for future work
- References.

In order to produce the material in this format it might be convenient to assemble information under headings and subsequently produce paragraphs which are built up into the required sections; 'introduction', etc. However it may sometimes be helpful to adopt the spidergram approach which was used to note down ideas for this appendix. In this approach a rectangle is drawn in the middle of a blank sheet of paper. One or two words describing the subject of the presentation are written into this rectangular block. A line is then drawn from each of the corners representing the main points which will form the basis of the presentation. Spider-like legs are then developed consisting of words or phrases which develop outwards from each of the central main points. Some words may be repeated in the different legs. 'Audience' and 'outcomes', for example, are seen to be present in three of the subject areas. In general, however, the legs represent different aspects of the main subject in the central rectangle.

The first draft would then be revised as many times as necessary to produce a polished text which was clear and as interesting as possible. Decisions would also be made on the relevant visual aids needed to illustrate and support the presentation. A short attractive handout summarizing the main points of the seminar would also be helpful. This would give your aim or objective and act as a guide to your presenta-

tion for the audience. It could be in the form of questions which were subsequently answered in your presentation. The handout should not only reinforce the presentation but also be useful for taking away as a record and reminder of the presentation.

Physical facilities

For groups of greater then 20 people it is usual to use a purpose-built lecture room for the presentation. This type of room is usually arranged with an overhead projector in the format indicated in Figure A6.2A. The head-on arrangement centres the audience attention on both the illustrations and

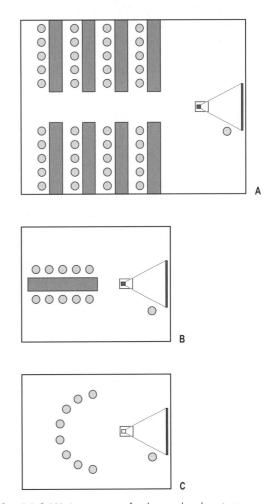

Fig. A6.2 (A) Arrangement for the overhead projector (OHP) with lecture theatre-type seating arrangement. **(B)** Table seating arrangement for use with small groups and the OHP. **(C)** Half circle seating arrangement for use with small groups and the OHP.

the presenter at the same time. A slide projector may also be in the central position of Figure A6.2A but situated further from the screen at the back of the lecture theatre with the controls near to the presenter. For groups of less than 20 people, ideally 12–15 people, the bench or table seating arrangement of Figure A6.2B is convenient. This encourages a good degree of interaction and provides a flat surface for note taking and consulting other documents. The half circle arrangement (Fig. A6.2C) also allows for easy discussion but if note taking is required each seat would need its own small table attached. Other arrangements of these basic configurations are obviously possible. Whichever small group arrangement is chosen the common requirement is for ease of interaction between presenter and participants and participant and participant.

VISUAL AIDS

A presentation is usually improved by the appropriate use of visual aids and these are included in Figure A6.1.

Writing directly

Writing and/or drawing on a blackboard with chalk has been the traditional visual aid used in teaching. It has the advantage of being cheap and widely available. It has now been replaced in the majority of higher education establishments by more effective methods. The whiteboard with coloured felt-tipped pens is now more commonly used. Whiteboards are suitable for informal meetings and discussions with groups of up to 20 people. The felt tips need to be kept capped when not in use or the pens rapidly dry out. Care also needs to be taken not to use permanent inks or the board cannot be cleaned without the use of the appropriate solvent.

Flipcharts, again with the use of coloured felt-tipped pens, are useful with small groups for presenting and recording textual material. They are especially useful in brainstorming sessions and the sheets can be torn off and displayed like posters around the room. Flipcharts are cheap but can be rather fragile and somewhat difficult to handle. Their final appearance, however, can look somewhat scrappy.

Projection

The overhead projector (OHP) plus acetate sheets and coloured felt-tipped pens have become the most popular method for presenting textual or graphical material. This is because of the great versatility of the OHP for use in a large number of situations and without the need for complete blackout facilities. Care needs to be taken to ensure that the seating positions allow all present to see the whole screen. In a smallish room it may be preferable for the presenter to sit next to the OHP when displaying the material. The OHP should ideally be used with an angled white screen to avoid distorting the picture. Although not ideal the OHP can be used with a light-coloured wall or flat white screen. In fact the versatility of the OHP is such that it is often used in less than ideal circumstances. This also applies to the preparation of the text on the acetate sheets for projection. It is not uncommon to see typewritten pages and tables copied directly onto the acetates. No one but the presenter is then able to read the text and possibly even they can only read it with difficulty. Figure A6.3 gives an indication of what an acetate should look like. The following guidelines should be helpful when preparing the acetates.

- The size of the letters should be a minimum of 6–7 mm in height. That is 24–28 point. This should be readable up to 15 m.
- When writing on the acetates by hand use suitable squared paper with the area to be used marked out as a template. The squares will be a guide to writing the right sized letters neatly.
- Try using the acetate in 'landscape' position with a 2.5 cm margin on all four sides. This will help to remove the temptation of including too much on the acetate!
- Have a maximum of 15–20 words per acetate sheet.
- When using graphs do not use more than five different lines per graph and try to use different colours for each line.
- Horizontal or vertical bar charts should not contain more than six bars or groups of bars.

> **PSEUDOMONAS AERUGINOSA**
>
> **Resistant Opportunistic Pathogen**
> - Burn wounds
> - Immunocompromised
> - Cystic fibrosis
> - Indwelling catheter
> - Corneal abrasions
> - Contaminant of non-sterile pharmaceuticals

Fig. A6.3   Sample text for use with an OHP.

- Pie charts should not contain more than six wedges. One floating wedge may be used to highlight a particular set of information (Figure A6.4).
- Purple, blue, dark green and black are the easiest colours to see. Do not use red and green for data that is to be compared or contrasted—it will cause difficulties for those who suffer from colour blindness.

Acetates can be used by revealing the whole sheet at one time or by progressively revealing the information by sliding a backing sheet down the acetate. It is also possible to build up an increasingly complex picture by using a sequence of overlays. There are some people who insist that the acetate slides should be revealed progressively and these people often switch off the projector between acetates. Both views appear somewhat unreasonable. It is best to decide from the content of the acetate whether it is best to reveal progressively or all at once. The life of the projector bulb is related to the number of times it is switched on and off, so why cut short the usable life of an expensive bulb? Rather than switch the projector on and off it is better to use blank coloured acetates between the acetates containing information.

Slides are another very versatile visual aid and can be used with large and small audiences. Producing the slides is more expensive than producing overheads and requires more skill, but good slides can be used repeatedly. High quality slides can be produced using computer graphic packages. Microsoft PowerPoint is very useful for producing presentations of high calibre (OHP or slides) and is very popular. Hard copies of the presentation are often used as handouts. PowerPoint can also be used directly from the computer via a projector. This can be a very useful technique if the hardware is available, allowing a variety of data sources to be used. However, users should beware of the danger of using too many colours or 'actions' because these will detract the listener from what is being said.

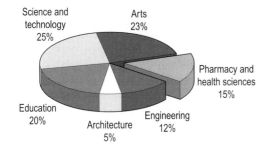

Fig. A6.4 Example of a pie chart—distribution of students by faculty.

Video presentations are not usually a suitable means for making small group or specifically academic presentations. To prepare a high-quality video presentation oneself is very difficult.

COMMUNICATION

This is the subject of Chapter 3, but in that chapter the emphasis is on one-to-one communication, especially between a pharmacist and a patient or co-worker. In this appendix the emphasis is on the communication skills required for making an effective oral presentation to a group of people who are fellow students, staff members, pharmacists and other health professionals.

Kinds of communication

Figure A6.1 indicates that there are several kinds of communication, written, oral, body language, visual, touch, participation and combinations of these. Estimates vary but it is likely that after 3 hours the average person will remember about 70% of a verbal presentation and possibly only 10% after 3 days. A visual presentation improves the retention rate to about 75% after 3 hours and 20% after 3 days. When the presentation consists of a mixture of verbal and visual media the retention improves to 85% after 3 hours and 66% after 3 days. This shows that it is important for a presenter to ensure that their audience have the opportunity to both hear and see what they are seeking to get across by using appropriate visual aids. Where possible the audience should also be given opportunities to interact with the speaker during the presentation as well as through questions at the end of the presentation. How all three aspects can be included should be considered at the time the text outline is being prepared. It should also be mentioned that it is important to keep the presentation short and simple. This will be referred to again in the section on 'Delivery'.

Another sobering thought about the means we use to communicate is that for most members of the audience the presenter's body language and the way they speak has a greater influence on their credibility with the audience than the content of what they say. In general a person who speaks fairly slowly in a medium or low tone without frequent extravagant gestures is perceived as a credible person. The stance of the presenter is also important. It is good to be as natural and relaxed as possible. Fixed stances like folding arms, placing hands on hips or clasping hands in front of the body act as a barrier to communication with the listeners.

Hands in pockets and fiddling with the contents of pockets can be considered sloppy and distracting, neither is continuously clicking a ballpoint pen an endearing habit. Sitting on the table provided for your notes etc., may be interpreted as indicating a superior and disrespectful attitude to your audience.

Engage with your audience

Think carefully how you will manage the first half minute of your presentation. This often sets the tone and influences the impact of the whole presentation. The object will be to attract the listeners' attention by using something which you know will be of interest to them. A quote from a well-chosen reference relating to your subject could be a good way of attracting their attention and easing them into your presentation at the same time. The quote could take the form of a shocking statistic related to the subject of your presentation. This would be especially so if you were going to be able to show that the statistic could be greatly improved. For example: 'Four million of the world's children die needlessly each year from diarrhoea. Oral rehydration fluids are simple to prepare and cheap and could save the majority of those lives. I am going to explain what oral rehydration consists of.'

Eye contact provides a useful link between you and your audience. This should consist of a few seconds contact with certain sympathetic members of your listeners. The eye contact indicates to you the level of interest and understanding of your audience. It answers the question 'How am I doing?' It enables you to adjust your delivery if necessary, vary your voice, or to even interpose a question, or ask the audience if they have a question.

Questions

A time for questions is usually included after the presentation has been completed but there is no reason why a question should not be asked by the speaker, or invited from the audience, during the course of the presentation. This promotes interaction between speaker and audience and helps to clear up misunderstandings before they result in restlessness amongst the participants and discussions between themselves. There are potential pitfalls in taking questions, however, and it would be good for the speaker to be aware of some helpful hints in answering questions.

Firstly listen carefully to the whole question. Keep your mind from wandering to thinking about the answer to the question while the questioner is still speaking. Worse still

don't second guess the questioner and start answering the question before it has been completed.

Secondly repeat the question clearly so that all can hear. This helps you to have time to think about the answer to the question. It also helps other people to understand the question, which everyone might not have heard clearly when it was asked initially, and it reassures the questioner that you have understood the question correctly.

Thirdly avoid having a dialogue with one questioner by breaking eye contact with the questioner as you complete your answer. If you do not know the answer to a relevant question then say that you will let them have an answer at some specific time later. Always seek to be calm and polite in answering questions and be relaxed enough to allow the final question time to develop into a discussion, with you as the moderator, if that seems helpful.

DELIVERY

Timing

This is where the mnemonic **KISS** is useful. **KISS** stands for Keep It Short and Simple (less politely expressed Keep It Short Stupid!). It is good advice and easy to remember. Failing to keep to the allocated time and inadequate preparation are the two main causes for poor presentations. KISS will help you to avoid the first and this appendix should encourage you to avoid the second.

Most presentations will be of a pre-agreed length of time. Knowing how much time is available means that the preparation must be geared to that time. When the first outline draft has been prepared as described in the section on 'Preparation' the delivery will need to be practised and modified until it fits the time available.

Recording the presentation on an audiocassette and listening to the playback is a good way to improve the delivery of the presentation and to tailor it to the allocated time.

Structure

In addition to the time for the presentation being stated it is quite likely that an indication may be given for the structure of the presentation. For a piece of research this would follow the headings: title, brief introduction, methods, key results, discussion (placing the work in context), conclusion and summary. This would be followed by an opportunity for the listeners to question the speaker. If the presentation is based on a literature review it might follow the headings: title, brief introduction (putting the subject in context), presentation of the relevant information, summary of the main points giving the advantages and disadvantages, followed by a time of questions and discussion. Key references for both types of presentation could be given on a handout.

Style

The style of the delivery is important and for a pharmaceutical topic the presentation should use precise language with a few apt illustrations, probably using an overhead projector. Vague language and unsubstantiated quotations should be avoided. Prompts as an aide-mémoire should be used and may take the form of numbered hand-held notes on filing cards or equivalent size pieces of strong paper. These will contain clearly written headings and key phrases. A full text is not really recommended but might be used as a handout. Overheads could contain the same headings and key phrases as the cards.

In addition to a well-thought-out, interesting, attention-grabbing introduction, the delivery should end with a well-prepared set of closing remarks. Some people keep saying that they are just about to finish but seem unable to do so. Just stop the presentation after the summary. If there is time for questions, however, and you wish to draw the question time to a close say, 'the next question will be the last question', then after you have answered it, stop.

In general the content of your presentation will be judged on its accuracy and usefulness and the delivery of your presentation will be judged on its clearness and its interest. Be positive and enjoy yourself.

Appendix 7

Key references and further reading

INTRODUCTION

This section includes guides to further reading and the references used in some chapters. Several books are referred to many times, especially pharmacopoeias and similar books. Others are important textbooks including the two companion volumes to this book. These have been grouped together in the first section. Following that there is a chapter by chapter listing of other suggested reading to expand on the individual chapters, and references cited within the chapters where appropriate. When using a pharmacopoeia, you must always use the information in the most recent edition. Sometimes the information you require, such as the formula for a medicine, may not be in the current edition. You then have to work back until you find the most recent edition in which it occurs.

FREQUENTLY USED REFERENCES

Ansel HC, Popovich NG, Allen LV. Pharmaceutical dosage forms and drug delivery systems, 7th edn. Malvern, USA: Williams & Wilkins; 2000.

Aulton ME. Pharmaceutics: the science of dosage form design, 2nd edn. Edinburgh: Churchill Livingstone; 2002.

British National Formulary, current edition. London: British Medical Association and Royal Pharmaceutical Society of Great Britain.

British Pharmaceutical Codex. London: Pharmaceutical Press; 1973.

British Pharmacopoeia, current edition. London: The Stationery Office.

Committee of Inquiry into Pharmacy: a report to the Nuffield Foundation. London: Nuffield Foundation; 1986.

Diluent Directories (Internal and External), current edition. St Albans: National Pharmaceutical Association.

European Pharmacopoeia, current edition and supplements. Saint Ruffine, France: Maisonneuve, SA.

Farwell J. Aseptic dispensing for NHS patients (The Farwell Report). London: The Stationery Office; 1995.

Handbook of Pharmaceutical Excipients, current edition. London: Pharmaceutical Press. [Gives technical details on many ingredients.]

Harman RJ. Patient care in community practice, 2nd edn. London: Pharmaceutical Press; 2002.

Lawson DG, Richards RME. Clinical pharmacy and hospital drug management. London: Chapman and Hall; 1982.

Martindale: the extra pharmacopoeia, current edition. London: Pharmaceutical Press.

Medicines Compendium, current edition. London: Datapharm Publications.

Medicines Control Agency. Rules and guidance for pharmaceutical manufacture. London: The Stationery Office; 2002.

Pharmaceutical Codex, 11th edn. London: Pharmaceutical Press; 1979.

Pharmaceutical Codex, 12th edn. London: Pharmaceutical Press; 1994.

Royal Pharmaceutical Society of Great Britain. Medicines, ethics and practice—a guide for pharmacists, current edition. London: RPSGB.

United States Pharmacopeia, current edition. Easton, PA: Mack.

Wade E, ed. Pharmaceutical handbook, 19th edn. London: Pharmaceutical Press; 1980.

Walker R, Edwards C. Clinical pharmacy and therapeutics, 3rd edn. Edinburgh: Churchill Livingstone; 2003.

PART 1: PHARMACY IN SOCIETY

Chapter 1: The contribution of pharmacy to today's health care provision

Clinical Resources Audit Group. Clinical pharmacy in the hospital pharmaceutical service: a framework for practice. Edinburgh: The Stationery Office; 1996.

Department of Health. Choice and opportunity. Primary care: the future. London: The Stationery Office; 1996.

Department of Health. Response to the report of the public inquiry into children's heart surgery at the Bristol Royal Infirmary 1984–1995. London: The Stationery Office; 2001.

Department of Health. Pharmacy in the future; implementing the NHS plan—a programme for pharmacy in the National Health Service. London: The Stationery Office; 2002.

Farwell I. The Bristol Royal Infirmary Inquiry (The Kennedy Report). London: The Stationery Office; 2001.

Royal Pharmaceutical Society of Great Britain. Pharmacy in a new age: the new horizon. London: RPSGB; 1996.

Scottish Executive. The right medicine: a strategy for pharmaceutical care in Scotland. Edinburgh: The Stationery Office; 2002.

Weller PJ, ed. Pharmacists' directory and yearbook, current edition. London: Royal Pharmaceutical Society of Great Britain.

Chapter 2: Social and behavioural aspects of pharmacy

FIP (International Pharmaceutical Federation) Standards for Quality of Pharmacy Services. Online. Available: http://www.fip.org

Gard P, ed. A behavioural approach to pharmacy practice. Oxford: Blackwell Science; 2000.

Harding G, Nettleton S, Taylor K. Sociology for pharmacists. London: MacMillan; 1990.

Lilja J, Larsson S, Hamilton D. Drug communication. How cognitive science can help the health professionals. In: Pharmaceutical Sciences No 24. Kuopio: Kuopio University Publications; 1996.

Marmot M, Wilkinson RG. Social determinants of health. Oxford: Oxford University Press; 1999.

Miller DF, Price JH. Dimensions of community health, 5th edn. Boston: McGraw-Hill; 1998.

Panton R, Chapman S. Medicines management. London: Pharmaceutical Press; 1998.

Quick JD. Management sciences for health: managing drug supply, 2nd edn. West Hartford, USA: Kumarian Press; 1997.

Sarafino EP. Health psychology—biopsychosocial interactions, 4th edn. New York: John Wiley; 2001.

Smith FJ. Research methods in pharmacy practice. London: Pharmaceutical Press; 2002.

Smith MC, Knapp DA. Pharmacy, drugs and medical care, 5th edn. Baltimore: Williams and Wilkins; 1992.

Smith MC, Wertheimer AI. Social and behavioural aspects of pharmaceutical care. New York: Pharmaceutical Products Press; 2002.

Taylor KMG, Harding G, eds. Pharmacy practice. London: Taylor & Francis; 2001.

Chapter 3: Communication skills for the pharmacist

Burnard P. Effective communication skills for health professionals, 2nd edn. London: Chapman & Hall; 1997.

Dickson D, Hargie O, Morrow N. Communication skills training for health professionals, 2nd edn. London: Chapman and Hall; 1997.

Ley P. Communicating with patients. London: Croom Helm; 1988.

Pease A. Body language, 2nd edn. London: Sheldon Press; 1997.

Tindall WN, Beardsley RS, Kimberlin CL. Communication skills in pharmacy practice, 4th edn. Baltimore, MA: Lippincott/Williams & Wilkins; 2002.

USP Medication Counseling Behaviour Guidelines. www.usp.org

Chapter 4: WHO and the essential medicines concept

1. World Health Organization. The world health report: making a difference. Geneva: World Health Organization; 1999.

2. World Health Organization. WHO medicines strategy: framework for action in essential drugs and medicines policy 2000–2003. Document reference WHO/EDM/2000.1. Geneva: World Health Organization; 2000.

3. World Health Organization. Revised drug strategy: WHO's work in pharmaceuticals and essential drugs. Document reference EB/RDS/RC/1. Geneva: World Health Organization; 1998.

4. World Health Organization. WHO as an organization. 2002. Online. Available: http://www.who.int/m/topicgroups/who_organization/en/index.html

5. World Health Organization. Report on infectious diseases: removing obstacles to healthy development. Document reference WHO/CDS/99.1. Geneva: World Health Organization; 1999.

6. World Health Organization. Report on infectious diseases: overcoming antimicrobial resistance. Document reference WHO/CDS/2000.2. Geneva: World Health Organization; 2000.

7. World Bank. World development report 2000/2001: attacking poverty. New York: Oxford University Press; 2000.

8. Quick JD. Management sciences for health: managing drug supply, 2nd edn. West Hartford, USA: Kumarian Press; 1997.

9. World Health Organization. The use of essential drugs. WHO Technical Report Series 895. Geneva: World Health Organization; 2000.

10. World Health Organization. Updating and disseminating the WHO Model List of Essential Medicines: the way forward. Document reference EB108/INF.DOC./2. Geneva: World Health Organization; 2001.

11. World Health Organization. The selection and use of essential medicines. WHO Technical Report Series. Draft report of the Expert Committee, including the 12th Model List of Essential Medicines. Geneva: World Health Organization; 2002. Online. Available: http://www.who.int/medicines/organization/par/edl/ expertcomm.shtml

12. World Health Organization. Health reform and drug financing: selected topics. Health economics and drugs, DAP series no 6. Document reference WHO/DAP/98.3. Geneva: World Health Organization; 1998.

13. World Health Organization. Global comparative pharmaceutical expenditures with related reference information. Health economics and drugs, EDM series no 3. Document reference EDM/PAR/2000.2. Geneva: World Health Organization; 2000.

14. World Health Organization. WHO's policy perspectives on medicines. The selection of essential medicines. Geneva: World Health Organization; 2002. Online. Available: http://www.who.int/medicines/library/edm_general/6pagers/ppm04emg.pdf

Chapter 5: Pharmacy management

Jones IF. Community pharmacy and the National Health Service. Pharm J 1998;261(suppl): NHS24–27.
Jones IF. Net profit from NHS dispensing (part 1). Independent Community Pharmacist. 1999; July.
Jones IF. Net profit from NHS dispensing (part 2). Independent Community Pharmacist. 1999; October.

PART 2: PRINCIPLES OF PHARMACY PRACTICE

Chapter 6: The principles and applications of quality assurance

Commission of the European Communities. The rules governing medicinal products in the European Community, vol IV: Good manufacturing practice for medicinal products. Luxembourg: The EU Commission; 1998.
Department of Health. Clinical governance in community pharmacy: guidelines on good practice for the NHS. London: The Stationery Office; 2001.
Goldberger F. Pharmaceutical manufacturing quality management in the industry. Evreaux, France: Ebur, 1991.

Chapter 8: Pharmaceutical calculations

Howard C, Ansel HC, Stoklosa MJ. Pharmaceutical calculations, 11th edn. Baltimore: Lippincott/Williams and Williams; 2001.
Rees JA, Smith I, Smith B. Introduction to pharmaceutical calculations. London: Pharmaceutical Press; 2000.
Rouse SH, Webber MG. Calculations in pharmacy, 3rd edn. London: Pitman Medical Publishing; 1968.

Chapter 9: Packaging

Dean DA, Evans ER, Hall IH. Pharmaceutical packaging technology. Andover, UK: Taylor and Francis; 2000.

Chapter 10: Storage and stability of medicines

Longland PW, Rowbotham PC. Room temperature stability of medicines recommended for cold storage. Pharm J 1989;243:589–595.
Lynch M, Lund W, Wilson DA. Chloroform as a preservative in aqueous systems. Pharm J 1977;219:501–510.
Rhodes CT. An overview of kinetics for the evaluation of the stability of pharmaceutical systems. Drug Dev Pharm Ind 1984;10:1163–1174.

Chapter 11: Labelling of dispensed medicines

Royal Pharmaceutical Society Working Party Report. Labelling of dispensed medicines. Pharm J 1990; 245:128–129.

Chapter 12: Principles and methods of sterilization

Annex 17 to the EU Guide to Good Manufacturing Practice. Brussels: The European Commission; 2001.
Health Technical Memorandum no 2010. Sterilization. London: The Stationery Office; 1966.
Kirk B, Hambleton R, Everett M. Computer aided autoclave monitoring. Pharm J 1982;299:252–254.
Report of a working party established by the Association of British Pharmaceutical Industry and others on the use of gamma radiation sources for the sterilization of pharmaceutical products. London: Association of British Pharmaceutical Industry; 1960.

Chapter 13: Sterile production areas

Beaney AM. Quality assurance of aseptic preparation service, 3rd edn. London: Pharmaceutical Press; 2001.
Commission of the European Communities. The rules governing medicinal products in the European Community, vol 1V: good manufacturing practice for medicinal products. Luxembourg: The European Commission; 2001.
Guidance for pharmaceutical manufacturers and distributors. London: The Stationery Office; 1997.

Chapter 14: Sterility testing

Guidance for pharmaceutical manufacturers and distributors. London: The Stationery Office; 1997.

SECTION 3: PHARMACEUTICAL PRODUCTS

Chapter 15: The prescription

Consultation on SOPs for dispensing. Pharm J 2001;266:616–619.
Department of Health. Review of prescribing, supply and administration of medicines, final report. London: The Stationary Office. Online. Available: http://www.doh.gov.uk
Drug Tariff, current edition. The Stationery Office. Online. Available: http://www.tso.co.uk
National Prescribing Centre. Prescribing analysis terms. Online. Available: http:// www.npc.co.uk
National Prescribing Centre. Signposts for prescribing nurses. Prescriber Users Bull 1999;1:(1).

Review of prescribing, supply and administration of medicines. Initial report. (Crown review). London: Department of Health; 1998.

Review of prescribing, supply and administration of medicines. Final report. (Crown review). London: Department of Health; 1999.

Chapter 24: Inhaled route

ABPI compendium of patient information leaflets, current edition. London: Datapharm Publications.

The British guidelines on asthma management. Thorax 1997;52(suppl 1).

British Thoracic Society. BTS guidelines for the management of chronic obstructive pulmonary disease. Thorax 1997;52 (suppl 5).

Chlorofluorocarbon (CFC) free inhalers. MeRec Bull 1998;9(5).

Inhaled corticosteroids: their role in chronic obstructive pulmonary disease. MeRec Bull 2000;11(6).

Inhaler devices: an update. MeRec Bull 1995;6(9).

The management of chronic obstructive pulmonary disease. MeRec Bull 1998;9(10).

Purewal TS, Grant DJW. Metered dose inhaler technology. Buffalo Grove, IL: Interpharm Press, 2002.

Royal Pharmaceutical Society of Great Britain Respiratory Disease Task Force. Practice guidance on the care of people with asthma and chronic obstructive pulmonary disease. London: RPSGB; 2000.

Chapter 25: Parenteral products

Akers MJ. Parenteral quality control: sterility, pyrogens, particulate and package integrity testing. New York: Marcel Dekker; 1994.

Avis KE, Lieberman HA, Lachman L. Pharmaceutical dosage forms: parenteral medications, vol 1, 2nd edn. New York: Marcel Dekker; 1992.

British Standard 2463 1989 Part 2. London: British Standards Institution.

Collentro WV. Pharmaceutical water: systems design, operation, and validation. Buffalo Grove, IL: Interpharm Press; 1999.

DeLuca PP, Boylan JC. Formulation of small volume parenterals. In: Avis KE, Lieberman HA, Lachman L, eds. Pharmaceutical dosage forms: parenteral medications vol 1, 2nd edn. New York: Marcel Dekker; 1992.

Demorest LJ, Hamilton JG. Formulation of large volume parenterals. In: Avis KE, Lieberman HA, Lachman L, eds. Pharmaceutical dosage forms: parenteral medications, vol 1, 2nd edn. New York: Marcel Dekker; 1992.

Levchuk JW. Parenteral products in hospital and home care pharmacy practice. In: Avis KE, Lieberman HA, Lachman L, eds. Pharmaceutical dosage forms: parenteral medications, vol 1, 2nd edn. New York: Marcel Dekker; 1992.

Turco S. Sterile dosage forms: their preparation and clinical application. Philadelphia: Lea & Febiger; 1994.

Williams KL. Endotoxins, pyrogens, LAL testing and depyrogenation. New York: Marcel Dekker; 2001.

Chapter 26: Ophthalmic preparations

Guidance for use of ophthalmic preparations in hospital and care homes. Pharm J 2001;267:307.

Chapter 27: Specialized services

Allwood M, Stanley AP, Wright et al. The cytotoxics handbook, 4th edn. Oxford: Radcliffe Medical Press; 2001.

Department of Health and Social Security. Breckenridge Working Party Report of the working part on addition of drugs to intravenous infusion fluids. HC (76)9. London: The Stationery Office; 1976.

Department of Health and Social Security. Guidance notes for hospitals on the premises and environment required for the preparation of radiopharmaceuticals. London: The Stationery Office; 1982.

Needle RA. Survey of hospital centralised intravenous additive services. Pharm J 1995;225:326–327.

Pharmaceutical Society Working Party Report, Guidelines for the handling of cytotoxic drugs. Pharm J 1983;230:230–231.

Sabra K, Wilson H, Ballelli J. The use of isolators in centralized IV additive services in hospital pharmacies. Hosp Pharm 1996;31:1257–1263.

Sampson CB. Textbook of radiopharmacy theory and practice, 2nd edn. Gordon and Breach Science Publishers; 1994.

Chapter 28: Parenteral nutrition and dialysis

Wood S. Home parenteral nutrition: quality criteria for clinical services and the supply of nutrient fluids and equipment. Maidenhead: British Association for Parenteral and Enteral Nutrition; 1995.

Chapter 29: Wound management, stoma and incontinence products

Anon. Modern wound management dressings. Prescribing Nurse Bull 1999; 1(2):5–8. Online. Available: http://www.npc.co.uk/nurse_pres.htm

Drug Tariff, current edition. London: The Stationery Office.

Elcoat C. Stoma care nursing. London: Baillière Tindall; 1986.

Gartley CB. Managing incontinence. London: Souvenir Press Educational and Academic; 1988.

Morgan DA. Wound management products in the Drug Tariff. Pharm J 1999;263:820–825.

Morgan DA. Formulary of wound management products, 8th edn. Surrey: Euromed Communications; 2000. With updates online. Available: http://www.euromed.uk.com/formulary.htm

SMTL dressings datacards. Online. Available: http://www.dressings.org

Thomas S. Wound management and dressings. London: Pharmaceutical Press; 1990.

Turner T. The healing process. Pharm J 1993;250:735–737.

World wide wounds at http://www.worldwidewounds.com.

Note

Many manufacturers have websites with information on specific products, e.g. http://www.smith-nephew.com

Chapter 30: Medical gases

British Standard EN 850 1997 London: British Standards Institution.

Grant WJ. Medical gases: their properties and uses. Aylesbury: HM&M Publishers; 1978.

Thomson G. Assessing the relative safety of domiciliary oxygen delivery systems. Pharm J 2002; 268: 540–542.

SECTION 4: USING PHARMACEUTICAL SKILLS IN CARING FOR PATIENTS

Chapter 31: Clinical pharmacy practice

Access to Health Records Act (1990) http://www.hmso.gov.uk/acts/acts1990/Ukpga_19900023_en_1.htm

Audit Commission. A spoonful of sugar. London: Audit Commission; 2001.

Clinical Resources and Audit Group. Clinical pharmacy in the hospital pharmaceutical service: a framework for practice. Report of a working group (Chairman, Cromarty JA). Edinburgh: The Scottish Office; 1996.

Data Protection Act (1998) http://www.hmso.gov.uk/acts/acts1998/80029_a.htm#1

Department of Health. Pharmacy in the future—implementing the NHS plan. A programme for pharmacy in the National Health Service. London: The Stationery Office; 2002.

Department of Health. Primary care: the future. London: NHS Executive; 1996.

Department of Health. Saving lives: executive summary. London: The Stationery Office, 1999.

Department of Health. The way forward for hospital pharmaceutical services. HC(88)54. London: The Stationery Office; 1988.

Field MJ, Lohr KN. Guidelines for clinical practice. From development to use. Washington: National Academy Press; 1992.

Hepler CD, Strand LM. Opportunities and responsibilities in pharmaceutical care. Am J Hosp Pharm 1990;47:533–543.

Kennedy I. The Bristol Royal Infirmary Inquiry (the Kennedy Report). London: The Stationery Office; 2001.

Marinker M. Controversies in health care policies. Challenges to practice. London: BMJ Publishing Group; 1994.

National Health Service and Community Care Act. London: The Stationery Office; 2002.

Patient Group Directions http://www.show.scot.nhs.uk/sehd/mels/hd1200107.htm

Pharmaceutical Services Negotiating Committee. Developing patient care: medicine management in community pharmacy. London: PSNC; 1999.

Royal Pharmaceutical Society of Great Britain. Pharmaceutical care: the future for community pharmacy. Report of the joint working party on the future role of the community pharmaceutical services. London: The Royal Pharmaceutical Society; 1992.

Royal Pharmaceutical Society of Great Britain. Flint J. Training for medicines counter assistants Pharmaceutical Journal 1996; 256: 858–859.

Scottish Executive. The right medicine: a strategy for pharmaceutical care in Scotland. Edinburgh: The Stationery Office; 2002.

Secretaries of State for Health WNIaS. Working for patients. CM 249. London: The Stationery Office; 1989.

Secretaries of State for Social Services WNIaS. Promoting better health. CM 249 London: The Stationery Office, 1987.

Secretary of State for Health, Social Security Wales and Scotland. Caring for people: community care in the next decade and beyond. London: The Stationery Office; 1989.

Chapter 32: Adverse drug reactions

Cox A, The Committee on Safety of Medicines' Yellow Card scheme. Pharmacy in Practice; 10:213–215

Dukes MNG, Aronson JK. Meyler's side effects of drugs, 14th edn. Amsterdam: Elsevier Science Publishers; 2000.

Jarernsiripornkul N, Krska J, Capps PAG, Richards RME, Lee A. Patient reporting of potential adverse drug reactions: a methodological study. Br J Clin Pharmacol 2002;53:318–25.

Jick H, Garcia Rodriguez LA, Perez-Gutthann S. Principles of epidemiological research on adverse and beneficial drug effects. Lancet 1998;352:1767–70.

Krska J, John DN, Hansford D, Kennedy EJ. Drug utilization evaluation of non-prescription H_2-receptor antagonists and alginate-containing preparations for dyspepsia. Br J Clin Pharmacol 2000;49:1–6.

Lee A. Adverse drug reactions. London: Pharmaceutical Press; 2001.

Mann RD. Prescription-event monitoring—recent progress and future horizons. Br J Clin Pharmacol 1998;46:195–201.

Medicines Control Agency. Online. Available: http://www.open.gov.uk/mca/mcahome.htm

Sinclair HK, Bond CM, Hannaford P. Over-the-counter ibuprofen: how and why is it used? Int J Pharm Pract 2000;8:121–127.

Stockley IH. Drug interactions—a source book of adverse interactions, their mechanisms, clinical importance and management, 6th edn. London: Pharmaceutical Press; 2002.

Chapter 33: Medicines information

Anon. An introduction to assessing medical literature. MeReC Briefing 1995;9:1–8.

Brazier H, McCabe G. Making the most of Medline. Hosp Med 1998;59(10):756–761.

Covell DG, Uman GC, Manning PR. Information needs in office practice: are they being met? Ann Intern Med 1985; 103:596–599.

Dukes MNG, Aronson JK. Meyler's side effects of drugs, 14th edn. Amsterdam: Elsevier Science Publishers; 2000.

Ely JW, Osheroff JA, Bell MH et al. Analysis of questions asked by family doctors regarding patient care. Br Med J 1999;319:358–361.

Ely JW, Osheroff JA, Ebell MH et al. Obstacles to answering doctors' questions about patient care with evidence: qualitative study. Br Med J 2002;324:710–713.

Gardner M. Information retrieval for patient care. Br Med J 1997;314:950–954.

Greenhalgh T. Assessing the methodological quality of published papers. Br Med J 1997;315:305–308.

Hands D, Judd A, Golightly P, Grant E. Drug information and advisory services—past, present and future. Pharm J 1999;262:160–162.

Impicciatore P, Pandolfini C, Casella N, Bonate M. Reliability of health information for the public on the world wide web: systematic survey of advice on managing fever in children at home. Br Med J 1997;314:1875–1881.

McKibbon KA. How to search for and find evidence about therapy. Evidence-Based Med 1996;March/April:70–72.

Malone P. Drug information technology and Internet resources. J Pharm Pract 1998;11:196–218.

Shaughnessy AF, Slawson DC, Bennett JH. Becoming an information master: a guidebook to the medical information jungle. J Fam Pract 1994;39:489–499.

Slawson DC, Shaughnessy AF. Obtaining useful information from expert based sources. Br Med J 1997;314:947–949.

Slawson DC, Shaughnessy AF, Bennett JH. Becoming a medical information master: feeling good about not knowing everything. J Fam Pract 1994;39:505–513.

Smith R. What clinical information do doctors need? Br Med J 1996;313:1062–1068.

Stockley IH. Drug interactions—a source book of adverse interactions, their mechanisms, clinical importance and management, 6th edn. London: Pharmaceutical Press; 2002.

Wright SG, LeCroy RL, Kendrach MG. A review of the three types of biomedical literature and the systematic approach to answer a drug information request. J Pharm Pract 1998;11:148–162.

Chapter 34: The evaluation of medicines

Bandolier. Online. Available: http:// www.jr2.ox.ac.uk/bandolier/

Cochrane Collaboration. Online. Available: http://www.cochrane.org/

Evidence Based Medicine. Online. Available: http://www.evidence-basedmedicine.com

Health Technology Board for Scotland. Online. Available: http://www.htbs.co.uk

Jarernsiripornkul N, Krska J, Capps PAG, Richards RME, Lee A. Patient reporting of potential adverse drug reactions: a methodological study. Br J Clin Pharmacol 2002;53:318–325.

Krska J, John DN, Hansford D, Kennedy EJ. Drug utilization evaluation of non-prescription H$_2$-receptor antagonists and alginate-containing preparations for dyspepsia. Br J Clin Pharmacol 2000;49:1–6.

McGavock H. Handbook of drug use research methodology, 1st edn. UK Drug Utilisation Research Group; 2000.

National Institute for Clinical Excellence. Online. Available: http://www.nice.org.uk

Sackett DL, Straus SE. Evidence-based medicine, 2nd edn. Edinburgh: Churchill Livingstone; 2000.

Scottish Intercollegiate Guidelines Network SIGN 50. A guideline developer's handbook. Online. Available: http://www.nhsis.co.uk/sign/guidelines/published/index.html

Sinclair HK, Bond CM, Hannaford P. Over-the-counter ibuprofen: how and why is it used? Int J Pharm Pract 2000;8:121–127

Chapter 35: Pharmacoeconomics

Brazier J, Deverill M, Green C. The use of health status measures in economic evaluation. In: Stevens A, ed. The advanced handbook of methods in evidence based healthcare. London: Sage; 2001:195–214.

Briggs A, Alastair G. Using cost effectiveness information. Br Med J 2000;320:246.

Cooke J. Pharmacoeconomics. In: Walker R, Edwards C, eds. Clinical pharmacy and therapeutics, 2nd edn. Edinburgh: Churchill Livingston; 1999:85–93.

Donaldson C, Gerard K. Economics of health care financing: the visible hand. Basingstoke: Macmillan; 1993.

Donaldson C, Hall J. Economic evaluation of health care: guidelines for costing (Discussion Paper 1). Westmead, New South Wales: Centre for Health Economics Research and Evaluation; 1991.

Donaldson C, Mugford M, Vale L. Evidence-based health economics. London: BMJ Books; 2002.

Drummond MF, O'Brien B, Stoddart GL, Torrance GW. Methods for the economic evaluation of health care programmes, 2nd edn. Oxford: Oxford Medical Publications; 1997.

Euroqol Group. EQ-5D homepage. Online. Available: http://www.euroqol.org/ 28 Jun 2002.

Evidence Based Medicine Working Group. Finding and using articles about an economic analysis. Online. Available: http://www.med.ualberta.ca/ebm/artecon.htm 27 Jun 2002.

Gateway. Online. Available: http://www.healtheconomics.com

Johannesson M, Aberg H, Agreus L, Borgquist L, Jonsson B. Cost-benefit analysis of non-pharmacological treatment of hypertension. J Intern Med 1991;230:307–312.

Kielhorn A, Graf von Schulenburg JM. The health economics handbook. Chester: Adis International; 2000.

Kristiansen IS, Eggen AE, Thelle DS. Cost-effectiveness of incremental programmes for lowering serum cholesterol concentration: is individual intervention worthwhile? Br Med J 1991;302:1119–1122.

Lowson K, Drummond M, Bishop J. Costing new services: long term domiciliary oxygen therapy. Lancet 1981;May 23:1146–1149.

Malek M. Glyceryl trinitrate sprays in the treatment of angina: a cost minimisation study. Pharm J 1996;257:690–691.

Malek M. Pharmacoeconomics. Pharm J 1996;256:759–61; 1997; 258:23–24,99–101.

Meltzer MI. Introduction to health economics for physicians. Lancet 2001;358:993–998.

Mooney G. Economics, medicine and health care, 2nd edn. Hemel Hempstead: Harvester Wheatsheaf; 1992.

O'Brien BJ, Heyland D, Richardson WS, Levine M, Drummond MF. How to use an article on economic analysis of clinical practice. Online. Available: http://www.cche.net/usersguides/economic.asp 27 Jun 2002.

Rittenhouse B. Uses of models in economic evaluations of medicines and other health technologies. London: Office of Health Economics; 1996.

Robinson R. Economic evaluation and health care. Br Med J 1993;307:670–673, 726–728, 793–795, 859–862, 924–926, 994–996.

Sinclair HK, Silcock J, Bond CM, Lennox AS, Winfield AJ. The cost-effectiveness of intensive pharmaceutical intervention in assisting people to stop smoking. Int J Pharm Pract 1999;7:107–112.

University of Aberdeen. Online. Available: http://www.abdn.ac.uk/heru/

University of York. Online. Available: http://www.york.ac.uk/res/herc

Chapter 36: Formularies and guidelines

AGREE (Appraisal of Guidelines, Research and Evaluation for Europe) guideline appraisal instrument. Online. Available: http://www.agreecollaboration.org/

Garvey G, Jappy B, Stewart D et al. Grampian Health Board's joint drug formulary. Br Med J 1990;301:851–852.

National Prescribing Centre. Area Prescribing Committees: maintaining effectiveness in the modern NHS—a guide to good practice. Liverpool National Prescribing Centre; 2000.

National Prescribing Centre. Implementing NICE guidance: a practical handbook for professionals. Oxford: Radcliffe Medical Press; 2001.

Scottish Intercollegiate Guideline Network SIGN 50. A guideline developer's handbook. Online. Available: http://www.nhsis.co.uk/sign/guidelines/published/index.html

Chapter 37: Responding to symptoms

Blenkinsopp A, Paxton P. Symptoms in the pharmacy, 4th edn. Oxford: Blackwell Science; 2001.

Edwards C, Stillman P. Minor illness or major disease? Responding to symptoms in the pharmacy, 3rd edn. London: Pharmaceutical Press; 2000.

Nathan A. Non-prescription medicines, 2nd edn. London: Pharmaceutical Press; 2002.

OTC Directory. Treatments for common ailments, current edition. London: Proprietary Association of Great Britain. [Updated annually.]

Chapter 38: Counselling

ABPI Compendium of patient information leaflets, current edition. London: Datapharm Publications. [Updated annually.]

Clinical Research and Audit Group. Counselling and advice on medicines and appliances in community pharmacy practice. Edinburgh; The Stationery Office; 1996.

Department of Health. National Service Framework for older people. London: The Stationary Office; 2000.

Department of Health. NHS Plan, a plan for investment, a plan for reform, London: The Stationary Office; 2000.

Primary Care Symposium. Pharm J 2001;267:474.

Royal Pharmaceutical Society of Great Britain Working Party Report, From compliance to concordance (Chairman, Marinker M). London: Royal Pharmaceutical Society; 1997.

Chapter 39: Health promotion

Andersen C. Guidance for the development of health promotion by community pharmacists. Pharm J 1998;261:771–775.

Department of Health. Pharmacy in the future—implementing the NHS plan. London: The Stationery Office; 2000.

Department of Health. Saving lives: our healthier nation white paper. London: The Stationary Office; 1999. Online. Available: http:// www.ohn.gov.uk/ohn

Department of Health. The NHS Plan. A plan for investment, a plan for reform. London: The Stationery Office; 2000.

National Service Frameworks. Online. Available: http://www.doh.gov.uk/nsf

Pharmacy Healthcare Scheme and Audit Unit. Online. Available: http://www.rpsgb.org.uk

Prochaska JO, DiClemente CC. Towards a comprehensive model of Change. In: Miller W, Heather N, eds. Treating addictive behaviours: processes of change. New York: Plenum; 1986.

Review of the UK and international evidence-base for pharmacy health development. Online. Available: http://www.rpsgb.org.uk/patientcare/

Chapter 40: Concordance and compliance

Clepper I. Noncompliance: the invisible epidemic. Drug Topics 1992;Aug 17:44,45,49,50,56,59,60,62,65.

Hayne McKibbon A, Kanani R. Systematic review of randomised trials of interventions to assist patients to follow prescriptions for medications. Lancet 1996;348(Aug 10):383–386.

Horne R, Weinman J, Hankins M. The beliefs about medicines questionnaire: the development and evaluation of a new method for assessing the cognitive representation of medication. Psychol Health 1999;14:1–24.

Ley P. Communicating with patients. London: Croom Helm; 1988.

Rivers PH. Compliance aids—do they work? Drug Therapy 1992;2:103–111.

Roberts K. Compliance. Pharm Update 1987;March:90,92,94–96,98–100.

Royal Pharmaceutical Society of Great Britain Working Party Report, From compliance to concordance (Chairman, Marinker M). London: RPSGB; 1997.

Task Force on Medicines Partnership. Medicines partnership from compliance to concordance. Online. Available: http://www.concordance.org

Chapter 41: Complementary/alternative medicine

Barnes J, Anderson LA, Phillipson JD. Herbal medicines. A guide for healthcare professionals, 2nd edn. London: Pharmaceutical Press; 2002.

Commission of the European Communities 2002/0008. Proposal for amending the directive 2001/83/EC as regards traditional herbal medicinal products. Brussels: The European Commission; 2002.

Department of Health. Government response to the House of Lords Select Committee on Science and Technology's report on complementary and alternative medicine. London: The Stationery Office; 2001.

Eisenberg DM, Davis RB, Ettner SL et al. Trends in alternative medicine use in the United States, 1990–1997. Results of a national follow-up survey. JAMA 1998;280:1569–1575.

House of Lords Select Committee on Science and Technology, Session 1999–2000, 6th report. Complementary and alternative medicine. London: The Stationery Office; 2000.

Kayne S. Complementary therapies for pharmacists. London: Pharmaceutical Press; 2002.

The Medicines for Human Use (Marketing Authorisations etc.) Regulations. (S1 1994/3144) 1994. London: The Stationery Office.

The Medicines for Human Use (Marketing Authorisations etc.) Amendment Regulations (S1 2000/292) 2000. London: The Stationery Office.

The Medicines (Aristolochia and Mu Tong etc.) (Prohibition) Order. (S1 2001/1841) 2001. London: The Stationery Office.

Mills S, Peacock W. Professional organisation of complementary and alternative medicines in the United Kingdom 1997. A report to the Department of Health. Exeter: University of Exeter; 1997.

Mintel 2001 Complementary medicines. Market Intelligence. London: Mintel International Ltd; 2001

Thomas KJ, Nicholl JP, Coleman P. Use and expenditure on complementary medicine in England: a population based survey. Complement Ther Med 2001;9:2–11.

Traditional ethnic medicines. Public health and compliance with medicines law. London: Medicines Control Agency, 2001 http://www.mca.gov.uk.

Zollman C, Vickers A. What is complementary medicine? Br Med J 1999;319:693–696.

Chapter 42: Substance use and misuse

Berridge V. Opium and the people. London: Free Association Books; 1998.

Department of Health. Drug Misuse and Dependence— Guidelines on Clinical Management. London: The Stationery Office; 1999.

DVLA. At a glance guide to medical aspects of fitness to drive. Swansea: DVLA; 1998.

Gelder M, Mayou R, Cowen P, eds. Misuse of alcohol and drugs. In: The shorter Oxford textbook of psychiatry, 4th edn. Oxford: Oxford University Press; 2001.

Gossop M. Living with drugs, 5th edn. Aldershot: Ashgate Publishing; 2000.

Gossop M, Marsden J, Stewart D. NTORS after five years: changes in substance use, health and criminal behaviour during the five years after intake. London: National Addiction Centre (Crown copyright); 2001.

Neale J. Drug users' views of substitute prescribing conditions. Int J Drug Policy 1999;10:247–258.

Roberts K, Bryson SM. The contribution of Glasgow pharmacists to the management of drug misuse. Hosp Pharmacist 1999;6:244–248.

Stimson GV, Des Jarlais DC, Ball A. Drug injecting and HIV infection. London: Taylor & Francis; 1998.

Walker M. Shared care of opiate misusers in Berkshire. Pharm J 2001;266:547–552.

Ward J, Hall W, Mattick R. Role of maintenance treatment in opioid dependence. Lancet 1999;353:221–226.

Wills S. Drugs of abuse. London: Pharmaceutical Press; 1997.

World Health Organization. Expert Committee on Drug Dependence. 28th Report. Geneva: World Health Organization; 1993.

Chapter 43: Clinical governance

Clinical Resource and Audit Group. Clinical pharmacy in the hospital pharmaceutical service: a framework for practice. Edinburgh: The Stationery Office; 1996.

Clinical Resource and Audit Group. Counselling and advice on medicines and appliances in community pharmacy practice. Edinburgh: The Stationery Office; 1996.

Clinical Resource and Audit Group. Clinical pharmacy practice in primary care. Edinburgh: The Stationery Office; 1999.

Dean B. What is clinical governance? Pharmacy in Practice 2000;10:182–184.

National Prescribing Centre. Pharmacy audit handbook; 2000. Online. Available: http://www/npc.co.uk/publications/audit/

NHS Executive and National Prescribing Centre. Competencies for pharmacists working in primary care, 1st edn; 2000. Online. Available: http://www/npc.co.uk/publications/CompPharm/

The Royal Pharmaceutical Society of Great Britain, Scottish Executive. Pharmacy audit support pack. Online. Available: http://www.rpsgb.org.uk

The Royal Pharmaceutical Society of Great Britain, Scottish Executive. Audit to excellence. Available as CD-ROM. Online. Available: http://www.rpsgb.org.uk

Appendix A1: Current UK pharmaceutical legislation

Appelbe GE, Wingfield J. Dale and Appelbe's pharmacy law and ethics, 7th edn. London: Pharmaceutical Press; 2001.

Merrills J, Fisher J. Pharmacy law and practice, 3rd edn. Oxford: Blackwell Science; 2001.

Appendix A2: National Health Service dispensing

Chemist and Druggist Directory. Tonbridge: Miller Freeman. [Use current edition.]

National Health Service England and Wales. Drug Tariff. London: The Stationery Office. [Published monthly—use current edition.]

National Health Service in Scotland. Drug Tariff. Edinburgh: The Stationery Office. [Published quarterly—use current edition.]

NPA Guide to the Drug Tariff and NHS Dispensing. St Albans: National Pharmaceutical Association. [Use current edition appropriate to home country.]

Appendix A4: Latin terms and abbreviations

Carter S. Dispensing for pharmaceutical students, 13th edn. London: Pitman Medical; 1975.

Appendix A6: Presentation skills

Bradbury A. The Sunday Times successful presentation skills. London: Kogan Page; 2000.

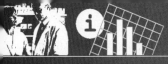

Subject Index

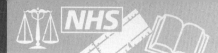

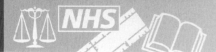

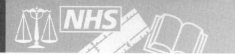

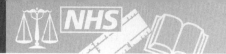

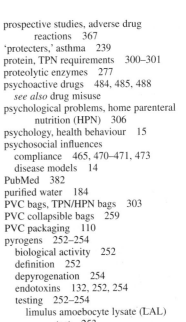

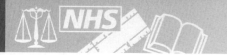

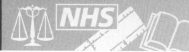

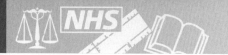